1978 YEAR BOOK OF MEDICINE®

THE 1978 YEAR BOOKS

The YEAR BOOK series provides in condensed form the essence of the best of the recent international medical literature. The material is selected by distinguished editors who critically review more than 500,000 journal articles each year.

Anesthesia
Drs. Eckenhoff, Bart, Brunner, Holley and Linde.

Cancer
Drs. Clark and Cumley.

Cardiology
Drs. Harvey, Kirkendall, Kirklin, Nadas, Paul and Sonnenblick.

Dentistry
Drs. Hale, Hazen, Moyers, Redig, Robinson and Silverman.

Dermatology
Drs. Malkinson and Pearson.

Diagnostic Radiology
Drs. Whitehouse, Bookstein, Gabrielsen, Holt, Martel, Silver and Thornbury.

Drug Therapy
Drs. Azarnoff, Hollister and Shand.

Endocrinology
Drs. Schwartz and Ryan.

Family Practice
Dr. Rakel.

Medicine
Drs. Rogers, Des Prez, Cline, Braunwald, Greenberger, Bondy and Epstein.

Neurology and Neurosurgery
Drs. De Jong and Sugar.

Nuclear Medicine
Drs. Quinn and Spies.

Obstetrics and Gynecology
Drs. Pitkin and Scott.

Ophthalmology
Dr. Hughes.

Orthopedics and Traumatic Surgery
Dr. Coventry.

Otolaryngology
Drs. Strong and Paparella.

Pathology and Clinical Pathology
Drs. Carone and Conn.

Pediatrics
Dr. Gellis.

Plastic and Reconstructive Surgery
Drs. McCoy, Dingman, Hanna, Haynes, Hoehn and Stephenson.

Psychiatry and Applied Mental Health
Drs. Romano, Freedman, Friedhoff, Kolb, Lourie and Nemiah.

Surgery
Drs. Schwartz, Najarian, Peacock, Shires, Silen and Spencer.

Urology
Dr. Grayhack.

The YEAR BOOK of Medicine®

1978

Edited by

DAVID E. ROGERS, M.D.
ROGER M. DES PREZ, M.D.
MARTIN J. CLINE, M.D.
EUGENE BRAUNWALD, M.D.
NORTON J. GREENBERGER, M.D.
PHILIP K. BONDY, M.D.
FRANKLIN H. EPSTEIN, M.D.

YEAR BOOK MEDICAL PUBLISHERS, INC.
CHICAGO • LONDON

Printed in U.S.A.

Library of Congress Catalog Card Number: CD38-25

International Standard Book Number: 0.8151-7436-5

Table of Contents

The material covered in this volume represents literature reviewed up to November, 1977.

Current Literature Quiz

The significant advances described in this YEAR BOOK introduce new diagnostic and therapeutic procedures useful for treating conditions seen frequently in your practice. The following questionnaire will test your familiarity with the current literature. References to the articles on which the questions are based are given in the back of the book.

1. Which of your patients should receive the newly released pneumococcal vaccine?
2. Your patient, a 48-year-old banker, is planning a hunting trip into the jungles of Central America. His last smallpox vaccination was 15 years ago. Should you vaccinate him?
3. What is currently thought to be the best antibiotic against the bacillus that causes legionnaires' disease?
4. Where is the reservoir of *Candida albicans* in patients with recurrent candidal vaginitis?
5. How long should antibiotic prophylaxis against rheumatic fever be continued?
6. How effective is Ara-A therapy in herpes simplex encephalitis?
7. Multi-drug-resistant strains of pneumococci have been found in which country?
8. How does infant botulism differ from the adult form of the disease?
9. How can the diagnosis of legionnaires' disease be established?
10. In treatment and prevention of recurrent urinary tract infection, what is the likely efficacy of: (a) methenamine mandelate (Mandelamine), (b) nitrofurantoin, (c) sulfamethoxazole-trimethoprim?
11. What is the likely etiology of clindamycin-associated pseudomembranous colitis? How might it be treated?
12. In treatment of nongonococcal urethritis, what is the likely efficacy of (a) spectinomycin, (b) sulfisoxazole, (c) tetracycline?
13. A lawyer's wife whom you treated for a small skin abscess a week ago complains of low back pain. She has some tenderness over the lower spine, a slightly diminished patella reflex on the right, no fever and a normal white blood cell count. What disease should you suspect? How do you make the diagnosis and treat the illness?
14. Should steroids be used in septic shock? If so, in what dose and for how long?
15. How valuable is liver biopsy in establishing a diagnosis in patients with fever of unknown origin?
16. What two genetically determined lung diseases are associated with hepatic dysfunction and chronic obstructive pulmonary disease (COPD)?
17. What two genetically determined diseases are associated with infertility and COPD?
18. Combined severe metabolic acidosis and mild respiratory acidosis or insufficient respiratory adjustment to metabolic acidosis should suggest deficiency in what ion or ions?

19. Are antibiotics advisable for patients with hypoxemic respiratory failure after aspiration of gastric contents?
20. How frequent is significant gastrointestinal bleeding in patients on controlled ventilation therapy?
21. What is the period of the day during which hospitalized asthmatics are most likely to die?
22. What is the best dosage of aminophyllin in patients with cirrhosis?
23. What two diseases are most frequently associated with pulmonary infiltrates and eosinophilia in asthmatics?
24. What percentage of vena cava umbrella filters cause complete occlusion of the vessel?
25. When sarcoid presents with the radiologic picture of metastatic malignancy, what is the likelihood of clearing?
26. What is the difference in time of onset, x-ray picture, treatment and prognosis between radiation fibrosis and radiation pneumonitis?
27. What percentage of cirrhotics with ascites have concomitant pleural effusion?
28. What is the prognosis of surgical treatment of chronic pancreatic pleural effusion and chronic pancreatic ascites?
29. Should liver, brain and bone scan be done as a routine component of preoperative evaluation in bronchogenic carcinoma?
30. What clinical parameters define aplastic anemia with a poor prognosis?
31. At what level should the hematocrit be maintained in patients with polycythemia vera, with the use of cerebral blood flow as the criterion?
32. What is the most effective mode of administration of available iron-chelating agents?
33. Do all blast transformations of chronic myelocytic leukemia arise from primitive granulocyte precursors?
34. Is mediastinal irradiation well tolerated in chronic lymphocytic leukemia?
35. What is the origin of the malignant cell in hairy cell leukemia?
36. What is the incidence and character of acute leukemia developing in patients with aggressively treated Hodgkin's disease?
37. Is Hodgkin's disease a monoclonal disorder?
38. Is it true that central nervous system involvement is quite rare in advanced non-Hodgkin's lymphoma?
39. Is "benign monoclonal gammopathy" a misnomer?
40. Is platelet cyclo-oxygenase deficiency the cause of the defective platelet function in Glanzmann's thrombasthenia?
41. Is plasmapheresis effective in thrombotic thrombocytopenic purpura?
42. Is the detection of the carrier state of hemophilia A and that of hemophilia B equally easy?
43. Are the indications for splenectomy early in the course of myeloid metaplasia clearly defined?
44. What are the consequences of the absence of cell membrane receptors that bind low-density lipoproteins?
45. Do oral contraceptives that contain "low-dose estrogens" increase cardiovascular disease mortality in young women?
46. What is the effect of alcohol consumption on blood pressure and on the incidence of coronary artery disease?
47. How does the effect of cigarette smoking on cardiac function differ between normal subjects and patients with coronary artery disease?
48. Is there a real association between earlobe creases and coronary heart disease, or is this simply related to age?
49. Are there significant differences between the effects of nitroprusside and

nitroglycerin on ischemic injury in patients with acute myocardial infarction?

50. In what time interval after experimental coronary occlusion must an intervention be applied in order to be effective in salvaging ischemic myocardium?
51. What are the effects of hyaluronidase in patients with acute myocardial infarction?
52. How can the new technique of transaxial tomography after the intravenous administration of radiolabeled palmitate be helpful in the study of patients with coronary artery disease?
53. What are the relative sensitivities of thallium-201 myocardial perfusion imaging and electrocardiography during exercise in detection of ischemic heart disease?
54. What are the clinical differences between patients with variant angina and normal coronary angiograms and those with variant angina with obstructive coronary artery disease?
55. What is the effect of coronary bypass grafting on survival of patients with chronic stable angina pectoris?
56. What are the relative advantages of internal mammary grafting versus saphenous vein bypass grafting in patients with ischemic heart disease?
57. How can patients with impaired left ventricular function who are candidates for coronary bypass surgery be divided into those in whom the impaired left ventricular function is due to scar and those in whom it is due to ischemia?
58. What are the relative advantages of porcine aortic valve xenografts and mechanical valvular prostheses?
59. What is the long-term prognosis of the mitral valve prolapse syndrome?
60. What are the indications for afterload reduction with agents that act on the arterial circulation versus those that act on the venous circulation?
61. What are the differences between the hemodynamic effects of inotropic agents and those of vasodilators in patients with severe heart failure?
62. What is the presumed mechanism of sudden death in patients with chronic bifascicular block?
63. How does a successfully treated episode of cardiac arrest affect the prognosis of acute myocardial infarction?
64. How do psychologic stress and β-adrenergic blockade affect electric stability of the ventricle?
65. What is diabetic cardiomyopathy?
66. How does restrictive cardiomyopathy differ from congestive cardiomyopathy?
67. What is the most frequent mechanism of cardiac death in patients with sarcoidosis of the heart?
68. What is the relationship between the renin-angiotensin and the kallikrein-bradykinin systems?
69. What is the mechanism of action of the antihypertensive agent clonidine?
70. What are the indications for pericardiectomy in uremic pericardial effusion?
71. What are the most frequent diagnoses in patients in whom heart transplantation has been carried out?
72. Do antacids accelerate the healing of duodenal ulcer disease? Does persistence of dyspepsia imply persistence of active ulceration?
73. Does early endoscopy in upper gastrointestinal bleeding alter outcome, i.e., morbidity and mortality?
74. Should all patients with gastric ulceration undergo serial gastroscopic examinations?

75. What is the mechanism of postgastrectomy steatorrhea?
76. What is the median incubation period for common foodborne bacterial enteritis?
77. What factors determine the cancer risk in patients with idiopathic ulcerative colitis?
78. What is the pathogenesis of vascular ectasias of the colon, a common cause of rectal bleeding in the elderly?
79. Does Gilbert's syndrome exist?
80. Does γ-globulin modify the course of posttransfusion hepatitis?
81. Does persistence of hepatitis B surface antigen (HB_sAg) influence the response to corticosteroids in chronic active liver disease?
82. Is ascitic fluid actually a good culture medium? Does this influence the development of spontaneous bacterial peritonitis in cirrhotics?
83. Is diuretic therapy in cirrhotic patients with ascites associated with an increased rate of complications?
84. Does cholecystectomy alter biliary lipid composition?
85. How effective are current tests in the diagnosis of pancreatic carcinoma?
86. What are the factors influencing the response to pancreatic enzyme therapy in exocrine pancreatic insufficiency?
87. Under what circumstances is section of the pituitary stalk likely to be useful in treating diabetic retinopathy? What about photocoagulation?
88. When ectopic ACTH syndrome occurs in patients with "nonendocrine tumors," is the excess ACTH always derived from the tumor? If not, where does it come from? Why?
89. Nonfunctioning thyroid masses in children are known to have a high risk of being malignant. Is this also true of functioning masses?
90. How should gas gangrene from aerobic organisms in diabetic patients be treated?
91. Describe three forms of androgen insensitivity and explain the cause of the defective response to androgens in each case.
92. A patient with insulinoma has normal serum concentration of human chorionic gonadotropin (hCG) and of both hCG-α and hCG-β. Does this rule out malignancy of the insulinoma?
93. Is it justified to use a kidney transplant to treat renal failure due to diabetic renovascular disease? What kind of kidney is likely to give the best results?
94. What evidence is there that treatment of diabetes improves the course of diabetic retinopathy?
95. Can a diagnosis of Cushing's syndrome be made from measurements of urinary steroids on any aliquot of urine less than a full 24-hour collection? What might be the advantages of a collection lasting less than 24 hours? Which hours would you use for the collection?
96. Does the plasma concentration of growth hormone always fall to normal when acromegalic patients have a clinical response to bromocriptine? to transsphenoidal adenomectomy?
97. Which single thyroid hormone concentration in plasma gives the best indication of adequate replacement treatment with thyroxine in myxedema?
98. Recurrent thyroid cancer usually indicates its presence by producing an indicator substance that can be measured in plasma. What is this substance? How reliable is its presence as an indicator of metastases?
99. How can one increase the accuracy of the fasting test for insulinoma?
100. How do you explain the impotence or amenorrhea of patients with a pituitary chromophobe adenoma?
101. What is the best treatment for Nelson's syndrome?

102. The renal biopsy of a 23-year-old man with mild proteinuria and intermittent hematuria shows granular deposits of IgA on immunofluorescence. What is the likelihood of progressive glomerulonephritis developing?
103. What is the long-term outlook for renal function in an adult with the nephrotic syndrome in whom proteinuria has declined to 2 gm per day and creatinine clearance has been normal for 3 years?
104. What is the most common carcinoma associated with nephrotic syndrome? How does the glomerular pathology differ from that seen in nephrotic syndrome associated with Hodgkin's disease?
105. Over the course of 3 weeks, a patient with lymphosarcoma develops progressive renal insufficiency. What are the possible causes and what would you do?
106. Name a cheap, safe and effective method to relieve uremic itching.
107. What is the relationship between ureteral reflux and late failure of transplanted kidneys?
108. A 55-year-old woman with unilateral hydronephrosis has a blood pressure of 210/110. How would you determine whether nephrectomy would relieve the hypertension?
109. Excessive production of prostaglandins might explain which symptoms of severe potassium depletion?
110. An 80-year-old woman with mild azotemia (blood urea nitrogen 42 mg/100 ml) and diabetes has a serum potassium level of 6.2 mEq/L, a bicarbonate level of 19 mEq/L and complete heart block. What are the factors that might be contributing to hyperkalemia? Can you suggest a simple treatment?
111. What are four causes of a reduced anion gap?
112. What is the reason for the elevated serum phosphate level in lactic acidosis? How does this feature help to distinguish lactic acidosis from diabetic ketoacidosis?
113. How can measurements of urinary cyclic adenosine monophosphate help in the diagnosis of hyperparathyroidism?
114. A 40-year-old man is referred because of recurrent calcium stones with normal serum calcium, phosphorus and electrolyte levels. He brings in a 24-hour urine sample collected while on his usual diet. What measurements would you suggest be made on that urine and how would the results guide your therapy?
115. What is the drug of choice to suppress urinary infection in a patient with recurrent gram-negative urinary infection and renal calculi?

PART ONE

INFECTIONS

DAVID E. ROGERS, M.D.

Introduction

In contrast to last year, this one has been a splendid success story for workers in the area of infectious disease. As promised, thanks to studies by many investigators, we have been able to give you, our readers, a much better picture of legionnaires' disease and how to treat it. Pneumococcal vaccine is now available – and this involves a wonderful tale of meticulous research and controlled trial leading to a scientific advance of benefit to mankind. The etiology of clindamycin-induced pseudomembranous colitis seems to have been unraveled – as well as an effective means to treat the disease. These and some other fine contributions appear on the following pages.

Again I am much in the debt of, and increasingly dependent on, my two Vanderbilt University colleagues, Drs. Zell McGee and William Schaffner. They have made the selections and we have pounded out the comments together. For the next several months I am again a reasonable expert in the field. As long as the publishers tolerate me, I will continue to take this yearly crash course.

DAVID E. ROGERS

Newly Appreciated Infections

► ↓ As my colleagues and I met in our annual seminar to sort out this year's selection of articles, there was no doubt as to which would lead the list. It is with great pleasure that we are able to present the reports of a clear triumph in legionnaires' disease. We refer not only to the isolation of the causative bacterium by Doctors McDade and Shepard of the Center for Disease Control, but also to the fine way local, state and federal health authorities were able to work together under chaotic circumstances. Despite overlapping jurisdictions, the glare of publicity, the anxiety of the populace, political interest and the elusive nature of the disease itself, a first-rate investigation was completed in short order. The system works. We fielded a large team of professionals and came up with answers. We should be proud of our resources for communicable disease control! – Ed. ◄

Legionnaires' Disease.—*I. Description of an epidemic of pneumonia.*—David W. Fraser, Theodore R. Tsai, Walter Orenstein, William E. Parkin, H. James Beecham, Robert G. Sharrar, John Harris, George F. Mallison, Stanley M. Martin, Joseph E. McDade, Charles C. Shepard, Philip S. Brachman and the Field Investigation Team[1] (Center for Disease Control, Atlanta, Ga.) describe the explosive, common-source outbreak of pneumonia caused by a previously unrecognized bacterium, which affected primarily persons attending an American Legion convention in Philadelphia in July, 1976. Twenty-nine of 182 cases were fatal. Eight epidemiologic surveys were carried out, including surveys of hotel guests and employees, a roommate survey, a legionnaire census and two case-control surveys.

About 80% of patients were hospitalized and 16% died. Typically illness began in patients a week after arrival at the convention and 3 days after returning home. Most hospitalized patients had preexisting illnesses. Chest radiographs were abnormal in 90% of patients and showed patchy interstitial infiltrates or areas of consolidation. Usually the illness progressed over 2–3 days; survivors had a remittent fever that broke by lysis. Individual patients seemed to improve after antibiotic therapy, but no antibiotic was clearly effective in the patients as a group. Pathologic findings included pneumonia and acute diffuse alveolar damage with many bacilli present in affected alveoli. The epidemic curve is shown in Figure 1. Spread of the bacterium appeared to be airborne. The source was not found, but epidemiologic analysis suggested that exposure may have occurred in the lobby of the headquarters hotel or in the area immediately surrounding the hotel. Many hotel employees appeared to be immune, suggesting that the agent may have been present in the vicinity, perhaps intermittently, for 2 or more years.

The shape of the epidemic curve suggests a continuing common-source exposure. Person-to-person spread seems not to have occurred.

---

(1) N. Engl. J. Med. 297:1189–1197, Dec. 1, 1977.

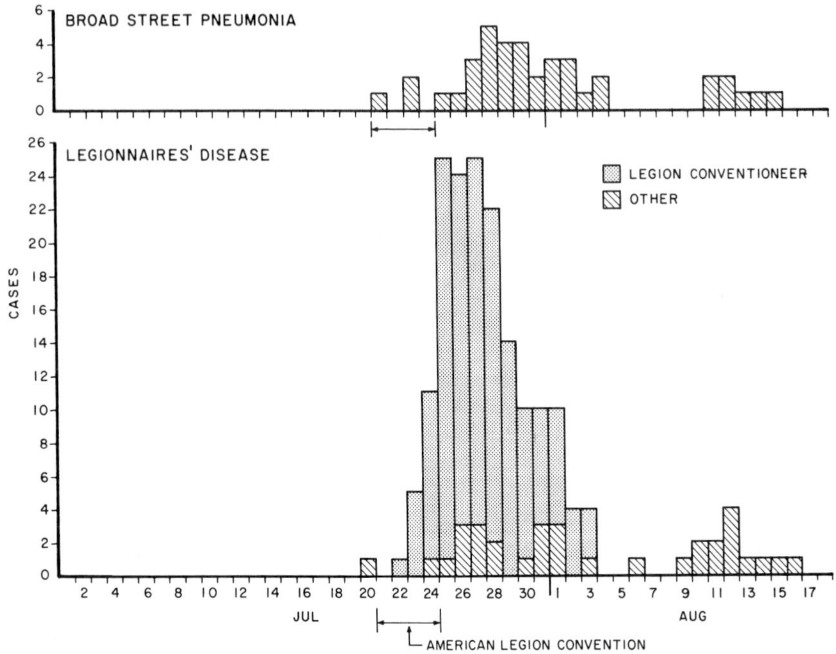

Fig 1.—Dates of onset of illness in cases of legionnaires' disease and cases of Broad Street pneumonia in Philadelphia, July 1–August 18, 1976. Dates of onset of 2 cases of legionnaires' disease are unknown. (Courtesy of Fraser, D. W., et al.: N. Engl. J. Med. 297:1189–1197, Dec. 1, 1977.)

Sporadic Cases of Pneumonia with Seroconversions to the Bacterial Agent of Legionnaires' Disease

Case No.	Age (Yr)	Sex	State of Residence	Date of Onset	Serum 1		Serum 2		Clinical Course
					*titer**	*day*	*titer**	*day*	
1	31	F	Vermont	8/10/76	<32/<32	8	256/256	31	Respiratory failure; death on 35th day.
2	62	M	Massachusetts	8/18/76	32/32	7	≥1,024/≥1,024	23	Fever (of 40.6°C) for 11 days
3	34	M	Michigan	8/19/76	<16/<16	3	≥512/≥512	21	Fever (to 41.7°C); respiratory-distress syndrome; recovery.
4	55	F	Massachusetts	9/07/76	<32/<32	3	512/512	50	Fever (of 40.6°C) for 5 days; respiratory & cardiac arrest.
5	32	M	Indiana	10/05/76	16/16	10	64/128	14	Pneumonia; respiratory failure; death on 14th day.
6	60	M	California†	1/03/77	16/16	10	2,048/2,048	20	Diffuse interstitial pneumonia, with renal failure; recovery.
7	60	M	Tennessee†	2/11/77					Respiratory & renal failure; death on 10th day.‡
8	31	M	Vermont	3/06/77	64/256	4	≥1,024/≥1,024	17	Fulminant broncho-pneumonia; temperature of 40.6°C; recovery with ventilatory support.
9	43	M	California†	4/01/77	64/64	5	1,024/1,024	15	Gastroenteritis; trilobar pneumonia; mechanical ventilation for 3 days; recovery.

*Titer against isolate 1/titer against isolate 2.

†Because these patients traveled during their incubation periods, they could have acquired the infection outside their state of residence.

‡Bacterium isolate from lung specimen.

Two previous outbreaks caused by this or a related bacterium also had the pattern of a continuing common-source airborne exposure.

II. Isolation of a bacterium and demonstration of its role in other respiratory disease.—McDade, Shepard, Fraser, Tsai, Martha A. Redus, Walter R. Dowle and the Laboratory Investigation Team[2] identified the etiologic agent of legionnaires' disease by examining serums and tissue specimens from victims of the outbreak.

A bacterium was isolated in guinea pigs from lung tissues in 4 fatal cases. The lungs of 4 of 6 patients examined yielded a gram-negative, non-acid-fast bacillus that could be transferred to yolk sacs of embryonated eggs. When yolk-sac cultures of the bacillus were used as antigen to survey suspected serums, with use of antihuman globulin fluorescent antibody, specimens from 101 of 111 patients meeting clinical criteria for legionnaires' disease showed diagnostic increases in antibody titers. Diagnostic increases were also found in 54 recent sporadic cases of severe pneumonia and, retrospectively, in stored serums from most patients in two other previously unsolved outbreaks of respiratory disease (table). Classification of the organism is incomplete.

It is concluded that legionnaires' disease is caused by a gram-negative bacterium that may be responsible for widespread infection.

Demonstration of the Agent of Legionnaires' Disease in Tissue is reported by Francis W. Chandler, Martin D. Hicklin and John A. Blackmon[3] (Center for Disease Control, Atlanta, Ga.). The putative causative agent of the epidemic of acute febrile respiratory disease occurring in Philadelphia in the summer of 1976 has been found to be a novel bacterium, not previously recognized as an agent of human disease. The organism was isolated from the lungs of 4 patients with legionnaires' disease and 1 with Broad Street pneumonia. Seroconversion to the agent occurred in both categories of patients. Study was made of lung tissue obtained at autopsy from 22 patients with legionnaires' disease and 4 with Broad Street pneumonia, including the 5 from whom the bacterium was isolated. Liver and spleen from guinea pigs inoculated with the agent of legionnaires' disease were also examined.

Small, blunt, pleomorphic, occasionally vacuolated bacilli were demonstrated by the Dieterle silver-impregnation method in 15 cases of legionnaires' disease and 3 of Broad Street pneumonia. Four of 5 patients from whom the agent of legionnaires' disease was isolated had positive findings. Organisms were consistently seen in areas of pneumonia and were most numerous within the necrotic cellular debris in affected alveoli and respiratory bronchioles (Fig 2). Organisms were both intracellular and extracellular. Where the organism was not seen, either the tissue samples were not representative or the diagnosis of legionnaires' disease was doubtful. No standard staining method was consistent in demonstrating the agent of legionnaires' disease.

The Dieterle silver-impregnation stain is the most sensitive method

(2) N. Engl. J. Med. 297:1197–1203, Dec. 1, 1977.
(3) Ibid., pp. 1218–1220.

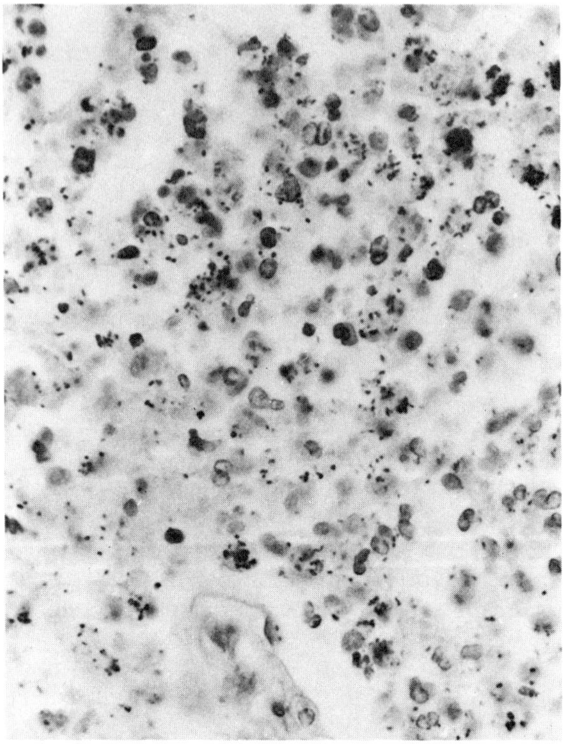

Fig 2.—Small, blunt, pleomorphic intracellular and extracellular bacilli in a respiratory bronchiole of a patient from whom the agent of legionnaires' disease was isolated. Dieterle silver-impregnation stain; reduced from ×600. (Courtesy of Chandler, F. W., et al.: N. Engl. J. Med. 297:1218–1220, Dec. 1, 1977.)

for demonstrating the agent of legionnaires' disease in histologic sections, but the specificity of the stain is not completely known.

► [Although we have discovered much about this disease, much remains yet to be learned. Obviously, our notions about it will have to be updated as new information comes along. As of this moment, I believe we can say the following:

Legionnaires' disease occurs both sporadically and in outbreaks. It has probably been around for some time. We do not yet know where the organism resides in nature nor why epidemics occur. Although the evidence points to airborne spread as the mode of transmission, exactly how this occurs remains a mystery. Person-to-person spread has not been documented in either the community or the hospital. Nevertheless, it seems prudent to place patients suspected of having this disease on respiratory isolation while they are hospitalized.

The clinical features of the disease are not sufficiently characteristic to be pathognomonic. Malaise, weakness, high fever, dyspnea, nonproductive cough, pleuritic chest pain, nausea, abdominal pain and diarrhea are all common. Chest examination usually reveals rales without signs of consolidation. Patients with underlying lung disease or a smoking history or both seem at greater risk. Rapidly deteriorating pulmonary function, anoxia and obtundation occur in the most seriously ill. Renal failure also can occur. On the basis of animal studies and a retrospective look at the Philadelphia experience, erythromycin appears to be the most effective antibiotic.

Diagnosis is made in one of three ways: (1) by serologic means, (2) by isolation of the organism and (3) by demonstration of the organism in tissue with the use of special stains. Serologic diagnosis is the most common method; paired acute and convalescent serums are necessary. Many state health department laboratories soon will have the capability of running these tests. To date, the organism has *not* been isolated from either sputum or blood. It has been recovered from pleural fluid and from postmortem lung tissue. Experience with lung biopsy specimens is as yet too limited to make any statements as to their value. Most hospital laboratories have received instructions as to the appropriate laboratory procedures required to isolate the agent. The organism can be demonstrated in tissue specimens by using the Dieterle silver stain and by fluorescent techniques (to date available only at the Center for Disease Control).

It must be obvious from the above that the laboratory is not yet able to provide immediate help in the diagnosis of legionnaires' disease. My colleagues who have seen 3 patients with confirmed diagnoses are still wrestling with the problem of which patients with undiagnosed pneumonia should be treated with erythromycin. They are collecting serum specimens on all such patients and, more often than not, treating with erythromycin.

We shall be following the story with great interest and will bring you further installments of this thriller. Tune in, same place, next year. . . . —Ed.] ◄

► ↓ We have included the following two articles on *Hemophilus influenzae* pneumonia because my 2 colleagues have seen what they characterize as a "flurry" of *H. influenzae* infections in adults during the past year. These articles call attention to a pathogen previously believed to be an extremely rare producer of disease in those over the age of 2 years. —Ed. ◄

Hemophilus influenzae **Pneumonia in Adults.** *Hemophilus influenzae* is known to cause serious infections in young children but is an uncommon cause of disease in adults. E. Dale Everett, Adolf E. Rahm, Jr., Roy Adaniya, Dennis L. Stevens and Theodore R. McNitt[4] report the findings in 18 cases of *H. influenzae* pneumonia seen in adults at Brooke Army Medical Center in the past 3 years. The diagnosis was based on an acute infiltrate seen on a chest film and a pure culture of *H. influenzae* from a transtracheal aspirate (TTA), blood cultures or empyema fluid. Two thirds of the patients were over age 50. Eleven patients had underlying lung disease, whereas 4 were healthy hosts (table).

Sputum production, cough, fever, chills and chest pains were the most common features. Only 1 patient had hemoptysis. All but 2 had rales, and 5 patients were afebrile on admission. The infiltrates had a lobar distribution, the lower lobes being involved most often. Eleven patients had white blood cell counts over 10,000/cu mm. Gram staining of TTA gave correct identification of the organism in 11 cases. Pure cultures of *H. influenzae* were obtained from all TTAs but from only 1 of 14 throat or sputum cultures. Of 15 patients with blood cultures done, only 1 had a positive culture. Ampicillin was used most often in

FEATURES OF PRESENT SERIES OF PATIENTS AND 30 REPORTED CASES*

Findings	No. (%) of Patients, Present Series	No. (%) of Patients, Literature
Underlying lung disease	11/18(61)	16/30(53)
Age, >50 yr	12/18(67)	21/30(70)
WBC count, >10,000/cu mm	11/18(61)	19/30(63)
Neutrophilic response	17/18(94)	20/21(95)
Pleural effusion	0/18(0)	7/30(23)

*Not recorded in all cases.

(4) J.A.M.A. 238:319–321, July 25, 1977.

therapy in doses of 2–8 gm daily. All patients except 1 treated with phenoxymethyl penicillin responded within 24–48 hours. One patient recovered without treatment. Generally treatment was continued for 10–14 days. Three patients died, 2 of oat cell carcinoma and 1 with progressive respiratory failure and A_2 influenza.

It is apparent that *H. influenzae* pneumonia in adults is more common than has been thought. Isolation of the organism from a reliable source is important with increasing reports of type b *Hemophilus* and nontypable strains resistant to ampicillin. Since the appearance of *H. influenzae* on gram stains of TTA specimens is virtually diagnostic, this procedure is recommended in patients with acute pneumonia where the cause is not apparent, along with cultures of the specimen, blood and pleural fluids.

Bacteremic *Hemophilus influenzae* Pneumonia in Adults: Report of 24 Cases and Review of the Literature. Recent reports indicate that the incidence of *H. influenzae* meningitis and bacteremia in adults is increasing but current texts devote little attention to *H. influenzae* pneumonia. David C. Levin, Marvin I. Schwarz, Richard A. Matthay and F. Marc LaForce[5] (Univ. of Colorado) reviewed 24 proved cases of *H. influenzae* pneumonia in adults, seen at three hospitals in Denver in 1970–74, and compared the features with those of 43 previously reported pneumonia cases, 29 of them associated with positive blood cultures for *H. influenzae.* All patients were over age 20. The study group included 16 men and 8 women with a mean age of 54; 19 patients were over age 40. Thirteen (54%) had a history of significant pulmonary disease (emphysema, tuberculosis, bronchiectasis). Twelve (50%) were chronic alcoholics and 4 had chronic liver disease. Other serious underlying disease was present in an additional 7 patients.

Fever was the most common complaint on admission, followed by cough, dyspnea and chills. The mean white blood cell count was 11,000/cu mm; 3 patients were leukopenic on admission. Initial sputum gram stains showed gram-negative coccobacillary organisms suggestive of *H. influenzae* in 12 of 16 patients. Sputum cultures were positive in only 6 of 17 patients and blood cultures in 23 patients. The two pleural effusions present on admission proved to be *H. influenzae* empyemas. Chest films showed diffuse bronchopneumonia on admission in 18 patients, and 9 had evidence of lobar consolidation, alone or combined with bronchopneumonia. Nineteen patients received ampicillin alone or with other antibiotics and 16 of them survived. All 5 patients treated with other antibiotics died within 5 days. Seven of 8 deaths were attributable to the infectious process; 3 deaths involved polymicrobial infection.

The high mortality in this series may be attributed to the advanced age of the patients and to the presence of associated illnesses. The 10-year review suggested a true increase in the incidence of *H. influenzae* pneumonia in adults. It is not clear whether the decrease in the prevalence of *H. influenzae* bactericidal antibodies observed in the older population is the cause of the current increase in *H. influenzae* pneumonia in adults.

(5) Am. J. Med. 62:219–224, February, 1977.

► [It seems appropriate to discuss this article and the preceding one together, for from them a picture of the syndrome of *H. influenzae* pneumonia emerges.

As observed in these two series (and this is bulwarked by the picture that developed in collective analysis of the 84 other cases reported since 1942), this is a disease of older people. The patients often are alcoholics with underlying pulmonary disease. Other unassociated serious disease—especially malignancy—is common. The clinical syndrome is indistinguishable from other bacterial pneumonias. Pleural involvement is quite common. For those not well trained in analyzing gram stains, the call may be missed on review of a straight sputum smear, but in the series presented by Everett et al., the gram-negative coccobacillary microbe was recognized in a high percentage of stained transtracheal aspirates. The actual incidence of bacteremia is unknown. The Colorado series was selected *because* of positive blood cultures. In the series of Everett et al., bacteremia was present in 1 of 15 cultures taken. Most patients responded well to ampicillin therapy but the incidence of ampicillin-resistant strains is rising, and I think it is fair to say that optimal treatment regimens are still in flux.

A few additional comments follow.

First, I wish that the authors had indicated the season of the year the cases were seen and whether influenza A was being observed simultaneously. Since 1892, it has been clear that *H. influenzae* infections in adults can be seen in association with influenza—indeed, it was this association that caused Pfeiffer to so label the microbe in the first place, believing it to be the causative agent of influenza.

Second, it is clear that sputum cultures are not very helpful in making the diagnosis. In the Colorado series of bacteremic patients, the organism was recognized in sputum cultures in only 6 of 17 cases. In the series of Everett et al., *H. influenzae* was isolated in pure culture from 18 of 18 transtracheal aspirates, but only 1 of 14 sputum cultures in the same patients. This may result from the fragile nature of the microbe, sampling errors, overgrowth of normal flora or failure to culture sputum specimens on chocolate agar. Thus it should be kept in mind that a negative *sputum* culture does not rule it out. Transtracheal aspirates look valuable.

Both groups of authors (and my colleagues) believe that *H. influenzae* infections in the adult may be on the increase. Some authors have speculated that prompt antimicrobial treatment of *H. influenzae* infections in children may result in lesser antibody response, leaving us with a susceptible adult population. Perhaps so. It is interesting to note that Norden recently screened a large adult population for bactericidal antibodies to *H. influenzae* and found them present in only 23%. In my day, it was almost 80% (J. Infect. Dis. 130:489, 1974).

One last comment—and it is one that I have made in past YEAR BOOKS. In the series by Everett et al., the proper diagnosis was missed on gram stain in 7 of 18 instances. The authors state that this mistake was usually caused by poor staining (decolorizing) leading to an erroneous call of pneumococcus—a gram-positive microbe. This mistake can be avoided if you place the specimen to be examined on one part of the slide, a bit of debris from between your own teeth on another section of the same slide and then stain the whole slide. Examine your own debris first. We all harbor both gram-positive and gram-negative microbes between our teeth, and you will rapidly come to recognize a properly stained smear from this personal reference point. It is particularly important in examining cerebrospinal fluid from patients with meningitis. A wrong call on a gram stain can be fatal.—Ed.] ◄

Group Y Meningococcal Disease in United States Air Force Recruits. Until 1963, nearly all meningococcal disease in United States military recruits was caused by group A *Neisseria meningitidis,* but subsequently group B and then group C organisms became predominant. In 1971, group C meningococcal infections began to disappear and presently the causative organism is group Y *N. meningitidis.* Gerald M. Koppes, Charles Ellenbogen and Ronald J. Gebhart[6] (Lackland Air Force Base, Texas) reviewed the findings in 88 Air Force recruits seen in 1971–74 with group Y meningococcal disease, 68 of whom had primary bacterial pneumonia.

(6) Am. J. Med. 62:661–666, May, 1977.

PREVALENCE OF SYMPTOMS AND SIGNS ON ADMISSION AMONG 68 PATIENTS WITH GROUP Y MENINGOCOCCAL PNEUMONIA*

Symptoms	Per Cent	Symptoms	Per Cent
Cough	100	Nausea and/or vomiting	34
Sore throat	66	Headache	23
Chest pain		Fever	100
Total	59	103°F	60
Pleuritic	33	105°F	14
Chills	59	Rales	96
Previous upper		Pharyngitis	79
respiratory tract		Cervical adenopathy	36
infection (3 weeks)	58	Dullness or egophoney	14
Dyspnea	19	Pleural friction rub	10
Hemoptysis	13	Cardiovascular	
Sweats	13	Pulse rate $\geq$130/min	7
Fatigue	56		

*Neither petechiae, purpura, 3d heart sound, friction rub or hypotension was present on admission.

In the group of 68 patients with group Y meningococcal pneumonia, 80% of 64 cultures of transtracheal aspirates grew only group Y *N. meningitidis*. The clinical features are summarized in the table. Blood cultures were positive in 15% of patients. Nine of 16 patients with pneumonia had transient elevations in serum glutamic-oxaloacetic transaminase. Patchy alveolar infiltrates were the most common x-ray finding. No large pleural effusions were seen.

Antibiotic therapy included procaine penicillin G and phenoxymethyl penicillin. The response to therapy was prompt; only 5 patients remained febrile after 4 days and all ultimately responded. Ten patients had meningococcemia due to group Y *N. meningitidis*. While all 10 were in shock, 9 had no cutaneous manifestations of petechia or purpura. One patient with preexisting neutropenia died. Six other patients had culturally proved meningitis, 4 of them with skin manifestations. The onset was abrupt in most cases and all patients were febrile. Respiratory findings were common in this group. Twelve patients responded favorably within 24–48 hours of the start of penicillin G therapy. All patients with shock responded rapidly to antibiotic therapy. *Neisseria meningitidis* sinusitis was diagnosed in 2 patients and arthritis in 1. One patient had an acute self-limited upper respiratory tract infection.

Group Y *N. meningitidis* has emerged as a predominant pathogen since 1970, causing either meningococcemia, meningitis or primary pneumonia. Group Y meningococcal pneumonia cannot be clinically distinguished from either nonbacterial or bacterial pneumonia due to other pathogens. There are epidemiologic similarities to group B and C disease. At present, group Y disease may be waning in importance. The apparent 4-year cycle of meningococcal serogroups has yet to be proved, but it prompts concern that a new serogroup could supersede group Y in the near future.

► [What a fascinating parasite, the meningococcus! As noted in this article, until 1963 virtually all meningococcal disease in military recruits was caused by group A meningococci. The clinical syndrome was predominantly that of meningitis, less frequently fulminant meningococcemia without meningitis but with florid skin manifestations. Although meningococcal pneumonia has been recognized for 60 years, it was an unusual clinical entity even during epidemics. In 1963, group A meningococcal infections began to disappear and group B infections emerged to take their place. About 4 years later, group B infections began to wane, and group C infections became predominant. In both instances, the clinical syndromes mimicked group A infections—meningitis and meningococcemia predominated. In 1970–71, group C meningococcal polysaccharide vaccine was introduced. However, even as the vaccine came into use, group Y meningococci began to replace group C as a cause of meningococcal disease. Thus meningococci have continued to pose disease problems among recruits.

This time, the clinical syndrome has been distinctly different. Pneumonia predominates 4:1 over bacteremic meningitis syndromes. Those patients with meningococcemia, despite shock or disseminated intravascular coagulation, fail to show the skin lesions that were so helpful diagnostically in meningococcal infections produced by A, B and C strains. The clinical manifestations suggest that group Y meningococci produce a more slowly progressive, less lethal disease, and this appears borne out by the mortality rate—1% compared with 4–7% generally reported with treated group B or C meningococcal infections.

The infections due to group Y meningococci are now on the decline. It sounds like the cycles seen with type A influenza, doesn't it? What comes next?—Ed.] ◄

Infant Botulism: Epidemiologic, Clinical and Laboratory Aspects. None of the 603 cases of botulism reported in California since 1899, one third of the United States total, occurred in an infant. Stephen S. Arnon, Thaddeus F. Midura, Susan A. Clay, Ronald M. Wood and James Chin[7] reviewed the 6 case histories of infant botulism documented to date in the United States. *Clostridium botulinum* organisms and toxin were identified in the feces of 6 infants, aged 5–20 weeks, who had clinical features consistent with botulism. Five lived in California and became ill within a 6-month period in 1976; 1 became ill in New Jersey in 1975. Three cases were type A and 3, type B botulism. No source of ingested toxin was found in any instance. The clinical findings included constipation, weak sucking and crying, cranial nerve deficits, generalized weakness and, on occasion, sudden apnea. An electromyographic pattern of brief, small, abundant motor unit potentials was observed.

The source of *C. botulinum* toxin in these cases is thought to have been in vivo gastrointestinal production following the ingestion of *C. botulinum* organisms. No ingested item common to all 6 cases was found, and none of the families knew or had any common associations with the other families. Botulism apparently can occur in infants who have not ingested preformed botulinal toxin. Examination of the feces, not just serum, is important in establishing the diagnosis of botulism. Electromyography may permit rapid substantiation of the clinical diagnosis. Only 1 infant received botulinal antitoxin, but all survived. The mechanism permitting recovery remains obscure. In some cases, the indolent onset may have allowed time for humoral antibody against botulinal toxin to develop. Studies are under way to explore the possibility that infant botulism may explain some cases of the sudden infant death syndrome.

► [Although we usually do not discuss pediatric infectious diseases in this section of the YEAR BOOK, I have selected this important article on infant botulism for two rea-

(7) J.A.M.A. 237:1946–1951, May 2, 1977.

sons. The first is nostalgia. I have twice had the opportunity to help investigate outbreaks of botulism and the disease has an irresistible fascination for me. Secondly, this newly recognized entity has raised several important points about the pathogenesis and diagnosis of botulism in all age groups.

To summarize, some "floppy" babies with constipation, weakness, hypotonia, ophthalmoplegia, ptosis, sluggish pupillary responses and a normal cerebrospinal fluid examination have been shown to have botulism. First recognized in California, cases have now been reported from around the United States (Vanderbilt University included; see Am. J. Dis. Child. 131:857, 1977).

Botulinus toxin has not been found in the serum of the babies (it is usually present in adults), but both *Clostridium botulinum* organisms and toxin have been found in stool (both findings also are common in adults).

In adults, botulism usually is thought to be caused by the ingestion of preformed toxin in food. In contrast, toxin has not been found in the food of these infants (indeed, some were exclusively breast-fed). Thus, it seems that these babies ingest *C. botulinum* spores from some source in their environment (still undetermined), the spores germinate in the gut, toxin is produced and absorbed and disease results. Soviet workers have for some years attempted to convince us that a similar mechanism is at work in some cases of adult disease, i.e., that prolonged illness could be due to continuing production of toxin in the gastrointestinal tract. I have been skeptical of this notion in the past, but now am much more receptive to the idea.

The specialized laboratory analyses for demonstrating both toxin and the organism are usually not available in your hospital. Call the state public health laboratory and the state epidemiologist for prompt assistance. While you are waiting for these results (24–48 hours), have a STAT electromyogram performed on the patient. It has now been shown that botulism produces quite characteristic changes highly suggestive of the diagnosis (enhanced and prolonged posttetanic facilitation, muscle fibrillation and many small-amplitude polyphasic motor unit potentials). — Ed.] ◄

Infections of Medical Progress

Septicemia in a Community Hospital, 1970 through 1973. Differences between patient populations in community and noncommunity acute-care hospitals may preclude the valid extrapolation of incidence data from studies in noncommunity hospitals. William E. Scheckler[8] (Univ. of Wisconsin) reviewed experience with septicemia at a 370-bed, acute-care general hospital in Madison, Wisconsin, in 1970–73. Of 61,481 patients admitted in the 4-year study period, 207 had septicemia documented by blood culture, which was an incidence of 34 cases per 10,000 admissions. Eighteen per 10,000 were gram-negative bacteremias, 12 per 10,000 were gram-positive bacteremias and 4 per 10,000 were mixed bacteremias or fungemias.

A total of 5–10% of blood cultures drawn in each of the 4 years grew an organism. Contaminants were identified in specimens from 52 patients. Septicemia as related to in-hospital mortality is given in the table. Primary bacteremia occurred in 20 of 209 episodes of septicemia in 207 patients. An average of 2.3 antibiotics was used to treat each septicemic patient. Prophylactic antibiotics had been instituted before the onset of septicemia in 16 of 70 patients with nosocomial septicemia. An additional 13 patients received antibiotics for another infection before the development of nosocomial sepsis. The organism isolated was sensitive to an antibiotic being given in 131 of 137 patients with community-acquired septicemia and in 61 of 70 with nosocomial septicemia. The average stay for all patients in the hospital was 7 days. Patients with community-acquired septicemia stayed an average of 18 days and those with nosocomial septicemia stayed an average of 33 days. Clinical shock or a systolic blood pressure below 100 mm Hg developed on the day of blood culture in 9.7% of the patients. Ten of the 16 patients with gram-negative septicemia died, and 3 of 4 with com-

INCIDENCE OF SEPTICEMIA AND NUMBER OF IN-HOSPITAL DEATHS*

	Disease Category			
	Nonfatal	Ultimately Fatal	Rapidly Fatal	Total
No. of patients with septicemia	149	38	20	**207**
No. of patients dead	14	19	17	**50**
No. (%) of deaths related to infection	13(8.7)	14(37.0)	15(75.0)	**42**(20.3)
Incidence of septicemia per 10,000 admissions	27	71	360	34

*St. Mary's Hospital Medical Center, 1970–73.

(8) J.A.M.A. 237:1938–1941, May 2, 1977.

munity-acquired streptococcal infections died. Frequency of and mortality from shock were associated with underlying disease.

Differences in the incidence of septicemia between community and noncommunity hospitals probably are related to differences in the frequency of underlying diseases. Extrapolation of rates of septicemia from noncommunity hospitals to the population of all acute-care hospital patients in the United States should be made with great caution, or not at all. The incidence of septicemia must be viewed in relation to the underlying diseases of the population being studied.

► [From my current vantage point, I have had the chance to examine our health-care system from a different view. In addition to my present concern for how office-based primary care is being delivered, my academic background has made me remain very interested in how hospitals function as community health care resources. Doctors who practice in several types of hospitals are quite sure that different hospitals serve different populations of patients. However, most opinions are based on anecdotal experience and not careful analysis.

Doctor Scheckler's study supports the thesis that there indeed are differences. He has demonstrated very nicely that, insofar as patients with sepsis are concerned, these three hospitals in Madison, Wisconsin (a community hospital, a Veterans Administration hospital and a university hospital), serve a different "mix" of patients. Only 1% of the septic patients at the community hospital had an underlying disease that was classified as "rapidly fatal"; at the university hospital this figure was 13%. The Veterans Administration hospital was in between. This would confirm my previously held notions regarding how doctors use hospitals—very sick patients and those with complex illnesses frequently are referred to university centers. Doctor Scheckler rightly cautions that data on the occurrence of sepsis acquired solely from academic centers can not be extrapolated willy-nilly to all acute-care hospitals. Along these lines, I was fascinated to see that very few instances of hospital-acquired sepsis in the community hospital could be traced back to infected Foley-catheterized bladders. This is a prominent cause of sepsis in studies from university and municipal hospitals. It looks as though the staff is doing a superior job of catheter care in that community hospital!

A similar study was published later in the year by Dr. Peter Gross, who practices in a New Jersey community hospital (Arch. Intern. Med. 137:1698, 1977). He also demonstrated a lower rate of gram-negative bacteremia than is usually reported from teaching hospitals. He made two other interesting points. He analyzed the experience with gram-positive bacteremia (much less studied of late) and showed that patients with gram-positive bacteremia had a *higher* mortality than patients with gram-negative bacteremia (42% vs. 27%). Many of these infections were community acquired and the major offending microbes were the old favorites: pneumococci and staphylococci. I was impressed that 4 of 5 patients with pneumococcal bacteremia who did *not* have a serious underlying disease died of their infection. These data provide yet another plug for the use of pneumococcal vaccine (discussed in The Chest, in this volume).

The effect of appropriate antibiotic therapy given within the first 24 hours after the onset of bacteremia was evaluated. Doctor Gross was able to confirm that choosing an appropriate antimicrobial does enhance survival—even among patients with an underlying disease that was classified as rapidly fatal. This is indeed encouraging. He states that aminoglycoside therapy was carefully adjusted with the use of frequent serum levels as a guide. I wonder whether this could be cited as a study of the benefits to be realized when a trained infectious disease person is available to help in the management of such seriously ill patients.

Doctors Scheckler and Gross are in the vanguard of a recent movement of young infectious disease specialists to full-time practice in community hospitals. In addition to their helping in the care of patients, I hope more of them will conduct similar careful studies to educate us all about the features of infectious illness in the populations they serve. Well done!—Ed.] ◄

Semiquantitative Culture Method for Identifying Intravenous Catheter-Related Infection. Catheter-related septicemia complicates up to 8% of venous cannulations and affects about 25,000 patients in the United States each year. In many past studies, the technique for catheter removal has not been standardized. Quantitative culture of the external catheter surface should distinguish contamination from infection more reliably than the broth-culture method. Dennis G. Maki, Carol E. Weise and Harold W. Sarafin[9] (Univ. of Wisconsin) report the results of a prospective clinical study of 250 venous catheters, cultured both by a semiquantitative technique and conventionally in broth. Venous catheters from unburned adult medical and surgical patients were cultured over a 4-month period. Semiquantitative cultures were done on sheep-blood agar plates that, with trypticase soy broths, were incubated at 37 C and subcultured after 72 hours.

Most of the 250 catheters, obtained from 198 patients, were from peripheral veins. Colony counts on semiquantitative plates were bimodally distributed; a small number of catheters yielded many colonies (Fig 3). Local inflammation was more frequent with catheters yielding 15 or more colonies, and, thus, 15 or more colonies on the plate equaled a positive result. In all, 19.6% of catheters were positive only in broth or yielded only 1 – 7 colonies on the plate, and none of these resulted in septicemia. Of 25 positive catheters, 4 produced septicemia (table). In each case, confluent growth of the infecting pathogen was demonstrated on semiquantitative culture. Local inflammation was present about 16 of 25 catheters that were positive on culture and about 30 of 225 that were negative, a significant difference. Rates of positive cultures and catheter-related septicemia increased significantly with the duration of catheter placement. A positive semiquantitative culture for *Staphylococcus aureus, Candida albicans* or *Klebsiella* species was as-

Fig 3.—Typical positive semiquantitative catheter culture. Original catheter segment has been placed on the plate for perspective. The plate shows confluent growth of *Staphylococcus aureus* and is from a catheter that produced septicemia. (Courtesy of Maki, D. G., et al.: N. Engl. J. Med. 296: 1305 – 1309, June 9, 1977.)

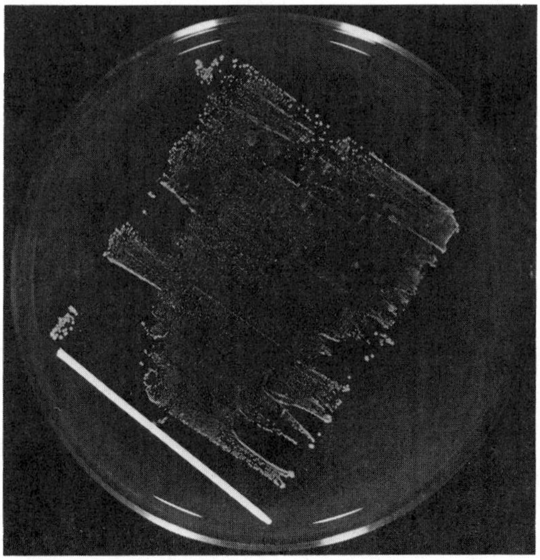

(9) N. Engl. J. Med. 296:1305 – 1309, June 9, 1977.

Relation of Results of Semiquantitative Culture to Catheter-Associated Inflammation and Septicemia

Datum	Culture Results	
	Negative	Positive*
No. of catheters	225	25
No. with inflammation	30 (13.3%)	16 (64%)†
No. with septicemia	0	4 (16%)‡

*≥ Fifteen colonies on primary plate.
†Chi-square = 32.6, $P < 0.001$.
‡$P = 0.008$ by Fisher's exact test.

sociated with septicemia in 4 of 7 instances. Of 37 catheters in 22 patients who were exposed to bacteremias from distant sites of infection unrelated to the catheter, 4 yielded the same species in broth culture. None gave a positive semiquantitative culture with the bloodstream pathogen. At least 1,000 colonies were present on semiquantitative culture in all 4 cases of catheter-related septicemia.

Semiquantitative culturing of venous catheters promises to facilitate the diagnosis of suppurative phlebitis, the most serious form of catheter-related sepsis. This method also holds promise for the investigation of new techniques of local asepsis in infusion therapy. A positive semiquantitative culture, rather than overt septicemia, can serve as the index of catheter-related infection in clinical trials.

► [Doctor Maki continues to make illuminating contributions to our understanding of the factors that influence the risk of infection complicating infusion therapy. Here he and his colleagues have applied a general concept; if you can quantify a previously qualitative observation, your ability to draw conclusions becomes much more powerful. Their conclusions make good sense; the more dense the microbial contamination of the intravenous catheter tip, the more likely it is to produce phlebitis and sepsis. The technique holds promise in helping to identify patients with suppurative phlebitis which is often not evident clinically. If a patient develops overwhelming septicemia (especially if it is staphylococcal), if a site of origin remains obscure and if the semiquantitative catheter culture is positive for the same microbial species and bacteremia persists despite therapy, one would be very inclined to proceed with exploratory venotomy.—Ed.] ◄

Transfusion-Associated Cytomegalovirus Mononucleosis. The occurrence of cytomegalovirus (CMV) infection as a consequence of blood transfusion has been documented. Phillip I. Lerner and James E. Sampliner[1] (Cleveland) encountered 3 patients in less than 1 year with transfusion-associated CMV mononucleosis after trauma. Both massive and limited-volume transfusions were involved. Hectic fever was a characteristic feature in these otherwise remarkably asymptomatic patients, without the classic features of heterophile-positive infectious mononucleosis. The illness developed several weeks after extensive thoracic or abdominal trauma surgery. Laboratory clues included atypical lymphocytosis, markers of altered immunity (cold agglutinins, rheumatoid factor) and moderate hepatic dysfunction. In 1 pa-

(1) Ann. Surg. 185:406–410, April, 1977.

tient, focal isotope defects in a spleen scan misleadingly suggested a septic complication. A false positive monospot test was obtained in this patient.

Failure to consider this self-limited viral infection may be a critical factor leading to unnecessary surgery. The spectrum of response to posttransfusion CMV infection ranges from asymptomatic seroconversion to a self-limited mononucleosis-like syndrome. High, often spiking, and long-lasting fever may dominate the clinical picture, usually without significant physical impairment. The features of classic infectious mononucleosis are lacking. Fatal disseminated CMV infection in adults appears limited, for the most part, to immunosuppressed patients. It is unlikely that effective screening measures can be developed from serologic testing only, because of the high incidence of positive reactors for CMV-CF antibody in the general population. Trauma and splenectomy may influence the course of postoperative viral infections acquired by transfusion. The diagnosis of CMV infection does not exclude the presence of an abscess. With an increasing number of cases of surgery for trauma and the extensive use of blood replacement therapy, many patients may be at risk.

► [We have included this article as a reminder. Cytomegalovirus was first shown to produce febrile illness after transfusion when the postperfusion syndrome ("postpump pyrexia") was defined. Since then it has been identified in a variety of circumstances, surgical and medical, after transfusions.

Nevertheless, the diagnostic problem remains—especially after surgery where unexplained spiking fever often signifies an undrained abscess. The diagnosis of CMV infection is serologic, which means that the complement-fixation titer may not rise for 2 weeks or more. That hardly helps one decide whether to go ahead with an exploratory laparotomy. The authors offer some diagnostic clues: high fever with relative bradycardia, the finding of atypical lymphocytes on peripheral smear, positive tests for cold agglutinins or rheumatoid factor, and mildly abnormal liver function studies. All this is fine but, as the authors take pains to point out, these features are not invariably present and in posttrauma circumstances they may be obscured by many other features. No panaceas here! Whoever said medicine was easy?—Ed.] ◄

► ↓ Renal dialysis and transplantation programs are now a common feature of the American medical landscape. The following two articles alert us to one viral and one bacterial infection that can complicate management of patients with renal transplants. Anogenital herpesvirus infections, although not usually life-threatening diseases, can be extraordinarily painful. Their recognition can spare the patient the administration of unnecessary antimicrobials. *Listeria monocytogenes,* on the other hand, can produce life-threatening disease and responds promptly to ampicillin therapy.—Ed. ◄

Atypical Herpesvirus Hominis Type 2 Infection in Uremic Patients Receiving Immunosuppressive Therapy. William J. Stone, Eric B. Scowden, Clarence L. Spannuth, Sandra P. Lowry and Robert H. Alford[2] (Vanderbilt Univ.) report unusual, initially misdiagnosed presentations of anogenital herpesvirus hominis (HVH)-2 infection in 3 male renal allograft recipients and another immunosuppressed patient with uremia. The latter patient had idiopathic thrombocytopenia. Painful, initially vesicular lesions developed in the anogenital region during immunosuppressive drug therapy and enlarged, coalesced and ulcerated. Initial misdiagnoses often led to inappropriate antimicrobial therapy. Routine cultures, sections and Tzanck

(2) Am. J. Med. 63:511–515, October, 1977.

RESULTS OF INITIAL VIROLOGIC STUDIES

Case No.	Specimen Received	Cells Used for Isolation	First Appearance of Cytopathic Effect
1	Skin biopsy	WI-38*	2 days
		HEK	2 days
2	Swab from scrotal vesicle	WI-38	1 day
		HEK	1 day
3	Swab from genital lesions	WI-38	2 days
4	Rectal swab	WI-38	2 days
		HEK	5 days

*WI-38, established strain of human fibroblasts; HEK, primary human embryonic kidney cells.

preparations were seldom helpful. The correct diagnosis was established within 18 – 48 hours by viral culture of swab or biopsy material. Isolated viruses were subsequently identified as HVH-2 by neutralization kinetics, infectivity titers and ability to plaque in chick embryo cells. Various treatments were ineffective; clinical improvement correlated best with a decreasing dose of immunosuppressive agents. The virologic findings are summarized in the table.

Man, 39, given a cadaveric renal transplant 3 years before, was admitted with steadily declining renal function. A biopsy specimen of the transplant a

Fig 4. – Necrotic, crater-like ulcerations are located on the dorsum of the penis and adjacent scrotum of the patient. (Courtesy of Stone, W. J., et al.: Am. J. Med. 63:511 – 515, October, 1977.)

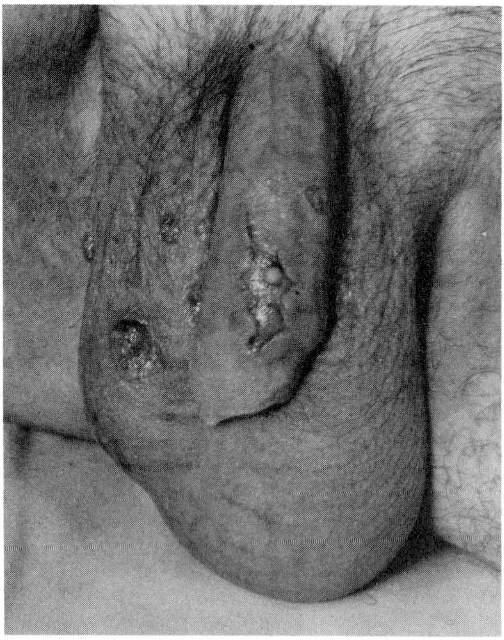

month earlier had shown findings compatible with chronic rejection. Immunosuppression consisted of 50 mg cyclophosphamide, 150 mg azathioprine and 10 – 60 mg prednisone daily. Deep ulcerations were present on the penis (Fig 4), scrotum and buttocks. The white blood cell count was 1900/cu mm with 88% neutrophils. The serum creatinine was 5.2 mg/dl and the blood urea nitrogen 132 mg/dl. Fever and tachycardia developed with a rise in the serum cytomegalovirus titer. Culture of the skin lesions showed *Candida albicans* and a *Corynebacterium* organism. The skin ulcers failed to respond to local nystatin or potassium permanganate therapy. Culture of a swab of the genital lesions yielded HVH-2. The ulcerations subsided after transplant nephrectomy and the cessation of immunosuppression, but the patient died of irreversible hypotension 11 weeks after admission. Autopsy showed no histologic evidence of disseminated HVH infection.

Prompt diagnosis of HVH infection is possible with use of current virologic methods. The major significance of the diagnosis of HVH-2 infection at present is in avoiding inappropriate antibacterial and antifungal therapy. Treatment of anogenital HVH-2 infections must remain symptomatic until effective specific antiviral chemotherapy is developed.

► [This is an instance where the virus diagnostic laboratory can produce clinically useful information within the same time span that we usually associate with bacteriologic diagnosis. Unfortunately, one's only therapeutic recourse is to reduce the dosage of immunosuppressive drugs. Fortunately, it sometimes works. – Ed.] ◄

***Listeria monocytogenes* Infection after Renal Transplantation.** Immunosuppressive therapy renders recipients of transplants susceptible to a variety of infections by opportunistic pathogens such as *Listeria monocytogenes*. Gerhard P. J. Schröter and Richard Weil III[3] (Univ. of Colorado) reviewed experience with *L. monocytogenes* infections in over 700 renal transplants done in 1962 – 76. About 20% were retransplants. Most grafts were from living donors. Immunosuppression was with azathioprine and prednisone. Most patients have received a course of heterologous antilymphocyte globulin since 1966. Cyclophosphamide replaced or was used with azathioprine in some patients in 1971 – 72. Most recipients of related kidneys had bilateral nephrectomy and splenectomy.

Thirteen cases of *L. monocytogenes* infection occurred. Nine male and 4 female patients aged 11 – 46 were affected. Seven had primary related grafts at the time of infection; 11 had had bilateral nephrectomy and splenectomy. Three patients were in chronic renal failure at the time of infection and 2 of them were on hemodialysis. The infections occurred 1 month to 7 years after initial transplantation. Seven patients had meningitis, whereas 6 had bacteremia alone. Two patients had signs of encephalitis; 2 had gastroenteritis and 2 had thrombophlebitis of the lower extremities. The isolated strains of *L. monocytogenes* were sensitive to a variety of antibiotics. Treatment was delayed for several days in 2 patients. Intravenously administered ampicillin in high doses was the treatment of choice, but only 4 patients received ampicillin alone. One patient died with acute cerebral edema and uncal herniation. No relapse has occurred in the 12 patients who re-

(3) Arch. Intern. Med. 137:1395 – 1399, October, 1977.

covered. Five patients died within 3 years after the infection of unrelated causes, whereas 5 are alive 4 years or longer after their infections.

Immunosuppression of organ transplant recipients can interfere with defenses against *L. monocytogenes* infections. The major effect of immunosuppressive agents may be on immunologically specific mediators of macrophage function, rather than on macrophage function itself. The recommended treatment is intravenous ampicillin.

► [All the patients with meningitis in the series had an acute onset of illness with fever, chills, headache and, usually, stiff neck. Central nervous system infection with a more insidious onset also has been described. In these persons encephalitic signs may predominate with impaired mentation. My Vanderbilt University colleagues have seen a renal transplant recipient with this presentation within the past year. This young transplant recipient had an enviably positive outlook on life. He was a voracious reader and, in particular, kept himself well informed on current events. His family first noted that he became disinterested in the *New York Times,* which he read daily. Within a day he became somewhat confused. Only then was low-grade fever discovered. On admission to the hospital he was extremely confused and combative. The diagnostic money was on cryptococcal disease. *Listeria monocytogenes* grew in cerebrospinal fluid culture. He was strikingly improved after 24 hours of ampicillin therapy. At morning rounds on the 3d day of therapy he was found reading the *New York Times* and grumbling that he had a lot of reading to catch up on. — Ed.] ◄

Pneumococcal Infections

► ↓ My long-time friend Bob Austrian has steadfastly pursued his investigations of the pneumococcus throughout his distinguished career. While others remained dubious, he demonstrated the continuing serious impact the pneumococcus has on morbidity and mortality in our population. He championed the idea of pneumococcal vaccine and has performed the major laboratory and clinical studies demonstrating its safety and efficacy. The following report can be considered the culmination of his work. The vaccine was tested in a very large population of South African gold miners. These men are recruited from remote villages and gathered together at the mines where they live and work in close proximity to each other. Pneumococcal infections are regularly epidemic among the recruits. I think you will find the results most convincing.—Ed. ◄

Prevention of Pneumococcal Pneumonia by Vaccination was reviewed by Robert Austrian, Robert M. Douglas, Gerald Schiffman, Albert M. Coetzee, Hendrik J. Koornhof, Stanley Hayden-Smith and Robert D. W. Reid.[4] Attempts have been made to reduce mortality from bacteremic pneumococcal pneumonia by development of polyvalent vaccines of pneumococcal capsular polysaccharides. Capsular polysaccharides of 15 individual types were prepared commercially and tested for antigenicity in volunteers, most in doses of 5–1000 μg. The safety of monovalent vaccines was readily demonstrable. A dose of 50 μg was found to be suitable for each capsular antigen.

Field trials were carried out in gold mining novices in South Africa, in whom pneumonia is epidemic and the pneumococcus is the prevalent cause. The attack rate of putative pneumococcal pneumonia was 90 per 1,000 man-years of exposure. Three trials that involved 12,000 young men were conducted with a polyvalent pneumococcal vaccine, a group A meningococcal vaccine or a saline placebo. A hexavalent vaccine was used in the first study and a tridecavalent vaccine containing 13 polysaccharide types in the two subsequent trials. The dose of each antigen was 50 μg. Protection against putative infection by individual pneumococcal types was significant. In all trials combined, the vaccines were 82.3% effective in preventing pneumococcal bacteremia caused by types included in them. Three types not included in the vaccines accounted for over half the remaining bacteremic infections. Eight of 10 bacteremic infections in vaccinees that were caused by included types were infections with pneumococcus type 1, and analysis of this antigen in vaccine showed 9 rather than 50 μg to be present per dose.

Polyvalent vaccines of pneumococcal capsular polysaccharides are safe and at least 78.5% effective in protecting against type-specific putative pneumococcal pneumonia. Their efficacy in preventing bacteremic infection with the same organisms was 82.3%. They should be

(4) Trans. Assoc. Am. Physicians 89:184–194, 1976.

useful in preventing disease in adults at an increased risk of a fatal outcome of pneumococcal infection, including subjects aged 50 and over, those with chronic systemic illnesses and those with asplenia or sicklemia.

► [Pneumococcal vaccine recently has been licensed for general use. The vaccine contains purified capsular polysaccharide from the 14 pneumococcal types (Numbers 1–4, 6, 8, 9, 12, 14, 19, 23, 25, 51 and 56) which together account for 80% of all bacteremic pneumococcal infections encountered in the United States.

The United States Public Health Service Advisory Committee on Immunization Practices has just issued (coincidence—it arrived in my mail today!) its guidelines for the use of this vaccine (*Morbidity and Mortality Weekly Report* 27:25, Jan. 27, 1978). To summarize:

1. Mass immunization of healthy individuals is *not* advised.
2. Closed populations (in nursing homes, residential schools, etc.) should be considered for immunization.
3. Patients with a special predisposition to pneumococcal infection are prime candidates for the vaccine: asplenic patients or those with splenic dysfunction (sickle cell disease, especially), diabetics and those with impaired cardiorespiratory, hepatic or renal systems.

In the vaccine trials, about half the recipients developed mild pain and erythema at the injection site for a day (it is best to warn your patients; aspirin should suffice). No serious adverse reactions have been reported to date.

Thus, pneumococcal vaccine should become widely used by all physicians engaged in primary care. Pneumococcal pneumonia was once called the "old man's friend." Life expectancy and its quality have increased since that adage was in common use. Bob Austrian and his vaccine are the new friends of all for whom the vaccine is recommended.—Ed.] ◄

Fulminant Pneumococcal Infections in "Normal" Asplenic Hosts. Surgical removal of the spleen is known to increase the risk of life-threatening pneumococcal infection, especially in patients with diseases that are themselves associated with depressed reticuloendothelial function. There remains debate as to whether splenectomy in otherwise normal persons is attended by an increased risk of fulminant pneumococcemia. Venu Gopal and Alan L. Bisno[5] (Univ. of Tennessee) report 5 cases of life-threatening pneumococcal infection in asplenic persons who were otherwise normal; 2 were adults. Only 3 of 8 asplenic subjects seen in 1972–76 with life-threatening pneumococcal infections had severe underlying diseases. A fourth patient was a boy with sinus histiocytosis, a pseudolymphomatous disorder generally associated with a benign prognosis. A fifth otherwise normal patient was referred.

With the inclusion of the present cases, 18 episodes of overwhelming postsplenectomy infection syndrome in subjects older than age 4 have been reported in 17 patients after splenectomy for traumatic rupture. Three other subjects had splenectomy incidental to abdominal surgery for benign conditions, 3 others had idiopathic splenic atrophy or infarction and 2 had asplenia as an isolated congenital defect. Thirteen of the 25 subjects were over age 20 at the time of infection, with a mean age of 27.7. The average interval between splenectomy and infection in 21 episodes was 5.6 years; 6 episodes occurred 10 or more years after splenectomy. The case-fatality rate in postsplenectomy cases was 71%. The mortality in patients with congenital asplenia or splenic atrophy was

(5) Arch. Intern. Med. 137:1526–1530, November, 1977.

80%. Four of the 8 serotypes of infecting pneumococci identified were type XII, 2 were type XXII and 2 were type XXIII.

The precise pathophysiologic mechanisms underlying fulminant pneumococcal infection in otherwise normal asplenic hosts remain to be elucidated. Splenectomy itself is associated with an increased risk of overwhelming pneumococcemia. The magnitude of the risk is low, but the mortality from these infections is high. Undiagnosed febrile episodes in asplenic persons should be treated promptly with antibiotics while the culture findings are being awaited, regardless of the patient's age or general state of health. The finding that a limited number of pneumococcal serotypes, particularly type XII, appear to predominate in these cases suggests that pneumococcal vaccine might be highly effective in preventing this syndrome in otherwise normal hosts.

► [Doctor Bisno has been prominent among those investigators who have delineated the syndrome of overwhelming pneumococcal infection in asplenic persons. All of us have been convinced that increased risk exists when splenectomy is performed in patients who have underlying conditions that themselves carry an increased risk of sepsis (such as Hodgkin disease and histiocytoses). Some have doubted, however, whether otherwise normal persons who undergo traumatic splenectomy share this risk. Doctor Bisno and his associate have compellingly marshalled their own experience and that in the literature which should convince everyone that they do.

Fortunately, pneumococcal vaccine contains capsular polysaccharide antigens of pneumococcal types 12 and 23, which have been most often associated with sepsis in such asplenic persons. The administration of pneumococcal vaccine should now become routine after splenectomy.

The article makes another telling point. In the asplenic host, pneumococcal sepsis is "characterized by abrupt onset, frequently without any perceptible focus of pneumococcal infection, fulminant course and high mortality despite prompt and appropriate antibiotic therapy." This means that such patients must be instructed to call you at the very first indication of fever. They should be examined, blood cultures obtained and vigorous empiric antibiotic therapy begun. Never suggest, "Take 2 aspirins and call me if you don't feel better." You may never get that call. – Ed.]

► ↓ During my medical adolescence, I witnessed the introduction of a wonderous array of new antimicrobial agents. I was deeply impressed with the power this gave the physician to intervene effectively at the bedside and in office practice. In my opinion, the use of antibiotics (along with insulin, vitamin B_{12} and a few other substances) still ranks high among the most elegant and incisive medical means to reverse a pathophysiologic process.

Since these early days, I have had to adjust (grudgingly) to the progressive development of antibiotic resistance among numerous bacterial species. The gram-negative bacilli have been particularly adept at this annoying trick. Staphylococci, of course, are now almost all resistant to penicillin – and some to methicillin and the cephalosporins as well. Recently, some strains of *Hemophilus influenzae* and the gonococcus have acquired plasmids that enable them to produce a β-lactamase, making them resistant to ampicillin and penicillin, respectively.

All this I endured stoically. However, I admit to having been shaken by this year's shocker: pneumococci resistant to penicillin! Is nothing sacred? – Ed. ◄

***Streptococcus pneumoniae* Resistant to Penicillin and Chloramphenicol.** P. C. Appelbaum, A. Bhamjee, J. N. Scragg, A. F. Hallett, Annette J. Bowen and Rosemary C. Cooper[6] (Natal Univ.) report 5 cases of systemic infection in young African children, 3 of them fatal, which were caused by strains of *S. pneumoniae* serotype 19A resistant to penicillin-cephalosporin and chloramphenicol. Three patients had

(6) Lancet 2:995–997, Nov. 12, 1977.

SENSITIVITY OF PNEUMOCOCCI TO ANTIMICROBIAL AGENTS

		M.I.C. range (mg/l)			M.B.C. range (mg/l)		
Antimicrobial agent	Disc sensitivity*	10^3 c.f.u./ml	10^4 c.f.u./ml	10^7 c.f.u./ml	10^3 c.f.u./ml	10^4 c.f.u./ml	10^7 c.f.u./ml
Benzylpenicillin	R	4–8	..	4–8	4–8	..	4–8
Methicillin	R	22–32	..	22–45	22–45	..	22–64
Ampicillin	PR	1–4	..	2–5	2–5	..	4–10
Carbenicillin	R	101–128	..	128–256	101–128	..	128–512
Cephalothin	PR	4–15	..	4–30	4–15	..	4–30
Cephamandole	PR	4–8	..	8–16	4–8	..	15–30
Tobramycin	R	..	16–32	..	..	..	..
Gentamicin	R	..	16–32	..	..	..	..
Neomycin	R	..	250–500	..	..	..	..
Streptomycin	R	..	>2000	..	..	..	..
Kanamycin	R	..	64–125	..	..	..	..
Chloramphenicol	R	9–37	..	18–37	18–37	..	37
Erythromycin	S	0·01–0·03	..	0·01–0·03	0·01–0·03	..	0·01–0·03
Tetracycline	S	0·1–0·4	..	0·1–0·8	0·1–0·4	..	0·1–0·8
Clindamycin	S	<0·004–0·08	..	0·01–0·02	<0·004–0·08	..	0·01–0·02
Co-trimoxazole	S	6–12	..	12–25	6–12	..	12–25
Rifampicin	S	..	..	..	..	..	..
Vancomycin	S	..	..	..	..	..	..

*R, resistant; PR, partially resistant; S, sensitive.

meningitis and 2, septicemia. Quellung reactions showed all organisms to be serotype 19A, or type 57 by the American classification. The results of antimicrobial susceptibility tests were similar for all the organisms and were uninfluenced by inoculum strength (table.) The pneumococci were sensitive to erythromycin, tetracylcine, clindamycin, rifampicin, vancomycin and co-trimoxazole. No β-lactamase was demonstrated in any of the organisms. Nasopharyngeal swabs from 188 ward contacts, 100 randomly selected women attending the antenatal clinic and 100 casualty department patients yielded no resistant pneumococci.

Three of these five infections developed in the hospital. All 5 patients had received penicillin or chloramphenicol, or both, for relatively long periods before or during their hospital stay. The sensitivity pattern of the strains involved differs from that of previously reported penicillin-resistant pneumococci. These cases add *S. pneumoniae* to the growing list of drug-resistant organisms which have appeared in recent years. If drug-resistant pneumococci become widespread, the treatment of *S. pneumoniae* infections will require reevaluation.

► [This early report from Durban, South Africa, is the tip of the iceberg of the problem in that country. From May to November, 1977, 15 children in Durban and Johannesburg have had meningitis or bacteremic pneumonia due to this multiply resistant pneumococcal strain. Many other hospitalized children have had the organism isolated from sputum or pharyngeal cultures. In contrast to the results reported in this article, carriers have since been identified among hospital personnel. Carriers also were found among people in the community who had contact with affected hospitals or with other known carriers. Several different antibiotic-resistance patterns have been documented among the pneumococcal isolates. The method of resistance remains speculative at present.

As you can imagine, intensive control activities were instituted. The dust has not settled, so their effectiveness is not yet known. I promise further reports on this front in future editions of the YEAR BOOK. To date, no other countries have reported the isolation of multiply resistant pneumococcal strains. The infectious disease fraternity and clinical microbiologists in the United States have been put on the alert. We shall see. . . .

It looks as if the licensure of pneumococcal vaccine has come none too soon. I wouldn't be surprised to learn that the manufacturer is working on a vaccine against these strains right now. – Ed.] ◄

Enteric Infections

► ↓ Second only to upper respiratory tract infections, gastroenteritis is the major cause of human discomfort, time lost from work and the like. Most diarrheal diseases are acute and self-limited. Some pose more serious medical problems. Here is a series of five articles about gastrointestinal infections that caught our eye this year. – Ed. ◄

Salmonella typhi **Infections in the United States, 1967–72: Increasing Importance of International Travelers.** The incidence of typhoid fever has declined markedly in the past 3 decades in the United States, but increases in the number of Americans traveling to endemic areas abroad heighten concern about the disease. Peter A. Rice, William B. Baine and Eugene J. Gangarosa[7] (Center for Disease Control, Atlanta, Ga.) report a change in the epidemiology of *S. typhi* infection in the United States in 1967–72 that emphasizes the importance of travel-associated typhoid. The Center for Disease Control has conducted nationwide surveillance of typhoid since 1962.

Salmonella typhi isolates were reported in 1967–72 from 3,661 persons in the United States, including 1,798 with clinical cases and 1,482 carriers. Of 1,418 evaluable clinical cases, 470 (33%) were travel associated. The age and sex distribution of indigenous cases is shown in Figure 5. There was no secular trend in the number of indigenous cases during this period. In contrast, there was a steady rise in the number of travel-associated cases of typhoid fever during this time. Thus, while in 1967 only 37, or 17%, of the 220 cases reported were travel associat-

Fig 5. – Indigenous cases of *Salmonella typhi* infection, by age and sex, United States, 1967–72. Ages unknown for 76 men, 44 women and 12 patients of unknown sex. (Courtesy of Rice, P. A., et al.: Am. J. Epidemiol. 106:160–166, August, 1977.)

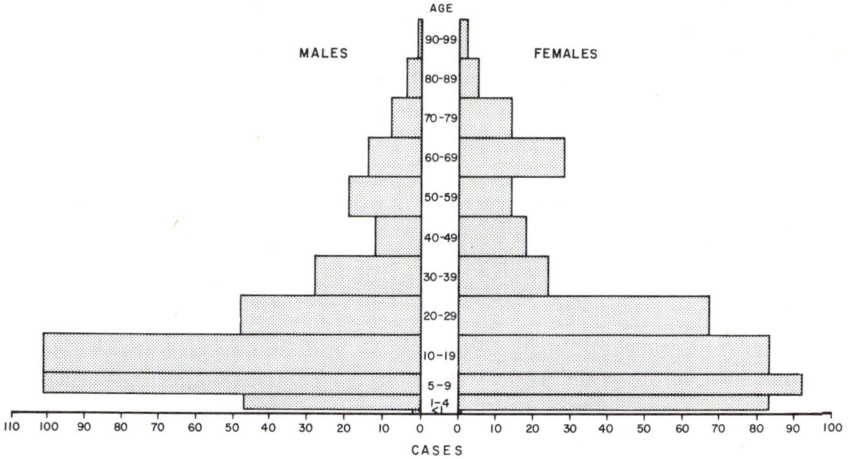

(7) Am. J. Epidemiol. 106:160–166, August, 1977.

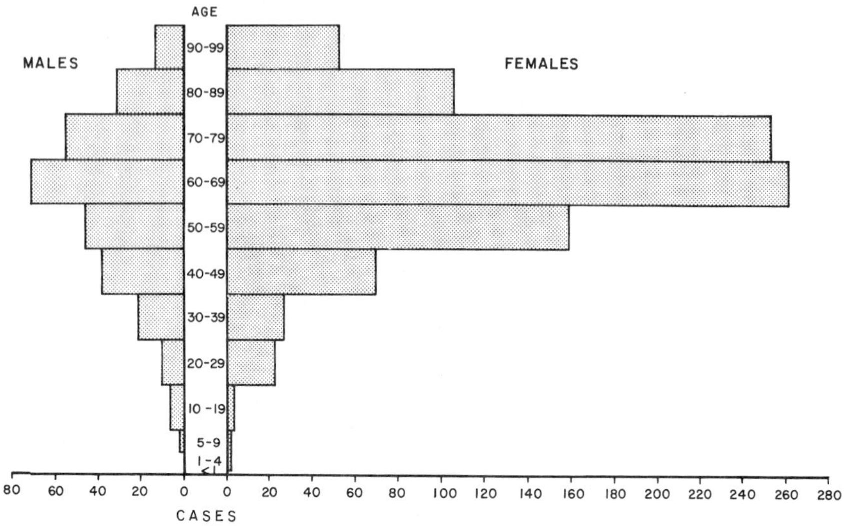

Fig 6.—*Salmonella typhi* carriers by age and sex, United States, 1967–72. Ages unknown for 59 men, 164 women and 8 patients of unknown sex. Sex unknown for 1 patient of known age. (Courtesy of Rice, P. A., et al.: Am. J. Epidemiol. 106:160–166, August, 1977.)

ed, 137, or 46%, of the 296 cases reported in 1972 were apparently contracted abroad. Only 8% of travel-associated cases were involved in recognized foreign outbreaks. Mexico, Italy and India accounted for 72% of the travel-associated cases. Most of the increase between 1967 and 1972 was due to cases associated with Mexico. The distribution of carriers is shown in Figure 6.

Persons with Hispanic surnames are at relatively high risk of acquiring typhoid. The increase in travel-associated cases is largely due to cases associated in some way with Mexico. Most indigenous cases have been in children or young adults and were not linked to recognized outbreaks. Most known typhoid carriers in the United States are elderly women. The typical patient with travel-associated typhoid was older and more likely to be male than his counterpart with indigenous disease, reflecting the demographic features of foreign travelers.

► [Although the number of cases is not large, the increase in travel-associated typhoid should be kept in mind in dealing with febrile members of our very mobile population. As noted by the authors, part of this increase appears to stem from the enormous increase in both legal and illicit travel between Mexico and the United States. An addendum to this article indicates that the proportion of cases associated with foreign travel remains high. During 1974, 1975 and 1976, the figures were 60%, 26% and 43%, respectively, of the cases reported.—Ed.] ◄

Paratyphoid Fever: Report of 62 Cases with Several Unusual Findings and Review of the Literature. With frequent and rapid world travel, paratyphoid fever (PTF) is now being seen in previously unexposed populations, and previous descriptions of the disease are of little value to the practicing physician. Roy A. Meals[8] (U. S. Air Force Hosp., Adana, Turkey) reports the findings in 62 cases occurring in a

(8) Arch. Intern. Med. 136:1422–1428, December, 1976.

healthy, homogenous population, American military personnel and their dependents living in southern Turkey. Of these, 54 patients had *Salmonella paratyphi B*, 6 had *S. paratyphi A* and 2 had both.

A seasonal incidence was observed, with 60 (97%) of the cases occurring between June and October. The most common initial symptom was fever (92%), with gastrointestinal or neurologic complaints. Five patients had intermittently spiking fevers with no other associated symptoms. All patients had oral temperatures of at least 38.5 C, with most (87%) having temperatures over 39.5 C. Frequently temperatures would spike every 6–8 hours, resulting in a characteristic febrile pattern useful in the diagnosis of PTF. Relative bradycardia was observed in most cases and only rarely did pulse rates exceed 100 beats per minute. Five patients had symptoms suggestive of meningitis, but cerebrospinal fluid was sterile and acellular. Other infrequent physical findings included liver enlargement (16%), papilledema, spleen enlargement, boggy prostate, rose spots and pulmonary ronchi.

Diagnosis was made from positive culture material. Blood cultures were positive in 59 of 62 patients. Stool cultures were positive in 21, 18 of whom had positive blood cultures. Stool cultures alone were positive in 3 patients. The white blood count was generally normal with a shift to the left. It was not helpful diagnostically. Liver function tests were frequently abnormal, with or without liver enlargement. Two patients had peripheral blood smears that were highly suggestive of acute leukemia. These findings returned to normal with recuperation from PTF.

Cloramphenicol is the drug of choice in treatment of PTF, with initial dosage of 50 mg/kg body weight/day in 4 divided doses, followed by 30 mg/kg/day when the patient becomes afebrile to complete a 10-day course. Ampicillin is an effective alternate drug.

Patients became afebrile within 1–9 days (average, 4.2 days) after initiation of treatment.

► [This is helpful in characterizing the clinical syndrome of *severe* bacteremic salmonellal infection in otherwise healthy young military personnel.

Bacteremic salmonellal infections are clinically indistinguishable from typhoid fever. Patients have chills, spiking temperatures that continue over some days, bradycardia, generally normal white blood cell counts with a polymorphonuclear leukocyte predominance, neurologic manifestations and few physical findings. Blood cultures are positive early. Positive stool cultures come later. Thus I disagree with the author that older descriptions of the disease are unhelpful. Read Osler on typhoid fever; it is the same syndrome. Secondly, I believe this article can give clinicians an extremely misleading picture of the spectrum of salmonellal infections as they actually occur in our American population. The patients described were those with gastroenteritis of longer than 48 hours' duration which was serious enough to take them to doctors, or patients with unexplained chills and fever who were admitted to the hospital.

The authors state that 11 patients with salmonellal gastroenteritis with "mild transient symptoms" were excluded from the study. I would have wished otherwise.

Salmonella other than *S. typhosa* are unselective little microbes that inhabit the guts and tissues of all kinds of creatures from birds to beasts to reptiles. Only the typhoid bacillus is fastidious enough to confine its infections to man. Because of their ubiquity, salmonellal infections are very common in human beings. Most of these infections are quite benign and self-limited. Most do not come to medical attention except during common-source epidemics. They produce short-lived gastroenteritis and flulike myalgias and do not generally require treatment. Indeed, this may be true of even those in patients with bacteremic disease, and Doctor Meals had 3 bacteremic patients who were well before blood culture results were known.

My own experience has led me to feel that the effectiveness of antimicrobial therapy, including chloramphenicol or ampicillin, in the treatment of salmonellal infections other than typhoid has not been convincingly established. Doctor Meals' data do not answer this question, but they give me pause. His patients became afebrile quite promptly after antimicrobials were started, and apparently relapses were not observed in this series. – Ed.] ◄

Epidemiologic Assessment of Relevance of So-Called Enteropathogenic Serogroups of *Escherichia coli* in Diarrhea is presented by Eugene J. Gangarosa and Michael H. Merson[9] (Center for Disease Control, Atlanta, Ga.). In the early 1950's, the concept evolved that certain serogroups of *E. coli,* designated enteropathogenic, are inherent enteric pathogens, and many clinicians regard diarrhea associated with these serogroups as a distinct clinical entity. Later evidence questioned the inherent virulence of enteropathogenic *E. coli,* particularly in sporadic cases of diarrheal disease in infants and adults. *Escherichia coli* enterotoxin-mediated diarrhea has been recognized in recent years, and there is good evidence that the enterotoxins are plasmid mediated. While there are no reports explaining definitively how the classic enteropathogenic strains cause diarrhea, it appears that these strains are not invariably pathogenic but may acquire virulence, as in the case of enterotoxigenic *E. coli.*

Serotyping of *E. coli* can be a useful epidemiologic tool in investigating outbreaks, but clustering of cases of diarrhea in which *E. coli* of the same serotype is isolated does not per se imply that a particular strain of *E. coli* is the cause. Routine serotyping to find the index case or cases in each outbreak is not necessary. Routine serogrouping of *E. coli* in sporadic cases of diarrhea, with the use of commercial antiserums currently available in the United States, is for practical purposes useless. Current methods of detecting enterotoxin are too time-consuming and technically difficult for routine laboratory use. Rowe et al. indicated that separate pools of antiserums prepared against selected enteropathogenic, enterotoxigenic and enteroinvasive strains may be useful for routine laboratory identification of *E. coli,* but this remains to be established definitively.

► [This is an important review, but it is difficult to summarize its findings in a short article. Let me tell you what I derived from it.

Current evidence suggests that strains of *E. coli* can cause enteric disease by one of two mechanisms. First, they can elaborate enterotoxin. Two types are recognized – one is heat labile (like cholera) and one is heat stable. Both are plasmid mediated – thus serotyping does not tell you whether you are dealing with a "meany" or a "cream puff" strain. Second, certain *E. coli* strains can cause actual mucosal invasion. However, why this occurs is not known, and the serotypes originally implicated in diarrhea do not invariably possess this capacity.

Like phage-typing of staphylococci, serotyping of *E. coli* can be a useful epidemiologic tool in investigating an outbreak but it does not seem helpful in surveillance or in determination of the etiology of diarrhea in specific cases.

Doctors Gangarosa and Merson politely suggest we are engaging in a lot of expensive busy work in such routine serotyping and recommend careful reassessment of current laboratory practices. Sounds reasonable to me! – Ed.] ◄

Trimethoprim-Sulfamethoxazole Compared to Ampicillin in the Treatment of Shigellosis. Recent reports have documented the

(9) N. Engl. J. Med. 296:1210 – 1213, May 26, 1977.

emergence of strains of *Shigella* organisms resistant to multiple antibiotics. Margan J. Chang, Lisa M. Dunkle, David Van Reken, Donald Anderson, Michael L. Wong and Ralph D. Feigin[1] (Washington Univ.) evaluated trimethoprim-sulfamethoxazole (TM-SM) in 20 children aged 1 – 12 years who presented in 1974 with features compatible with dysenteric shigellosis. All had a history of fever, abdominal pain and diarrhea and stool cultures positive for *Shigella* organisms. None had received antibiotic therapy in the week before admission. Ampicillin was given for 5 days in a dose of 100 mg/kg daily in four oral doses and TM-SM for 5 days in doses of 20 – 25 mg SM per kg and 4 – 5 mg TM per kg in two divided oral doses.

Nineteen children had *Shigella* organisms cultured from the initial stool swab. Twelve infections were due to *S. sonnei* and 7 to *S. flexneri*. Eleven children received TM-SM and 8 received ampicillin. The groups were comparable in severity of disease and duration of fever before admission. Children treated with TM-SM had significantly fewer stools during a 5-day hospital period. Stool cultures remained positive longer in the ampicillin-treated patients. One bacteriologic failure occurred in the TM-SM group. Three of 4 ampicillin-treated patients did well clinically despite the presence of isolates resistant to ampicillin, whereas 1 patient improved when changed to TM-SM therapy. A marked reduction in sensitivity of *S. sonnei* to ampicillin was observed from 1970 to 1975. Sensitivity to streptomycin and tetracycline also declined, whereas sensitivity to sulfasoxazole increased. The isolates were generally sensitive to chloramphenicol and nalidixic acid during the 6-year review period.

This limited trial confirms other observations indicating that TM-SM is the best program currently available for treating dysenteric shigellosis in areas where multiple antibiotic resistance of *Shigella* is common.

► [This study contained too few patients to prove definitively the superiority of trimethoprim-sulfamethoxazole over ampicillin therapy, but it does serve as a good vehicle to alert phsycians to the increasing incidence of ampicillin-resistant strains of *Shigella*.

The authors report that increasing ampicillin resistance has been reported from Dallas, St. Louis and the District of Columbia. The District of Columbia data have been particularly striking. Between 1964 and 1966, 5% of *Shigella* organisms were ampicillin resistant; in 1968, 11%; in 1969, 40%; in 1970, 70%; and in 1971, 95%! (See Ross et al.: J.A.M.A. 221:45, 1972.)

I would currently manage *Shigella* infections occurring in the United States with combined TM-SM therapy. – Ed.] ◄

Location of Food Consumption and Travelers' Diarrhea. Travelers' diarrhea usually develops within 2 weeks of the traveler's arrival in a foreign country. It is worldwide in distribution, but is more prevalent in tropical and subtropical countries with poor sanitation and hygiene. The disease is characterized by acute watery diarrhea and often nausea, cramps, chills or fever, and it generally lasts 2 – 3 days. Microbial pathogens have been believed to be the etiologic agents but this has been difficult to document definitively.

W. S. Tjoa, H. L. DuPont, P. Sullivan, L. K. Pickering, A. H. Hol-

(1) Pediatrics 59:726 – 729, May, 1977.

guin, J. Olarte, D. G. Evans and D. J. Evans, Jr.[2] attempted to correlate locations of food consumption with the development of enteric infection in a student population of 280 attending summer school in Mexico in the summer of 1975. A total of 260 completed the 30-day study. The population included 49 newly arrived students from the United States, 132 full-time United States students and 79 Latin American students. Diarrhea was defined as more than twice the usual number of unformed stools within 12 hours plus either fever, nausea, vomiting, abdominal cramps or malaise.

Diarrhea was associated with eating meals at local restaurants and the school cafeteria. It occurred in 13 of 29 (45%) United States summer students who ate more than half their meals at these sites, compared with 3 of 20 of those who usually ate in a private home. Shigella infection was more frequent in the former group (31% vs. 5%). Food-consumption sites were not related to diarrhea or *Shigella* isolation in the acclimatized student groups who had been in Latin America for a year or longer. Toxigenic *Escherichia coli* infection was related to eating at the cafeteria and public restaurants. Diarrhea was also more frequent in students who ate food obtained from street vendors. Studies of food samples from the sources implicated showed wide-

FOOD AND WATER CULTURES FROM CHOLULA AND PUEBLA (TOWN AND CITY ADJACENT TO SCHOOL IN MEXICO ATTENDED BY 280 STUDENTS PROSPECTIVELY ENROLLED IN STUDY)

Location	Description of food	Bacteria isolated
Open market	Marinated Beef	Klebsiella, *Pseudomonas species*
	Chile Pepper	Klebsiella, *Pseudomonas species*
	Ice Blocks (2)	Shigella C., Klebsiella, *Escherichia coli*
Meat (butcher's) shop	Sausage (cooked)	Klebsiella
Street vendors (4)	Tortilla with sauce	Klebsiella, *Pseudomonas species*
	Fruit	Klebsiella, *Pseudomonas species*
	Watermelon	*Salmonella species*
	Custard	Klebsiella, *Pseudomonas species*
Field (growing wild)	Mushroom	Shigella B
Restaurant #1	Tap water	Negative
	Pork steak	Enterobacter
Restaurant #2	Salad	Klebsiella, *Pseudomonas aeruginosa*
School cafeteria	Hamburger (cooked)	Shigella B
	Raw beef patties	Shigella B, Paracolon, *Klebsiella sp.*
	Chopped meat	Klebsiella
	Raw liver	Paracolon, Citrobacter, Klebsiella
	Catsup and salad dressing	Klebsiella
	Environmental surfaces	Klebsiella, Pseudomonas, Paracolon, Enterobacter
School clinic and dormitories	Bottled water	Negative
	Tap water	Negative
	Bottled water	Negative
	Tap water	Negative

(2) Am. J. Epidemiol. 106:61–66, July, 1977.

Sexually Transmitted Infections

► ↓ Although the epidemic of gonorrhea may have reached its peak nationally, the number of new cases each year is continuing to rise in some states, and the number of cases each year is still shockingly high. Even though therapy is more than 95% effective, the number of cases that fail on therapy is so large that treatment failure in these infections occurs more frequently than in all but two of the reportable communicable diseases. The spread of penicillin-resistant gonococci has not been nearly the problem we feared it would be (1977 YEAR BOOK, p. 25); however, infections with these oganisms are still occurring in isolated clusters and demand the vigilance of practicing physicians.

The need for a gonococcal vaccine is great. Fortunately, the chances of the development of an effective one are improving. Various fractions of gonococci have been partially or completely purified: (1) pili, which may aid attachment to mucosal surfaces; (2) lipopolysaccharide, which seems to participate in the serum bactericidal reaction and may damage mucosal cells; (3) capsules, which appear to be antiphagocytic; and (4) outer membrane proteins, the biologic function of which is unknown. It will take much more study to determine which of these or possibly other factors from gonococci are important in the pathogenic process so that one or more can be selected for use in a trial vaccine. Another problem in selecting an antigen for use in a vaccine is choosing one which does not vary from strain to strain. For instance, there are a number of serotypes of gonococcal pili so that any vaccine using pili would have to be multivalent. There are many other problems to be solved and questions to be answered, but it promises to be an interesting saga.

Meanwhile, the emphasis on research in sexually transmitted diseases by the National Institute of Allergy and Infectious Diseases is reaping benefits in other areas. We know, for instance, that the number of cases of nongonococcal urethritis equals or is greater than the number of cases of gonococcal urethritis. In white men with urethritis, the etiology is nongonococcal in about 70% of cases (1974 YEAR BOOK, p. 74; and 1975 YEAR BOOK, p. 67). *Chlamydia trachomatis* has been isolated from about 40% of patients with nongonococcal urethritis (1976 YEAR BOOK, p. 74) and seems to be one of the etiologic agents of this syndrome. However, in previous studies, *Ureaplasma urealyticum* organisms (formerly called "T-strain" mycoplasmas) were isolated with equal frequency from patients with nongonococcal urethritis and from patients without urethritis. Thus, there was little support for a role of ureaplasmas in nongonococcal urethritis. The following study provides a more incisive analysis of data on the isolation of chlamydiae and ureaplasmas in nongonococcal urethritis. In addition, it makes use of the sensitivity of chlamydiae to sulfisoxazole but not spectinomycin and the sensitivity of ureaplasmas to spectinomycin but not sulfisoxazole to make inferences about the role these organisms play in the infection. – Eds. ◄

Differential Response of Chlamydial and *Ureaplasma*-Associated Urethritis to Sulphafurazole (Sulfisoxazole) and Aminocyclitols. Nongonococcal urethritis (NGU) is the most common sexually transmitted disease in men. W. R. Bowie, J. F. Floyd, Y. Miller, E. R. Alexander, J. Holmes and K. K. Holmes[3] (Univ. of Washington) evaluated the response to treatment in 91 men who were randomly treated for NGU.

Chlamydia trachomatis (C) can be isolated significantly more often from the urethra of men with NGU than from men with gonorrhea or

(3) Lancet 2:1276–1278, Dec. 11, 1976.

Clinical Improvement* of Urethritis after Treatment with Sulphafurazole or Aminocyclitol

Treatment	No. improved/no. treated			
	C+U+	C+U−	C−U+	C−U−
Sulphafurazole	2/6	7/7	5/19	0/5
Aminocyclitol	1/8*	0/6	9/11†	3/6
		$P<0.002$	$P<0.05$	

*Improvement was assessed 7 – 14 days after start of treatment and indicates complete disappearance of urethral discharge or a change in the character of the discharge from purulent to clear, with less than 20 leukocytes in each of five 400× microscopic fields of the first voided urine sediment.

†Analysis limited to cases in which *Ureaplasma* was eradicated.

without urethritis, and serologic evidence indicates that onset of NGU is related temporally to recent acquisition of *C. trachomatis* infection. In white men with *Chlamydia*-positive (C+) and *Chlamydia*-negative (C−) NGU, *Ureaplasma urealyticum* (U) is isolated from the urethra more often and in higher concentration from men with C− NGU than from men with C+ NGU.

Initial urethral cultures were positive for *C. trachomatis* in 36 of 91 (40%) men. *U. urealyticum* was recovered from 21 of 36 (58%) C+ and 42 of 55 (76%) C− men. Among white men having a first episode of urethritis, *U. urealyticum* was recovered from 20 of 21 (95%) C− men and 5 of 8 (63%) C+ men. Ureaplasma infection was present in 26 of 47 (55%) men with recurrent infection.

Patients were treated with sulfisoxazole, 500 mg orally 4 times per day for 10 days, or with an aminocyclitol (streptomycin or spectinomycin), 2 gm intramuscularly for 1–3 doses at 12-hour intervals. The clinical response to therapy is illustrated in the table. Among men with C+U− NGU, treatment with sulfisoxazole produced clinical improvement in every patient, but treatment with aminocyclitols did not produce improvement in any patient. Among men with C−U+ NGU, clinical improvement occurred in 5 of 19 given sulfisoxazole and in 9 of 11 given aminocyclitol and from whom *Ureaplasma* organisms were eradicated. Initial treatment with either antimicrobial alone failed in 11 of 14 (79%) C+U+ cases and 8 of 11 (73%) C−U− cases.

Chlamydia-positive, *Ureaplasma*-negative NGU responds significantly better than C−U+ NGU to therapy with sulfisoxazole, which is active against *C. trachomatis* but relatively inactive against *U. urealyticum* in vitro. Conversely, C−U+ NGU responds significantly better than C+U− NGU to therapy with aminocyclitols, which are active against *U. urealyticum* but not *C. trachomatis* in vitro. *Ureaplasma*-associated NGU responds only if the aminocyclitol eradicates the *U. urealyticum* from the urethra.

► [This study supports previous evidence that chlamydiae play an etiologic role in nongonococcal urethritis (NGU). Most importantly, it also provides the following evidence that suggests an etiologic role for *U. urealyticum:* (1) *U. urealyticum* was recovered from 95% of *Chlamydia*-negative white men having their first episode of urethritis (vs. colonization of 40–60% of normal persons in previous studies); (2) in patients whose urethral cultures were positive only for *U. urealyticum,* 9 of 11 (82%) improved clinically with eradication of the organism, and none of 8 showed improvement if ureaplasmas were not eradicated; and (3) if both chlamydiae and ureaplasmas were present, treatment for chlamydiae led to improvement in only 33% vs. 100% improvement if ureaplasmas were not present initially.

A different type of evidence has been provided by Taylor-Robinson et al. (Quart. J. Med. 183:309, 1977), who reported the occurrence of urethritis in 2 volunteers who received intraurethral inoculation of ureaplasmas. The ureaplasmas multiplied in the urethra, and dysuria, pyuria and an immunologic response occurred. Therapy with tetracycline resulted in elimination of ureaplasmas and gradual disappearance of signs and symptoms. Considered together, this evidence strongly suggests that ureaplasmas cause at least some cases of NGU.

A number of questions remain to be answered about NGU. For instance, there are at least eight distinct serotypes of *U. urealyticum;* do some serotypes simply colonize and other serotypes cause disease? What causes those 10% of cases in which no etiologic agent is found? Still, it should be comforting to the clinician to know that in treatment of NGU, tetracycline works in most cases. – Ed.] ◄

► ↓ The following article helps define which microorganisms are the most likely causative agents in a relatively frequent genitourinary problem, acute epididymitis. The answer, as you might have guessed, is not simple; different microbes are involved in different age groups. – Ed. ◄

Etiology of Acute Epididymitis. James P. Harnisch, E. Russell Alexander, Richard E. Berger, George Monda and King K. Holmes[4] (Seattle) studied the association between acute epididymitis and those agents implicated as causes of nongonococcal urethritis in 24 men with symptoms suggestive of acute epididymitis. Symptoms were present for less than a month and no patient had taken antibiotics during the preceding month. Diagnosis of epididymitis was made on the basis of tenderness and swelling confined to the epididymis.

Microbiologic evaluation included urethral cultures for isolation of *Neisseria gonorrhea, Ureaplasma urealyticum, Chlamydia trachomatis,* cytomegalovirus and herpes simplex virus. In all patients without urethritis, urine cultures were performed for isolation of gram-negative aerobic bacteria.

Six men were more than age 45, and the other 18 were less than age 32. *Escherichia coli, Klebsiella* organisms or *Pseudomonas aeruginosa* were isolated from urine specimens from 4 of the 6 men over age 45, but from none of 6 men under age 32. Of the other 2 men over age 45, 1 had *U. urealyticum* infection and the other had no pathogen isolated. Of the 18 men under age 32, 13 (72%) were infected with *C. trachomatis* or *N. gonorrhea,* or both. Among the other 5, 3 had urethritis. *Ureaplasma urealyticum* was recovered from 2 patients with and 1 patient without urethritis.

These findings suggest that acute epididymitis in older men usually is associated with coliform or *Pseudomonas* bacteriuria, whereas in younger men it is usually associated with urethritis caused by sexually transmitted organisms, including *N. gonorrhea, C. trachomatis* and possibly *U. urealyticum.*

Asymptomatic Gonorrhea in Men: Caused by Gonococci with Unique Nutritional Requirements. The proportion of heterosexual men with gonorrhea who lack signs and symptoms of urethritis is high

(4) Lancet 1:819–821, Apr. 16, 1977.

among infected men brought to treatment because they were named as sexual contacts of infected women. It is not clear whether host or gonococcal factors, or both, determine whether symptomatic urethritis occurs. In some areas of the United States, isolates from patients with disseminated gonococcal infection (DGI) have unique nutritional requirements for arginine, hypoxanthine and uracil on chemically defined mediums. George Crawford, Joan S. Knapp, Judith Hale and King K. Holmes[5] (U.S.P.H.S. Hosp., Seattle) undertook a case-control study to determine whether gonococci whose nutritional requirements include arginine, hypoxanthine and uracil ($Arg^-Hyx^-Ura^-$) were also associated with asymptomatic gonorrhea in men without DGI who are not sex partners of patients with DGI.

Study was made of 25 asymptomatic heterosexual men who had other venereal diseases or were named as contacts of women with gonorrhea. None had had sexual exposure within a week before treatment. Control subjects with symptomatic gonococcal urethritis were matched with the study patients for age and race. The $Arg^-Hyx^-Ura^-$ strains were recovered from 24 of the 25 study patients and from 10 of 25 symptomatic control patients, a significant difference. The difference between symptomatic black and white men was not significant.

These findings may help explain reported racial differences in the incidence of gonorrhea; a larger study has shown a much higher rate of isolation of $Arg^-Hyx^-Ura^-$ strains in whites than in blacks. Symptom-producing non-$Arg^-Hyx^-Ura^-$ strains may be transmitted more efficiently or eliminated less efficiently among nonwhite than among white populations. Symptomatic infections in whites may tend to be treated promptly, thus eliminating non-$Arg^-Hyx^-Ura^-$ strains from the population. Infections with symptom-producing strains may have a better chance of transmission in nonwhite populations because patients wait longer to seek therapy. Control of gonorrhea in nonwhites may require earlier treatment of men with ignored symptoms, whereas in whites the further control of disease may depend more on reducing the reservoir of strains that persist because of their ability to cause asymptomatic infection.

► [This is an extremely provocative article. It is of note that the $Arg^-Hyx^-Ura^-$ strains, which predominate in asymptomatic infection, have a number of other biologic properties that distinguish them from strains causing symptomatic gonorrhea. For instance, they are more resistant to killing by human serum and they are much more sensitive to penicillin.

The fact that a gonococcal infection is asymptomatic should in no way be interpreted as its being less serious. Quite the contrary, most men with asymptomatic gonococcal infection continue to be culture positive (documented for at least 165 days!) and continue to be sexually active. Thus, they are an important reservoir for gonococcal infection in the community. Moreover, these same $Arg^-Hyx^-Ura^-$ strains that are associated with asymptomatic infection in men cause most cases of disseminated gonococcal infections in women. Previous studies (1975 YEAR BOOK, p. 66) have shown that about 2% of a large group of men considered sexually active had asymptomatic gonococcal infection. Hein et al. (J. Pediatr. 90:634, 1977) performed screening cultures on 2,064 asymptomatic but sexually active boys aged 12–16 and isolated *Neisseria gonorrhoeae* from 40, or 1.9%. One wonders if we shouldn't be doing routine cultures for gonococci in asymptomatic but sexually active young men. — Ed.] ◄

---

(5) Science 196:1352–1353, June 17, 1977.

Anorectal Gonococcal Infection is discussed by Eric J. Klein, Larry S. Fisher, Anthony W. Chow and Lucien B. Guze.[6] Anorectal gonococcal infection is common in women and in homosexual men. It is often asymptomatic but may present with acute or chronic symptoms that mimic other causes of proctitis, and the diagnosis can easily be missed unless gonorrhea is considered. Anorectal involvement is common in women with uncomplicated gonorrhea. The mode of infection in such women is unclear. Male patients are almost exclusively homosexuals who are infected by rectal intercourse (table). Most patients have no, or only minimal, symptoms. The proctoscopic features of anorectal gonorrhea are nonspecific. The diagnosis should not be based on the gram stain alone. Incorporation of the delayed fluorescent antibody technique with routine culture methods has enhanced the diagnosis of anorectal gonorrhea. False positive results are uncommon except for cross-reactivity with meningococci and other *Neisseria* species.

Currently recommended treatment regimens for uncomplicated gonorrhea appear to be effective for anorectal gonorrhea in women. Procaine penicillin and probenecid are preferred. A test of cure should be done 7–14 days after the completion of therapy; multiple sites in addition to the rectum should be cultured. The results of treatment of men are comparatively discouraging. Variable results have been obtained with spectinomycin and kanamycin. Controlled studies are urgently needed to establish effective regimens for anorectal gonococcal infection in men. At present, no less than currently recommended doses of penicillin or ampicillin plus probenecid should be used. Education of both the medical profession and the gay community and diligent contact tracing of all homosexual cases appear to be the only effective means of controlling the increasing incidence of anorectal gonococcal infection at present.

► [This article rightly emphasizes that patients with symptoms of proctitis should have anorectal cultures. In those male patients with gonococcal proctitis who are homosexual, it is important to perform cultures from the pharynx as well as tests of cure for infection in both areas, because it is harder to eradicate gonococcal infection from these sites than from the urethra. Additionally, it is especially critical in these patients to be sure that all sexual partners are treated. – Ed.] ◄

Prevalence of Anorectal Gonorrhea among Homosexual Men Attending Venereal Disease Clinics

Author(s)	Year	Area	Patients	Patients with Anorectal Gonorrhea
			no.	%
Scott and Stone	1966	London	82	44
Pariser and Marino	1970	Virginia	56	55
Owen and Hill	1972	Louisiana	79	41
Harnisch, Wiesner, and Holmes	1972	Seattle	138	28

(6) Ann. Intern. Med. 86:340–346, March, 1977.

► ↓ In addition to the role that homosexuals play as a reservoir for gonorrhea, they are also a major reservoir for syphilis. The currently recommended treatment schedules for syphilis were reviewed in the 1977 YEAR BOOK (p. 28), and the following article raises concern about the efficacy of some of the regimens for syphilis of the central nervous system. – Ed. ◄

Persistence of *Treponema Pallidum* Following Penicillin G Therapy: Report of Two Cases. Edmund C. Tramont[7] (Walter Reed Army Med. Center) has encountered 2 patients in whom *Treponema pallidum* was isolated from cerebrospinal fluid despite treatment with currently recommended amounts of penicillin G benzathine.

CASE 1. – Man, 62, was found to have a weakly reactive Venereal Disease Research Lab (VDRL) test confirmed by reactive fluorescent treponemal antibody absorption (FTA-ABS) and treponemal immobilization tests. He was treated with 1,200,000 units of penicillin G benzathine intramuscularly 3 times weekly for 3 consecutive weeks. Two weeks after therapy, motile spirochetes were observed in the cerebrospinal fluid. Inoculation of 0.5-ml aliquots of cerebrospinal fluid into rabbits resulted in testicular infection. He was retreated with 9,600,000 units of aqueous penicillin G benzathine intravenously daily for 10 days. Except for persistent positive FTA-ABS and FTA-unabsorbed tests, findings of further cerebrospinal fluid examinations at 3 and 6 months were normal and aliquots failed to infect rabbits.

CASE 2. – Man, 45, had a maculopapular rash. Ten days later he received tetracycline for a perirectal abscess. One month later he was found to have a positive VDRL test, confirmed by positive FTA-ABS and *Treponema pallidum*-immobilizing tests. He was treated with 4,800,000 units of penicillin G benzathine intramuscularly. Rabbits injected with aliquots of his cerebrospinal fluid became infected. He was then treated with 20 million units of aqueous penicillin G benzathine intravenously daily for 3 weeks. Cerebrospinal fluid obtained after this therapy no longer infected rabbits.

The initial antibiotic therapy failed to rid these 2 patients of spirochetes. These findings raise important considerations in the treatment of neurosyphilis in adults.

► [This article underscores the importance of checking patients for neurosyphilis and performing tests of cure rather than simply treating with a regimen said to be adequate. The failure of penicillin in these 2 patients is bothersome. One patient received what should have been an adequate total dose, though it was not given strictly by current guidelines (1977 YEAR BOOK, p. 28; and Ann. Intern. Med. 85:94, 1976). The other patient received an inadequate dosage for neurosyphilis. Current regimens prescribe 2,400,000 units of benzathine penicillin G intramuscularly weekly for 3 weeks. Data elsewhere in this volume (Hieber and Nelson, in the Chapter Therapy of Infections) indicate relatively low levels of penicillin (usually less than 1 μg/ml) in patients with inflamed meninges despite daily doses of penicillin equivalent to 17,000,000 units a day in an adult. Therefore, I share Doctor Tramont's concern about whether the recommended 2,400,000 units once per week will provide adequate levels of penicillin in brain tissue and cerebrospinal fluid, especially if there is little inflammation of the meninges. This concern seems borne out by a study of penicillin concentrations in the cerebrospinal fluid of neurosyphilis patients treated with recommended doses of benzathine penicillin G intramuscularly. Twelve of 13 patients had no detectable penicillin in the cerebrospinal fluid (J.A.M.A. 236:2208, 1976). It may be that intravenous regimens are preferable for primary treatment of neurosyphilis. Most authors are agreed that intravenous regimens are indicated for retreatment. – Ed.] ◄

(7) J.A.M.A. 236:2206 – 2207, Nov. 8, 1976.

Urinary Tract Infections

► ↓ Methenamine mandelate (Mandelamine), nitrofurantoin and sulfonamides (with or without trimethoprim) all have been used for the treatment and long-term supression of chronic urinary tract infections. In the following two articles these drugs are evaluated. . .with some discouraging results. – Ed. ◄

Lack of Effect of Methenamine in Suppression of, or Prophylaxis against, Chronic Urinary Infection. Bernardo Vainrub and Daniel M. Musher[8] (Houston) felt that methenamine was ineffective in patients for whom it is most often prescribed. The drug frequently is prescribed for patients with chronic urinary infection with or without indwelling catheters, despite seemingly clear evidence of a lack of effect. The effect of the drug in a small homogeneous group of subjects with a high rate of chronic urinary infection, paraplegics or quadriplegics, was examined. Thirty-two male inpatients were included in the study and 9 were studied on two or more occasions. All had had many documented episodes of urinary infection and had or had previously had a urinary catheter present. None had evidence of ureteral obstruction and all had a serum creatinine of 1.2 mg/dl or below. Twenty-seven episodes of established bacteriuria were treated with 1 gm methenamine and ascorbic acid every 6 hours. A prophylactic study included 15 episodes in patients initially having uninfected urine.

No suppressive or prophylactic effect of the treatment was observed in any of the patients. No significant changes in urinary colony-forming units or white blood cells were observed in the suppression study, regardless of the urinary pH and regardless of whether or not indwelling catheters were present. The regimen was ineffective prophylactically both in patients with indwelling catheters and those on intermittent catheterization. No changes in flora or bacterial counts were observed during methenamine treatment when urine obtained from the catheter collecting bag was used.

These findings suggest that methenamine should not be used in patients with indwelling catheters. Continued use of this drug, either in the absence of an observed effect on bacterial colonization or if a transient initial effect is followed by recolonization, should be discouraged.

► [These poor results with methenamine mandelate, even when urine pHs were ≤ 6, parallel those in a study in the 1976 YEAR BOOK (p. 40) in which patients receiving this drug as a chronic suppressant frequently required interim therapy with other antimicrobials. Its poor performance and the danger of metabolic acidosis being induced while an attempt is made to acidify the urine raise serious questions about whether it is simply a placebo for the doctor rather than treatment for the patient. – Ed.] ◄

Long-Term Treatment with Sulfamethoxazole-Trimethoprim (Bactrim) and Nitrofurantoin in Chronic Urinary Tract Infections: Controlled Clinical Trial. Several controlled clinical trials

(8) Antimicrob. Agents Chemother. 12:625–629, November, 1977.

Results of a 1-Year Trial with S-T vs. Nitrofurantoin

	S/T		Nitro-furantoin		
Urine sterile during 12 months uninterruptedly = successful treatment	12		1		treatment
Sterility of the urine only temporary = therapeutical failures	3	4	7	10	failures due to inefficacy or side-effects
Stop of treatment due to side-effects	1*		3†		
Evaluable collective	16		11		
Death during treatment (death unrelated to treatment)	1		2		

*Occurrence of fever.
†Vomiting, 2 patients; parasthesia, 1 patient.

have shown sulfamethoxazole-trimethoprim (S-T) to be more effective than the sulfonamides alone in the treatment of urinary tract infections, and long-term nitrofurantoin therapy has prevented bacteriuria in patients with recurrent urinary tract infections. Jørgen Scherwin and Per Holm[9] evaluated these agents in patients with recurrent urinary tract infections with respect to the frequency with which the urine could be kept sterile for 1 year. Consecutive patients without indwelling catheters and with a serum creatinine level below 2 mg/100 ml were included in the study if there was significant bacteriuria due to a strain sensitive to both agents. Patients received two tablets of 400 mg sulfamethoxazole and 80 mg trimethoprim each twice daily for 1 week and then half these doses, or 100 mg nitrofurantoin 4 times daily and then 50 mg 3 times daily. If the serum creatinine was 1.6–2 mg/100 ml, the dose of nitrofurantoin was 100 mg 3 times daily initially and then 50 mg twice daily.

Thirty patients with a median age of 82 were included in the study. Seventeen received S-T and 13, nitrofurantoin. One nitrofurantoin patient was withdrawn because of vomiting. Only 1 patient on nitrofurantoin completed a year of treatment with persistently sterile urine, compared with 12 of the 17 patients treated with S-T, a significant difference. The results are given in the table. A small but significant increase in serum creatinine occurred during S-T treatment.

The urine was maintained sterile for 1 year much more often with S-T therapy than with nitrofurantoin in this study of patients with chronic urinary tract infection. The study is viewed as a pilot trial, and the results are encouraging and justify more sophisticated studies on greater numbers of patients.

► [Not only did nitrofurantoin do a poor job, but the side effects associated with its use occurred more frequently than with sulfamethoxazole-trimethoprim (S-T). The best of the three drugs tested appears to be S-T. Further studies are needed to determine if the maintenance dose of 800 mg sulfamethoxazole and 160 mg trimethoprim per day is more than necessary. In a study of prophylaxis of recurrent urinary tract infection in women, a single dose of 200 mg sulfamethoxazole-40 mg trimethoprim at bedtime was quite effective (1975 YEAR BOOK, p. 91). However, those patients might have had a shorter period of risk per 24 hours than the patients in this study by Scherwin and Holm. – Ed.] ◄

(9) Chemotherapy 23:282–288, 1977.

Candidal Infections

► In preceding editions of the YEAR BOOK we have commented on the emergence of *Candida albicans* as a cause of infections complicating prolonged broad-spectrum antibiotic treatment. Once regarded as a "nuisance" organism, it has earned our respect as a cause of sepsis (1974 YEAR BOOK, p. 59), cystitis, renal abscesses, endocarditis and esophageal moniliasis (1977 YEAR BOOK, p. 49). We are devoting this chapter to infections produced by this ubiquitous yeast.

The first article discusses the gut as the microbiologic reservoir of the organism and describes its role in seeding the vagina to produce recurrent vaginal moniliasis, an exceedingly common problem.—Ed. ◄

Recurrent Vaginal Candidiasis: Importance of an Intestinal Reservoir. Vaginitis caused by *Candida albicans* has become one of the most troublesome forms of vaginitis because it is so often a recurrent problem. Mary Ryan Miles, Linda Olsen and Alvin Rogers[1] (Michigan State Univ.) obtained evidence that the intestine acts as a reservoir for *C. albicans* and that minor alterations in the milieu of the host may facilitate a change from commensal to parasite in or on mucocutaneous surfaces. Studies were done in healthy nonpregnant women aged 18–20 who presented with three or more episodes of vaginitis. Of 98 patients included in the study, 51 (52%) were found to harbor *C. albicans* in both the vagina and fecal material, whereas 46 were *Candida* free in both sites. One patient was stool positive but vagina negative for *C. albicans* (table). In no case was *Candida* previously isolated from the vagina of a patient who subsequently proved to be yeast free.

There is no evidence that *C. albicans,* once part of the fecal flora, ever leaves the host spontaneously. The findings support the view that a cure of vaginitis is not possible without prior eradication of *C. albicans* from the gut. The concept of the gut as a reservoir may apply to other forms of candidiasis as well and to the immunologic phenomena observed in some cases.

► [Well and good! There was 100% correlation between the presence of *C. albicans* in the vagina and that in the stool. As the authors acknowledge, we have been aware of the gastrointestinal reservoir of this yeast for some time. The intimate relationship between stool carriage and recurrent vaginal candidiasis deserved reemphasis. Unfortunately, the article stops short of exploring some provocative questions. If many women harbor candida in the stool, why do only some develop recurrent vaginitis? If simple

Correlation between Presence or Absence of *C. albicans**

C albicans	Vagina, Positive No. (%)	Vagina, Negative No. (%)
Stool, positive	51 (98)	1 (2)
Stool, negative	0 (0)	46 (100)

**Candida albicans* isolated from stool and vagina of 98 patients with recurrent vaginitis.

(1) J.A.M.A. 238:1836–1837, Oct. 24, 1977.

"spillover" is involved, could something as simple as the mechanical use of toilet tissue after urination facilitate vaginal contamination? I know some gynecologists who swear that an anterior-to-posterior swipe is preferable to the reverse. Second, sexual practices might make a difference; direct inoculation via hand or penis might be involved. Lastly, because recurrence is so common and the gut is the reservoir, would a low-dose oral nystatin regimen have a beneficial effect in reducing recurrence rates? Okay, authors, you have us hooked! How about some follow-up? – Ed.] ◄

► ↓ The following are two articles concerning more serious *Candida* infections from the infectious disease unit of the University of California School of Medicine, Los Angeles. – Ed. ◄

***Candida* Peritonitis: Report of 22 Cases and Review of the English Literature.** Although the incidence of focal and generalized candidal infections has been increasing rapidly in recent years, peritonitis due to *Candida* has not been commonly described. Arnold S. Bayer, Michael J. Blumenkranz, John S. Montgomerie, Jeffrey E. Galpin, Jack W. Coburn and Lucien B. Guze[2] report their experience with 22 patients and review 12 cases in the literature.

Table I summarizes the clinical and laboratory features of 31 patients with positive peritoneal cultures for *Candida*. The findings in 9 patients suggested peritoneal contamination rather than frank peritonitis, and the cultures from these patients were only transiently positive. Twenty-two patients had characteristic clinical findings of intra-abdominal sepsis due to *Candida* peritonitis. The infection was acquired during peritoneal dialysis in 10 patients and was associated with gastrointestinal surgery or perforation in 12.

In the peritoneal dialysis group, patients had received dialysis from 2 days to 1.5 years before acquiring peritonitis. All patients were persistently febrile, had leukocytosis and cloudy or purulent peritoneal

TABLE 1. – CLINICAL AND LABORATORY FEATURES OF 31 PATIENTS WITH *Candida* ISOLATED FROM PERITONEAL FLUID

	Contamination (9 cases)	Peritonitis (22 cases)
Underlying process		
Peritoneal dialysis	9	10
Gastrointestinal surgery or perforation	0	12
Fever $\geq$ 38°C*	0	20
Peritoneal signs*	0	22
Abnormal plain films of the abdomen (adynamic ileus* and/or free intraperitoneal air)	0/4	13/13
Peripheral leukocytosis* $\geq$ 12,000 white blood cells/mm^3	0	22
Turbid or purulent peritoneal fluid*	0	22

*The incidence of these features is significantly different between the two groups (P<0.001) as determined by the χ^2 method with Yates correction factor.

(2) Am. J. Med. 61:832–840, December, 1976.

fluid. Six of the 10 patients had received antibiotics within 3 weeks before developing peritonitis. Therapy consisted of continuous peritoneal lavage in 4 patients, and 6 patients required antifungal drugs. The infection was cleared in 9 of these patients. In 1 patient peritoneal lavage could not be maintained because of a viscid peritoneal exudate, and *Candida* peritonitis was still present antemortem.

In 12 patients who had *Candida* peritonitis associated with surgery, infection followed perforation of an abdominal viscus in 10. In the other 2, candidiasis complicated gastrointestinal surgery. An anastomotic or suture line leak was demonstrated in both. Eight of 10 patients with a perforation were treated by operative repair with drainage of the infected peritoneal fluid and all survived. The 2 patients who were not treated surgically died. In 2 patients with postoperative suture line leaks, disseminated candidiasis developed and they died de-

TABLE 2.—*Candida* Peritonitis Results of Treatment—Present Series plus Literature Cases*

Therapy	No. Patients	Infection Cured
Group I—Associated with Peritoneal Dialysis		
None	1	0
Continuous peritoneal dialysis alone	4	4
Peritoneal dialysis + amphotericin B intravenously	2	2
Peritoneal dialysis + amphotericin B intravenously and intraperitoneally†	4	3
Peritoneal dialysis + gentian violet intraperitoneally	1	1
	12	10
Group II—Associated with Gastrointestinal Surgery or Enteric Perforation		
None	3	0
Peritoneal dialysis alone	1	0
Peritoneal dialysis + gentian violet intraperitoneally	1	0
Surgical repair and drainage alone	11	9
Surgical intervention plus postoperative amphotericin B systemically	4	4
Amphotericin B intravenously alone	1	1
	21	14

*In 1 case from the literature, insufficient data prevented assessment of therapy.

†Two patients also received 5-fluorocytosine orally.

spite surgical drainage of an abscess. Systemic antifungal agents were not administered to either of these patients.

The results of treatment in both present and previously described patients are summarized in Table 2. The 12 previously reported cases were quite similar in terms of patients' general clinical characteristics, systemic response to infection, laboratory data, antecedent antibiotic therapy and association with gastrointestinal surgery, perforation or peritoneal dialysis.

If untreated, mortality is high in *Candida* peritonitis, but when abdominal drainage, surgical repair or antifungal therapy, or a combination, was provided, mortality was low and was comparable to that in patients with bacterial peritonitis.

► [An additional point: *Candida* species other than *Candida albicans* were commonly recovered from these episodes of peritonitis: *C. tropicalis, C. guilliermondi* and *C. parakreusii.* Clinical microbiology laboratories generally are now more skilled in speciating *Candida* isolates than they used to be. Although their names may still be unfamiliar to many clinicians, these yeasts should not be dismissed as inconsequential. These isolates have the same implications as isolates of *C. albicans.*

The patients were not treated according to a protocol, so various regimens were used. The lesson from Table 2 is that "washout" peritoneal dialysis with short-course antifungal therapy gives best results. – Ed.] ◄

***Candida* Meningitis: Report of Seven Cases and Review of the English Literature.** The incidence of candidal infections, both focal and generalized, has increased rapidly in recent years, but meningitis due to *Candida* organisms has been uncommonly described. Arnold S. Bayer, John E. Edwards, Jr., James S. Seidel and Lucien B. Guze[3] (Univ. of California, Los Angeles) report experience with 7 such cases and a review of 21 cases previously reported in the English literature. The authors' cases were encountered in 1970 – 75.

The authors' series included 3 adults and 4 infants; 3 infants were under age 3 months. All 7 patients had serious underlying diseases; 3 had renal failure. All the patients were persistently febrile and had typical symptoms of meningitis. One patient had papilledema and 2 had focal neurologic deficits. All patients exhibited a peripheral leukocytosis and neutrophilia and all had cerebrospinal fluid pleocytosis, though in most cases the white blood cell count was below 50 cells per cu mm. Lymphocytic predominance was noted in 5 patients. Cerebrospinal fluid cultures yielded *C. albicans* in 5 patients and *C. tropicalis* in 2. All patients were receiving systemic antibiotics for bacterial infection. One of the 2 given systemic steroids had disseminated candidal infection. Three of the 4 patients not given specific antifungal therapy died shortly after diagnosis, whereas 1 recovered completely after ventricular aspirations and replacement of an infected ventriculoperitoneal shunt. Two patients were cured by antifungal drug therapy, whereas 1 died with sterile cerebrospinal fluid. All 3 surviving patients had normal psychomotor findings at follow-up. Two of three autopsies showed obvious widespread disseminated candidiasis.

The results of treatment of candidal meningitis are summarized in the table. Mortality is high in untreated cases but relatively low when

---

(3) Medicine (Baltimore) 55:477 – 486, November, 1976.

THERAPY OF *Candida* MENINGITIS

Type	Number	Mycologic cure	Survival
Inadequate or no therapy	11	1	1
Amphotericin B intravenously alone	6	5	5
Amphotericin B intravenously and intrathecally	3	3	1
Parenteral iodides	3	1	1
Parenteral gentian violet	1	1	1
Parenteral iodides and gentian violet	3	2	2
Repeated ventricular aspirates	1	1	1
	28	14	12

adequate and appropriate antifungal therapy is given. Factors associated with a poor prognosis include a diagnostic delay exceeding 2 weeks, a cerebrospinal fluid glucose below 35 mg/100 ml and the presence of intracranial hypertension and focal neurologic deficits.

► [The lessons here are basically the same as those previously noted. This is a much more ominous infection (57% of all patients described in the literature have died), so prompt recognition and treatment are imperative. The recent addition of 2 infants successfully treated with a combination of amphotericin B and 5-fluorocytosine (Chesne et al.: J. Pediatr. 89:1017, 1976) provides a cautiously optimistic outlook for future patients with this disease. – Ed.] ◄

Bacterial Endocarditis

Infective Endocarditis: Review of 125 Cases from the University of Washington Hospitals, 1963–72. Lawrence L. Pelletier, Jr., and Robert G. Petersdorf[4] (Univ. of Washington) reviewed 125 cases of infective endocarditis (IE) seen between 1963 and 1972. An average of 12.5 cases occurred annually among three hospitals during this 10-year period. *Streptococcus viridans* infections constitute a decreasing percentage of total infections, whereas *Staphylococcus aureus* is emerging as the predominant organism. Overall mortality was 36.8%; gram-negative bacillary endocarditis resulted in a higher mortality than other types of endocarditis. There were more men than women in the study due to the high percentage of drug addicts, but there was no difference in mortality between the sexes. Mortality was higher at both age extremes.

An apparent portal of entry was present in 63% of cases of IE (Table 1). Drug addiction and prior cardiac surgery were the most common causes of IE development. About 30% of cases were acquired in the hospital or within 30 days after discharge. Preexisting heart disease was evident in 72% of patients. Eighteen patients were drug addicts and *S. aureus* was present in 10 of these patients; 6 had evidence of preexisting heart disease. About half the patients received antibiotics before admission; in them diagnosis was frequently delayed. The physical findings are summarized in Table 2. The prevalence of congestive heart failure (CHF) was 67% and 60% of these had CHF for the first

TABLE 1.—Source of Infection

Source	No.	(%)
Parenteral drug addiction	19	(15)
Recent heart valve surgery	12	(10)
Dental focus[1]	11	(9)
Others[2]	10	(8)
Urinary tract[3]	8	(6)
Wound infection[4]	6	(5)
AV shunt or phlebitis	6	(5)
Skin (non-addicts)[5]	5	(4)
Female genital tract[6]	3	(2)

[1]Streptococcal organisms, 7; culture negative, 2; anaerobes, 2.
[2]Pneumococcus, 6; *S. aureus*, 1, *Neisseria* mucosa, 1; non-group A β-hemolytic streptococci, 1; *Bacteroides corrodens*, 1.
[3]Enterococcus, 3; *S. epidermidis*, 2; gram-negative, 2; *S. aureus*, 1.
[4]*S. aureus*, 5; *S. epidermidis*, 1.
[5]*S. aureus*, 4; group A β-hemolytic streptococci, 1.
[6]*S. viridans*, 1; enterococcus, 1; culture negative, 1.

(4) Medicine (Baltimore) 56:287–313, July, 1977.

TABLE 2.—PHYSICAL FINDINGS IN 125 EPISODES OF IE

Physical Signs	Positive Finding #	(%)
Heart murmur	109	(89)
Fever (>100.5F°)	85	(77)
Embolic episode[1]	63	(50)
Skin manifestations[2]	61	(50)
Splenomegaly	35	(28)
Septic complications[3]	24	(19)
Mycotic aneurysms[4]	23	(18)
Proven glomerulonephritis	19	(15)
Clubbing[5]	15	(12)
Retinal lesions	11	(9)

[1]Number of clinically recognized embolic episodes: brain, 25; lung, 17; coronary artery, 8; extremity, 8; spleen, 8; eye, 3; gut, 4.
[2]Petechiae, 43; splinter hemorrhages, 16; Osler's nodes, 15.
[3]Pneumonia, 17; prosthetic valve dehiscence, 10; meningitis, 7; arthritis, 4; splenic abscess, 3; brain abscess, 1; pancreatitis, 1; perinephric abscess, 1; phlebitis 1.
[4]Sinus of Valsalva, 17; cerebral artery, 5; hepatic artery, 1.
[5]New finding, 10; congenital heart disease associated, 5.

time during the course of IE. Persistent CHF led to cardiac surgery in 16 of 34 patients. Ten patients with CHF died either as a result of it or of complications of cardiac surgery. Anemia was common and latex agglutination tests were positive in about half the patients studied. The erythrocyte sedimentation rate was significantly higher in survivors than in patients who died.

All blood cultures were positive in 68% of patients, wereas in 13%, cultures were persistently negative; in the latter group mortality was 50%. Overall, more than a third of the patients died of complications of IE (Table 3). Most deaths were related to hemodynamic events secondary to valve destruction, aneurysm formation or embolism. About 20% of patients had adverse reactions to antibiotic therapy; 11 of 90 courses of therapy were discontinued due to severe toxic reactions. There were 16 cases of IE in patients with prosthetic heart valves, with

TABLE 3.—CAUSE OF DEATH

Cause of death	Number	(%)
Congestive heart failure	37	(79)
Surgical deaths	12	(26)
Acute cardiac infarction	10	(21)
Embolic episodes	6	(13)
Mycotic aneurysm rupture	6	(13)
Arrhythmia	6	(13)
Sepsis	4	(8)
Prosthetic valve dehiscence	4	(8)
Other*	3	(6)

*Pulmonary embolus, 1; left ventricular perforation, 1; superinfection, 1.

a mortality of 43.8%. The mean duration of follow-up of 106 patients was 29 months. Relapses occurred after treatment in 19% of 90 patients, whereas 54% of 63 patients had persistent heart failure. Reinfection of the endocardium with another organism occurred in 3 of 63 patients.

Since the leading cause of death in this series was congestive heart failure due to valvular dysfunction, early surgical intervention should be considered in such patients despite the high risks.

► [A short article cannot really do justice to this careful review of infective endocarditis as it is in 1977. It should be read by all internists.

In many ways, it is a sad story—a mirror held up to our changing society that makes one wonder whether all of our changes, technologic and cultural, represent progress.

When I went to medical school in 1944, 95% of patients with bacterial endocarditis were infected with *Streptococcus viridans* and most had underlying rheumatic heart disease. By the mid-1960's, we had dramatically reduced the incidence of rheumatic heart disease. Enterococci and staphylococci caused 25–40% of the infective endocarditis seen on our services, but recovery of 80–even 85–of each 100 patients with endocarditis was not uncommon. Now drug addicts have replaced those patients with rheumatic heart disease. As emphasized by Doctors Pelletier and Petersdorf, theirs is a selective experience that encompasses those patients seen in a university hospital, a county hospital and a Veterans Administration hospital. Thus they see many more drug addicts and those referred for cardiac surgery than would be the case in a community hospital. Be that as it may, this experience could be duplicated in most urban centers.

So where are we now? First, the predominant microbe (and a mean one) is *Staphylococcus aureus*. Drug addiction and cardiac surgery were the most common antecedents. Overall mortality was a distressing 36.8%. Deaths resulted from congestive heart failure, embolism, ruptured mycotic aneurysms, complications of cardiac surgery or superinfection due to resistant microorganisms.

The authors make a strong case for earlier surgical intervention in patients manifesting failure due to valve dysfunction. This is also the authors' recommendation in the following article. Oh, to return to the more bucolic days of the mid-1960's!—Ed.] ◄

Prosthetic Valve Endocarditis: The Case for Prompt Valve Replacement is made by Jeffrey R. Saffle, Pierce Gardner, Stephen C. Schoenbaum and Wayne Wild.[5] The overall mortality rate for patients with prosthetic valve endocarditis remains high, leading to the consideration of prompt valve replacement as a potential treatment. The mortality is related to onset and causative organism (Table 1). The outcomes of valve replacement and antibiotic therapy are compared in Table 2. The mortality has been reduced in patients having valve replacement for late-onset prosthetic valve endocarditis. The authors have treated 6 consecutive patients, 3 with early onset and 3 with late-onset endocarditis, by valve replacement before completion of a course of antibiotics. All were febrile at the time of operation. All survived operation, 1 dying later of noninfectious causes. One patient had post-pericardiotomy syndrome. Four patients have lived for over a year, and 1 is well 4 months after valve replacement. All patients received antimicrobials for at least a month postoperatively.

Patients at a high risk of dying can now be identified on the basis of onset of infection, causative organism, hemodynamic status and the presence of septic emboli. At least 70% of patients in recent series were at high risk, but only about 20% were managed by valve replacement. Analysis of previous reports together with the authors' experience in-

(5) J. Thorac. Cardiovasc. Surg. 73:416–420, March, 1977.

TABLE 1.—PROSTHETIC VALVE ENDOCARDITIS: MORTALITY BY ONSET AND CAUSATIVE ORGANISM*

Organism	*Early onset (deaths/ cases)*	*Late onset (deaths/ cases)*	*Total (deaths/ cases)*
Staphylococcus epidermidis	7/13	3/7	10/20 (50%)§
Staphylococcus aureus	13/15	8/10	21/25 (84%)
Streptococcus, viridans group	2/2	4/18	6/20 (30%)
Group D streptococci	3/4	3/12	6/16 (37%)
Other streptococci†	–	3/9	3/9 (33%)
Gram-negative bacilli	13/15	3/12	16/27 (59%)
Candida species	7/8	2/2	9/10 (90%)
Other‡	2/3	2/4	4/7 (56%)
Totals	47/60 (78%)	28/74 (38%)	75/134 (56%)

*One hundred thirty-four cases of endocarditis occurred in 131 patients in three reviewed series.

†Other streptococci consisted of the following: group C streptococci, 1 case; group K streptococci, 1 case; group B streptococci, 2 cases; unclassified streptococci, 5 cases.

‡Other organisms: *Corynebacterium xerosis,* 2 cases; diphtheroids, 2 cases; micrococcus, 3 cases.

§Figures in parentheses are mortality rates.

TABLE 2.—OUTCOME OF VALVE REPLACEMENT VERSUS ANTIBIOTIC THERAPY ALONE FOR PROSTHETIC VALVE ENDOCARDITIS IN PATIENTS SURVIVING AT LEAST 1 WEEK AFTER DIAGNOSIS*

	Early onset		*Late onset*		*Total*	
Series	*Medical (deaths/cases)*	*Valve replacement (deaths/cases)*	*Medical (deaths/cases)*	*Valve replacement (deaths/cases)*	*Medical (deaths/cases)*	*Valve replacement (deaths/cases)*
Mayo Clinic	11/13	–	11/21	1/7	22/34	1/7
University of Oregon	18/21	1/1	5/16	0/5	23/37	1/6
Mass. General Hospital	7/11	2/4	4/11	1/5	11/22	3/9
Totals	36/45 (80%)	3/5 (60%)	20/48 (42%)†	2/17 (12%)†	56/93 (60%)†	5/22 (23%)†

*As compiled from three reviewed series.

†$P<0.05$.

dicates that prompt valve replacement is feasible and should be standard therapy for prosthetic valve endocarditis in all patients who are not in the lower-risk group, i.e., those with late-onset infections due to organisms associated with low mortality and in whom there are no other indications for surgical intervention, such as congestive heart failure, valve dysfunction, emboli or refractory infection.

► [This article is fraught with methodologic pitfalls that one could drive a truck through, but it fits my prejudices. I am not sure that prompt valve replacement can be stated to be "standard therapy" without further study, but alas, it looks like the only way to go.—Ed.] ◄

Prevention of Bacterial Endocarditis is outlined by Edward L.

Kaplan, Bascom F. Anthony, Alan Bisno, David Durack, Harold Houser, H. Dean Millard, Jay Sanford, Stanford T. Shulman, Max Stillerman, Angelo Taranta and Nanette Wenger[6] (Committee on Prevention of Rheumatic Fever and Bacterial Endocarditis of the American Heart Association). Bacterial endocarditis remains one of the most serious complications of cardiac disease. Prophylaxis is recommended in those situations most likely to be associated with bacteremia. Generally, parenteral antibiotic administration is preferred when practical, especially for patients at high risk. The highest level of oral health must be maintained in patients at risk, and prophylaxis is recommended with all dental procedures likely to cause gingival bleeding, including routine professional cleaning. Prophylaxis is also indicated for surgery on any infected or contaminated tissues. Prophylaxis may be elected to cover dental and surgical procedures in patients with indwelling cardiac pacemakers. Prophylaxis is not necessary in diagnostic cardiac catheterization and angiography. Antibiotic doses used to prevent recurrence of acute rheumatic fever are inadequate for preventing bacterial endocarditis.

Adults having dental procedures and upper respiratory tract surgery should receive 1 million units of aqueous crystalline penicillin G mixed with 600,000 units procaine penicillin, intramuscularly, 30–60 minutes before the procedure and then 500 mg penicillin V orally every 6 hours for 8 doses. Oral therapy is with 2 gm penicillin V before the procedure and then 500 mg every 6 hours for 8 doses. Allergic patients may be given vancomycin or erythromycin. An alternative regimen consists of aqueous penicillin G with procaine penicillin G, plus 1 gm streptomycin intramuscularly before the procedure and then penicillin V orally. Adults having genitourinary or gastrointestinal surgery or instrumentation should be given 2 million units of penicillin G parenterally, or 1 gm ampicillin plus 1.5 mg gentamicin per kg or 1 gm streptomycin intramuscularly. Penicillin-allergic patients may be given vancomycin plus streptomycin.

► [It makes eminently good sense to believe that antimicrobial prophylaxis given in situations commonly associated with bacteremia should reduce the incidence of bacterial endocarditis in those with valvular and intravascular abnormalities predisposing to this infection. However, it's important to recognize that we have absolutely no *proof* that this prophylaxis will work in man. Fortunately the nice studies of Durack, Petersdorf and their associates, using an experimental animal model which permits consistent induction of endocarditis with microbes commonly producing disease in man, have allowed testing of this thesis. The bottom line is that prophylaxis does prevent endocarditis in animals under these controlled circumstances. Thus we have the recommendation outlined here (for those who want to see the experimental evidence see Durack, D. T., and Petersdorf, R. G.: J. Clin. Invest. 52:592, 1973; and Durack, D. T., et al.: J. Lab. Clin. Med. 90:171, 1977).

It, however, does seem somewhat worrisome to make such sweeping recommendations on the basis of what works in modest numbers of rabbits. Implementing these recommendations will require giving lots of potent and expensive antimicrobials in very significant dosages to thousands of people. Don't misunderstand me—I see no easy alternative, but the authors are talking of millions of dollars and some potentially harmful side effects on fairly shallow evidence. I am sure they agonized over it.—Ed.]

---

(6) Circulation 56:139A–143A, July, 1977.

Prevention and Prophylaxis of Infection

Smallpox Vaccination. J. Michael Lane[7] (Center for Disease Control, Atlanta, Ga.) points out that smallpox vaccination has been dropped just when the media have been criticizing the profession for lack of attention to preventive medicine and that some patients and physicians do not understand the reasons for ceasing routine smallpox vaccination. For practical purposes, infection results only from contact with patients in the acute phase of the disease; there is no carrier state and no animal reservoir. When smallpox is gone, it is gone permanently. Smallpox eradication data are accurate, and we can be confident that the disease is gone from everywhere except Somalia, on the horn of Africa. Smallpox is a dramatic and highly visible disease. The World Health Organization has suggested that 2 years elapse between the last known case in a given country and an official declaration of a smallpox-free state.

In no area of the United States is smallpox vaccination now required for entry into school. Vaccination is no longer required for any United States citizen reentering the United States after foreign travel or for aliens entering the United States. There are serious complications of vaccination and, in view of the virtually nonexistent benefits arising from vaccination at present, these risks cannot be ignored. The major vaccine manufacturers still have plenty of vaccine on hand and in production, and no shortage is anticipated. Patients must realize that physicians are not generalizing from smallpox vaccine to other immunizing agents. Many children in the United States remain unimmunized against polio, diphtheria, pertussis, tetanus and particularly measles and rubella.

► [The extraordinarily successful story of the World Health Organization's campaign to eradicate smallpox from the globe has not received the publicity it deserves. As of this writing, an intensive field surveillance effort is being geared up to search out the last remnants of smallpox in the remote desert regions of Somalia—the last focus of smallpox transmission anywhere on the face of the earth. This is a monumental achievement and is a vivid testimony to what international cooperation in health can accomplish. It is also an achievement in which American medicine can take special pride. Epidemiologists from the Bureau of Smallpox Eradication of the Center for Disease Control in Atlanta, Georgia, were the chief architects of the eradication strategy and also spent untold months "in the trenches" supervising the details of work in the field.

However, all this remote international activity does cause an occasional quandary for the practicing physician in his office. Should international travelers be vaccinated against smallpox? If smallpox exists only in Somalia's hinterland, there is, obviously, no risk to travelers going to Paris, New Delhi, Tokyo or Rio de Janeiro. Because smallpox vaccination does pose occasional risks (postvaccinial encephalitis) and frequent discomfort (florid "takes" with fever and tender arms), is vaccination necessary?

There are two answers to this question. Clinically, the answer is "no." However,

(7) J.A.M.A. 237:2419–2420, May 30, 1977.

we must also consider the regulations of the ministries of health of the various countries of the world. In recognition of the diminishing reservoir of smallpox in the world, vaccination for entry into the United States has not been required for years. However, other countries are moving more slowly. You do not want your patient to encounter difficulties when he gets off the airplane in Bombay and is faced with an adamant health official. I have recently read of 2 physicians (without vaccinations) traveling on official duty out of the White House who were placed in quarantine abroad. They were released barely in time to make their appointment with the local head of the government.

After discussion with the Atlanta experts, we recommend the following procedure if you do not wish to vaccinate your patient. On your office letterhead, write a short note "to whom it may concern" that your patient, Mr. or Mrs. A. B. Jones, has a medical condition that is a contraindication to smallpox vaccination. A specific diagnosis is not necessary; the entirely valid contraindication is the aforementioned risk-benefit analysis. Sign the letter. Have the patient take the letter to the local health department where it can be validated with an official stamp. Then staple the letter into the yellow International Certificate of Vaccination.

This is not a new procedure; it has always been in effect and has been used for such contraindications as eczema, pregnancy and other conditions. The experts in Atlanta tell us they have never heard of a traveler with such a validated letter experiencing difficulties. I believe this is a practical solution for the few remaining years before the World Health Organization can certify that there is no human being on the earth with smallpox. – Ed.] ◄

Prevention of Rheumatic Fever is reviewed by Edward L. Kaplan, Alan Bisno, Warren Derrick, Richard Facklam, Leon Gordis, Harold B. Houser, W. Ham Jackson, H. Dean Millard, Stanford T. Shulman, Angelo V. Taranta and Lewis W. Wannamaker[8] (Committee on Rheumatic Fever and Bacterial Endocarditis of the Council on Cardiovascular Disease in the Young of the American Heart Association). The prevention of initial attacks of rheumatic fever requires accurate recognition and proper treatment of streptococcal upper respiratory tract infections. Treatment should be started as soon as a definite diagnosis is made; however, it has been shown that a short delay does not significantly interfere with rheumatic fever prevention. Penicillin is preferred for nonallergic patients, in the form of intramuscular benzathine penicillin G. The oral antibiotic of choice is penicillin G. Recurrent rheumatic fever is prevented by continuous prophylaxis, perhaps for life. Prophylaxis should be continued even after prosthetic heart valve implantation. The most effective regimen consists of intramuscular injections of 1.2,000,000 units of benzathine penicillin G every 4 weeks. Successful oral prophylaxis depends on patient compliance.

When a patient continues to harbor group A streptococci, continued treatment is not necessary if repeated infections from other sources are ruled out, except in rheumatic patients or rheumatic families. Many physicians choose not to treat asymptomatic carriers with antibiotics. Family contacts of high-risk patients should be cultured and treated if positive. In lower-risk situations, the benefit of treating family contacts is undefined, but it seems prudent to culture family contacts who have upper respiratory symptoms and to treat those who have positive cultures.

► [The Committee on Rheumatic Fever and Bacterial Endocarditis of the American

(8) Circulation 55:1–4, January, 1977.

Heart Association periodically updates its recommendations. This is its latest reassessment of rheumatic fever prevention. It is a carefully worded three-page statement which we could not include *in toto* because of space limitations.

To highlight a few points: (1) The drug of choice for the *treatment* of group A streptococcal upper respiratory infections is intramuscular benzathine penicillin G. Drug companies vigorously push prepackaged formulations of benzathine penicillin mixed with shorter-acting penicillins. They offer no advantage; avoid them. In penicillin-allergic patients, use erythromycin. (2) The drug of choice for rheumatic fever *prophylaxis* is likewise intramuscular benzathine penicillin G, given at 4-week intervals. Sulfadiazine (oral) is satisfactory for penicillin-allergic patients (assuming adequate compliance).

A somewhat new recommendation is given concerning the *duration* of rheumatic fever prophylaxis. Ideally, it should be lifelong, but the committee has recognized that many patients do not continue prophylaxis once they have reached adulthood. Indeed, the risk of rheumatic fever recurrence diminishes with increasing age. The committee offers no cutoff age because data do not exist to help them make a recommendation. It should be emphasized that some adults are at increased risk of streptococcal infection and that pains should be taken to continue them on prophylaxis, *i.e.,* those persons in regular contact with children: parents of young children, school teachers, physicians, nurses and allied health personnel. Also at risk are all persons who are from disadvantaged circumstances.

As if to emphasize the foregoing recommendations, a study was published in 1977 which analyzed recurrences and sequelae of rheumatic fever in a metropolitan area (Quinn et al: J.A.M.A. 238:1512, 1977). Doctor Quinn has studied streptococcal infections and rheumatic fever in this population for over 20 years, accumulating some excellent observations. Since the subjects were not part of a special protocol, the findings provide a realistic insight into what actually happens in a community. His team found that younger subjects' compliance with prophylaxis was more complete, intramuscular benzathine penicillin was clearly superior to oral medication in preventing recurrences and black persons were at greater risk of rheumatic fever, carditis and the development of rheumatic heart disease than were whites. These results add further weight to the committee's recommendations.

The committee's report made me reflect again on the diagnosis of streptococcal pharyngitis. Since all studies reveal the fallibility of using clinical criteria to distinguish between streptococcal and nonstreptococcal pharyngitis, their emphasis on the use of the throat culture for diagnosis is appropriate. Increasing numbers of physicians (especially pediatricians) seem to be doing throat cultures in their offices. However, most patients with pharyngitis still do not have their throats cultured. There must be many reasons for this, including cost and physician interest (or lack of it).

Let's face it, the diagnostic approach to a sore throat hasn't improved in over 30 years. Biomedical science ought to be able to provide us with a quick, easy and reliable test. Sometimes the things that look very simple turn out to be anything but that.

Lastly, I note that the recommendations were published in *Circulation,* the journal sponsored by the American Heart Association. I doubt whether many primary care physicians subscribe to it. I wonder how the American Heart Association expects to get this information into the hands of the doctors who really ought to read it. Surely there are better ways to disseminate such documents (also the one on prevention of bacterial endocarditis) in 1977. Fortunately, the incidence of rheumatic fever is declining. Perhaps it is, as Osler said of tuberculosis, "a social disease with medical manifestations." – Ed.] ◄

Therapy of Infections

► ↓ Gram-negative infections continue to be a major cause of death in hospitalized patients. In a distressing proportion of these patients the infections result from indwelling intravenous catheters or Foley catheters, some of which may have been left in place for the convenience of the physician or nursing staff. Other less obvious acts on the part of physicians, such as the use of immunosuppressive drugs, cytotoxic drugs or "broad-spectrum" antibiotics, also predispose patients to gram-negative infections. To complicate matters further, organisms that are resistant to our mainstays of therapy for severe gram-negative infections, gentamicin and tobramycin, are appearing with increasing frequency in the hospital environment (1977 YEAR BOOK, p. 40; and Schaberg et al.: J. Infect. Dis. 134:181, 1976).

The first four articles in this chapter deal with the therapy of gram-negative infections, including sepsis. The first two are concerned with amikacin, a newer aminoglycoside that is active against a wide spectrum of gram-negative bacilli, including *Pseudomonas,* as well as organisms resistant to gentamicin and tobramycin. Amikacin has been shown to be effective in gram-negative infections, but the following two articles take the important step of determining by controlled trials whether or not amikacin is as effective as gentamicin and whether it is or is not more toxic. — Ed. ◄

Controlled Comparison of Amikacin and Gentamicin. Infections due to enteric gram-negative bacilli are a major cause of morbidity and mortality in hospitalized patients. Gentamicin, the drug currently used most often to treat these infections, is nephrotoxic and ototoxic. Initial trials have suggested that amikacin is effective for serious gram-negative infections, including those due to gentamicin-resistant organisms. Craig R. Smith, Kenneth L. Baughman, Corwin Q. Edwards, John F. Rogers and Paul S. Lietman[9] (Johns Hopkins Med. Inst.) conducted a prospective, randomized, double-blind study of these drugs in patients with a diagnosis of possible severe gram-negative infections. Of 174 patients entered in the study, 103 were excluded as not having gram-negative infection. Enteric gram-negative bacilli were pathogenic in 71 patients, 39 of them treated with amikacin and 32 with gentamicin. An initial dose of 2 mg gentamicin per kg or 8 mg amikacin per kg was given intravenously over 30 minutes and subsequent doses were adjusted to maintain 1-hour plasma levels of 5 – 10 μg gentamicin per ml or 20 – 40 μg amikacin per ml. Penicillin was given until a gram-negative pathogen was isolated. Treatment was continued until the patient was afebrile for 4 days.

Amikacin was effective in 10 of 12 bacteremias, 21 of 24 urinary tract infections, 2 of 5 pneumonias and 4 of 6 other serious infections. Gentamicin was effective in 12 of 15 bacteremias, 15 of 18 urinary tract infections, 2 of 4 pneumonias and all 3 other serious infections. The two treatment groups were similar in age, severity of underlying illness, presence of shock and type of infection. The results are summarized in the table. The development of possible and definite nephrotox-

(9) N. Engl. J. Med. 296:349 – 353, Feb. 17, 1977.

Clinical Response of 32 Patients Treated with Gentamicin and 39 Patients Treated with Amikacin

Response	Gentamicin		Amikacin	
	no.	*%*	*no.*	*%*
Cure	14	44	20	51
Response	11	34	10	26
Total favorable	25	78	30	77
Failure	1	3	4	10
Death	6	19	5	13
Total adverse	7	22	9	23
Colonization	7	22	7	18
Superinfection	2	6	4	10

icity was similar in the two groups and the frequencies of auditory toxicity were also similar.

These findings indicate that amikacin is effective in the treatment of severe gram-negative infections and is no more ototoxic or nephrotoxic than gentamicin. Effective serum drug levels were obtained in most patients with normal renal function. Monitoring of serum drug levels with frequent dosage changes may have been responsible for the high favorable response rate and low rates of toxicity obtained in this trial.

► ↓ The following article deals with a slightly different use of amikacin and gentamicin. It previously has been shown that patients with an inadequate number of circulating white blood cells have a better chance of surviving gram-negative sepsis if gentamicin is combined with carbenicillin. Presumably, synergistic activity between these two drugs helps kill *Pseudomonas,* the most frequent cause of sepsis in leukopenic patients. This article compares the efficacy of amikacin-carbenicillin with that of gentamicin-carbenicillin in a group of patients who have a maximal risk of death from gram-negative sepsis.—Ed. ◄

Comparative Efficacy and Toxicity of Amikacin-Carbenicillin versus Gentamicin-Carbenicillin in Leukopenic Patients: Randomized Prospective Trial. William K. Lau, Lowell S. Young, Robert E. Black, Drew J. Winston, Stuart R. Linné, Ralph J. Weinstein and William L. Hewitt[1] (Univ. of California, Los Angeles) performed a prospective single-blind study comparing amikacin and gentamicin therapy in 157 leukopenic patients seen in 1974–76 with neoplastic disease or a marrow failure syndrome. Patients received either 7.5 mg amikacin per kg every 8 hours plus 100 mg carbenicillin per kg every 4 hours or gentamicin in an intravenous loading dose of 2 mg/kg followed by 1.5 mg/kg every 8 hours in addition to carbenicillin. The indications for treatment were fever and evidence suggestive of gram-negative bacillary infection. A total of 155 courses of amikacin were given to 112 patients and 140 courses of gentamicin to 98 patients.

Response rates in proved and possible bacterial infections are given in Table 1. Total response rates in the two treatment groups did not differ significantly. Response rates in cases of aerobic gram-negative bacillus bacteremia were also similar. Antimicrobial synergism and

(1) Am. J. Med. 62:959–966, June, 1977.

TABLE 1.—RESPONSE RATES IN PROVED AND POSSIBLE (CLINICALLY SUSPECTED BUT UNDOCUMENTED) BACTERIAL INFECTIONS

	Amikacin	Gentamicin	Total
Proved infections (no. of courses)	50	47	97
Positive response rate (%)	72.0	83.0	77.3
Possible infections (no. of courses)	92	84	176
Positive response rate (%)	77.2	70.3	73.9
Over-all response rate (%)	75.3	74.7	75.1

TABLE 2.—AGENTS IN COMBINATION: ANTIMICROBIAL SYNERGISM AND OUTCOME

	Total (no.)	Lived (no.)	Died (no.)	Mortality (%)
A. Synergism	22	18	4	18
B. Addition, not synergism	9	5	4	44
C. Inhibition by only one drug	7	2	5	71
D. Not inhibited by two drugs	2	0	2	100
P value				
A versus B + C + D	<0.01			
A versus B + C	<0.05			

outcome are outlined in Table 2. Significant ototoxicity was documented in 20% of amikacin courses and 13.6% of gentamicin courses; the difference was not significant. Nephrotoxicity was associated with elevated blood drug levels in both treatment groups. Age and total drug dose were not significant factors in amikacin nephrotoxicity but previous exposure to aminoglycosides was significantly associated. There were 10 superinfections in the amikacin group and 7 in the gentamicin group. Superinfection was the primary cause of death in 11 of 17 patients.

Improved survival in both treatment groups in this study was associated with the use of drug combinations that interacted synergistically in vitro. No significant differences between the two regimens in ototoxicity and nephrotoxicity were observed. For patients with infections due to an organism susceptible to both amikacin and gentamicin, a regimen incorporating carbenicillin and either drug is equally effective. Empiric use of amikacin is indicated when there is a reasonable possibility of infection due to gentamicin-resistant organisms.

► [These studies indicate that the effectiveness of amikacin is equal to that of gentamicin in patients with even the most severe gram-negative infections. The ototoxicity and nephrotoxicity of amikacin equal that of gentamicin. In this study by Lau et al., 2 patients with bacteremia caused by gentamicin-resistant but amikacin-sensitive organisms received therapy with gentamicin; both died even though they were also receiving carbenicillin. Because of concern that amikacin-resistant organisms may be selected if the drug is used excessively, most workers are trying to reserve the use of amikacin for those cases in which gentamicin-resistant gram-negative bacilli are known or suspected to be present.—Ed.] ◄

Metronidazole and Anaerobic Sepsis. Metronidazole has long been used as an oral treatment of trichomoniasis and is effective in several types of anaerobic infection, but its use in severely ill patients has been limited because no parenteral preparation was available until recently. Susannah J. Eykyn and Ian Phillips[2] (London) evaluated intravenous and oral metronidazole in severely ill patients with anaerobic sepsis. When possible, metronidazole was given as the sole antimicrobial agent, but many patients also received other agents. Metronidazole was given intravenously as a buffered isotonic 0.5% aqueous solution in a dose of 500 mg in about 20 minutes every 8 hours. The 2 children treated received 250 mg every 8 hours. The oral dosage was 400 mg every 8 hours for adults and 200 mg every 8 hours for children. The dose was not reduced for 4 patients in renal failure but 3 were on hemodialysis and 1 was recovering from acute renal failure.

Fifty patients aged 6 – 80 were given metronidazole; 18 were treated intravenously only, 10 orally and 22 by both routes. Twenty-four patients received metronidazole only. All patients tolerated the drug well. Clinical responses to treatment are summarized in the table. Twenty of the 24 patients given metronidazole only had good responses, but 13 had operations. Three of the patients who failed to respond were severely ill from underlying disease or bronchopneumonia and 2 of them died. Mixed cultures were grown from 18 patients. In 7 of these, sepsis was due to aerobic bacteria; 5 had wound infections and 2 had septicemia. Anaerobes were isolated from all 44 cultures made, alone in 5 cases and with aerobes in 39. *Bacteroides melaninogenicus* was isolated from 10 of 14 specimens of pus that fluoresced bright red in ultraviolet light. Serum concentrations of metronidazole were measured within 48 hours of intravenous infusion in 10 patients and after 48 hours in 8. The mean peak and trough serum concentrations were 27.4 and 15.5 mg/L, respectively. Three patients in renal failure had peak concentrations of up to 28 mg/L.

These findings suggest that metronidazole is safe and highly effective for the treatment of severe anaerobic sepsis and that the intravenous preparation is well tolerated and of particular use in severely ill patients, especially after major surgery.

► [This study, done in England, confirms earlier work by Talley et al. (Antimicrob. Agents Chemother. 7:672, 1975). It indicates the clinical efficacy of both oral and intravenous metronidazole (Flagyl) in anaerobic infections. This is not as yet an approved use of the drug in the United States. Although its spectrum of activity is limited to obligate anaerobes, the action of metronidazole on these organisms is bactericidal, whereas that of clindamycin and chloramphenicol is bacteristatic. Therefore metronidazole might be more effective than clindamycin or chloramphenicol in the therapy of anaerobic endocarditis or of infections in patients with diminished host defenses.

Most anaerobic infections are treated with clindamycin or chloramphenicol despite the threat of pseudomembranous colitis (see the article by Rifkin et al. in the chapter Complications of Therapy) with the former and fatal aplastic anemia with the latter. In this regard, the safety of both the oral and parenteral preparations of metronidazole are of interest.

Although high concentrations of metronidazole can be achieved with oral therapy and the drug diffuses well to all tissues, a parenteral preparation is needed in many pa-

(2) Br. Med. J. 2:1418 – 1421, Dec. 11, 1976.

BACTERIA ISOLATED, SURGICAL DRAINAGE AND CLINICAL RESPONSE IN PATIENTS TREATED WITH METRONIDAZOLE ALONE AND WITH OTHER ANTIBACTERIALS

Bacteria isolated	Treatment with metronidazole alone			Treatment with metronidazole and other antimicrobials		
	Good response		Poor response	Good response		Poor response
	With drainage	Without drainage		With drainage	Without drainage	
Anaerobes alone	3	1		1		
Anaerobes and aerobes	8	6	4	11	4	6
No culture*	2			3	1	
Total patients	13	7	4	15	5	6

*All patients had intra-abdominal sepsis.

tients with serious anaerobic infections. We look forward to further studies which will define better the place of Flagyl in the treatment of anaerobic infections. – Ed.] ◄

► ↓ The following article presents compelling evidence that steroids in high doses for a short period are a useful adjunct to other modes of therapy of septic shock. – Ed. ◄

Steroids in Treatment of Clinical Septic Shock. William Schumer[3] (Chicago Med. School, North Chicago, Ill.) reports both a double-blind prospective study and a retrospective study done to determine the efficacy and safety of steroids in the treatment of septic shock. The prospective study involved 172 patients admitted consecutively in septic shock in 1967–75. Patients received saline, 3 mg dexamethasone (DMP) per kg in saline or 30 mg methylprednisolone (MPS) per kg in saline as a single bolus infusion over 10–20 minutes at the time of diagnosis. If necessary, the infusion was repeated once after 4 hours. Chloromycetin was used early in the study period and gentamicin and clindamycin subsequently. The retrospective study included 328 patients seen in 1967–76 with septic shock, 168 of whom received DMP or MPS (60 and 108 patients, respectively). Age and sex distributions

Fig 7. – Mortality in relation to severity of shock of untreated and steroid-treated patients in the prospective study. (Courtesy of Schumer, W.: Ann. Surg. 184:333–341, September, 1976.)

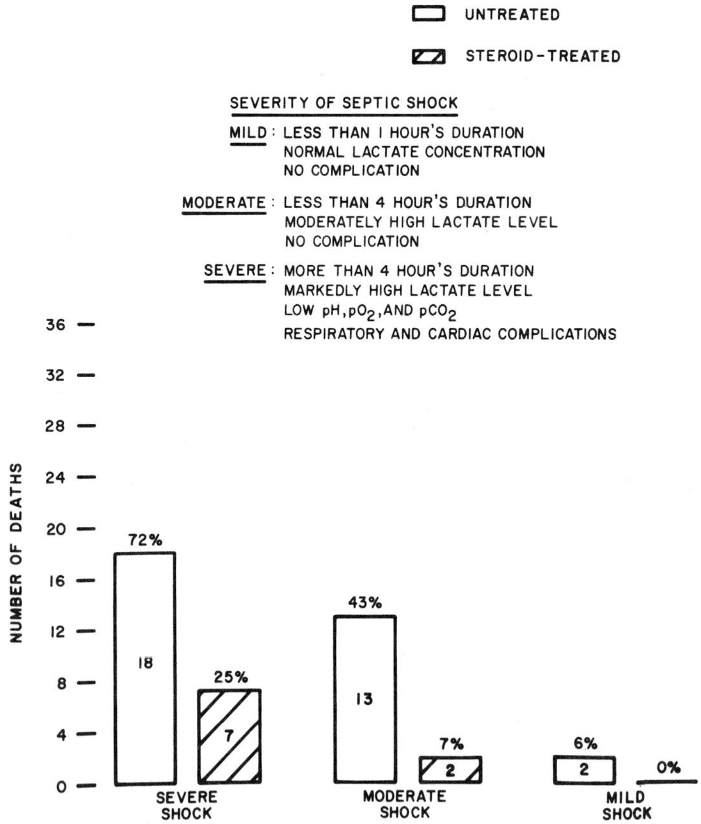

(3) Ann. Surg. 184:333–341, September, 1976.

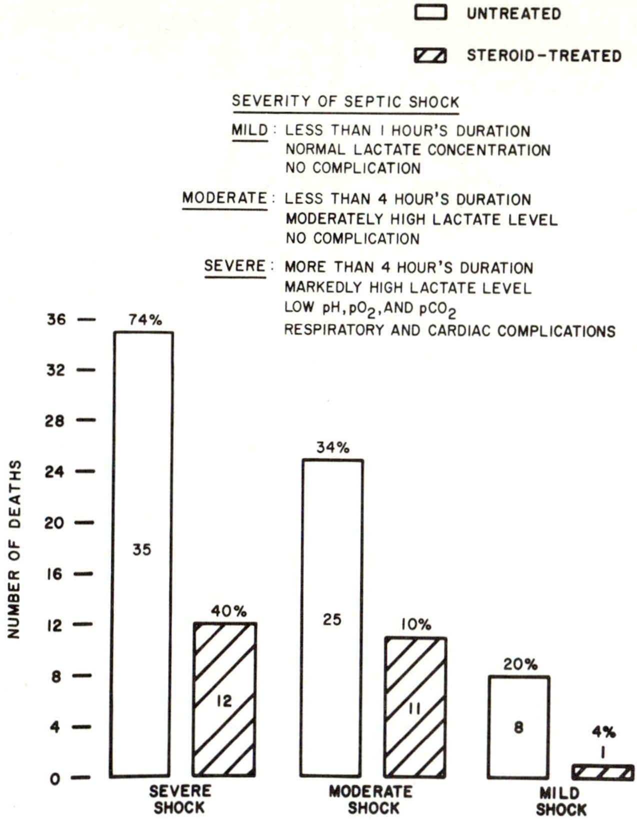

Fig 8. – Mortality in relation to severity of shock of untreated and steroid-treated patients in the retrospective study. (Courtesy of Schumer, W.: Ann. Surg. 184:333–341, September, 1976.)

were comparable in the steroid-treated and control groups in both studies.

In the prospective study, mortality was 38.4% in placebo patients and 10.4% in those given steroids. In the retrospective study the respective mortalities were 42.5% and 14%. Mortality was related to age in only placebo patients in the prospective study but in both patient groups in the retrospective study. Mortality is related to the severity of shock in Figures 7 and 8. Underlying conditions significantly affected mortality in both studies. Differences in complication rates between steroid-treated and control patients in both studies were not significant. No arrhythmia occurred in any steroid-treated patient in either study. The overall complication rate was 6% in both studies. In only 1 patient did the steroid appear to compound septic shock.

Extrapolation of results of animal studies indicates that steroid alone cannot protect the septic patient efficiently. Early steroid administration is adjunctive to other measures for septic shock, including antibiotics, fluid replacement and correction of acid-base imbalance.

► [It has been extraordinarily difficult to prove that steroids are of use in septic shock. There have been very many studies with conflicting answers conducted over the past

20 years. Doctor Schumer seems to have provided extremely convincing evidence that they do reduce mortality. Next, I hope he will tackle the problem of whether or not they are of use in sepsis not complicated by shock. – Ed.] ◄

► ↓ The following article is most timely. Every 2 or 3 weeks my colleagues at Vanderbilt University are called on to decide what therapy should be given a patient who has a serious infection with staphylococci or streptococci but who is allergic to penicillin. The nature of the patient's illness and his penicillin allergy – whether he fainted when given an injection of penicillin or had a frank anaphylactic reaction – can help decide if the 15% risk of an allergic cross-reaction entailed with giving a cephalosporin, such as Keflin, is warranted. Another frequently considered option is desensitization or making the patient temporarily tolerant to penicillin (Green et al.: Ann. Intern. Med. 67:235, 1967; and Zolov et al.: J. Allergy 39:107, 1967). This procedure is time-consuming, delays initiation of effective therapy and carries some risk itself. Vancomycin usually is considered but sometimes is passed by in this situation because of its toxicity. The following article presents the case for giving vancomycin stronger consideration. – Ed.

Vancomycin: A Second Look is taken by Anthony L. Esposito and Richard A. Gleckman[4] (Boston). With the introduction of methicillin sodium into clinical practice in 1960, vancomycin hydrochloride stopped being used. It was known to be a difficult antibiotic to tolerate and had produced irreparable harm in some patients that included deafness and renal failure. A second look, however, is indicated because of improvements in the manufacturing process, reports of methicillin-resistant staphylococci causing serious disease and confirmation of the efficacy of vancomycin in the treatment of life-threatening infections due to *Staphylococcus aureus, Streptococcus viridans* and enterococci.

Untoward reactions to vancomycin have been reduced by the use of more purified material and careful attention to details of infusion. Vancomycin may be useful in patients considered penicillin allergic who have severe infections. Vancomycin is of proved value in the treatment of serious staphylococcal infections. Most patients with endocarditis and pneumonia have been cured with vancomycin. Infections of the skin, including wound infections have responded in 90% of cases. Virtually all cases of parotiditis and enterocolitis have been treated successfully. Vancomycin also appears to be useful in the treatment of staphylococcal meningitis. A single weekly infusion has been useful in patients with restricted venous access who received long-term hemodialysis. Vancomycin, alone or with streptomycin, has cured *S. viridans* and enterococcal endocarditis in penicillin-allergic patients.

Vancomycin therapy is not invariably successful. Evaluation of vestibular function and audiometric testing are important in patients given this antibiotic. Sequential evaluation of renal status to determine drug dosage is mandatory in institutions without access to serum antibiotic determinations.

► [Two possible new indications for therapy with vancomycin are described in this Section (see the article by G. F. Rifkin et al. in the chapter Complications of Therapy and one by P. C. Appelbaum et al. in the chapter Pneumococcal Infections). – Ed.] ◄

Pharmacologic Evaluation of Penicillin in Children with Purulent Meningitis. The dose of penicillin G used to treat meningitides should be based on known amounts needed to create bactericidal con-

(4) J.A.M.A. 238:1756–1757, Oct. 17, 1977.

centrations in the cerebrospinal fluid (CSF). J. Patrick Hieber and John D. Nelson[5] (Univ. of Texas Southwestern Med. School) studied the relation of serum to CSF levels of penicillin during acute purulent meningitis in infancy and childhood. Studies were done in 24 patients with group A streptococcal or meningococcal meningitis, with an age range of 2 weeks to 11 years. Only 1 patient was under age 1 month. Patients were begun on 100 mg chloramphenicol per kg, intravenously, daily and 250,000 U aqueous penicillin G per kg daily in 6 divided doses infused in 15 minutes. Chloramphenicol was stopped when the organism was identified. Serum and CSF specimens were assayed for penicillin activity within 36 hours.

The pharmacokinetics of serum penicillin were similar on all 3 study days (Fig 9). Mean peak CSF concentrations were 0.8–1.1 μg/ml, 30–60 minutes after infusions on all 3 days. The mean CSF level, as a percentage of the simultaneous serum level, declined from 18.4% on day 1 to 4.9% on day 10. Both serum and CSF levels correlated with bactericidal titers against the patient's pathogen. The entry of penicillin into the CSF correlated closely with the usual measures of meningeal inflammation. There was a strong negative correlation between the CSF-to-serum glucose ratio and the CSF penicillin concentration. The CSF protein level correlated with both the absolute CSF level and the percentage of the simultaneous serum concentration in the CSF.

These observations are consistent with those made in animal models

Fig 9.—Serum *(open circles)* and cerebrospinal fluid *(closed circles)* penicillin concentrations in acute bacterial meningitis (mean values). (Courtesy of Hieber, J. P., and Nelson, J. D.: N. Engl. J. Med. 297:410–413, Aug. 25, 1977.)

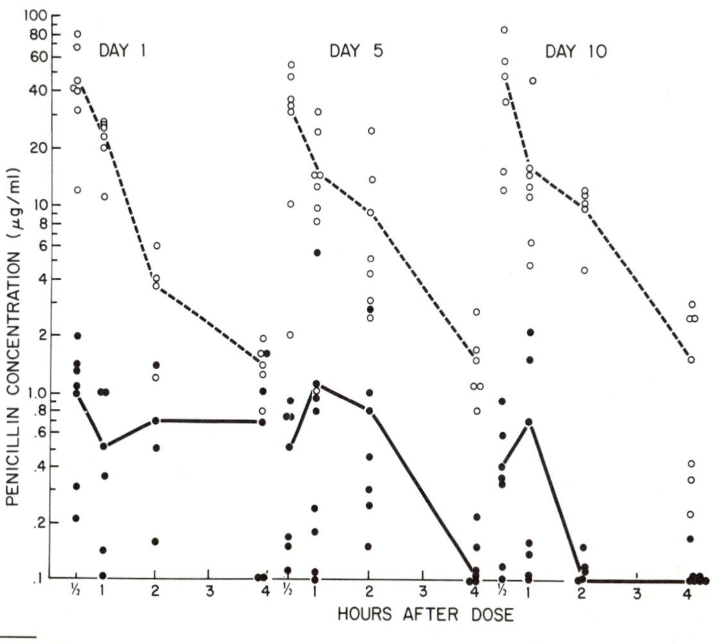

(5) N. Engl. J. Med. 297:410–413, Aug. 25, 1977.

of purulent meningitis, in which the sustained elevation of CSF penicillin early in the process is due to increased permeability of the blood-CSF barrier and to decreased clearance by a partially inhibited organic acid pump. All the present patients recovered uneventfully. The treatment schedule used appears to be adequate for pneumococcal, group A streptococcal and meningococcal meningitis in pediatric patients. Higher doses may be needed with an organism having an unusually high minimal inhibitory concentration to penicillin, and monitoring of CSF penicillin levels may be indicated in such cases.

► [Over the past few years there has been much work done to establish the pharmacodynamics of those antimicrobials used to treat gram-negative (1976 YEAR BOOK, p. 34) and gram-positive meningitis. Such data are critical if we are to be sure that CSF concentrations are well above the minimal inhibitory or bactericidal concentration of the antimicrobial for the infecting organism. In this study of penicillin and in a recent study of nafcillin (Kane et al.: Ann. Intern. Med. 87:309, 1977) there has been troublesome variation in both the absolute amount of the penicillin that reached the CSF and in the serum-CSF ratio. Some patients who had high serum levels had borderline or inadequate CSF levels. Whereas this may not be a serious problem in infections with pneumococci or group A streptococci, which are quite sensitive to penicillin, it may well be a problem with *Hemophilus influenzae* infections, which require greater concentrations of ampicillin, or *Staphylococcus aureus* infections, which require greater concentrations of nafcillin or oxacillin for their control. It is clear that the CSF concentrations of any of the penicillins achieved with a given systemic dose decrease as the patient improves. Thus, with clinical improvement one should increase, not decrease, the systemic dose in order to maintain the desired level of antimicrobial in the CSF.—Ed.]

► ↓ In the 1977 YEAR BOOK (p. 57) we reviewed a controlled study of the use of adenine arabinoside in the therapy of herpes zoster in immunocompromised patients. It seemed to work and we sounded a cautiously optimistic note. Well, as you have gathered from all the notices in the news media, there is another oasis in the desert of antiviral chemotherapy. Adenine arabinoside also seems of benefit in the treatment of herpes simplex encephalitis.—Ed. ◄

Adenine Arabinoside Therapy of Biopsy-Proved Herpes Simplex Encephalitis: National Institute of Allergy and Infectious Diseases Collaborative Antiviral Study is reported by Richard J. Whitely, Seng-jaw Soong, Raphael Dolin, George J. Galasso, Lawrence T. Ch'ien, Charles A. Alford and the Collaborative Study Group.[6] Encephalitis due to herpes simplex virus is considered the most common cause of sporadic fatal encephalitis in the United States. Idoxuridine was gaining acceptance until controlled studies showed clear-cut toxicity without efficacy. Adenine arabinoside was found to be effective for the systemic treatment of zoster infections in immunocompromised persons. It has now been evaluated in patients with evidence of an acute febrile encephalopathy and cerebrospinal fluid findings compatible with viral infection. Patients received adenine arabinoside intravenously in a dose of 15 mg/kg daily over 12 hours or a placebo. Patients with a positive brain biopsy specimen from which virus was isolated received drug or placebo for 10 days; treatment was stopped after 5 days in patients with a negative biopsy specimen to avoid possible drug toxicity.

Mortality data are given in the table. Adenine arabinoside significantly reduced the mortality of proved herpes simplex encephalitis

(6) N. Engl. J. Med. 297:289–294, Aug. 11, 1977.

Summary of Mortality* Data in Patients Treated with Adenine Arabinoside (Ara-A) and Placebo

Biopsy	Ara-A			Placebo		
	Total studied	Dead	Mortality rate %	Total studied	Dead	Mortality rate %
Positive†	18	5	28	10	7	70
Negative	11	1	9	11	3	27
Totals	29			21		

*Mortality calculated at 1-month interval after onset of therapy by χ^2 analyses. Statistical evaluation: Ara-A vs. placebo, biopsy positive, P = 0.03; Ara-A vs. placebo, biopsy negative, P = 0.27; biopsy negative vs. biopsy positive, placebo, P = 0.05; biopsy positive (Ara-A) vs. biopsy negative (placebo), P = 0.98; biopsy positive (placebo) vs. biopsy negative (Ara-A), P = 0.005.

†One case positive at autopsy was negative at biopsy.

from 70% to 28% and significance was further enhanced when the data were adjusted for increased severity. The prognosis depended on both treatment and the level of consciousness at the time of therapy (Fig 10), but duration of disease before biopsy was not a determinant of the outcome. Progression of the disease was quite variable. The treated and placebo groups were generally comparable in age, sex, cerebral edema, alteration of consciousness and seizures. Localization was seen by brain scan and was more frequently found in patients with positive biopsy specimens. All the brain isolates were herpes simplex type 1. Adverse clinical reactions were not identified at dosage used and there were no serious adverse effects of therapy on marrow, liver or renal function. No patient had absolute granulocytopenia and only 2 had thrombocytopenia, with no evidence of bleeding.

Adenine arabinoside has a good therapeutic index for the treatment of type 1 herpes simplex encephalitis, but it must be given early in the course of infection, before the advent of coma. It should be coupled with brain biopsy to avoid the unnecessary treatment of nonresponsive en-

Fig 10.—Relation between outcome and state of consciousness at time of initiation of adenine arabinoside *(Ara-A)* or placebo therapy in biopsy-proved herpes encephalitis. (Courtesy of Whitley, R. J., et al.: N. Engl. J. Med. 297:289–294, Aug. 11, 1977.)

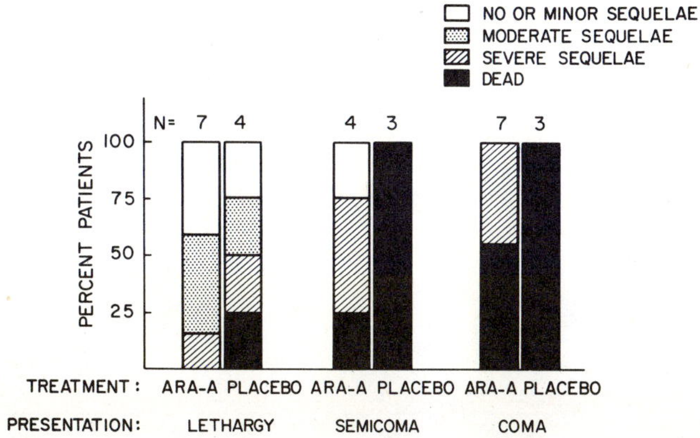

cephalitides that can mimic herpes simplex. Hopefully more precise definition of the drug's action on viral replication at the molecular level will lead to the development of even more specific and potent chemotherapeutic agents.

► [This is an article that should be read by all of you. In addition to the demonstration of therapeutic effect, two other features are worthy of special emphasis. In the doses used, adenine arabinoside was unaccompanied by serious side effects. Second, the most important prognostic indicator was the patient's state of consciousness on admission to the hospital. For maximum benefit, the decision to give the drug must be made speedily.

The authors strongly recommend brain biopsy before therapy is started. This immediately became a debatable point on rounds at Vanderbilt University and elsewhere (see letters to the editor, N. Engl. J. Med. 297:1288, 1977). Adenoside arabinoside is not toxic and it does not affect the course of other encephalitides adversely (St. Louis, eastern equine, etc.). Because brain biopsy in severely ill patients is not without risk and because the biopsy might miss the involved area, is biopsy really necessary in routine clinical practice? There is no doubt that it was a critical requirement of the investigation, but my colleagues are far from convinced that the risk-benefit equation now invariably requires biopsy. I agree. – Ed.] ◄

Complications of Therapy

► ↓ Clindamycin was enthusiastically welcomed as an alternative to chloramphenicol for the treatment of anaerobic infections. However, the enthusiasm was soon dampened by reports of pseudomembranous colitis associated with clindamycin in up to 10% of cases (1975 YEAR BOOK, p. 97). This complication is characterized by fever, watery diarrhea, lower abdominal pain and a typical picture on endoscopy (1977 YEAR BOOK, p. 79). It is associated with prolonged morbidity and even death in some patients. As pointed out in the 1977 Year Book (p. 79), other antibiotics, such as ampicillin and lincomycin, also are associated with the syndrome. The pathogenesis of the syndrome has never been understood, though cholestyramine was said to have a salutary effect. Recently, various research groups have independently reported results that suggest the cause of this syndrome . . . and a means for treating it! – Ed. ◄

Antibiotic-Induced Colitis: Implication of a Toxin Neutralized by *Clostridium sordellii* Antitoxin. Pseudomembranous colitis has long been recognized as a complication of antimicrobial therapy. The pathogenesis has remained unclear but a heat-labile toxin found in the feces of affected patients was implicated by Larson et al. G. D. Rifkin, F. R. Fekety, J. Silva, Jr. (Univ. of Michigan), and R. B. Sack[7] (Johns Hopkins Univ.) have demonstrated a similar toxin and its neutralization by polyvalent clostridial antitoxin in hamsters with clindamycin-induced ileocecitis. Toxin has now been demonstrated in the feces of 2 patients with antibiotic-associated colitis.

The toxin found in the feces of these patients was heat labile, was rapidly lethal for hamsters, increased vascular permeability in rabbit skin and was cytotoxic for cells in tissue culture. It was neutralized by *C. sordellii* antitoxin, but not by antitoxins prepared against other clostridia, *Escherichia coli* toxin or *Vibrio cholerae* toxin. These features are identical to those of the toxin implicated in antibiotic-induced colitis in the hamster. One patient improved rapidly after oral vancomycin therapy, concomitantly with disappearance of the toxin from the stool.

These findings confirm the presence of a heat-labile toxin or toxins in the feces of patients with pseudomembranous colitis induced by clindamycin or ampicillin. The toxin(s) appears to be derived from *C. sordellii*. Hopefully this report will stimulate microbiologic and toxicologic studies of all cases of pseudomembranous colitis in order to define more clearly the role of *C. sordellii* and possibly other toxin-producing organisms in this disease.

► [This study suggests that during therapy with clindamycin or ampicillin, certain of the bowel flora are inhibited, thus allowing *Clostridium sordellii* and perhaps other clostridia to multiply and elaborate a toxin that is responsible for the local and systemic manifestations of the pseudomembranous colitis syndrome. Bartlett et al. (J. Infect. Dis. 136:701, 1977) have also isolated a clostridial strain that causes the syndrome in hamsters. Bacteria-free supernatant fluid from this strain also produced the syndrome. The colitis could be prevented by gas gangrene antitoxin.

---

(7) Lancet 2:1103 – 1106, Nov. 26, 1977.

The clostridial strains that elaborate the toxin are resistant to clindamycin but inhibited or killed by vancomycin. Vancomycin therapy was associated with a prompt decrease in symptoms in the patient with pseudomembranous colitis described above. In addition, Bartlett et al. (Gastroenterology 73:772, 1977) found that clindamycin or lincomycin therapy produced lethal enterocolitis in 65 of 67 hamsters, but when vancomycin was administered in conjunction with the clindamycin, no animals died in a group of 49 so treated. Similar protection of hamsters from clindamycin-induced colitis by oral vancomycin has been reported by Browne et al. (Johns Hopkins Med. J. 141: 183, 1977).

These studies indicate the need for trials of vancomycin therapy of pseudomembranous colitis in human beings. The implications of these studies for the use of vancomycin as prophylaxis during clindamycin therapy are much less clear—it sounds like it could get dreadfully complicated.—Ed.] ◄

► ↓ The controversy over whether oxacillin and nafcillin are superior to methicillin in the therapy of serious staphylococcal disease has brewed for years. The following article may settle the argument on grounds other than efficacy.—Ed. ◄

Nephropathy Associated with Methicillin Therapy: Prevalence and Determinants in Patients with Staphylococcal Bacteremia. Methicillin sodium has been implicated as a cause of acute interstitial nephritis but the complication is considered rare. Charles M. Nolan and Robert S. Abernathy[8] (Univ. of Arkansas) sought evidence for this adverse drug reaction in 105 consecutive patients with bacteremia due to *Staphylococcus aureus,* including 81 who received methicillin or a cephalosporin parenterally as primary antibiotic therapy. Antibiotic-associated nephropathy was diagnosed on the basis of proteinuria and hematuria with a sterile urine culture and no catheter present, an otherwise unexplained fever or skin rash and blood eosinophilia and improvement in the renal and extrarenal findings after withdrawal of the antibiotic.

Fifty-two patients received methicillin as primary therapy, whereas 29 received a cephalosporin, usually cephalothin. The groups were comparable in age and frequencies of endocarditis, drug addiction and hospital-acquired bacteremia. Antibiotic-associated nephropathy occurred in 9 (17%) of 52 patients receiving methicillin but only 1 (3%) of 29 patients receiving a cephalosporin. Eosinophilia was present in 7 of

FREQUENCY OF METHICILLIN NEPHROPATHY ACCORDING TO LENGTH OF TREATMENT AND TYPE OF INFECTION

Group	Frequency of Nephropathy*
Treatment over 10 days	
Endocarditis	7/16 (44%)†
Nonendocarditis	2/11 (18%)†
Treatment 10 days or less	
Endocarditis	0/3
Nonendocarditis	0/19

*Numerator, cases of nephropathy; denominator, cases treated. Omitted from the total treated are the 2 patients with other types of adverse drug reaction and a patient with antibiotic failure.

†Not significantly different (P = 0.17, Fisher's exact test).

(8) Arch. Intern. Med. 137:997–1000, August, 1977.

these patients and fever in 6. Of the 10 patients, 6 had evidence of deteriorating renal function, whereas 4 had no change in renal function. Nephropathic reactions to methicillin were correlated with endocarditis and with treatment for over 10 days but not with a history of intravenous drug abuse. The findings are summarized in the table. Two methicillin-treated patients had adverse reactions without renal involvement. These reactions consisted of fever and leukopenia and occurred in patients with endocarditis.

The ability to diagnose drug-induced renal disease has recently been advanced by the use of immunofluorescent techniques to detect drug-derived haptens, immunoglobulins and complement in renal biopsy tissue. Renal biopsy often facilitates the decision regarding whether to continue methicillin therapy. Prompt discontinuance of the drug seems prudent when early signs of nephropathy are detected, because the renal damage in antibiotic-induced acute interstitial nephritis, though usually transient, may be irreversible.

► [Somehow, the suggestion that doing a renal biopsy will facilitate the decision regarding whether or not to continue methicillin therapy helps me make the decision to stop using methicillin therapy entirely. This study, which shows a much higher frequency of nephritis with methicillin than with cephalosporins, parallels previous studies showing a higher frequency of nephritis with methicillin than with oxacillin. Reports of an inordinately high incidence of failure of cephalosporin therapy in serious staphylococcal disease makes me wary of a change to those drugs. However, there is no evidence that oxacillin and nafcillin are any less effective than methicillin, and they cause nephritis much less frequently. The way completely to avoid the risk of methicillin nephritis seems clear. – Ed.] ◄

► ↓ Many practicing physicians were trained in the days before we knew anything about plasmids and sexual transmission of multiple antibiotic resistance among microorganisms. When they hear about these transmissible loops of DNA, they ask, "Gee, do you think I'm making those things in all the patients I'm giving tetracycline to for their acne?" The following article answers the questions with an emphatic "Yes!" – Ed.

Changing Patterns of Plasmid-Mediated Drug Resistance during Tetracycline Therapy. Problems related to the increasing prevalence of infectious multiple-drug resistance have serious implications for the health of human beings throughout the world. Certain antibiotics, notably tetracycline, have a great potential for selection of bacteria with R plasmid-determined drug resistance and such bacteria may also be resistant to other drugs. J. K. Møller, A. Leth Bak, A. Stenderup, H. Zachariae and H. Afzelius[9] (Univ. of Aarhus) studied the drug resistance patterns and frequency of R plasmids in *Escherichia coli* isolated from otherwise healthy persons who received low oral doses of tetracycline for acne vulgaris for varying periods. None of the 88 patients had received other antibiotics in the past 6 months. An oral dose of 250–500 mg tetracycline daily was given for 2 weeks, followed by 250 mg daily in most cases. Eighteen patients were not yet treated, whereas 13 had been treated for 7 days, 16 for 1 month and 41 for longer periods. Fecal cultures were obtained and all resistant *E. coli* were tested for transfer of resistance to the *E. coli* K-12 strain J53-1.

The results are given in Tables 1 and 2. The percentage of patients with resistant *E. coli* increased from 50% before treatment to 88% in

(9) Antimicrob. Agents Chemother. 11:388–391, March, 1977.

TABLE 1.—FREQUENCY OF MULTIPLE-RESISTANT *E. coli* FROM PATIENTS WITH ACNE VULGARIS TREATED WITH TETRACYCLINE

Duration of Treatment	No. and % of Multiply*† Resistant Strains
Before treatment	0 of 18 (0%)
1 week	0 of 13 (0%)
4 weeks	6 of 16 (38%)
More than 4 weeks	20 of 41 (49%)

*t (Rank test), 4.02, 2P<0.01%.
†Strains resistant to three or more of the following drugs: tetracycline, sulfonamide, streptomycin, trimethoprim, chloramphenicol, kanamycin, nalidixic acid, ampicillin and gentamicin.

TABLE 2.—PATTERNS OF RESISTANCE IN *E. coli* FROM PATIENTS BEFORE AND AFTER TREATMENT WITH TETRACYCLINE

Before Treatment	Treatment for: 1 Week	4 Weeks	More than 4 Weeks
Sensitive (9)*	Sensitive (4)	Sensitive (4)	Sensitive (5)
Su† (1)	Su (1)	Tc (4)	Tc (9)
Tc (6)	Tc (6)	Tc-Su (1)	Tc-Su (2)
Tc-Su (1)	Tc-Ap (2)	Tc-Sm (1)	Tc-Ap (3)
Su-Sm (1)		Tc-Su-Sm (4)	Tc-Sm (3)
		Tc-Su-Sm-Ap (1)	Tc-Su-Sm (10)
		Tc-Su-Sm-Cm-Ap (1)	Tc-Su-Sm-Ap (2)
			Tc-Su-Cm-Ap (1)
			Tc-Su-Sm-Cm-Ap (3)
			Tc-Su-Tp-Sm-Ap (1)
			Tc-Su-Tp-Sm-Cm-Km (1)
			Tc-Su-Sm-Cm-Km-Ap (1)

*Number in parentheses is number of patients.
†Tc, tetracycline; Su, sulfonamide; Tp, trimethoprim; Sm, streptomycin; Cm, chloramphenicol; Km, kanamycin; Ap, ampicillin; Nx, nalidixic acid; Gm, gentamicin.

the group treated for over 4 weeks. The respective frequencies of R plasmids in the resistant bacteria were 63% and 83%. No multiple-resistant *E. coli* were found in patients before or after 1 week of treatment but such organisms were found in about half the patients treated for over 4 weeks. Most bacteria isolated in patients treated for 4 weeks or longer were either monoresistant or multiple-resistant *Proteus mirabilis* or *Streptococcus fecalis* when only susceptible *E. coli* were present.

Long-term tetracycline therapy is associated with an increasing frequency of R plasmid-determined resistance and with a progressive tendency for this resistance to be multiple. Patients may harbor multiply drug-resistant bacteria at a low concentration before treatment or may acquire them during treatment, or drug resistance may be transferred from the anaerobic bacteria that constitute most enteric bacteria in the bowel flora. If only certain antibiotics can preferentially select multiple resistance, a limitation in use of these drugs should be recommended.

► [This article and the first one in this chapter clearly focus on the havoc we raise for our fellow human beings when we manipulate their flora with antimicrobials. But the chain of ecologic disturbance does not stop with the person treated. Petrocheilou et al. (Antimicrob. Agents Chemother. 12:219, 1977) have documented the spread to other persons of multiply resistant *Escherichia coli* that arose during tetracycline treatment of acne. This should be kept in mind when one considers the administration of tetracycline or any other antimicrobial to any patient. – Ed.] ◄

Miscellaneous

Infections due to *Staphylococcus aureus*. Daniel M. Musher and Suzanne Olbricht McKenzie[1] (Baylor College of Medicine) reviewed the findings in 123 patients seen in a 5-year period in 1971–76 with infection due to *S. aureus*. There were 122 men and 1 woman. Fifty-six patients had soft tissue infections and 42 had bacteremia; 32 patients had osteomyelitis and 20 had pneumonia.

The soft tissue infections were generally quite severe even when localized to a particular site. Forty-four of the 56 patients had identifiable local factors that had predisposed to infection by breaking the integrity of the skin. Identification of *S. aureus* as a cause of soft tissue infection was surprisingly easy. Sources of sepsis are given in Table 1. The superficial soft tissue infections included impetigo, ecthyma and infection superimposed on skin diseases; the deep infections included cellulitis, fasciitus, boils and abscesses. Thirteen of the 56 patients with soft tissue infections had bacteremia. Thirty-two patients had osteomyelitis, 20 of them adjacent to an area of open trauma, previous surgery or soft tissue infection. Of 20 patients with pneumonia due to *S. aureus,* 11 had aerogenous and 9 had hematogenous infections. The relationship between blood culture results and the likelihood of endocarditis is shown in Table 2.

The pathogenesis of staphylococcal infections is not completely understood. Various underlying diseases appear to predispose to severe infection. The diagnosis is usually not difficult to make. The tendency for purulent collections to form usually requires a combined medical and surgical approach to treatment. Deaths have usually been attributable to destruction of vital tissues or to underlying diseases. Clini-

TABLE 1.—INFECTED FOCI AS SOURCE FOR STAPHYLOCOCCAL SEPSIS IN 42 PATIENTS

Extravascular focus		16
Cellulitis, abscess, decubitus ulcer	10	
Burns	1	
Osteomyelitis	2	
Pneumonia	3	
Intravascular focus		9
Intravenous catheter site	4	
Arteriovenous shunt	5	
Presumed intravascular focus		12
Heroin addiction	10	
Arteriovenous fistula	2	
No focus		15
Total		52

(1) Medicine (Baltimore) 56:383–409, September, 1977.

TABLE 2.—RELATIONSHIP BETWEEN NUMBER AND POSITIVITY OF BLOOD CULTURES AND LIKELIHOOD OF ENDOCARDITIS IN 41 PATIENTS

	Patients	Patients with all cultures positive	Total number cultures done	Percent positive
Definite endocarditis	15	13	78	94
Probable endocarditis	5	4	27	89
No evidence of endocarditis	21	17	88	88
Total	41	34	193	91

cal studies to evaluate various semisynthetic penicillins, dosage and duration of therapy are in progress. *Staphylococcus aureus* having very high minimum bactericidal concentrations for semisynthetic penicillins have begun to appear and it may be only a matter of time before these isolates are seen as common pathogens in the United States.

► [A short article cannot really do justice to this review, the original of which contains 229 references. I guess I like it because it refers to so much of the previous work done by me and my colleagues when the staphylococcus was the major focus of my laboratory! It is a good review article.

Table 2 requires some explanation. Doctors Musher and McKenzie attempted to determine whether the *number* of positive blood cultures could help establish a diagnosis of endocardial involvement and found it did not. Those patients without apparent endocarditis were just as commonly bacteremic as those with probable heart valve involvement. However, their data did not permit them to determine whether a continuous or steady-state bacteremia was helpful in making this differentiation—in many cases multiple blood cultures were taken during a short period before therapy was started. Also, as far as I could tell, they did not do pour plates which would have permitted quantitation of the *level* of bacteremia. Almost 40 years ago, Dr. Paul Beeson showed that patients with endocarditis have a surprisingly constant number of bacteria in the bloodstream at all times. This quantitation might have helped.

The authors did find—as have a number of other recent students of staphylococcal disease—that patients with no obvious focus for their disease who acquired their infection outside the hospital were more likely to have endocarditis than those with an obvious primary focus or those who developed infection while in the hospital. It appears that making this important differentiation can now be aided by measurement of serum antibodies to teichoic acid. Elevated levels strongly suggest the diagnosis of endocarditis.

These authors—and others—are now cautiously making decisions regarding management by the following ground rules: (1) If an easily treatable focus of recent origin is thought to be responsible for the bacteremia; (2) if there is no evidence of endocarditis on careful study; (3) if the patient has normal host defense mechanisms; and (4) if levels of serum antibodies to teichoic acid are not evaluated; they will treat for 1–2 weeks rather than the 6–8 weeks formerly used. I think this makes good sense.

To get the latest data on staphylococcal disease, my colleagues recently consulted with Dr. Richard E. Dixson, a former student who now runs the hospital infection unit at The Center for Disease Control, Atlanta, Georgia. He reports that there have been clusters of methicillin-resistant staphylococci appearing on the scene. So far, burn units have been the source of these strains. One should be on the lookout for such infections. Most can be treated with vancomycin (see the article by A. L. Esposito and R. A. Gleckman in the chapter Therapy of Infections.—Ed.] ◄

Spinal Epidural Abscess. Epidural abscess continues to defy the diagnostic skills of physicians. David Schlossberg and Jonas A.

TABLE 1.—SUMMARY OF SIX CASES OF SPINAL EPIDURAL ABSCESS

Patient Number	*Age/Sex*	*History of Trauma*	*Infection*	*Fever*	*Elevated Peripheral WBC*	*CSF Protein (mg/100 ml)*	*CSF WBC/cu mm (% polys)*	*Results of Laminectomy*	*Etiology**	*Other Associated Disease*	*Definitive Diagnostic Procedures*
1	43/M	—	—	+	+	82	2(0)	Full recovery	α-hemolytic *Streptococcus*	Alcoholism	Myelography
2	30/M	+	—	—	—	56	4(0)	Improvement	*Staphylococcus aureus*	None	Myelography
3	58/F	—	+	+	+	218	3(67)	No improvement	*Staphylococcus aureus*	Diabetes	Myelography
4	43/M	+	+ (Bronchitis)	+	+	186	6(50)	No improvement	*Staphylococcus aureus*	None	Myelography
5	51/M	—	—	—	—	1852	280(90)	No improvement	Culture negative	Alcoholism	Myelography
6	46/M	—	+ (*E coli* bacteremia)	—	+	Not available	Not available	No improvement	Culture negative	Alcoholism	Myelography

*Results of cultures of abscess material are shown except in patient 1 where streptococci were grown from blood only and patient 4 where staphylococci were recovered from blood as well as from abscess material.

TABLE 2.—Common Misdiagnoses of Spinal Epidural Abscess

Acute Epidural Abscess:	Meningitis
	Perinephric abscess
	Rheumatoid spondylitis
	Acute back strain
	Transverse myelitis
	Acute poliomyelitis
	Spontaneous extradural hematomas
	Hematomyelia
	Polyneuritis
	Uncomplicated vertebral osteomyelitis
Chronic Epidural Abscess:	Polio
	Tumors (intradural, extramedullary, extradural)
	Embolus
	Spinal vessel thrombosis
	Vertebral osteomyelitis
	Chronic meningitis
	Pott's disease with compression myelitis

Shulman[2] (Emory Univ.) report 6 recent cases of spinal epidural abscess (Table 1). Helpful clues that were overlooked included a history of prior trauma in 2 patients and a history of another site of infection in 3. Fever was absent in 3 patients and peripheral neutrophilia was lacking in 2. Symptoms of 2 patients with severe alcohol abuse were misinterpreted as complications of alcoholism.

Spinal epidural abscess is often manifested by fever, leukocytosis, local spinal tenderness and neck stiffness. A previous infection at a distant site is common. Spinal ache is almost always present, usually in the thoracic area. Fever, however, is not always present. A stiff neck is frequently present. Common misdiagnoses of spinal epidural abscess are listed in Table 2. The distinction from transverse myelitis can be extremely difficult. The absence of back pain is strong evidence against abscess and transverse myelopathy progresses more rapidly. If vertebral osteomyelitis is demonstrated, epidural abscess is almost certain. Positive blood cultures strongly suggest an abscess. The danger of lumbar puncture in suspected epidural abscess is overrated. If no pus is found and the subarachnoid space is entered, manometrics should be done; a complete or partial block is nearly always found. Staphylococci are the most common causative organisms. Most epidural abscesses occur in a midthoracic or lower lumbar location.

Rapid diagnosis and treatment are essential, since the degree of recovery is proportional to the extent of the neurologic deficit present before operation. Only 1 of the present 6 patients recovered fully. Even with appropriate and rapid surgery, one third of survivors have significant neurologic deficits postoperatively. Antibiotic therapy should also be given. It is usually safe to begin with an antistaphylococcal drug such as oxacillin. This therapy should be expanded if there is reason to suspect another pathogen, especially in the urinary tract, or with an underlying disease known to predispose to infection with a specific pathogen.

(2) South. Med. J. 70:669–673, June, 1977.

► [Doctors Schlossberg and Shulman have clearly presented the difficulties in diagnosing epidural abscesses as well as a picture of the devastating consequences which result if an early diagnosis and prompt surgical drainage are not obtained. However, early in the course the only two clues the physician may have are back pain and a recent history of an infection. The back pain may have followed a fall or some other minor injury and may be attributed to a mechanical problem. The infection is often an insignificant pimple or furuncle. Note that some of their patients had neither fever nor an elevated peripheral white blood cell count, even when the disease was advanced. The diagnosis is suspected more readily if there are the additional signs of neck stiffness and changes in the reflexes. If the disease has progressed such that there is back pain plus clear-cut weakness or paralysis, spinal epidural abscess should be a major diagnostic consideration.

My colleagues have taken issue with the suggestion that suspicion of the disease should prompt a lumbar puncture. There is agreement that cerebrospinal fluid should be obtained, but their concern is that putting a needle through the abscess on the way to the subarachnoid space may convert a staphylococcal abscess to staphylococcal meningitis. After conversations were held with the chronologically senior author of the article, the following seems to be the most reasonable approach to diagnosis. If there is only back pain, tenderness and possibly neck stiffness, lumbar puncture is indicated. The benefits of early diagnosis are considered to outweigh the risk of converting an abscess to meningitis. Cerebrospinal fluid abnormalities, even limited to an elevated protein level, should prompt a myelogram, preferably by the lateral cervical route to avoid putting another needle through the possible abscess. If there is weakness or paralysis so that it is clear that a myelogram will be done anyway, a neurosurgeon should be contacted and the initial cerebrospinal tap via the lateral cervical approach should be combined with a myelogram. In either instance, if there are cerebrospinal fluid or myelographic abnormalities, or if the patient shows other signs of infection, therapy should be begun with oxacillin or nafcillin. The dose should be high (200 mg/kg/day) because of the relatively poor diffusion of these drugs into the cerebrospinal fluid, even with inflamed meninges (Ann. Intern. Med. 87:309, 1977). Clearly, spinal epidural abscess should be considered a medical emergency and all haste made in securing the diagnosis and establishing surgical drainage. – Ed.] ◄

Changed Spectrum of Purulent Pericarditis: 86-Year Autopsy Experience in 200 Patients. Purulent pericarditis continues to be a diagnostic and therapeutic problem. Peter G. Klacsmann, Bernadine H. Bulkley and Grover M. Hutchins[3] (Johns Hopkins Med. Inst.) compared the autopsy findings in 145 patients seen in 1889–1943 with purulent pericarditis (group 1) with those in 55 patients seen since 1943 (group 2). Inadequate histologic material was available for review in 18 cases. The two groups were separated by the time at which penicillin became available for general use.

Male patients comprised 67% of group 1 and 55% of group 2. The median age was 20 for group 1 and 49 for group 2, although the age ranges were similar in the two groups. The diagnosis was made antemortem in 30% of patients seen before 1944 but in only 18% of those seen later. In the early period, purulent pericarditis contributed to the death of 41% of patients and tamponade was present in 26%. In the more recent period, pericarditis contributed to death in 35% of cases and tamponade was present in 18%. The organisms isolated are shown in the table. Primary infectious disease was present in 86% of group 1 patients; most of these had pneumonia. Since 1943, primary infectious disease was associated with only 22% of patients and major underlying disease was present in 78% of patients. Myocardial abscesses were present in 11% of group 1 patients and 18% of group 2 patients. Preexist-

(3) Am. J. Med. 63:666–673, November, 1977.

Purulent Pericarditis: Organisms Isolated*

Organisms	1889–1943 No.	%	1944–75 No.	%
Gram-positive				
Pneumococcus	62	51	6	9
Staphylococcus	23	19	15	22
Streptococcus	12	10	9	13
Gram-negative				
Proteus, Escherichia coli, Pseudomonas, Klebsiella	3	2	22	32
Salmonella-Shigella	1	1	3	4
Neisseria meningitidis	3	2	2	3

*Group 1, 1889–1943, 122 isolates in 114 patients; group 2, 1944–75, 69 isolates in 53 patients.

ing aseptic pericarditis may have been a predisposing condition in 47% of group 2 cases. Autopsy evidence of associated infection was widespread, especially before 1944. Bacterial pneumonia was present in 72% of group 1 patients and in 33% of group 2 patients.

Purulent pericarditis is now less likely to be seen in children or young adults with pneumonias or other primary infectious diseases but rather in debilitated adults with chronic disease or malignancy or after thoracic surgery. Not only have there been changes in age and source of infection but also incidence has declined and the etiologic agent has altered. The *pneumococcus* has been replaced as the predominant agent by the *Staphylococcus* and gram-negative aerobic bacilli. Perhaps the best way of reducing the mortality from purulent pericarditis is to maintain a high index of suspicion in patients presenting in typical clinical settings.

► [This is really a fine article. It shows the payoff of meticulous attention to careful observations, recording of findings and maintaining of specimens for retrospective study, a tradition at Johns Hopkins Hospital since it opened its doors in 1889. The incidence, age and sex distribution, predisposing events and the microbes producing purulent pericarditis have all changed dramatically since penicillin ushered in a new era in medicine. It is not a common disease. Of the 40,000 autopsies done at Johns Hopkins Hospital since 1889, purulent pericarditis was found in only 200. Furthermore, it seems to be only about one-third as common now as in the preantimicrobial era. Though it was formerly largely a complication of pneumococcal pneumonia in young men, women are now getting their share—clearly an unwanted accompaniment of equal opportunity. I like the explanation for the former sex differential given by Doubleday in 1888, and quoted by these authors: "The lord of creation is more exposed to weather in earning his daily bread and more addicted to the cup that cheers and inebriates than the female portion of the race."

But to return to the business at hand—most worrisome is the frequency with which the diagnosis is missed antemortem. It was diagnosed in only 1 of every 5 patients. Clearly recognition is important. The disease is virtually 100% fatal when missed. About 60% of patients recover if the diagnosis is made and appropriate surgical-medical treatment initiated.—Ed.] ◄

Fever of Unknown Origin: Assessment of the Value of Percutaneous Liver Biopsy. There is a widely held belief, with little evidence to support it, that liver biopsy is helpful in arriving at a diagnosis in patients with fever of unknown origin (FUO). Douglas P. Mitchell, Thomas E. Hanes, Anastacio M. Hoyumpa, Jr., and Steven Schenker[4]

(4) Arch. Intern. Med. 137:1001–1004, August, 1977.

ASSESSMENT OF THE VALUE OF PERCUTANEOUS LIVER BIOPSY IN 43 PATIENTS WITH FEVER OF UNKNOWN ORIGIN

Group	No. of Patients (%)	Hepatomegaly*	Abnormal Results From Liver Function Test,† No. of Patients (%)
1	6 (13.9)	4/6 (66.6)‡	6/6 (100)
2	11 (25.6)	3/11 (27.3)	8/11 (72.7)
3	26 (60.5)	5/26 (14.2)	20/26 (76.9)

*As judged by clinical examination.

†Any one of SGOT, alkaline phosphatase or bilirubin levels greater than the normal limit.

‡Significantly higher incidence of hepatomegaly ($P<0.05$) than in groups 2 and 3.

(Vanderbilt Univ.) reviewed experience with percutaneous liver biopsy in the diagnosis of FUO at one institution in a 12-year period. A FUO was defined as an illness of at least 3 weeks' duration with a temperature above 38.3 C on several occasions and no established diagnosis after at least 1 week of hospital study. Forty-three patients (10% of all with FUO) had liver biopsy in the course of FUO in 1963–75. No complications of biopsy occurred.

The findings are summarized in the table. In 6 patients (group 1), abnormal biopsy findings were helpful in the diagnosis and often the treatment of the febrile illness. In 11 patients (group 2) the findings were definitely abnormal but not helpful in diagnosis and management. In 26 patients (group 3) the biopsy findings were normal or the changes were trivial and nonspecific. Group 1 patients had hepatomegaly about 3 times as often and abnormal liver function tests 25% more often than the other two groups combined, but the overlap was substantial. Two group 1 patients had tumor, 2 had alcoholic hepatitis and 1 each had amebiasis and tuberculosis. The group 2 patients exhibited nonspecific hepatitis of varying severity. No firm diagnosis was substantiated by repeated studies or the subsequent course in 15 group 3 patients. Two of 7 diagnostic laparotomies yielded a definite diagnosis. Of the 28 patients followed for more than 6 months after liver biopsy, 85% survived. The mean follow-up was 40.3 months.

Liver biopsy may be helpful in diagnosing FUO but only in a very few cases. A surprisingly large number of patients with FUO are undiagnosed, but the overall prognosis is relatively good. A prospective study of the role of liver biopsy in the diagnosis of FUO in a larger group of cases is warranted, in view of new diagnostic techniques and the small percentage of patients with FUO who undergo biopsy.

► [In their now-classic article published in 1961 (Medicine (Baltimore) 40:1, 1961), Doctors Petersdorf and Beeson were quite enthusiastic about liver biopsy as a helpful adjunct in the diagnosis and management of fever of unknown origin. Most of us have faithfully followed their advice when faced with the frustrating and worrisome problem of a patient with ominous persistent fever that remains undiagnosed over a reasonable period. In retrospect, my own experience would more closely resemble that reported by Doctor Mitchell and his colleagues. The batting average has been low. Unfortunately, ancillary data—whether the liver is enlarged or liver function tests abnormal—doesn't help much in predicting payoff from biopsy. Perhaps some of the new technologies that give us a better look at the liver may help in this dilemma.

Fever of obscure origin remains a very frustrating problem for physicians. In the current series, only 40% of the cases were *ever* diagnosed. In most series (except for Petersdorf and Beeson who claimed eventual diagnosis in 93%), only 50–60% are satisfactorily resolved. I cannot quite agree that the overall prognosis is relatively good with or without diagnosis. Of the 43 patients, 16 were dead when the article was written.—Ed.] ◄

Atypical Radiographic Appearance and Clinical Presentation of Pulmonary Tuberculosis are discussed by Chen Fah Lian and Arvin Edward Robinson[5] (Duke Univ.). Exposure to tuberculosis is more widespread than has been realized. A more mobile society results in inadvertent exposure to persons who are unaware of their illness. It is not uncommon that patients with atypical radiographic or clinical features of this disease are present in a general hospital setting. Review was made of the findings in 14 patients with unusual presentation of pulmonary tuberculosis who were referred from general hospitals. Tuberculosis tends to occur in predisposed persons, such as infants, the aged and those in lower socioeconomic groups. Other susceptible groups include patients with debilitating diseases, diabetes, chronic alcoholism, silicosis and those on long-term steroid therapy.

Parenchymal changes are slightly more common in the upper lobes in primary pulmonary tuberculosis. A 1–7-cm area of consolidation with ill-defined margins may be seen, often associated with node enlargement. Airways may be compressed or eroded, and pleural effusion may be present. Reinfection typically presents as an ill-defined coalescence in the apical and posterior segments of the upper lobes. Cavitation is common. Scattered pulmonary nodules are an unusual presentation. Lower-lobe infiltrates are uncommon (Fig 11). Isolated involvement of the anterior segment of either upper lobe is unusual in adult

Fig 11.—Nonspecific left lower lobe pneumonia in a woman aged 61 years. (Courtesy of Lian, C. F., and Robinson, A. E.: South. Med. J. 69:1317–1322, October, 1976.)

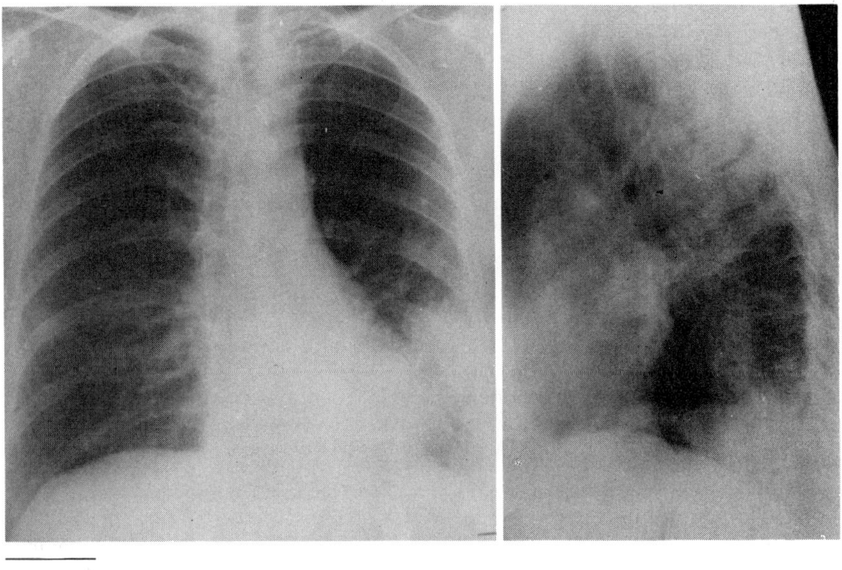

(5) South. Med. J. 69:1317–1322, October, 1976.

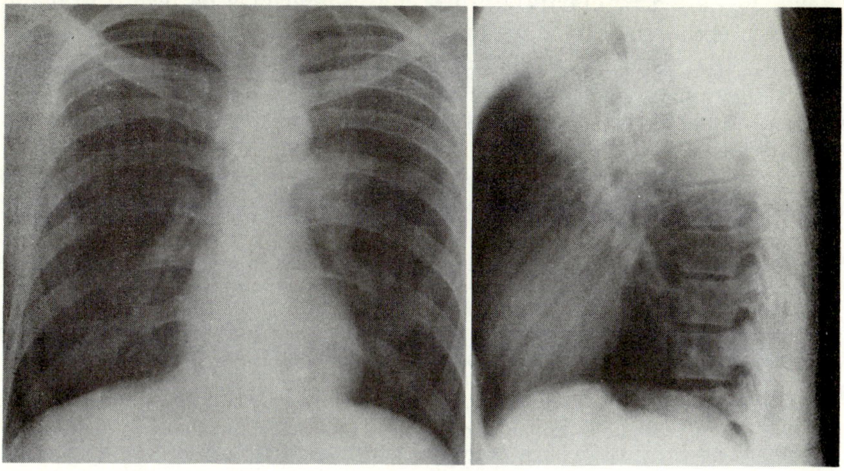

Fig 12.—A perihilar consolidation that simulates a tumor mass in a man aged 27 years. (Courtesy of Lian, C. F., and Robinson, A. E.: South. Med. J. 69:1317–1322, October, 1976.)

tuberculosis. Perihilar infiltrative disease may simulate a neoplasm (Fig 12). The presence of a primary tumor does not lessen the possibility of tuberculosis superimposed on a debilitated state or related to suppressive therapy.

► [Unlike old soldiers, tuberculosis refuses to fade away. This study reminds us that tuberculosis should still be considered in the differential diagnosis of pneumonia—especially if the pneumonia does not respond to penicillin.—Ed.] ◄

Gas Gangrene Complicating Open Forearm Fractures: Report of Five Cases. Norman F. Fee, Andrew Dobranski and Ranjit S. Bisla[6] encountered 5 cases in a 5-year period of fractures of both forearm bones compounded by small lacerations or puncture wounds and complicated by severe clostridial infection and myonecrosis. Review of the English literature yielded 8 similar cases. Extensive soft-tissue damage was described in most of these; only 3 cases were in children. Four of the present injuries were in children and the result of falls from a height. The proximal fragment protruded and presumably was contaminated by soil containing clostridiae. The wounds were relatively small and deceptively innocuous in appearance. Initial management had consisted of cleaning the skin, excision of serrated borders and loose closure of small puncture wounds after the fracture was set. Symptoms of gas gangrene evolved insidiously in all cases. Pain was followed by chills, tachycardia and other evidence of toxemia and the skin became brownish and crepitant. A gram stain of the fluid exudate that showed gram-positive rods confirmed the diagnosis.

Local cleaning of the wound may suffice in some injuries with pinhole openings but more aggressive treatment should occasionally be considered, especially when the type of soil contamination is suspect. Such management includes adequate visualization of the bone ends, meticulous débridement and thorough irrigation. The wounds should

(6) J. Bone Joint Surg. [Am.] 59-A:135–138, January, 1977.

never be closed primarily. Splints may sometimes be useful to avoid tissue anoxia. In fully developed gas gangrene, all involved muscle should be excised. Prophylaxis with antibiotics is of proved value in gas gangrene. The use of passive immunization with polyvalent gas-gangrene serum is controversial. Hyperbaric oxygenation has been widely accepted. Three to five exposures lasting 60–90 minutes should be given at 8- to 12-hour intervals. Hyperbaric oxygen is indicated in all cases of gas gangrene.

► [This article was included largely to keep the clinical syndrome of gas gangrene in physicians' consciousness. It is a rare but thoroughly dreadful infection that requires very prompt diagnosis and very aggressive management if intervention is to be genuinely effective.

The article overstates what other than excisional therapy can do—particularly with established gas gangrene. When tissue death occurs and local anaerobic conditions obtain, I doubt that antimicrobials, antiserum or hyperbaric oxygen makes much difference, although I would use all three if available. Scream for the surgeon! These cases require swift decompression and débridement. All involved muscle must be excised. Three of these 5 patients (all children) required surgical removal of their arms above the elbow before the process was brought under control.—Ed.] ◄

Communitywide Outbreak of Giardiasis with Evidence of Transmission by a Municipal Water Supply. In recent years giardiasis has been recognized in epidemic gastrointestinal illness with increasing frequency. Peter K. Shaw, Richard E. Brodsky, Donald O. Lyman, Bruce T. Wood, Charles P. Hibler, George R. Healy, Kenneth I. E. MacLeod, Walter Stahl and Myron G. Schultz[7] report a large communitywide outbreak of giardiasis which occurred in 1974–1975 in Rome, New York, a city of about 50,000 in central New York State. A total of 350 residents had laboratory-confirmed giardiasis in a 7-month period. A household survey showed an overall attack rate for giardiasis of 10.6%.

Symptoms of patients with stool-positive *Giardia lamblia* infection are given in the table and the duration of episodes of diarrheal illness is shown in Figure 13. Many episodes were rather lengthy and over

SYMPTOMS OF 183 PATIENTS WITH STOOL-POSITIVE CASES OF *Giardia lamblia* INFECTION, ROME, NEW YORK, OCTOBER 1, 1974, TO MAY 5, 1975

Symptoms	*no.*	%
Diarrhea	169	92
Cramps	128	70
Nausea	107	58
Fever	51	28
Vomiting	42	23
Fatigue	36	20
Headache	35	19
Weight Loss	23	13
Bloating	17	9
Flatus	11	6
Anorexia	4	2
Constipation	1	1

(7) Ann. Intern. Med. 87:426–432, October, 1977.

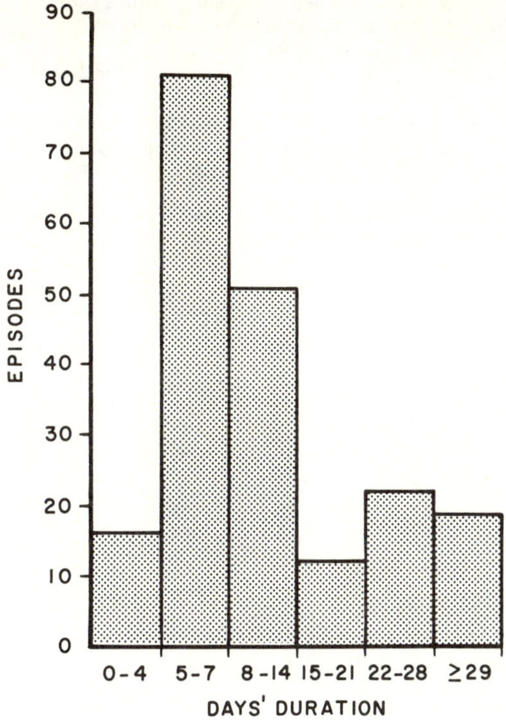

Fig 13.—Diarrheal illness, 201 episodes, by duration, Rome, New York, October 1, 1974, to May 5, 1975. (Courtesy of Shaw, P. K., et al.: Ann. Intern. Med. 87:426–432, October, 1977.)

half lasted more than a week. A significant association was found between illness and the use of water from the city system, rather than water drawn from home wells. The presence of human settlements in the city's watershed suggested that the water supply could have been contaminated by untreated human waste. The infectivity of municipal water was confirmed by production of giardiasis in specific pathogen-free dogs fed sediment samples of raw water obtained from an inlet of a city reservoir. Microscopic study of the sediments uncovered a *G. lamblia* cyst in one sample. Of 645 stool specimens submitted by persons surveyed, 3.4% were found to contain *G. lamblia* cysts.

Water conclusively has been shown to be an efficient vehicle for transmission of giardiasis and in the present outbreak the municipal water was implicated as the vehicle. This is the largest epidemic of giardiasis to be recorded in the United States. Chlorination procedures in Rome clearly were inadequate to prevent waterborne transmission of giardiasis. Study is needed to find other methods, such as sedimentation-filtration techniques, that will help protect communities from outbreaks of waterborne protozoan diarrheal illness.

► [Imagine practicing in a city of 50,000 and having 10% of the population develop a prolonged gastrointestinal illness characterized by diarrhea, cramps, nausea and a miscellany of other symptoms! That is what *Giardia* in the municipal water supply can do!

Many physicians are now aware that if their patients plan to spend a fascinating vacation touring the Soviet Union, they may return with an unwanted fellow traveler: *Giardia lamblia.* The risk is greatest if their itinerary includes Leningrad. (Beware of the water, Tovarich!)

In the spirit of détente, epidemiologists at the Center for Disease Control, also have documented several outbreaks of giardiasis in the United States. Several municipal water supply systems have been implicated as sources. In Colorado, campers and backpackers have become ill. A search among forest creatures turned up beavers as the probable source of contaminated mountain streams. Sorry, we have no information on Russian beavers.

The favored treatment is metronidazole (Flagyl), 250 mg 3 times daily for 10 days (a shorter regimen is 2 gm daily for 3 days). —Ed.] ◄

PART TWO

THE CHEST

ROGER M. DES PREZ, M.D.

Introduction

The editor would first like to reacknowledge that this section is a collaborative effort with Dr. Robert Goodwin, Professor of Medicine at Vanderbilt University and Chief of the Pulmonary Disease Section at the Veterans Administration Hospital, Nashville, and to express gratitude for his generous and enthusiastic participation since 1972.

One of the problems of attempting to put this section together year after year is that one's selections and comments are inevitably modified by what has been included in previous YEAR BOOKS. It would be the best of all worlds to assume that all readers were conversant with everything that had gone before and that, therefore, there was no need to repeat. On the other hand, it is impossible to operate with the assumption that each section year by year should be complete, or nearly so, in itself. There is not that much really new in a year's time, and some things must be repeated in order to place new knowledge in an intelligible context. We have elected to take a middle road, referring quite a bit to things covered in the past and also repeating some material and concepts in the hope of making the section worth reading in itself, but substantially enriched if referrals to previous volumes are pursued.

ROGER M. DES PREZ

Chronic Lung Disease and Other Conditions

► ↓The term "chronic obstructive lung disease" (COPD) includes so much that it tends to muddy precise thinking in terms of what is actually going on. Probably in the biggest patient group, COPD begins with some abnormality in the small (under 2 mm) conducting airways. However, the causes of small airways disease are multiple and often additive, such as bronchitis (abnormal secretions and inflammation—see 1976 YEAR BOOK, pp. 121 and 122), bronchitis plus bronchospasm, bronchitis plus loss of elastic recoil (1973 YEAR BOOK, p. 99) or all of the above in combination. Small airways disease and inflammation, when chronic, often progresses to peribronchiolar fibrosis, centrilobular emphysema and anatomical changes resulting in permanent mismatching of ventilation and perfusion (1972 YEAR BOOK, p. 107), but this is not always the case. The pathogenesis of panlobular emphysema and bullous emphysema is less well understood; homozygous α_1-antitrypsin disease is one condition that leads to destruction of lung support tissue and this sort of change, but loss of elastic recoil also tends to collapse small airways and eventually to cause inflammation therein. It is likely that there are many metabolic and infectious processes that may lead to panlobular emphysema.

Perhaps more importantly from a clinical and therapeutic point of view, there are many things more or less misdiagnosed as COPD when the actual problem is with the respiratory muscles, the upper airways, the respiratory control apparatus or peripheral nerves. These, when recognized, are discernibly different, but the fact is that they often are not recognized clearly. Addition of pulmonary edema, either cardiogenic or noncardiogenic (osmotic, or capillary leak, or alveolar and bronchial damage from noxious inhalants such as smoke or water), to underlying small airways disease may produce a situation that is complicated and difficult to analyze. Small degrees of left ventricular failure may present as respiratory failure with hypoxemia and carbon dioxide retention in patients with substantial underlying chronic bronchitis or emphysema or both (1973 YEAR BOOK, p. 134; 1974 YEAR BOOK, p. 110; and Burk and George: Acute respiratory failure in chronic obstructive pulmonary disease: Immediate and long-term prognosis, Arch. Intern. Med. 132:865, 1973). Patients with relatively minor degrees of baseline bronchitis, emphysema or both may present in respiratory failure with severe obstruction and ventilation-perfusion mismatching on the basis of viral infection of the lower respiratory tract. In the absence of some more precise system of classification, it would seem advisable to attempt to qualify the term "COPD" with some attempt to define pathogenic mechanisms and their interaction.—Ed. ◄

Pulmonary Abnormalities in Intermediate α_1-Antitrypsin Deficiency. Studies to date have not established conclusively that intermediate deficiency of α_1-antitrypsin (AAT) is an important risk factor in the pathogenesis of chronic obstructive pulmonary disease.

William J. Hall, Richard W. Hyde, Robert H. Schwartz, Govind S. Mudholkar, D. Robert Webb, Y. P. Chaubey and Phillip L. Townes[1] (Univ. of Rochester) compared lung function in subjects with the MZ and MS Pi (protease inhibitor) types of AAT with the findings in type MM control subjects matched for age, sex and smoking history. Type MZ subjects typically have 55–60% of normal serum AAT levels and type MS subjects, 80–85% of normal values. All subjects in the study

(1) J. Clin. Invest. 58:1069–1077, November, 1976.

MAXIMAL EXPIRATORY FLOW RATES ($\dot{V}_{max}$) EXPRESSED AS PERCENTAGE OF ABSOLUTE LUNG VOLUME AT 75%, 50% AND 25% OF THE VITAL CAPACITY IN NONSMOKING MZ SUBJECTS COMPARED TO MM CONTROLS MATCHED FOR AGE, SEX AND SMOKING HISTORY

	$\dot{V}_{max}$ (% absolute lung volume)					
	75%		50%		25%	
	MZ	MM	MZ	MM	MZ	MM
			s^{-1}			
1	1.18	1.50	0.60	0.91	0.31	0.65
2	1.20	1.50	0.60	0.80	0.31	0.67
3	1.14	1.42	0.60	0.80	0.22	0.40
4	1.12	1.38	0.60	0.75	0.25	0.60
5	1.16	1.43	0.56	0.77	0.31	0.59
6	0.95	1.32	0.60	0.72	0.24	0.40
7	0.75	1.32	0.45	0.80	0.18	0.55
8	1.06	1.41	0.57	0.74	0.31	0.50
9	0.93	1.47	0.65	0.85	0.25	0.62
10	1.06	1.34	0.62	0.90	0.28	0.76
11	1.50	1.55	0.93	0.90	0.45	0.53
12	0.80	1.12	0.48	0.52	0.25	0.29
13	0.89	1.44	0.55	0.89	0.23	0.58
14	1.15	1.98	0.48	1.20	0.16	0.75
15	1.23	1.33	0.74	0.75	0.51	0.50
Mean	1.08*	1.43	0.60*	0.82	0.28*	0.56

*$P < 0.01$ for MZ-MM pairs.

were lifelong nonsmokers randomly selected from a population in which the prevalence of intermediate AAT deficiency had been determined. None of the subjects reported respiratory symptoms.

Residual volume was elevated in both the MS and MZ subjects, compared to MM controls. Values for single-breath diffusing capacity were not significantly different in any group. Individual data for each MZ-MM pair are given in the table. No significant differences in airway resistance at any measured frequency were observed between either MS-MM or MZ-MM pairs. Increased frequency dependence of pulmonary resistance was observed in MZ subjects compared to MM controls, but no such difference was noted in the MS-MM pairs.

These findings suggest that detectable mechanical abnormalities are present in subjects with the MZ phenotype, even in the absence of established risk factors such as cigarette smoking and high air pollution. The clinical significance of these physiologic abnormalities remains unclear. Prospective studies are needed to determine if these subjects eventually will develop symptomatic lung disease. Others recently have indicated that cigarette smoking may be the significant determinant of development of chronic obstructive pulmonary disease in MZ heterozygotes.

► [The importance of this article is that it demonstrates defects in function tests generally regarded as indicating disease in the small conduction airways in asymptomatic nonsmoking patients with intermediate (MZ heterozygous) levels of α_1-antitrypsin deficiency. The fact that abnormalities of flow rates and frequency dependence of dynamic compliance are due to changes in the peripheral airways has been demonstrated clearly by Niewoehner et al. (Peripheral airways as a determinant of ventilatory function in the human lung, J. Clin. Invest. 60:139, 1977).

The pivotal importance of dysfunction or obstruction of the small conducting airways in the pathogenesis of chronic obstructive lung disease was discussed at some length in the 1976 YEAR BOOK (pp. 119–122). It seems worthwhile, in order to emphasize the clinical importance of such studies from a conceptual point of view, to repeat some of this. The first change in the garden variety of chronic bronchitis complicating cigarette smoking, as well as probably other forms of atmospheric contamination, is decrease in the number of Clara cells in the small, ciliated airways and increase in the number of mucous-secreting cells. The Clara cells elaborate a protein secretion with low viscosity in which cilia move easily. The few mucous glands present in health in these small airways provide a thin layer of sticky material which floats on top of the low-viscosity protein secretion (hypolayer) in which the cilia move. When mucous glands increase at the expense of Clara cells, the hypolayer becomes stickier, and therefore maladapted to integrated ciliary motion, and removal of secretions from the small airways deteriorates.

The change implied in this article is some loss of pulmonary elasticity which leads to a tendency to small airways collapse or at least some narrowing in caliber because the small conducting airways are held open, so to speak, by the intrinsic elasticity of the pulmonary supporting tissue. When this loss of distending force is combined with intrinsic disease of the small airways due to smoking or other factors, COPD often results (Larson et al.: Smoking and intermediate α_1-antitrypsin deficiency and lung function in middle-aged men, Br. Med. J. 2:922, 1977).

It is now clear that allergic asthma has its most important effects on the small conducting airways even though we usually define the severity of asthma by tests which reflect obstruction in larger airways (FEV, etc.) and are not sensitive to small airways disease. When small airways tests are monitored, it has been shown that measurable abnormalities persist for days or weeks after signs of large airway bronchospasm have disappeared (1973 YEAR BOOK, pp. 181 and 182). The clinical importance is twofold: (1) one can have considerable dysfunction due to the mechanisms which lead to asthma without any measurable abnormalities in the tests we usually use to define asthma and without wheezing, and (2) asthmatics should be treated vigorously for a week or two after they appear to be well if treatment is intended to restore a normal situation as much as possible. Viral infections may also cause prominent small airways disease which may be difficult to detect by the usual function tests and may persist for several weeks (1977 YEAR BOOK, p. 138).

Thus genetic factors, irritation of the airways by noxious inhalants, the effects of allergens and viral infection all may have an impact on the same region of the air conducting system, producing few clinical signs but, when prolonged, possibly leading to permanent anatomical changes and chronic obstructive lung disease.

Homozygous antitrypsin deficiency is associated not only with emphysema, but also with cirrhosis (with liver cells containing PAS-positive inclusions), bronchiectasis (Scott et al: α_1-antitrypsin deficiency with diffuse bronchiectasis and cirrhosis of the liver, Chest 71:535, 1977), and, one article suggests, Webber-Christian disease, whatever that is (Rubenstein et al.: α_1-antitrypsin deficiency with severe panniculitis, Ann. Intern. Med. 86:742, 1977). From a clinical point of view, phenotyping does not contribute to patient care; determination of α_1-antitrypsin concentration by immunodiffusion (simple, commercially available technique) suffices for diagnosis in the intermediate (heterozygous) deficiency states. The hemozygous state can be diagnosed by absence of the α_1-globulin peak on electrophoresis (1974 YEAR BOOK, p. 207). – Ed.] ◄

Cystic Fibrosis: New Outlook; 70 Patients above 25 Years of Age were studied by H. Shwachman, M. Kowalski and K.-T. Khaw[2] (Children's Hosp. Med. Center, Boston). The patients were followed for 2–28 years. Two thirds of the patients were men. A family history of

(2) Medicine (Baltimore) 56:129–148, March, 1977.

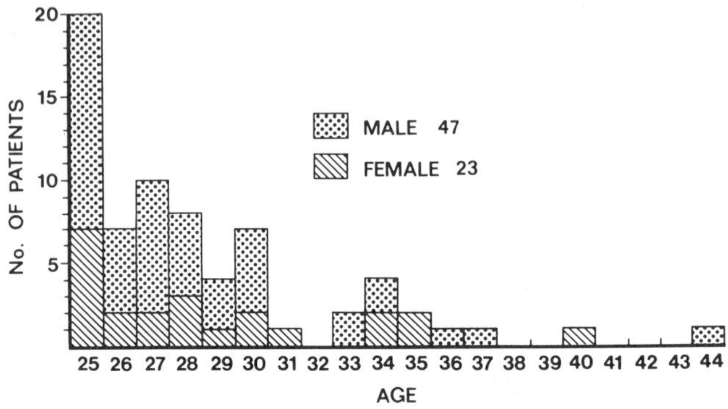

Fig 1.—Age and sex distribution of 47 men and 23 women aged 25 years or more with cystic fibrosis. (Courtesy of Shwachman, H., et al.: Medicine (Baltimore) 56:129–148, March, 1977.)

cystic fibrosis (CF) was present in 41.5% of the cases. The age distribution is shown in Figure 1 and the distribution of affected children in the 67 families with CF in Table 1. Many patients were diagnosed as having other conditions before referral (Table 2). The operations done before correct diagnosis are summarized in Table 3. The results of sweat tests initially and on recent testing are given in Figure 2.

Presently, 10% of the patients are considered to be in excellent condition, 37% are in good condition, 39% are mildly affected, 13% are moderately affected and 1% is severely affected. Forty-two patients (60%) are married. None of the 24 married men has fathered children. All patients except 1 are able to work. Six patients have been hospitalized for meconium ileus and complications. The average number of hospitalizations for the 70 patients is 4.1. Many patients with a de-

TABLE 1.—Distribution of Affected and Healthy Children in 67 Families with Cystic Fibrosis

No. children per family	1	2	3	4	5	6	7	8	12	Total
No. of families	4	12	20	15	5	2	7	1	1	67
Total no. of children	4	24	60	60	25	12	49	8	12	254
No. of children with CF	4	13	28	25	10	7	16	3	4	110
No. of healthy children	0	11	31	35	15	5	33	5	8	143

TABLE 2.—Other Conditions Treated

Diagnosis	Total	Mean length of treatment (yrs)
Celiac Disease	15	4-6/12
Bronchiectasis	6	7-6/12
Bronchial Asthma	5	3-8/12
Tuberculosis	3	1
Histoplasmosis	1	1-6/12
Delay in Sexual Maturation	2	1

TABLE 3.—HOSPITALIZATIONS AND SURGICAL PROCEDURES BEFORE DIAGNOSIS

Reason for Hospitalization	No. of Hospitalizations		
	CHMC	Other Hosp.	Total
Diagnostic admission	6	14	20
Lower pulmonary infections—(pneumonia)	1	35	36
Bronchiectasis	3	5	8
Bronchial asthma		1	1
Pulmonary tuberculosis		3	3
Lung atelectasis	1		1
Lobectomy		1	1
Myocarditis	1		1
Meconium ileus, repair, complication	3	2	5
Chronic diarrhea, failure to thrive	2	9	11
Cirrhosis		5	5
GI bleeding		1	1
Fecal impaction		2	2
Diabetes		2	2
Acute recurrent pancreatitis		3	3
Abdominal pain, appendectomy		4	4
Abdominal pain, laparotomy		2	2
Inguinal hernia repair		3	3
Jaundice		1	1
Orchidopexy		1	1
Salt depletion		4	4
Nasal polypectomy	1	8	9
Miscellaneous, unrelated to CF	2	4	6
	20	110	130

Fig 2.—Quantitative pilocarpine iontophoresis sweat tests. (Courtesy of Shwachman, H., et al.: Medicine (Baltimore) 56:129–148, March, 1977.)

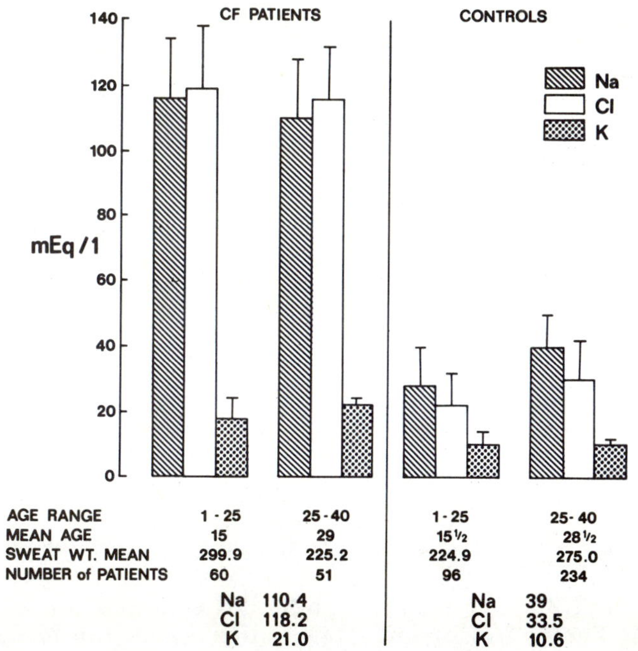

pressed P_{O_2} and evidence of moderate obstructive lung disease are able to function.

The frequency of symptomatic sinusitis was relatively low. The most common intestinal complication was fecal impaction, which occurred in 12 patients. Rectal prolapse occurred in 5. Two patients acquired portal hypertension secondary to hepatic cirrhosis. Two had recurrent acute pancreatitis. Six patients now have clinical diabetes and require insulin therapy. Three patients had duodenal ulcer disease. Five had symptoms related to salt depletion.

The goal has been to recognize CF as early in life as possible and to provide comprehensive medical care to these patients. The internist should take a more active role in the management of patients with CF, providing them with the care generally available in pediatric centers.

► [Only a small portion of the information in this large and definitive study could be presented here. Stern et al. (Cystic fibrosis diagnosed after age 13: Twenty-five teenage and adult patients including 3 asymptomatic men, Ann. Intern. Med. 87:188, 1977) also emphasize that this malady may not manifest itself in childhood. Their group of 25 comprised 3.4% of their total cystic fibrosis population. Nineteen had measurable pulmonary functional derangement, although in only 10 was this the presenting complaint. Fifteen had *Pseudomonas* and 11 had *Staphylococcus aureus* recovered from sputum. The sinuses were opacified in all 22 patients in whom sinus films were obtained. Delayed menarche, aspermia and oligospermia were frequent but not invariable features. Three patients were asymptomatic except for infertility and 4 presented with hepatic disease.

The hepatic process in cystic fibrosis begins with inspissated plugs in bile ducts, develops into biliary cirrhosis, may produce portal hypertension with esophageal varices, hypersplenism or both and generally is spotty so that hepatic parenchymal function is preserved. Portal decompression by shunting, therefore, has a more favorable prognosis than in the usual case of cirrhosis (Stern et al.: Symptomatic hepatic disease in cystic fibrosis: Incidence, course and outcome of portal systemic shunting, Gastroenterology 70:645, 1976). In the study by Stern et al. (ibid.) the incidence of hepatic involvement was 15 of 693 patients—2.2%. Thirteen of the 15 had symptoms related only to portal hypertension. Ten of the 13 had hypersplenism, 6 had variceal bleeding and 3 developed both. Only 2 manifested ascites. Two of the 15 had symptoms principally related to hepatocellular dysfunction. The results of portal decompression by shunting were very good. Postoperative encephalopathy was not observed and in many patients good health seemed to have been restored completely. Many of these patients were teenagers or young adults, alcoholism was not a feature and HAA studies were negative.

The nature of the fundamental defect in cystic fibrosis is a matter of current investigation. All agree that there is a substance or substances in the serum of cystic fibrosis patients which interrupt or disorganize ciliary action and modify secretory processes, but there is no agreement as to what that substance or substances are. The most attractive (to us) hypothesis postulates that the basic defect is the absence of an enzyme which normally inactivates a family of membrane-active molecules; the "ciliary dyskinesia factor" demonstrable in serum, according to this hypothesis, actually constitutes an abnormal accumulation of normal substances (Conover et al.: On the nature of the defect in cystic fibrosis, Texas Rep. Biol. Med. 34:45, 1976).

Corey et al. (Five- to 7-year course of pulmonary function in cystic fibrosis, Amer. Rev. Respir. Dis. 114:1085, 1976) record an exponential decline in the rate of forced expiration (FEV 25–75) somewhat less than in a population of ordinary patients with COPD, with many patients remaining stable (see also Boat and Petty: Chronic bronchitis and cystic fibrosis: Two chronic obstructive lung diseases of adults, ibid. 116:1, 1977; and Case 26-1977, Case records of the Massachusetts General Hospital, N. Engl. J. Med. 296:1519, 1977).—Ed.] ◄

Immotile Cilia Syndrome: Congenital Ciliary Abnormality as Etiologic Factor in Chronic Airway Infections and Male Sterili-

ty. Men with totally immotile but otherwise apparently normal spermatozoa were recently found to have sperm tails with no dynein arms, and mucociliary transport in the tracheobronchial tract was found to be extremely slow in 2 of the 3 men who were studied. Rune Eliasson, Björn Mossberg, Per Camner and Björn A. Afzelius[3] (Karolinska Inst., Stockholm) examined mucociliary clearance and the ultrastructure of respiratory cilia and sperm tails in 6 men and 1 woman. Five men presented with only immotile but otherwise normal spermatozoa. Two of these patients were found to have Kartagener's syndrome, and 2 others were selected for this reason. All patients had a history of chronic or recurrent upper and lower airway infections, and otitis was common. Bronchiectasis had been demonstrated in 3 patients. All patients had barren marriages. Lung clearance studies were done with an aerosol of Teflon particles tagged with ^{99m}Tc.

Retention of particles was significantly higher in the patients than in healthy subjects. A normal cilium or sperm tail is illustrated in Figure 3. The patients showed complete absence of dynein arms in their sperm tails, but the axoneme was otherwise normal. Dynein arms were nearly absent in cilia from the nasal and bronchial mucosae in the woman and 2 men, and the respiratory cilia were irregularly oriented. All patients had slow and probably absent mucociliary transport.

These observations are compatible with the postulate that immotility of embryonic cilia results in situs inversus in about half the cases. Impaired mucociliary transport predisposes to the development of obstructive lung disease, but other factors may be required for this complication to develop. The present patients lived comparatively normal lives, and all were professionally active. Infections tended to be most severe in late childhood and adolescence. These observations may be

Fig 3.—Cross section of cilium or of central portion of sperm tail. Assembly of 9 outer microtubular doublets and 2 central microtubules is held together by three kinds of connections: dynein arms, nexin links and spokes. Dynein arms are believed to be responsible for motility. (Courtesy of Eliasson, R., et al.: N. Engl. J. Med. 297:1–6, July 7, 1977.)

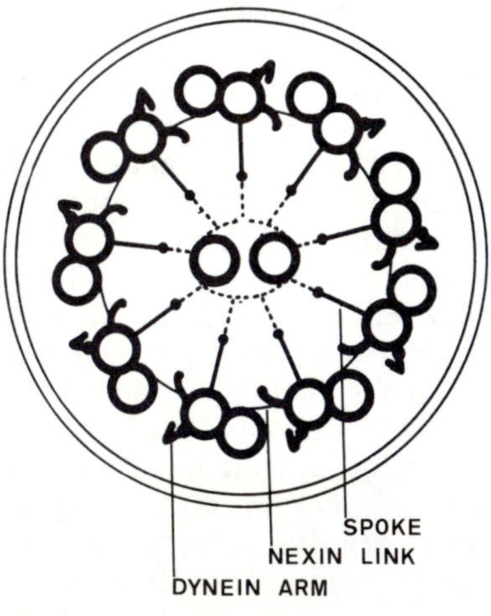

(3) N. Engl. J. Med. 297:1–6, July 7, 1977.

related to the fact that patients with Kartagener's syndrome can reach an advanced age.

► [Like α_1-antitrypsin deficiency, Kartagener's syndrome is a congenital lesion that may present with sinusitis, chronic obstructive pulmonary disease (COPD) and infertility. The situs inversus is thought to be due to malfunction of embryonic cilia and need not be present in all cases. The defect is in the dynein arms. This may not be useful information, but it is gratifyingly elegant.

Egbert et al. (Kartagener's syndrome: Report of a case with mesangiocapillary glomerulonephritis, Arch. Pathol. Lab. Med. 101:95, 1977) report this renal complication in a single well-studied and autopsied case. They suggest that the renal lesion is a consequence of the chronic infection and offer some support for this speculation. Their discussion indicates that situs inversus occurs in 1 in 10,000 persons, 12–25% of whom have bronchiectasis and sinusitis. "Patients with Kartagener's syndrome have repeated upper respiratory tract infections, pneumonia, sinusitis, nasal polyposis, otitis media, productive cough and hemoptysis leading to eventual respiratory and cardiac failure. Ninety percent....develop symptoms as children...(but) an 88-year-old patient (has been described)."

Turner and Stanley (Fragile lung in the Marfan syndrome, Thorax 31:771, 1976) discuss another uncommon hereditary disorder with pulmonary manifestations. The 2 patients who were the subjects of the report both presented with spontaneous pneumothorax and both had upper lobe bullous emphysema, loss of elastic recoil, decreased expiratory flow rates at low lung volumes and a defect in carbon monoxide transfer factor. The authors noted that the clinical manifestations of Marfan's syndrome (hyperextensibility of joints, aortic dissection, subluxation of lenses) all were in organs with high collagen content and that collagen constitutes more than 10% of lung dry weight. They quote that in 10% of patients with Marfan's syndrome some type of pulmonary disorder occurs, one third of which is pneumothorax. Other pulmonary disorders include bronchiectasis, increased susceptibility to pneumonia, pectus excavatum and pectus carinatum and kyphoscoliosis with resulting cor pulmonale and respiratory failure. "An important clinical point is that the acute chest pain and breathlessness of pneumothorax should not be confused with aortic dissection, which is the commonest cause of death...."

Kueppers et al. (Familial prevalence of chronic obstructive pulmonary disease in a matched-pair study, Am. J. Med. 63:336, 1977), in a careful study, report detectable COPD not due to intermediate α_1-antitrypsin deficiency to be 2–3 times as frequent in close relatives of COPD patients as in controls. They review the literature which largely confirms this as yet poorly understood but definite familial clustering.—Ed.] ◄

Chronic Pulmonary Complications of Early Influenza Virus Infection in Children. Pulmonary sequelae after influenza virus infections in infancy and early childhood have rarely been described. Lourdes R. Laraya-Cuasay, Adamadia DeForest, Dale Huff, Harold Lischner and Nancy N. Huang[4] (Temple Univ.) followed 3 male patients who had influenza virus A infection at ages 5, 24 and 42 months, respectively, and had chronic pulmonary sequelae. Varying degrees of interstitial fibrosis, bronchial and bronchiolar erosions and metaplasia, obliterative bronchiolitis and interstitial chronic inflammatory infiltration were found on lung biopsy. Influenza A Hong Kong/68 (H_3N_2) virus was isolated from the lung tissue of 1 patient 8 weeks after the onset of illness; this is the longest persistance of infectious virus in lung tissue to be reported. Persistent radiographic changes included peribronchial thickening, interstitial densities, bronchiectasis, obliterative bronchiolitis and segmental atelectasis. Lung function tests showed an obstructive restrictive pattern with deterioration after exercise and mild improvement after bronchodilation.

---

(4) Am. Rev. Respir. Dis. 116:617–625, October, 1977.

Summary of Lung Biopsy Findings

	Patient AM	Patient JM	Patient TH
Day of Illness	52	166	51
Findings			
Bronchial and bronchiolar erosions and metaplasia	Mild	Moderate	0
Obliterative bronchiolitis	0	Mild	Severe
Peribronchial lymphoid follicles	0	Mild	0
Interstitial chronic inflammatory infiltrate	Moderate	Moderate	Mild
Interstitial fibrosis	Mild	Moderate	Mild
Intra-alveolar macrophages and/or pneumocytes	Moderate	Mild	Mild
Cultures for bacteria, fungi, and mycoplasma	Sterile	Sterile	Sterile
Virus culture	Positive	Negative	Negative

Findings in the lung biopsy specimens from these patients are summarized in the table. The findings in 2 patients were similar to those identified by others as "obliterative bronchiolitis." Progression of the obliterative changes with cicatrization, episodic obstruction by retained secretions and secondary infections could explain the fluctuating clinical course in these cases. Influenza infection was confirmed serologically in all 3 patients. Apparently influenza virus infection may be more serious in infants and young children than has been recognized and may contribute to the pathogenesis of unexplained interstitial pneumonitis, pulmonary fibrosis, obliterative bronchiolitis and bronchiectasis.

► [Although this article primarily discusses children, the literature cited suggests that similar mechanisms may obtain in adults as well. – Ed.] ◄

Arterial Blood Gas Tensions, Hydrogen Ion and Electroencephalogram during Sleep in Patients with Chronic Ventilatory Failure. Hypoxia, hypercapnia and acidosis occur during sleep in normal man and may be exaggerated in patients with chronic ventilatory failure. A. G. Leitch, L. J. Clancy, R. J. E. Leggett, P. Tweeddale, P. Dawson and J. I. Evans[5] (Edinburgh) examined arterial blood gas tensions and the EEG during sleep in 10 patients with severe chronic ventilatory failure and cor pulmonale secondary to chronic airways obstruction. The 8 men and 2 women had a mean age of 58.6 years. All had severe airways obstruction, with a mean FEV_1 of 0.57 L and a mean Pa_{O_2} of 6.8 kPa (57 mm Hg). All had polycythemia and pulmonary hypertension. The steady-state ventilatory response to inhaled CO_2 was markedly reduced in 7 of 8 cases. All patients were clinically stable at the time of the study. Patients slept in a quiet room on the nights of EEG and blood gas studies.

The findings are given in Table 1 and shown in Figures 4 and 5. The arterial P_{O_2} fell significantly during sleep; the mean maximal fall for the group was 1.2 kPa (9.2 mm Hg). The rise in P_{CO_2} during sleep was not significant, and the arterial pH did not change significantly. The

(5) Thorax 31:730–735, December, 1976.

TABLE 1.—SUMMARY OF VALUES

Subject	Air 1	2	3	4	5	6	7	8	9	10	Mean	SEM	P*	O₂ 6	9
Po_2 values															
Control	7·6	7·6	7·5	7·5	7·3	7·3	6·5	6·5	6·3	5·7	6·98	0·21		11·5	10·3
Lowest sleep	6·5	6·9	5·6	6·7	6·1	6·0	5·9	4·8	4·7	4·7	5·78	0·27	< 0·001	8·4	10·5
Mean sleep	7·0	7·3	6·6	7·0	6·4	7·0	6·4	5·1	5·2	5·1	6·31	0·28	< 0·001	11·0	11·5
Post sleep	7·1	6·8	7·3	7·9	6·7	7·2	7·6	5·3	5·6	5·6	6·70	0·28	NS	8·9	10·0
Pco_2 values															
Control	7·2	6·3	8·1	6·4	6·9	7·7	7·9	9·5	8·5	8·7	7·71	0·32		8·4	7·9
Highest sleep	8·4	6·8	9·2	7·1	7·7	8·4	8·3	9·3	9·3	9·2	8·36	0·29	< 0·001	11·1	8·5
Mean sleep	7·9	6·6	8·8	6·5	7·4	8·1	7·8	8·8	8·9	8·6	7·94	0·28	NS	9·6	8·0
Post sleep	7·3	6·5	8·4	6·3	7·1	8·0	6·9	8·7	8·9	8·3	7·63	0·29	NS	9·6	8·4
pH values															
Control	36	—	41	40	—	40	35	46	46	43	40·9	1·5		46	46
Highest sleep	42	—	44	43	—	45	36	45	49	43	43·3	1·3	< 0·05	56	46
Mean sleep	40	—	43	41	—	43	35	43	46	42	41·6	1·1	NS	51	45
Post sleep	40	—	39	40	—	42	30	42	47	41	40·1	1·7	NS	49	46

Inspired Gas: Air (subjects 1–10, Mean, SEM, P*); O_2 (subjects 6, 9).

*P values refer to significance of differences from control or presleep values.

TABLE 2.—ANALYSIS OF SLEEP IN PATIENTS AND CONTROLS OF SIMILAR AGE*

	Mean Values±SD (10 patients)	Range (10 patients)	Mean Values±SD (10 normals)	Values breathing Air		Values breathing Oxygen	
				Subject 6	Subject 9	Subject 6	Subject 9
Time in bed (min)	429·9±27·2	381 – 458	—	447	407	443	448
Total sleep time (min)	304·2±62·5	233 – 444	376·7±35·6	371	284	386	377
% sleep	70·5±11·9	60 – 97·4	91·0± 6·0	83	69·8	87·1	84·2
Delay to sleep (min)	27·5±29·6	1·3 – 40	7·9± 5·4	24	55	34	47
Delay to first REM sleep (min)	101·8±36·4	50 – 165	74·7±29·5	75	106	13	99
% awake	30·9±18·3	3·8 – 53·9	6·2± 5·3	13·9	22·7	2·7	3·5
Stage 1	7·4± 5·0	2·8 – 16·3	6·0± 2·2	13·0	12·1	3·0	6·4
Stage 2	55·6±10·8	40·2 – 71·3	50·8±11·7	44·2	68·1	61·7	54·3
Stage 3	10·6± 5·1	2·2 – 18·2	7·2± 2·8	5·8	14·3	5·2	17·5
Stage 4	10·0± 6·9	0 – 18·9	8·0±10·5	11·1	0	1·2	12·2
Stage 5 (REM)	15·5± 8·7	0·6 – 26·7	21·9± 4·3	23·5	0·6	27·9	8·8
Shifts/s	17·0± 4·9	7·0 – 22·8	7·1± 1·6	17·6	20·1	16·9	12·7

*Also shown are individual data for 2 subjects breathing air and breathing oxygen at 2 L/minute by nasal cannulae.

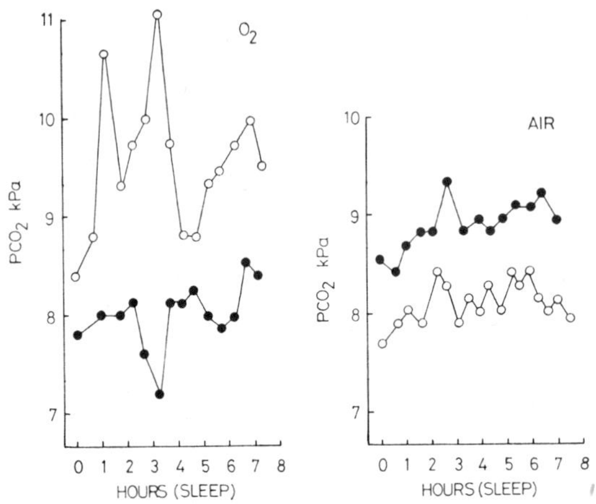

Fig 4.—Changes in arterial P_{CO_2} overnight in 2 patients when breathing oxygen (2 L/minute) and air. Mean sleep P_{O_2} was 7.0 and 5.2 kPa on air and 11.0 and 11.5 kPa on oxygen for the 2 patients, respectively. (Courtesy of Leitch, A. G., et al.: Thorax 31:730–735, December, 1976.)

addition of 2 L oxygen per minute by nasal catheter to the inspired air restored patients to normoxia. Sleep was disturbed in these patients (Table 2). The only consistent sleep change produced by oxygen therapy in the 2 patients treated was a marked reduction in time spent awake.

Hypoxemia and hypercapnia are limited in these patients by the presence of an active hypoxic drive to breathing. If the changes in blood gas tensions during sleep are due to hyperventilation from an active hypoxic drive to breathing, the hyperventilation may explain the poor sleep patterns noted in patients with severe respiratory dis-

Fig 5.—O_2–CO_2 diagram. *Hatched lines,* alveolar-arterial O_2 differences of 2, 4 and 6 kPa; *solid circles,* controls; *open circles,* patients. Most patients show an increase in alveolar-arterial oxygen partial pressure difference with sleep, indicating a worsening V/Q ratio. (Courtesy of Leitch, A. G., et al.: Thorax 31:730–735, December, 1976.)

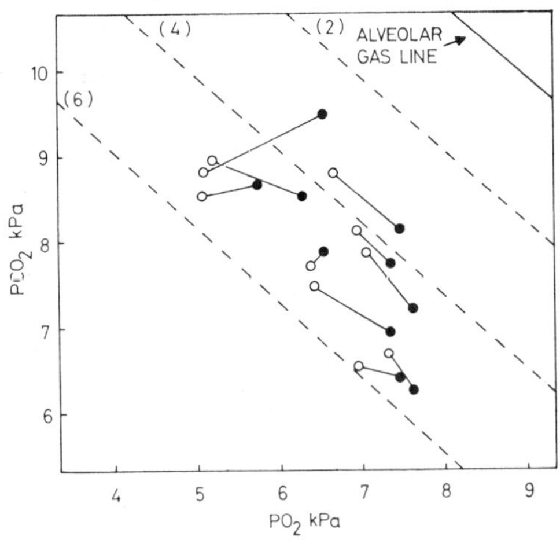

ability. Further trials of long-term oxygen therapy are warranted to determine whether large changes in H^+ and P_{CO_2} during sleep are deleterious and, if so, to select the most appropriate inspired oxygen concentration for these patients at night.

► [The abbreviation "kPa" stands for kilopascal and is a unit of pressure that apparently has something scientific to recommend it. Practically, the conversion factor from kPa to mm Hg (or torr) is 7.5. To convert kPa to cm H_2O rather than mm Hg, multiply by 10.2. This seems like just more confusion, but you have to know this in order to read some articles from England, such as this one.

This article makes several points. (1) Nocturnal hypoxemia can be very severe in these patients and causes sleep disturbance and EEG abnormalities. Also, it causes serious systemic and pulmonary hypertension and cardiac rhythm disturbances. (2) Most patients avoid more serious hypoxia and hypercapnia at night because of an intact hypoxic drive to respiration. (3) Administration of low-flow oxygen at night (2L/minute) is beneficial in most, but in some may seriously aggravate hypercapnia and acidosis. This needs to be assessed individually in each patient before a program of nocturnal oxygen therapy is embarked on.

A similar study from the University of Florida made somewhat more extensive observations with the use of an ear oximeter in 10 patients with severe obstructive lung disease (Flick and Block: Continuous in vivo monitoring of arterial oxygenation in chronic obstructive lung disease, Ann. Intern. Med. 86:725, 1977). Seven of the patients had manifested acute respiratory failure in the past. Daytime monitoring revealed reductions in arterial oxygen saturation when the patients urinated or ate and after nebulization of bronchodilator aerosol. (These interesting facts have no therapeutic implications.) Nighttime studies revealed that Sa_{O_2} decreased as patients went to sleep and, in addition to this baseline decrease, the tracings repeatedly showed steep declines lasting from a few seconds to up to an hour. The mean decrease in Sa_{O_2} from daytime level to the nighttime nadir in these patients was 25%. Measurement of Pa_{O_2} during the periods with low Sa_{O_2} "repeatedly showed levels below 40 mm Hg in 7 of the 10 patients and below 30 mm in 1 patient." The Pa_{CO_2} changed relatively little, increasing 5 mm Hg on the average. When oxygen at 2 L/minute was given to these patients, the mean nocturnal decline was much less (11%) and the Pa_{O_2} fell below 50 mm Hg in only 1 patient during sleep. The mean pH did not change during oxygen therapy in this group of 10 patients (in clear contrast to the study by Leitch et al., in which 1 patient developed serious hypercapnia and acidosis after being put on low-flow oxygen).

The study by Flick and Block should make one cautious about using single randomly obtained arterial gas samples to guide therapy because there is really no way of knowing when these periods of extreme hypoxemia might occur either during the day or during the night. The greatest decreases in Sa_{O_2} at night were seen in those patients with the most compromised FEV_1 (expressed as percent of FEV) and those with elevated Pa_{CO_2} values. It should be emphasized again that although all 10 of the patients studied by Flick and Block tolerated 2 L oxygen at night without untoward effect, 1 of the patients presented by Leitch et al. did become hypercapnic and acidotic. Both studies agreed that the mechanism of these hypoxic dips was usually intermittent worsening of the matching of ventilation to perfusion rather than alveolar hypoventilation.

The severity of the hypoxemia noted is indeed frightening. One wonders why the patients all don't die of arrhythmias, severe pulmonary hypertension, systemic hypertension, hypercoagulability and other bad consequences of serious hypoxemia and its attendant hyperepinephrinemia. – Ed.] ◄

Portable Oxygen and Exercise Tolerance in Patients with Chronic Hypoxic Cor Pulmonale. Breathlessness is the main symptom limiting exercise in patients with chronic hypoxic cor pulmonale, and even partial correction of the severe arterial hypoxemia that develops on exercise can reduce the minute ventilation and improve exercise tolerance. R. J. E. Leggett and D. C. Flenley[6] (Edinburgh) studied

(6) Br. Med. J. 2:84–86, July 9, 1977.

19 men and 7 women having chronic hypoxic cor pulmonale with pulmonary hypertension during bicycle and treadmill exercises when they breathed air and 30% oxygen. A single-blind study of the effects of oxygen provided by a patient-carried supply of liquid oxygen, the Union Carbide Oxygen Walker, was carried out. All patients were clinically stable at the time of study. In 16 patients the distance walked in 12 minutes on the level was determined at gas flows of 2 or 4 L air or oxygen per minute.

The mean Pa_{CO_2} fell from 6.9 to 6 kPa (51.7 to 45.0 mm Hg) on exercise, but the Pa_{CO_2} rose from 6.9 to 7.5 kPa. Minute ventilation was reduced on exercise in 12 of 15 patients breathing 30% oxygen, compared with air breathing at the same level of exercise. Carrying the oxygen walker when breathing oxygen did not increase the distance walked in 12 minutes over that found when breathing air alone, at an oxygen flow rate of 2 L per minute. All patients who wheeled the walker on a trolley increased their walking distance to a significant degree when breathing oxygen compared to when breathing air.

Oxygen during exercise can benefit severely hypoxic patients by permitting a small increase in the distance walked within a given time period. Wheeling an oxygen walker on a light-weight trolley will allow these breathless patients to derive benefit from oxygen during exercise, in addition to the benefit already obtained from having a portal oxygen supply providing oxygen therapy at least 15 hours a day.

► [This article was selected because it did have some good measurements indicating that the gain of portable oxygen therapy may in some instances be more apparent than real and to introduce, somewhat reluctantly, the whole subject of out-of-hospital oxygen therapy for the patient with chronic obstructive lung disease. Who should be treated in this manner remains a vexing and unsolved problem compounded by the expense involved (most often borne by third parties and, therefore, regretably of no concern to the patient or his doctor), the tremendous placebo effect and the understandable urge of the doctor to do something in the face of relentless breathlessness. The notion that oxygen is good for you has received a great boost by television shots of football heroes inhaling a quick fix on the sidelines. If it is good for those fellows, it must be good for everyone.

This article states on the basis of good evidence that increased exercise tolerance in the patients was offset by the increased work of carrying the portable oxygen device. It is maintained, probably rightly, that the improvement in general condition that results from being able to exercise a little is itself a worthwhile goal, but the gains must be marginal in most cases. Another study by Leggett et al., attempting to define objectively who should receive this expensive therapy (Long-term domiciliary oxygen therapy in cor pulmonale complicating chronic bronchitis and emphysema, Thorax 31:414, 1976), reported data on 10 patients, all of whom had pronounced hypoxemia (25–50 mm Hg), polycythemia, a history of decompensated cor pulmonale, and measured pulmonary artery hypertension. Polycythemia and pulmonary hypertension were improved in some of the patients receiving oxygen for at least 15 hours daily, but not in those receiving it for 12 hours a day. The concept that oxygen therapy has to be prolonged (15 hours daily) to result in objective benefit has been made by several others (summarized by Block, A. J.: Low-flow oxygen therapy: Treatment of the ambulant patient, Am. Rev. Respir. Dis. [Suppl.] 110:71, 1974). Although this sort of data does not speak to prolongation of life, it is possible to maintain that episodes of extreme nocturnal hypoxia with their attendant episodes of arrhythmia are serious and avoidable risks. This, however, remains to be established.

At present the following seem defensible statements. (1) The indications for chronic oxygen therapy at home are not yet established on firm grounds. Solid comparative studies should be available in 2 years or so. (2) Most would confine its use to patients with cor pulmonale refractory to the usual methods of treatment, severe (less than 55 mm Hg) hypoxemia, polycythemia and demonstrated severe obstructive lung disease who do not smoke and who have had optimum in-patient hospital treatment. Even in this group, the physician should attempt to reach some rational decision as to whether benefit actually has resulted, as not all such patients will be helped. (3) When low-flow oxygen is used, carbon dioxide retention is not a contraindication to use. However, some device should be added for most patients to prevent their increasing the flow rate beyond that prescribed. (4) Some other conditions, such as advanced interstitial lung disease and advanced cardiac failure, may be improved symptomatically by home oxygen therapy. (5) Its intermittent use to relieve breathlessness in the patient without cor pulmonale is a practice to be deprecated as wasteful, potentially harmful, a little magical and inevitably psychologically addicting. The ATS Council has provided a somewhat more enthusiastic set of recommendations (Oxygen Administration in the Home, ibid. 115:897, 1977).

The whole field of rehabilitation of the chronic lung disease patient was reviewed in a balanced presentation by Lertzman and Cherniak (Rehabilitation of patients with chronic obstructive pulmonary disease, ibid. 114:1145, 1976). One recent study from Scotland (McGavin et al.: Physical rehabilitation for the chronic bronchitic: Results from a controlled trial of exercises in the home, Thorax 32:307, 1977) demonstrated that unsupervised progressive and regular stair-climbing exercises produced measurably increased work performance and well-being while not changing ventilatory function, heart rate on exercise or body weight. This form of treatment is certainly nonwasteful, nonharmful, nonmagical and nonaddicting. It is nice to know it is also helpful.—Ed.] ◄

Prospective Study of Controlled Oxygen Therapy: Poor Prognosis of Patients with Asynchronous Breathing. If factors predictive of a successful outcome with controlled oxygen therapy could be identified on admission, some patients might be spared intubation and assisted ventilation. Robert Gilbert, Kumar Ashutosh, J. Howland Auchincloss, Jr., Shamsuddin Rana and David Peppi[7] (State Univ. of New York, Syracuse) attempted to develop methods of predicting success or failure of controlled oxygen therapy on admission.

Thirty-two patients with chronic obstructive airway disease were studied during 36 episodes of acute respiratory failure. Thirty-one episodes were associated with a Pa_{CO_2} above 45 mm Hg. Eleven episodes were treated by oxygen before arterial blood was drawn. Patients were studied within 24 hours of admission while receiving controlled oxygen therapy with a 24 or 28% Venturi mask. Separate movements of the chest (rib cage) and the abdomen (diaphragm) were recorded with an electromagnetic ventilation monitor. The various types of magnetometric tracings are shown in Figure 6, both the severely and mildly abnormal patterns were considered abnormal.

The patients in 25 episodes recovered without need for intubation and assisted ventilation. Two of the 9 intubated patients and 2 patients who were not intubated died. Seven intubated patients recovered after a prolonged period of assisted ventilation. All 11 patients who were failures and only 16 of the 25 who were successes had low diaphragms on the chest film. No other x-ray or ECG feature was significantly different in the two groups.

Seven of 12 episodes associated with asynchronous breathing resulted in failure, whereas 20 of 23 associated with normal synchronized breathing were successes. The predictive value of the breathing pattern, forced inspiratory volume (FIV_1) and Pa_{CO_2} is shown in the table.

---

(7) Chest 71:456–462, April, 1977.

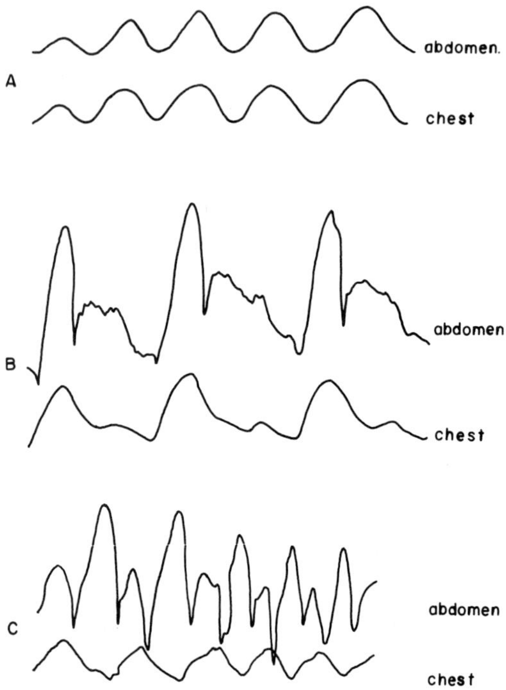

Fig 6.—Three types of magnetometric tracings. Spirometric signal, representing air flow at mouth, was omitted for simplicity. In all cases, air flow signal was synchronous with chest movement signal. In both chest and abdominal signals, upward deflection represents expansion—coils on front and back moving away from each other. Upward deflection of chest signal represents inspiration. **A,** synchronized breathing pattern, seen in all normal subjects and most patients with chronic obstructive airway disease. **B,** moderately asynchronous pattern: Chest and abdomen move together in inspiration and early expiration; later, in expiration, extra movements are seen in abdomen which do not correspond to chest movements or flow of air. **C,** severely asynchronous pattern: Extra abdominal expansion in expiration is greater than inspiratory expansion. (Courtesy of Gilbert, R., et al.: Chest 71:456–462, April, 1977.)

Statistical Analysis of 35 Episodes

Two-by-Two Array and Factors	Successes	Failures	Sensitivity, percent	Specificity, percent	Efficiency, percent	P Value
Array 1					77	0.02
Synchronous breathing	20	3	80	70		
Asynchronous breathing	5	7	70	80		
Array 2					77	0.01
Synchronous breathing and $FIV_1 > 650$ ml	18	1	72	90		
Not both	7	9	...	...		
Array 3					86	0.001
Asynchronous breathing and $PaCO_2 \geq 60$ mm Hg	2	7	70	92		
Not both	23	3	...	...		

The breathing pattern alone correctly predicted the outcome in 77% of the episodes. Adding an FIV_1 above 650 ml to a synchronous breathing pattern increased the specificity to 90%, but the efficiency was not improved. Adding a Pa_{CO_2} of 60 mm Hg or above to an asynchronous breathing pattern increased the specificity for prediction of failure to 92%, with no loss in sensitivity. The efficiency of this combination in prediction of success or failure was 86%. Multiple regression analysis using these factors led to the correct classification of 92% of patients.

There is definitely a risk to intubation and assisted ventilation, but no morbidity or mortality was attributable to the procedures in the present study. Immediate intubation is not yet recommended for patients admitted in respiratory failure with asynchronous breathing and a high Pa_{CO_2}; however, if any deterioration occurs during controlled oxygen therapy, intubation should be instituted earlier than in patients in a more favorable category on admission.

► [The poor prognostic import of this pattern of breathing was initially pointed out by the same authors in an article in the 1976 YEAR BOOK, page 122. This article by Gilbert et al. extends these observations in a clinically useful way. Careful measurement of the contributions of thoracic muscles and diaphragm to breathing is a relatively new area of research (see Sharp et al.: Thoracoabdominal motion in chronic obstructed pulmonary disease, Am. Rev. Respir. Dis. 115:47, 1977). O'Connell and Campbell (Respiratory mechanics in airways obstruction associated with inspiratory dyspnea, Thorax 31:669, 1976) point out that COPD patients who experience difficulty with inspiration are generally worse by all measurable parameters than those who experience difficulty largely with expiration (this, of course, does not apply to patients with central airways obstruction). This sensation of inspiratory difficulty is due largely to inefficiency of the depressed diaphragm (Rochester et al.: Diaphragmatic energy expenditure in chronic respiratory failure, Am. J. Med. 63:223, 1977). Refined history taking and refined physical examination can provide considerable information concerning the extent of disability and probable therapeutic requirements in COPD with acute-on-chronic respiratory failure. – Ed.] ◄

Amyotrophic Lateral Sclerosis Presenting with Respiratory Failure: Diaphragmatic Paralysis and Dependence on Mechanical Ventilation in Two Patients. A few cases of amyotrophic lateral sclerosis (ALS) have been reported in which exertional dyspnea was the original symptom. Gary B. Fromm, Peggy J. Wisdom and A. Jay Block[8] (Univ. of Florida) report the first 2 cases in which respiratory failure that recessitated mechanical ventilation was the initial symptom of ALS. The correct diagnosis was made only after multiple unsuccessful attempts to wean the patients from ventilatory support.

Man, 68, became short of breath, restless and tachypneic; mechanical ventilation was considered necessary. Attempts over the next 4 weeks to wean him from ventilation failed. The only pertinent physical finding was dullness over the lower left lobe; no neurologic abnormalities were noted. Intermittent mandatory ventilation was being used at a rate of 12/minute with no positive end-expiratory pressure. The FI_{O_2} was 0.4. Chest films showed bilateral patchy lower lobe infiltrates. The patient was afebrile and alert on treatment with gentamicin, heparin and positive end-expiratory pressure to 12 cm water. His arterial blood gases improved in the next 3 weeks, but attempts to wean the patient from respiratory support failed because of severe respiratory acidosis. Distal limb weakness was then noted, with wasting of the interosseous muscles. Chest fluoroscopy showed paradoxic diaphragmatic movement on the

(8) Chest 71:612–614, May, 1977.

right and no movement on the left. The patient died about 2 weeks later, after ALS was diagnosed.

Autopsy showed pulmonary congestion with bilateral pneumonia. Loss of anterior horn cells was most marked in the cervical spinal cord. No corticospinal tract demyelination was noted, and the cortex and brain stem were normal.

The other patient, a man aged 69, presented in acute respiratory distress 6 months after lung function tests had indicated airway obstruction. Muscle weakness with fasciculations was noted shortly afterward, and autopsy showed both extensive bronchopneumonia and loss of anterior horn cells in the spinal cord.

Segmental atrophy and limb weakness are the usual initial manifestations of ALS, although one fourth of the patients have bulbar paralysis. A disease of motor neurons that leads to respiratory muscle weakness and diaphragmatic paralysis, such as ALS, should be considered when respiratory support must be continued for reasons that are not clear.

► [Blythe et al. (Bilateral diaphragmatic paralysis in association with neurogenic disease, Arch. Intern. Med. 137:1455, 1977) report a case presenting with cor pulmonale, severe respiratory acidosis at night, a greatly decreased vital capacity (1.3 L) and no evidence of obstruction. The problem was only present in the supine position. Neurologic examination revealed proximal muscle weakness greater in the shoulder than the pelvic girdle. Weakness and atrophy of hand muscles also developed later. The neurologic diagnosis was never clear. In addition to ALS, as recorded in this article by Fromm et al., bilateral diaphragmatic paralysis has been noted to complicate the Guillain-Barre syndrome, neuralgic amyotrophy (brachial plexus neuropathy), recent tetanus immunization, postinfectious phrenic neuritis and poliomyelitis. Sandham et al. (Acute supine respiratory failure due to bilateral diaphragmatic paralysis, Chest 72:96, 1977) record a case they believe to have been due to blunt thoracic trauma sustained in a traffic accident. – Ed.] ◄

Blunted Respiratory Drive in Congenital Myopathy. Limited ventilatory capacity commonly is detected in patients with neuromuscular disorders, but respiratory failure usually occurs only in those with profound muscular weakness. David J. Riley, Teodoro V. Santiago, Ronald P. Daniele, Burton Schall and Norman H. Edelman[9] describe 2 adult patients with mild to moderate weakness due to nonmyotonic congenital myopathies who presented with severe chronic respiratory failure. Marked insensitivity of the respiratory center to carbon dioxide was present in both cases, suggesting a central cause of hypoventilation.

Muscle weakness alone could not account for respiratory insufficiency in these cases because static respiratory pressures were not impaired markedly, ventilation during exercise was normal and daytime ventilation was normal if ventilatory assistance was provided at night. The arterial blood gases are given in the table. Both patients had markedly blunted ventilatory responses to carbon dioxide (Fig 7). Hypoxic ventilatory drive was, at least qualitatively, intact. Morphometric studies showed the number of alveoli to be slightly less than predicted, but the mean alveolar size was only 57% of expected.

It is not likely that selectively severe involvement of the respiratory

(9) Am. J. Med. 63:459–466, September, 1977.

ARTERIAL BLOOD GASES*

Date	PO_2 (mm Hg)	pH	PCO_2 (mm Hg)	F_{IO_2} (%)	Comment
				Case 1	
3/14/70	41	7.20	75	21	Admission, rest (minute ventilation = 5.2 liters/min)
3/14/70	70	7.32	48	21	Voluntary hyperventilation (minute ventilation = 15.6 liters/min)
5/5/70	76	7.35	44	21	After treatment, awake
5/5/70	58	7.24	60	21	Asleep
5/26/70	92	7.35	46	21	Discharge
8/14/72	85	7.41	42	21	Two years after discharge
				Case 2	
3/23/71	40	7.33	93	24	Admission, rest (minute ventilation = 7 liters/min)
3/23/71	70	7.38	73	24	Voluntary hyperventilation (minute ventilation = 14 liters/min)
4/27/71	82	7.39	44	21	After treatment, awake
4/27/71	53	7.22	69	21	Asleep
5/4/71	79	7.40	42	21	Discharge
1/14/75	69	7.39	46	21	Three and a half years after discharge

*F_{IO_2} = fraction of inspired oxygen.

muscles explains these cases. Nonchemical sensory input, especially from skeletal muscle receptors, may be important in regulating ventilation. Certain myopathic processes may reduce sensitivity to carbon dioxide by altering afferent input to the central nervous system from skeletal muscles. Whatever the cause of the blunted ventilatory response to carbon dioxide, hypercapnic ventilatory drive appears to be of major importance only during sleep. Use of the cuirass respirator at night allowed oxygenation to be achieved without danger of hypercapnia in the present cases. The treatment proved effective in preventing pulmonary hypertension and cor pulmonale, and patient acceptance was good. This simple approach should be considered in patients with neuromuscular disorders and central depression of respiration who hypoventilate at night.

Fig 7.—Ventilatory responses to inhalation of carbon dioxide of both patients. End-tidal CO_2 (ordinate) is plotted against minute ventilation (abscissa). Shaded area represents normal predicted values of Weil et al., 1975. (Courtesy of Riley, D. J., et al.: Am. J. Med. 63:459–466, September, 1977.)

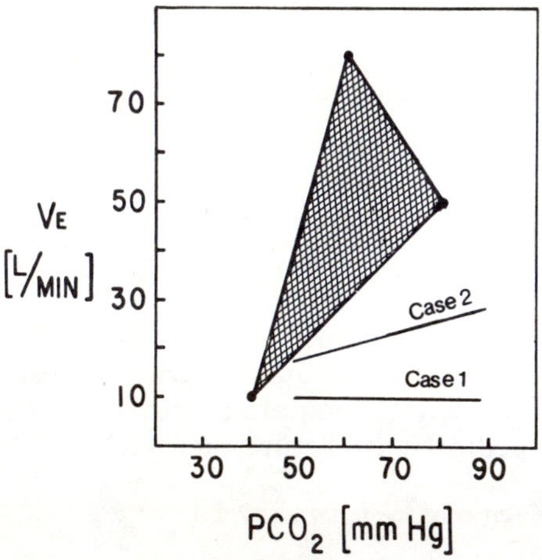

Acute Respiratory Failure Associated with Hypophosphatemia. Hypophosphatemia is being recognized increasingly as a cause of several systemic disorders, and therapeutic advances have created iatrogenic causes of hypophosphatemia. John H. Newman, Thomas A. Neff and Philip Ziporin[1] (Denver) report data on 2 patients in whom ventilatory failure was responsive to inorganic phosphate.

An alcoholic woman aged 58 with chronic obstructive lung disease was seen after a grand mal seizure; she improved on intravenous glucose and potassium therapy. The next day the serum inorganic phosphate level fell from 3.2 to 0.9 mg/100 ml and respiratory arrest occurred, necessitating intubation. Generalized areflexia and muscle weakness were noted. Potassium phosphate led to a lessening of the muscle weakness and a doubling of the forced vital capacity. Another alcoholic woman, aged 43, reported being unable to move for 2 days and exhibited decreased muscle strength and tone, with a serum phosphate level of 0.9 mg/100 ml. Ventilatory failure necessitated intubation and mechanical ventilation. Much improvement occurred within hours of phosphate replacement, and support was not necessary when the inorganic phosphate level reached 2.9 mg/100 ml.

These findings are typical of previously reported cases of hypophosphatemic syndromes. Both patients were alcoholic and both received infusions of 5% glucose on admission. One received antacids by nasogastric tube. Both patients had ventilatory collapse and required mechanically assisted ventilation. Hyporeflexia and marked generalized paresis were noted as the serum inorganic phosphate level dropped, with no worsening of mental status. The triose phosphate precursors of 2,3-diphosphoglycerate (DPG) build up in phosphate-depleted cells; the limiting step may be determined by the unavailability of inorganic phosphate for the synthesis of 2,3-DPG. Both of the present patients responded dramatically to intravenous phosphate repletion. In patients who can eat, phosphate deficiency can be corrected with milk products or with sodium biphosphate and sodium phosphate given by mouth.

► [The subject of hypophosphatemia recently has been reviewed extensively by Knochel (The pathophysiology and clinical characteristics of severe hypophosphatemia, Arch. Intern. Med. 137:203, 1977), although he did not mention respiratory failure as a problem. The clinical situations most prominently associated with hypophosphatemia are diabetic ketoacidosis, especially during recovery, alcoholism in a hospitalized patient and hyperalimentation without phosphate supplementation (this last is probably no longer a problem as phosphate supplementation is quite routine). The major clinical consequences listed are red blood cell dysfunction due to decreased erythrocyte 2,3-DGP and the consequent increased avidity of hemaglobin for oxygen, hemolysis, leukocyte dysfunction, platelet dysfunction, central nervous system dysfunction and rhabdomyolysis. The occurrence of acute renal failure in alcoholic rhabdomyolysis is not a rare event. – Ed.] ◄

Cricoarytenoid Arthritis and Airway Obstruction in Juvenile Rheumatoid Arthritis. Cricoarytenoid arthritis, estimated to be present in 26% of adults with rheumatoid arthritis, has been mentioned only once in the pediatric literature. Jerry C. Jacobs and Robert M.

(1) N. Engl. J. Med. 296:1101–1103, May 12, 1977.

Hui[2] (Columbia-Presbyterian Med. Center) describe a young boy with polyarticular febrile-onset juvenile rheumatoid arthritis who developed airway obstruction associated with arthritis of a cricoarytenoid joint, necessitating emergency tracheostomy.

Boy, aged 3 years 3 months, was hospitalized with a temperature of 40.5C, a generalized pink rash and polyarthritis which was not controlled with aspirin, 70 mg/kg/day. Inspiratory stridor developed about 2 weeks later. Dexamethasone therapy for 6 days was followed by prednisone for 6 days. The respirations became progressively labored, and hypopharyngeal hyperexpansion was noted. A tracheostomy was performed, and aspirin dosage was increased to 140 mg/kg/day, producing a salicylate level of 22 mg/100 ml. The arthritis improved, the tracheostomy tube was removed and he was discharged.

However, stridor recurred within 24 hours, and the patient was readmitted. Dexamethasone was again administered. The sedimentation rate was 118 mm/hour, the antinuclear anbodies (ANA) test was weakly positive. Laryngoscopy showed a fixed left cricoarytenoid joint, preventing normal motion of the posterior segment of that vocal cord. Aspirin was given to produce a salicylate level of 26 mg/100 ml, requiring 150 mg/kg/day. He was discharged on this regimen. In the succeeding 9 months, he required small doses of steroids and was admitted for viral meningoencephalitis and for pericarditis. The voice remains hoarse, but airway obstruction has not recurred.

Most adults with this manifestation of rheumatoid arthritis have inspiratory stridor. Some patients report fullness in the throat on swallowing or referred pain in the ear. The diagnosis is made by direct laryngoscopy. Laryngeal symptoms may be exacerbated with intercurrent respiratory infection and worsened by sedatives. Steroids may provide adequate relief; tracheostomy can probably usually be avoided in affected children. A severe rebound may occur if anti-inflammatory drugs are precipitately withdrawn. Stridor in an arthritic child may be due, at least in part, to laryngeal arthritis.

► [This article from the pediatric literature was selected simply because of the subject, as the condition is far more important in adults than in children. Our interest in it was stimulated by a rheumatoid patient with severe laryngeal stridor and breathlessness carried in our clinics for a long period as chronic obstructive pulmonary disease. Involvement of the cricoarytenoid joint occurs to one degree or another in as many as one fourth to one third of patients with rheumatoid arthritis, although in most patients symptoms are not marked (Lofgren and Montgomery: Incidence of laryngeal involvement in rheumatoid arthritis, N. Engl. J. Med. 267:193, 1962). The cases which have been reported ordinarily presented as emergencies because the basic cause of respiratory difficulty was not recognized initially, usually because of a coexistent upper respiratory infection or pneumonia (Smith and Shine: Rheumatoid arthritis of the cricoarytenoid joint: A report of a case presenting as a serious medical emergency, Ann. Intern. Med. 60:473, 1964). The condition is worse when the arthritis is worse, but can cause serious trouble when other manifestations of arthritis appear quiescent. Suggestive symptoms include pain in the ear, a sense of foreign body in the throat, difficulty swallowing, pain on swallowing, pain on talking, dyspnea on exertion and stridor, especially at night, but the condition may be advanced in the absence of all of these. Some cases appear to have been benefited with anti-inflammatory drugs, but those which have been published usually are serious enough to require tracheostomy and unilateral arytenoidectomy. In the past, diagnosis usually has been made by laryngoscopy both to establish the presence of upper airway obstruction and to rule out neurologic paralysis of the cords, edema and tumor. Now one should be able to sus-

(2) Pediatrics 59:292–294, February, 1977.

pect upper airway obstruction and to quantitate the defect by use of inspiratory and expiratory spirometry with flow volume curves (see 1977 YEAR BOOK, p. 107). – Ed.] ◄

► ↓ The hypoventilation-somnolence-cor pulmonale syndrome was first recognized in very fat people and blamed on the constricting effects of the fat on the chest cage, with resultant hypoventilation. It quickly became clear, however, that just fat per se was not enough to produce pathologic hypoventilation and that there was usually some other contributory factor such as hypothyroidism, considerable underlying bronchitis and emphysema, or defects in respiratory control (see 1976 YEAR BOOK, pp. 125–127; and Kronenberg: Acute respiratory failure and obesity with normal ventilatory response to carbon dioxide and absent hypoxic ventilatory drive, Am. J. Med. 62:772, 1977). Next it became established that the daytime somnolence characteristic of the syndrome might be due to one or another of two quite different causes: first, carbon dioxide retention with its known effects in producing decreased levels of consciousness, and, second, sleep deprivation, or at least deprivation of the most satisfactory levels of sleep due to intermittent obstruction to inspiration at night, producing arousal. Probably more or less at the same time it was realized that a short fat neck was not the only mechanism capable of producing intermittent airways obstruction at night (1975 YEAR BOOK, p. 136; Conway et al.: Hypersomnolence and intermittent upper airways obstruction: Occurrence caused by micrognathia, J.A.M.A. 237:2740, 1977; Imes et al.: Retrognathia and sleep apnea: A life-threatening condition masquerading as narcolepsy, 237:1596, 1977; and Licht et al.: Tonsillar hypertrophy in an adult with obesity-hypoventilation syndrome, Chest 70:672, 1976).

The following article was chosen because of the wide variety of subtle clinical symptoms that it attributes to sleep deprivation. This is probably a very important and often misdiagnosed condition which should be recognized and treated. The idea of averting divorce by tracheostomy is enchanting. – Ed. ◄

Sleep Apnea Syndrome due to Upper Airway Obstruction: A Review of 25 Cases is presented by Christian Guilleminault, Frederic L. Eldridge, Ara Tilkian, F. Blair Simmons and William C. Dement[3] (Stanford Univ.). Twenty-one of the 25 patients were referred to a sleep disorders clinic with excessive daytime somnolence. All patients were men; the average age was 44.3 years. Five men were of normal weight; 16 were 16% or more overweight. Ten patients had been diagnosed as narcoleptics and 4 as having pickwickian syndrome. Ten patients had taken methylphenidate, alone or with amphetamine, and 3 had received thyroid medication.

The major symptoms are given in the table. All patients had noisy pharyngeal snoring during sleep, with apneic periods lasting 20 seconds or longer. Five patients had had excessive daytime somnolence for over 10 years and 6 for 5–10 years. Hypnagogic hallucinations were reported by 10 patients, and automatic behavior occurred daily in 11. Fifteen patients reported difficulty in maintaining attention and inability to concentrate, even when wide awake. The families of 16 patients reported disturbing personality changes. Six patients had seen psychiatrists for anxiety and depression, and 2 broken marriages had resulted. Twelve patients reported impotence. Eleven spouses had noted abnormal behavioral outbursts. Eleven patients had recurrent morning headaches, and 2 reported intermittent nocturnal enuresis.

Hypertension was noted in 14 patients. All daytime EEGs were normal. "Obstructive sleep apnea" was recorded by respiratory monitoring during sleep in 86% of the apneic episodes. Sleep apnea was associated with rises in systemic and pulmonary arterial pressure.

---

(3) Arch. Intern. Med. 137:296–300, March, 1977.

MAJOR CLINICAL SYMPTOMS*

Patient	Snoring	Abnormal Motor Activity During Sleep	Excessive Daytime Sleepiness	Personality Changes	Deteriorating Intellectual Capacity	Hypertension	Sexual Problems	Abnormal Outbursts	Morning Headaches	Hypnagogic Hallucinations and Automatic Behavior	Nocturnal Enuresis
1	+	+	+	+	+	+	+	+	+	+	−
2	+	+	+	+	+	+	+	−	+	+	−
3	+	+	+	+	+	+	+	+	−	+	−
4	+	+	+	+	+	+	+	+	−	+	−
5	+	+	+	+	+	+	+	+	−	−	−
6	+	+	+	+	+	−	−	−	+	+	−
7	+	+	+	+	+	−	+	+	−	−	−
8	+	+	+	+	+	−	−	−	+	−	+
9	+	+	+	+	+	+	−	+	−	−	−
10	+	+	+	+	+	+	−	−	−	+	−
11	+	+	+	+	−	−	+	+	+	−	−
12	+	+	+	+	+	−	+	−	+	−	+
13	+	+	+	+	−	−	+	+	+	−	−
14	+	+	+	+	−	−	+	+	−	+	−
15	+	+	+	−	+	+	−	+	+	+	−
16	+	+	+	−	−	+	+	−	+	−	−
17	+	+	+	−	+	+	−	−	−	+	−
18	+	+	+	−	+	+	−	−	−	+	−
19	+	+	−	−	+	+	−	−	+	−	−
20	+	+	−	+	−	−	−	+	+	−	−
21	+	+	+	−	−	+	−	−	−	−	−
22	+	+	+	+	−	−	−	−	−	−	−
23	+	+	−	−	−	+	−	−	−	−	−
24	+	+	−	−	−	−	+	−	−	−	−
25	+	+	+	−	−	−	−	−	−	−	−

*Plus sign indicates present, and minus sign indicates absent.

Dieting resulted in no improvement except in a patient with few sleep apnea episodes. Aminophylline therapy was not helpful. Eight patients underwent tracheostomy and positioning of a permanent tracheal valve; all symptoms disappeared during 4–26 months after the procedure. Two of 5 untreated patients had worsening of their symptoms. Two patients have died, 1 in relation to marked hypoxia during sleep.

The causes of predominantly upper airway obstructive sleep apnea are not clear. Hypothetically, a dysfunction of the central nervous system is most likely, but peripheral factors may also be involved. If sleep apnea can be diagnosed before life-threatening conditions develop, less drastic treatment than tracheostomy may be possible.

► [Tilkian et al. have published a very helpful and thorough study in which the hemodynamic effects of sleep apnea were recorded and correlated with arterial blood gas measurements (Hemodynamics in sleep-induced apnea, Ann. Intern. Med. 85:714, 1976). The pivotal change was extreme hypoxia, and the other changes were regarded as secondary to this. Normal persons tend to lower their systemic blood pressure during sleep. In 9 of the 12 subjects studied, systemic hypertension was noted and correlated with the number and duration of apneic episodes and the attendant hypoxemia with increased sympathetic discharge. When the apneic episodes were widely spaced, pressures tended to return to their daytime normal, but when they followed more closely one on the other, the effect on blood pressure was cumulative, and persisting hypertension resulted. Pulmonary artery pressure also rose substantially during apneic periods. Apnea was associated with bradycardia, attributed by the authors to enhanced vagal discharge, and tachycardia was seen in the postapneic period. Thus the pathogenesis of cor pulmonale is clear; moreover, untoward effects on left ventricular function might be anticipated in persons who already have some systemic hypertension as a baseline. It should be emphasized that these hemodynamic studies apply equally well to chronic obstructive pulmonary disease patients without apneic episodes as a prominent feature but who develop serious hypoxemia at night.

The same authors (Tilkian et al.: Sleep-induced apnea syndrome: Prevalence of cardiac arrhythmias and their reversal after tracheostomy, Am. J. Med. 63:348, 1977) looked at cardiac rhythm during apneic episodes in 15 patients. They recorded extreme bradycardia (under 30 beats a minute) in 6, asystole for periods up to 6.3 seconds in 5, 2d-degree atrioventricular block in 2, complex premature ventricular beats in 10 and ventricular tachycardia in 2. Serious arrhythmia can cause sudden death in this group of patients (1975 YEAR BOOK, p. 136). — Ed.] ◄

Pulmonary Edema

► ↓ A totally satisfactory definition of the adult respiratory distress syndrome (ARDS) or acute respiratory failure is not available, because although the pathogenesis in some instances is relatively straightforward, in others it is more complicated. Insofar as it is defined as a clinical state with arterial hypoxemia which cannot be corrected with high concentrations of oxygen, pulmonary arteriovenous shunting with multiple areas of microatelectasis, and stiff lungs, it is clear that advanced interstitial or alveolar pulmonary edema, or both, from hydrostatic causes (heart failure) meets this definition. Some have equated noncardiogenic pulmonary edema due to increased permeability of the pulmonary microvasculature or to loss of vascular oncotic pressure, or to both factors, with ARDS. However, this does not take into account clinical situations which have all of these physiologic characteristics but are due to diffuse infection, typically viral, involving the smallest airways or to diffuse pulmonary injury initiating on the alveolar side of the alveolocapillary membrane such as drowning, diffuse aspiration of gastric contents, smoke injury or prolonged exposure to high concentrations of oxygen. Several other themes run through the multiple causes of the ARDS: specifically high levels of circulating catecholamines, intravascular coagulation, the probably related occurrence of platelet-leukocyte thrombi which come to lodge in the pulmonary microvasculature, hypocapnia, loss of pulmonary surfactant which causes small airways collapse—whatever the initiating cause—bacterial sepsis, and circulating immune complexes with effects on platelets, coagulation and the complement system. High concentrations of circulating catecholamines are thought to be of critical importance in pulmonary edema after cerebrovascular accidents, pulmonary edema complicating pheochromocytoma (Munk et al.: Pheochromocytoma presenting with pulmonary edema and hyperamylasemia, Can. Med. Assoc. J. 116:357, 1977), the ARDS after prolonged hypotension and, it seems reasonable to assume, in ARDS after amitriptyline overdosage (Lindstrom et al.: Respiratory distress syndrome and thrombotic, nonbacterial endocarditis after amitriptyline overdose. Acta Med. Scand. 202:203, 1977), since this drug prevents reuptake of catecholamines into neurosecretory granules. Kersten et al. (The nature of failure of pulmonary adaptation to atelectasis, Surgery 82: 90, 1977) have provided good evidence that the usual physiologic mechanism by which blood is redirected away from atelectatic areas of the lung is prevented by administration of epinephrine or norepinephrine, thus increasing arteriovenous shunting. The catecholamine story gets further complicated by the fact that epinephrine is a potent platelet-aggregating agent and for this reason, and probably others, states associated with high levels of circulating catecholamines in effect tend to hypercoagulability and diffuse intravascular coagulation. It should be emphasized that the case of amitriptyline overdosage mentioned above was also complicated by thrombotic nonbacterial endocarditis, a condition generally regarded as an indicator of accelerated intravascular coagulation. (See 1974 YEAR BOOK, p. 131, for further discussion of epinephrine.)

A review by Pardy and Dudley (Posttraumatic pulmonary insufficiency, Surg. Gynecol. Obstet. 144:259, 1977) focuses on the importance of hepatic reticuloendothelial compromise in the causation of acute respiratory failure. Their thesis runs as follows. Interposition of the liver between the gut and the remainder of the circulation protects the lungs; the evidence for this consists of a variety of clinical states and experimental situations such as cirrhosis, hepatic resection for trauma, and liver transplantation in which respiratory failure is frequently seen. Shock both increases absorption of toxic materials such as endotoxin and vasoactive peptides from the gut and decreases hepatic reticuloendothelial activity. The liver normally not only clears toxins from the circulation but also removes procoagulant substances such as thromboplastin which are always forming at a slow rate. In situations of compromised hepatic reticuloendothelial activity, these are thought to bypass the liver and go to the lung. Again the theme of hypercoagulability and platelet-leukocyte thrombi is prominent. Myrvold and Svalander (Pulmonary microembolism in early experimental septic shock, J. Surg. Res. 23:65, 1977) emphasize the role of platelet and leukocyte thrombi, particularly the latter (see also 1973 YEAR BOOK, pp. 108–110).

The untoward effects of hypocapnia in contributing to the overall process are discussed by Askanazi et al. (The role of carbon dioxide in the development of pulmonary insufficiency, J. Thorac. Cardiovas. Surg. 74:118, 1977). Hypocapnia causes bronchospasm (probably an overshoot of a normal regulatory mechanism by which ventilation is decreased in underperfused areas), increased arteriovenous shunting, decreased cardiac output and cerebral hypoperfusion. (See also 1975 YEAR BOOK, p. 150, and 1974 YEAR BOOK, pp. 124–128). Maintenance of normocapnia was found to be beneficial.

The role of surfactant depletion in the pathogenesis of ARDS was reviewed in part in an article on experimental pancreatitis which will be referred to in the section on pleural disease (J. Surg. Res. 22:566, 1977).

In summary, at present, at least, it is appropriate to regard ARDS as a result of a number of different abnormalities, often acting in concert, and to attempt, as much as possible, to think in terms of possible basic pathogenic mechanisms appropriate to the individual case and to avoid the probably overly simplistic thinking which the all-inclusive term ARDS tends to foster. — Ed. ◄

Clinical Significance of Pulmonary Function Tests: Pulmonary Function after Uncomplicated Myocardial Infarction is discussed by Charles A. Hales and Homayoun Kazemi[4] on the basis of review of the literature and the findings in patients hospitalized at the Massachusetts General Hospital during 1968–74. Derangement of lung function after myocardial infarction is related to severity of hemodynamic dysfunction. The reported reduction in vital capacity (VC) in congestive heart failure correlates well with severity of failure. The VC was reduced in the 1st week after acute infarction in 78 patients without congestive failure. Serial studies in 12 of these patients showed a VC of 83% of predicted 2–4 weeks after infarction, not signif-

Fig 8. — First section of diagrammatic representation of sequence of events following acute myocardial infarction leading to pulmonary dysfunction. At time of acute myocardial infarction, left ventricular end-diastolic *(LV-END)* pressure is elevated, resulting in increased pulmonary venous pressure. The elevation of pressure may last only a few hours. Increased venous pressure results in transudation of fluid into lung, first about the pulmonary venules and then about the extra-alveolar arterioles and their accompanying bronchioles. (Courtesy of Hales, C. A., and Kazemi, H.: Chest 72:350–358, September, 1977.)

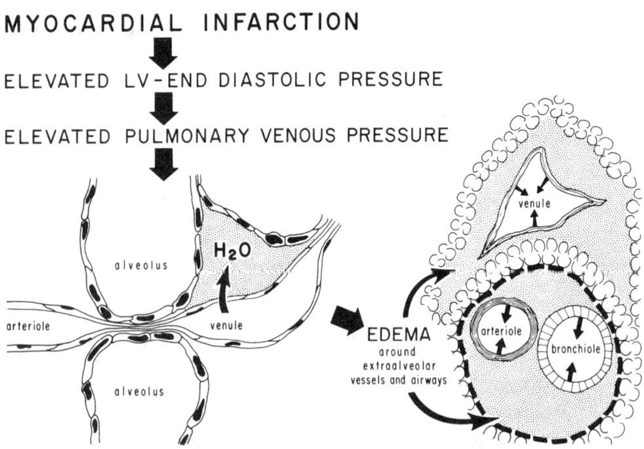

(4) Chest 72:350–358, September, 1977.

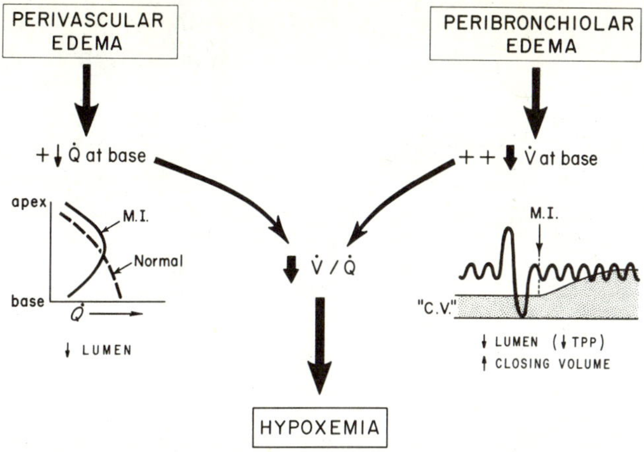

Fig 9. – Second section of diagrammatic representation of sequence of events following acute myocardial infarction *(MI)* leading to pulmonary dysfunction, showing effect of perivascular and peribronchiolar edema on distribution of perfusion *(Q̇)* and ventilation *(V̇)*. Because of perivascular edema in dependent parts of lung, there is relative hypoperfusion of pulmonary base and shift of perfusion toward apex with patient in erect position. Because of reduction in transpulmonary pressure *(TPP)* and peribronchiolar edema, small airways tend to collapse at higher than normal pulmonary volumes, i.e., increased closing volume *(CV)*. If CV becomes greater than functional residual capacity, some airways are closed during tidal breathing, causing areas of low ventilation, which, like perfusion, are in dependent parts of lung; however, ensuing relative reduction in perfusion leads to areas of low V̇/Q̇ ratio and hypoxemia. (Courtesy of Hales, C. A., and Kazemi, H.: Chest 72:350–358, September, 1977.)

icantly different from the 81% found on admission. The forced expiratory volume in the 1st second (FEV_1) and maximum expiratory flow rate also are reduced with pulmonary congestion.

An increased closing volume and frequency dependence of resistance are common after infarction, even in the absence of apparent pulmonary congestion. Total lung capacity is reduced as the degree of conges-

Fig 10. – Third section of diagrammatic representation of sequence of events following acute myocardial infarction leading to pulmonary dysfunction. As edema worsens, there is intra-alveolar and interstitial edema and vascular engorgement. These can cause lungs to become "stiff," with reduction in compliance, *VC* and total lung capacity. Intra-alveolar and interstitial edema can cause alveolar collapse, increasing right-to-left shunting and increased alveolar-arterial oxygen difference *($A\text{-}aDo_2$)* with patient breathing 100% oxygen. Interstitial edema and vascular engorgement can increase airway resistance, leading to reduction in flow rates, and also can increase residual volume *(RV)* and *CV*. (Courtesy of Hales, C. A., and Kazemi, H.: Chest 72:350–358, September, 1977.)

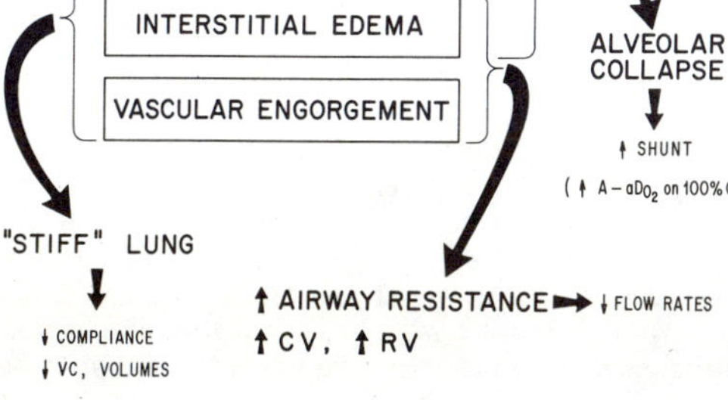

tion worsens. Arterial hypoxemia and an increased alveolar-arterial oxygen pressure gradient are common after infarction. The hypoxemia is attributable to both increased venous admixture and ventilation-perfusion imbalance.

The physiologic abnormalities noted in the lung after myocardial infarction tend to occur together and to improve together with time. They are related directly to severity of left ventricular dysfunction and subsequent pulmonary congestion. Accumulation of pulmonary edema fluid after infarction probably is initiated by increase in pulmonary capillary and venous hydrostatic pressure secondary to increased left ventricular end-diastolic pressure (Fig 8). Persisting interstitial edema reduces the diameter of extra-alveolar vessels and increases resistance to blood flow at the bases (Fig 9). Early interstitial edema also may cause increased trapping of air in the lung via collapse of small airways at higher-than-normal levels (Fig 10). With further edema, pulmonary volumes and flow rates become abnormal and, in florid pulmonary edema, the lung can become overwhelmed with serious impairment of oxygen transfer, and occasionally even impaired elimination of carbon dioxide.

► [This is the most comprehensive article we have seen concerning the pulmonary effects of congestive heart failure. It is focused on minor degrees of left ventricular dysfunction, but the same principles apply to more severe heart failure. To restate the sequence, left atrial hypertension, whether due to increased left ventricular end-diastolic pressure or to mitral valve disease, leads to pulmonary capillary hydrostatic hypertension. This increases the normal flow of fluid from the pulmonary microvasculature to the interstitial space and the pulmonary lymphatics. This increase in interstitial fluid or pressure, or both, leads to early closure of small airways which is more marked at the bases of the lungs (since the pulmonary veins have no valves and, therefore, the hydrostatic pressure is always greater in the dependent portions of the lungs). Collapse of small airways at the bases of the lungs during normal breathing ("closing volume" greater than functional residual capacity) produces the auscultatory sign of fine inspiratory rales at the bases of the lungs, accentuated by coughing and confined to the latter part of inspiration (see 1975 YEAR BOOK, p. 134). The attendant hypoxia (airways, not vascular) in the prematurely closed small airways leads to vascular spasm of the associated arterioles; this increase in precapillary vascular resistance in the lower lung fields causes redistribution of blood flow to the upper lung zones and the radiographic picture of upper lobe venous distention (see Bohr: The pulmonary hypoxic response: State of the field, Chest [Suppl.] 71:244, 1977). When the situation is more critical and there is a tendency to airways hypoxia involving more and more of the lung, the rise in pulmonary vascular resistance becomes generalized and right heart failure supervenes. Following a different set of consequences of increased fluid filtration at the capillary-interstitial interface, increased lung lymph flow makes the pulmonary lymphatics prominent which show up as Kerley's lines "B," "A," "C," "D-1" and "D-2" (see 1976 YEAR BOOK, p. 134) and as hilar clouding or indistinctness. Also, small pleural effusions at the bases or in the fissures usually appear.

The increased resistance to airflow in the patients studied in this article by Hales and Kazemi was attributed to small airways narrowing due to interstitial pulmonary edema. This may or may not be the case, but others feel that there is an active bronchospastic component to airflow obstruction in heart failure. An article by Wolf (Cardiac asthma, its origin, recognition and management, Ann. Allergy 37:250, 1976) reviews some of the older literature. We have always taught that left ventricular failure often makes itself known by its breathing pattern in that it is one of the few conditions in which obvious hyperventilation is associated with obvious obstruction to expiration. An older clinician of our acquaintance used to refer to the breathing of the patient in heart failure as "waltz-time breathing, one count in and two counts out." In one old article, crude kymographic measurements actually were made of this phenomenon (Heyer, H. E.: Abnormalities of the respiratory pattern in patients with cardiac dyspnea, Am. Heart J.

32:457, 1946), and similar data appear in another article of the same vintage (Plotz: Bronchial spasm in cardiac asthma, Ann. Intern. Med. 26:521, 1947). In the 1976 YEAR BOOK (p. 138), some experimental evidence was discussed indicating that increased airways resistance as a result of left atrial hypertension is reversed by inhalation of either β-adrenergic or atropine-like aerosols. From this it seems reasonable to postulate that bronchi become irritated when wet; it is well established that any type of bronchial irritation may result in vagally mediated bronchospasm. An article 2 decades ago by Cherniack et al., who used flow-volume loops, provided what still seems to us excellent evidence that the increased work of breathing in recumbancy in patients with heart failure is due to increased resistance to airflow in expiration, or, in other words, to bronchospasm (Circulation 15:859, 1957; and 1976 YEAR BOOK, p. 137). The promptness with which these changes were seen makes it likely that there is at least some active bronchospasm involved. This, incidentally, constitutes the best physiologic explanation for orthopnea known to us. Two other recent articles on the same subject are by Luepker et al. (Detection of pulmonary edema in acute myocardial infarction, Am. J. Cardiol. 39:146, 1977) and Biddle et al. (Hypoxemia and lung water in acute myocardial infarction, Am. Heart J. 92:692, 1976). – Ed.] ◄

► ↓ In the 1976 YEAR BOOK, pp 131 – 133, the work of Brigham and associates concerning the differentiation of hydrostatic (cardiogenic) and leaky capillary pulmonary edema was discussed at some length. To briefly restate what they found in their sheep model, pulmonary edema (increased pulmonary lymphatic flow) caused by left atrial hypertension was associated with a relative decrease in the lymph protein content due to molecular sieving (whatever that means), and this increase in the oncotic gradient between the intravascular and extravascular compartments, tending to hold fluid in the vessels, provided some protection against the effects of an increased hydrostatic gradient which tends to push fluid out of the vessels. It is of substantial interest that this has now been largely confirmed clinically (Figueras and Weil: Increases in plasma oncotic pressure during acute cardiogenic pulmonary edema, Circulation 55:195, 1977). In contrast to hydrostatic pulmonary edema, leaky capillary pulmonary edema caused by injection of *Pseudomonas* bacteria or by histamine produced an increase in both the volume and the protein content of pulmonary lymph, an intrinsically much more unstable situation. The work which led to the following article was initially undertaken to test the notion that aspirin might inhibit histamine-induced pulmonary edema. The finding that the converse was actually the case was rendered even more interesting by a case of salicylate overdosage with extensive pulmonary edema on our service at that time. This article pulls together the scattered but impressive clinical evidence that aspirin-induced pulmonary edema is observed and provides a reasonable explanation of why it happens in the sheep model. – Ed. ◄

Salicylate Pulmonary Edema: Mechanism in Sheep and Review of Clinical Literature. Ronald E. Bowers, Kenneth L. Brigham and Patty Jill Owen[5] (Vanderbilt Univ.) were led by several clinical reports of salicylate-induced pulmonary edema to study the effects of aspirin infusion on lung fluid balance in awake sheep. Left atrial pressure was raised by 15 – 20 cm water in 9 sheep. Sixteen aspirin studies were done in 12 sheep by infusing a solution of sodium acetyl salicylate in buffer at rates delivering 300 – 1,200 mg aspirin per hour. Aspirin control studies were performed with a solution of buffer alone. The blood was incubated with sodium ^{51}Cr-chromate and the cells were reinjected.

Lymph flow doubled with an average increase in left atrial pressure of 14 cm water, and the lymph protein concentration declined both absolutely and relatively to plasma. Lung lymph flow in aspirin studies and increased-pressure studies is shown in Figure 11. The lymph flow increase was similar with both interventions. The decrease

(5) Am. Rev. Respir. Dis. 115:261 – 268, February, 1977.

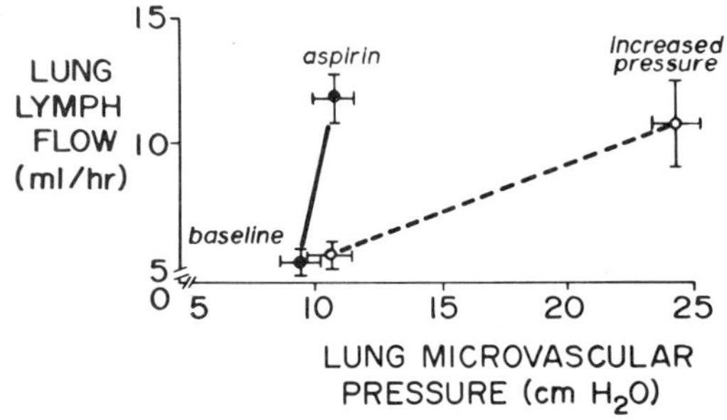

Fig 11.—Average steady-state lung lymph flow as function of estimated microvascular pressure (left atrial pressure + 0.4 [pulmonary artery pressure—left atrial pressure]) for 16 aspirin studies and 9 increased-pressure studies. Bars are mean ± SE. (Courtesy of Bowers, R. E., et al.: Am. Rev. Respir. Dis. 115:261–268, February, 1977.)

in the lymph-plasma protein concentration ratio was significantly greater after the mechanical pressure increase than after aspirin. The arterial Po_2 fell significantly on aspirin infusion and the pH increased. The ratio of extravascular lung water to dry weight of the bloodless lung was significantly elevated by aspirin infusion. Control infusions did not significantly alter the arterial blood gases, blood pH, vascular pressure or lung lymph flow.

Intravenous salicylate infusion in sheep can cause pulmonary edema. The edema apparently results from an increase in permeability of lung exchanging vessels to fluid and protein. Salicylate did not cause heart failure or substantial increases in pulmonary vascular pressures. Aspirin may cause edema in human beings even in doses considered to be therapeutic for some diseases, and pulmonary edema may be more common in salicylate overdosage. Both experimental and clinical data warrant a high index of suspicion of salicylate edema.

► [The levels of salicylate in these sheep were not determined routinely but when they were measured were not very high, but of the order of 10–15 μg/ml (Bowers, personal communication). It seemed reasonable to ask whether this was an easily observable phenomenon in normal individuals. Two Vanderbilt University medical students, Christopher Jackson and Philip Bressman, in a study which may or may not be published, measured all of the tests of small airways which could be done at our hospital including volume of isoflow, closing volumes and flow volume loops, in a group of young male Mormons (a remarkably homogeneous experimental group because of their avoidance of bad habits) before and after giving them sufficient aspirin to raise their salicylate levels to between 20 and 30 μg/ml and to make them feel fairly waffly. The results were negative. Measurements of lung water unfortunately were not done. Levine (Ventilatory stimulation by sodium salicylate: Role of thoracic receptors, J. Appl. Physiol. 41:639, 1976) arranged a preparation in dogs in which the carotid bodies and heads were cross perfused from normals. These dogs responded to injection of salicylate into the body circulation (head excluded) with a substantial increase in ventilation (118%). Injection so as to reach the head but not the body (spinal cord intact) resulted in a much smaller (23%) increase in ventilation. From this the author concluded that thoracic receptors were very important in mediating salicylate-induced hyperventilation; it is reasonable to postulate that increased lung water and interstitial receptors (J receptors) sensitive to the volume or pressure of interstitial lymph are involved.

Some other articles concerning noncardiogenic pulmonary edema are those by Sklar and Timms (Codeine-induced pulmonary edema, Chest 72:230, 1977), Sakar and Munshi (Postictal pulmonary edema, Postgrad. Med. 61:281, 1977) and Oswalt et al.

(Pulmonary edema as a complication of acute airway obstruction, J.A.M.A. 238:1833, 1977).—Ed.] ◄

Alterations of Gas Exchange Apparatus in Adult Respiratory Insufficiency Associated with Septicemia. Marianne Bachofen and Ewald R. Weibel[6] (Univ. of Berne) used a postmortem transthoracic injection method to fix lung tissues from 9 patients who died in different stages of acute respiratory distress syndrome due to septicemia; an ultrastructural and morphometric analysis was done. Small regions of lung were fixed in situ by multiple transcutaneous lung injections of stained glutaraldehyde solution within 10–20 minutes after death. Infraclavicular, medioaxillary and paravertebral sites usually were injected. The patients had no evidence of cardiac or respiratory ailments in their histories. All had respiratory distress syndrome during the course of their disease.

The normal appearances in Figure 12 are contrasted with those of acute-phase damage in Figure 13. Initially a widespread interstitial and alveolar edema was observed, with relatively well-preserved capillary endothelium and no large endothelial gaps. Local destruction of the squamous epithelium, often covered by hyaline membranes, and a rapid proliferation of type II epithelial cells were observed. In the subacute stage, cuboidal transformation of the epithelium and fibrotic changes in the interstitium predominated. The extent of fibrotic changes in lung architecture was not clearly related to the time course of the disease, but thickening of the air-blood barrier, estimated by morphometric analysis, mirrored the disturbances of gas exchange and lung mechanics. A considerable volume increase was observed in the acute stage and a further but highly variable augmentation in the

Fig 12.—Normal interalveolar septum of the human lung. Note that the gas exchange barrier is extremely thin on one side of the septum *(arrows)*. **Inset,** transition from thick to thin blood-gas barrier, where epithelial and endothelial basement membrane become fused *(fBM)*. *A,* alveolar space; *C,* capillary; *EC,* erythrocyte; *EP₁*, type I squamous epithelial cell; *IN,* interstitium; *BM,* basement membrane; *PE,* pericyte; *EP₂*, type II granular epithelial cell. (Courtesy of Bachofen, M., and Weibel, E. R.: Am. Rev. Respir. Dis. 116:589–615, October, 1977.)

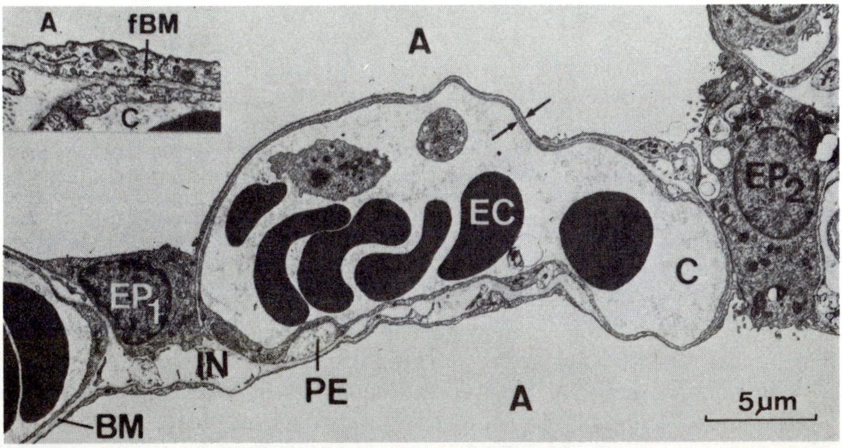

(6) Am. Rev. Respir. Dis. 116:589–615, October, 1977.

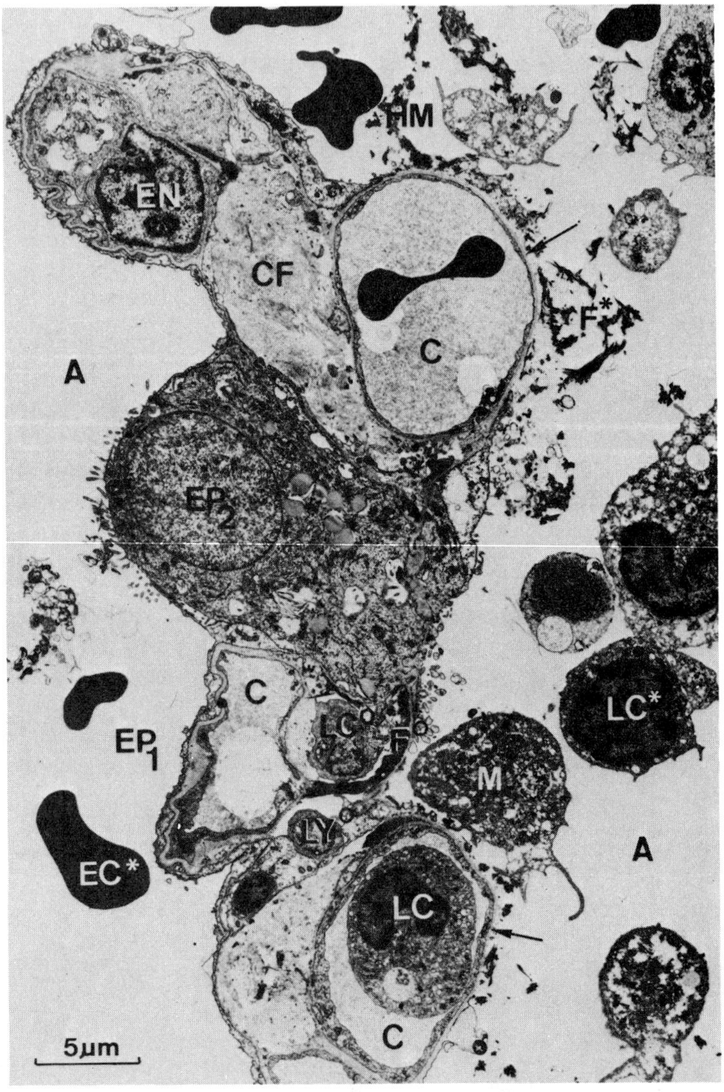

Fig 13. – Alveolar and interstitial edema in a patient who died 24 hours after onset of acute respiratory failure due to septicemia. Interstitial blood constituents are marked with degree sign and blood cells and fibrin in the alveolar space with asterisk. Arrows indicate areas of destroyed type I squamous epithelial cell. *HM,* hyaline membrane; *EN,* endothelium; *CF,* collagen fibers; *C,* capillary; *A,* alveolar space; EP_2, type II granular epithelial cell; EP_1, type I squamous epithelial cell; *LC,* leukocyte; *F,* fibrin; *LY,* lymphocyte; *EC,* erythrocyte. (Courtesy of Bachofen, M., and Weibel, E. R.: Am. Rev. Respir. Dis. 116:589–615, October, 1977.)

subacute phase in patients with the most serious gas-exchange disturbances. The findings are illustrated in Figure 14.

The nonspecificity of the lesions seen in the acute and subacute stages indicate a uniform, characteristic reaction pattern of the lung that does not reflect the type or route of the damaging agents. Thus it appears questionable whether lung biopsy specimens obtained from

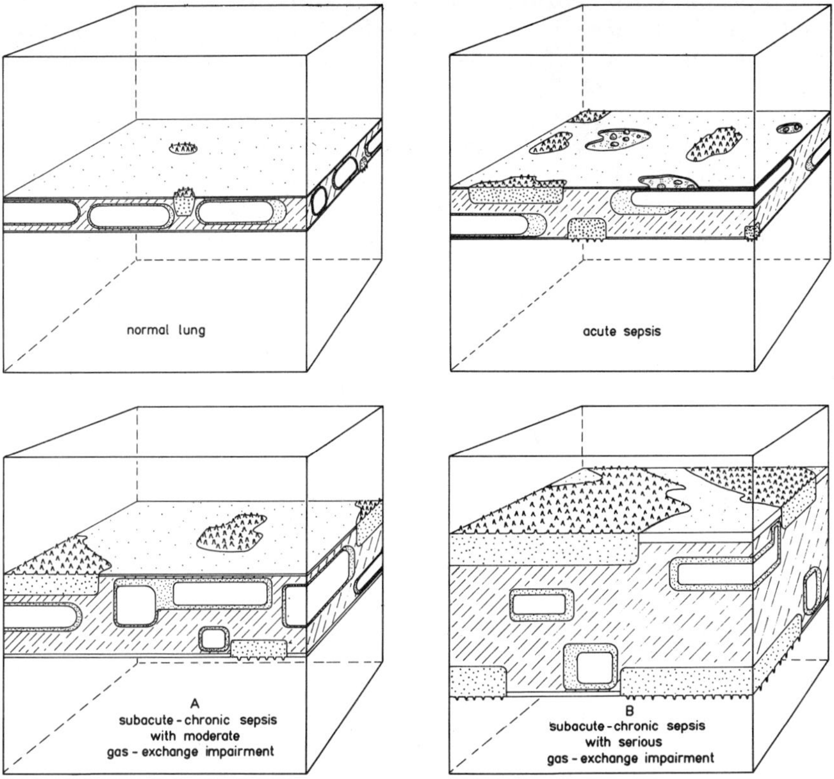

Fig 14. – Schematic reconstruction of normal and diseased interalveolar septa based on the morphometric data of the three patient groups in comparison to a normal lung. (Courtesy of Bachofen, M., and Weibel, E. R.: Am. Rev. Respir. Dis. 116:589–615, October, 1977.)

patients with acute respiratory distress syndrome can contribute to diagnosis of the underlying disease.

► [This very impressive morphological analysis has to be read in the original to be appreciated. It calls to mind an article by Guze written 15 years or so ago that indicated that hypocapnia and hypoxemia were prominent early findings in all cases of gram-negative septicemia, a point more recently emphasized by Vito et al. (Sepsis presenting as acute respiratory insufficiency, Surg. Gynecol. Obstet. 138:896, 1974). As emphasized in past YEAR BOOKS, the synergistic effect of systemic infection and hemodynamic factors (heart failure) in producing pulmonary edema should always be kept in mind, particularly so when, as is often the case in cirrhotics and debilitated persons, oncotic factors (hypoalbuminemia) also favor increased movement of water from the capillaries to the pulmonary interstitium.

The prognosis of the individual case of acute respiratory failure cannot be predicted at present. Some patients get completely well and some die no matter how well treated. There is accumulating evidence that at least one factor determining outcome is the degree to which the microvasculature is permanently damaged. Zapol and Snider (Pulmonary hypertension in severe acute respiratory failure, N. Engl. J. Med. 296:476, 1977) indicate that persisting elevation of the pulmonary vascular resistance is associated with a poor outcome. Case 22-1977 of the Case Records of the Massachusetts General Hospital (ibid., p. 1279) was the case of a patient with fatal acute respiratory failure secondary to trauma who at post mortem demonstrated "diffuse vascular obstruction with pulmonary vascular thrombosis or microembolism and diffuse interstitial fibrosis. . . ." – Ed.] ◄

Pulmonary Aspiration of Gastric Contents. Lincoln J. Bynum and Alan K. Pierce[7] (Univ. of Texas Health Science Center, Dallas) reviewed the records of 227 patients given a diagnosis of "aspiration pneumonia" in 1969–74, including 50 in whom aspiration of gastric contents was documented by witnessing the episode, seeing gastric contents in the airways at intubation or recovering gastric contents by suction from an endotracheal tube. The most common underlying disorders were sedative drug overdosage, general anesthesia and cerebrovascular accident. Tracheal intubation was performed in 94% of the 17 patients presenting with shock or apnea and in 52% of the others. The respective mortality rates were 59% and 12%.

Mortality rates were 48% for patients with an initial (a/A) P_{O_2} of 0.50 or below and 14% for those with higher values. Progressive radiographic clearing was observed in 62% of cases, with resolution of infil-

TABLE 1.—Results of Sputum Bacteriologic Studies in 21 Patients with Potentially Pathogenic Organisms in Cultures after Aspiration of Gastric Contents

	Infected patients (n = 13)		Uninfected patients (n = 8)	
	(no.)	*(%)*	*(no.)*	*(%)*
Gram-positive	2	15	0	0
Gram-negative	5	39	7	88
Gram-positive and negative	6	46	1	12
Streptococcus pneumoniae	3		1	
Staphylococcus aureus	5		0	
Enterococcus sp.	2		0	
Pseudomonas aeruginosa	4		2	
Proteus sp.	4		0	
Escherichia coli	3		0	
Klebsiella-Aerobacter sp.	2		4	
Citrobacter sp.	1		0	
"Gram-negative rod"	1		1	

TABLE 2.—Effect of Antimicrobial Drugs and Corticosteroids on Infection and Mortality in 54 Patients with Aspiration of Gastric Contents*

	Infected	Not Infected	Survived	Died
Antimicrobial drugs (total)				
Treated	12	29	29	12
Untreated	1	8	7	2
Antimicrobial drugs (prophylactic)				
Treated	12	25	24	13
Untreated	1	12	12	1
Corticosteroids				
Treated	10	23	21	12
Untreated	3	14	15	2

*Figures indicate number of patients in each category. There were no significant differences among groups by chi-square analysis.

(7) Am. Rev. Respir. Dis. 114:1129–1136, December, 1976.

trates in a mean of 4.5 days. Six patients had brief courses ending in death, and 13 showed early clearing and later developed new or extending infiltrates. Infection developed in 13 patients after aspiration. The results of sputum bacteriologic study are given in Table 1 and the effects of antimicrobial drugs and steroids on infection and mortality in Table 2. Antimicrobial drugs were given to 41 patients, prophylactically to 37. Intubation and ventilatory support were used in 33 cases. Parenteral steroids were used from the outset in 33 patients; most patients received the daily equivalent of 100–400 mg hydrocortisone. Fourteen (28%) of 50 patients died a mean of 7.2 days after aspiration. Patients who died were older than survivors, had a higher rate of shock or apnea and showed greater impairment of gas exchange initially.

Aspiration of gastric contents apparently produces a distinctive clinical syndrome that is easily distinguished from other aspiration-related lung disease. There is little clinical overlap with aspiration of oropharyngeal contents or of a foreign body. Awareness of the features of this condition should facilitate its diagnosis and permit more rational management.

► [The term "a/A P_{O_2}" simply means the ratio of arterial to calculated alveolar oxygen tension (see 1977 YEAR BOOK, p. 105, for calculation of alveolar oxygen). Assuming a Pa_{CO_2} of 40 on room air, an a/A P_{O_2} of 0.5 would mean a Pa_{O_2} of 45 mm Hg or less.

The first purpose of this article was to distinguish aspiration of gastric contents from other syndromes of "aspiration pneumonia," specifically anaerobic pleuropulmonary infections including abscess and empyemas due to aspiration of oropharyngeal material and localized bronchial obstruction due to aspiration of foreign bodies. The gastric acid aspiration syndrome was always associated with some compromise of consciousness. Ninety percent of those in whom anesthesia was a factor were patients having emergency operations or procedures. The onset was almost immediate, 1 or 2 hours within the event, with fever, tachypnea, rales and serious hypoxemia. The x-ray abnormalities in some cases resembled diffuse pulmonary edema but in 20% were unilateral and in 38% were confined to one lobe, most frequently the right lower lobe. The clinical courses could be grouped into three patterns, quick death (12%), gradual progressive improvement over 4–6 days (62%), and a biphasic pattern with initial clinical and x-ray improvement followed by new infiltrates and worsening symptoms, this last representing superinfection, usually with nosocomial gram-negative bacteria. The authors felt that steroids were not helpful and that antibiotics should be used only when superinfection had been demonstrated. They could not comment on the efficacy of intubation and ventilatory support.

Wynne and Modell have also reviewed this subject (Respiratory aspiration of stomach contents, Ann. Intern. Med. 87:466, 1977). They comment on the importance of the pH of the aspirates, those with values over 2.5 causing much less trouble. (It seems reasonable that preoperative patients may soon be treated with cimetidine since the preoperative use of oral antacid has been recommended.) The importance of surfactant destruction by acid was stressed. They advised against bronchoscopy unless aspiration of particulate material was suspected and advised against lavage in any event. They commented on the dangers of nasogastric tubes which can function inefficiently and compromise esophageal sphincters, favoring aspiration. The evidence that steroids help was reviewed and rejected, as was the case for prophylactic antibiotics. Stewardson (Pulmonary aspiration, an update, Arch. Surg. 112:1192, 1977) has also reviewed the subject in a crisp, somewhat more surgical style with the same conclusions except for advocation of the use of albumin (which is controversial; see Lowe et al.: Crystalloid vs. colloid in the etiology of pulmonary failure after trauma: A randomized trial in man, Surgery 81:676, 1977) and early intervention with intubation and positive end-expiratory pressure. For more discussion of steroids and albumin see the 1977 YEAR BOOK (pp. 138–141). Wolfe et al. (Diagnosis of gastric aspiration by fiberoptic bronchoscopy, Chest 70:458, 1976) indicate that diffuse erythema of the subsegmental bronchi is a fairly specific finding for acid aspiration. Irwin et al. (Food asphyxiation in hospitalized patients, J.A.M.A. 237:2744, 1977) discuss this quite different problem in chronically hospitalized patients, which is often misdiagnosed as myocardial infarction until autopsy. – Ed.] ◄

Continuous Positive Airway Pressure versus Positive End-Expiratory Pressure in Respiratory Distress Syndrome. Dhiraj M. Shah, Jonathan C. Newell, Robert E. Dutton and Samuel R. Powers, Jr.[8] (Albany Med. College), with technical assistance from Chandler M. Ralph, compared the respiratory and hemodynamic effects of the sequential use of continuous positive airway pressure (CPAP) and positive end-expiratory pressure (PEEP) in 9 adults with respiratory distress syndrome who could maintain spontaneous ventilation with a tidal volume about 300 ml and a Pa_{CO_2} below 45 torr. Measurements were made in 11 instances with each patient on 5 or 10 cm water CPAP or PEEP and in 9 instances with each patient on the ventilator without PEEP. A tidal volume of 12 – 15 ml/kg was used, with a level of CPAP identical to the level of PEEP being administered. The patients had had multiple injuries requiring intubation, mechanical ventilation and increased inspired oxygen.

Initially the mean physiologic shunt was 16%, the mean functional residual capacity (FRC) 1,920 ml, the mean cardiac index 4.2 L per minute per sq m of body surface and the mean Pa_{CO_2} 32 torr on ventilation without PEEP. With the change from PEEP to CPAP the mean Pa_{O_2} rose from 113 to 130 torr and the mean shunt fell from 14% on PEEP to 11%. The cardiac index rose on CPAP in 9 instances but increased on PEEP in only 2 instances; there was no change in mean cardiac index. Changes in oxygen delivery and consumption were not significantly different with CPAP and PEEP (table). The FRC did not increase significantly with PEEP The mean pulmonary wedge pressure rose from 5 torr on PEEP to 8 torr on CPAP.

Hemodynamic Data under Condition of Continuous Positive Airway Pressure (CPAP), Mechanical Ventilation without Positive End-Expiratory Pressure (O PEEP) and Mechanical Ventilation with Positive End-Expiratory Pressure (PEEP)*

Case No.	*CI (L/min/sq. M. body surface area)* CPAP	O PEEP	PEEP	*PAP (torr)* CPAP	O PEEP	PEEP	*PWP (torr)* CPAP	O PEEP	PEEP	*Oxygen delivery (ml./min.)* CPAP	O PEEP	PEEP	*$\dot{V}O_2$ (ml./min.)* CPAP	O PEEP	PEEP
1	4.3	3.9	3.0	16	14	17	5	2	4	1,808	1,629	1,237	274	231	197
2	5.7	6.7	5.2	21	17	18	10	5	8	1,345	1,341	1,067	290	238	194
3	3.2	2.7	3.1	20	12	15	9	3	6	912	769	887	133	115	144
4	4.8	—	4.5	24	—	27	13	—	13	1,270	—	1,177	320	—	257
5	3.2	3.9	4.2	20	18	20	5	5	5	838	1,157	1,157	201	236	281
6	5.1	4.8	4.4	20	18	19	8	4	6	1,076	1,016	940	304	260	237
7a	4.2	—	4.1	16	—	9	10	—	6	1,069	—	1,081	204	—	201
7b	4.4	—	3.6	12	—	9	9	—	4	1,113	—	935	213	—	193
8a	3.3	4.2	5.7	13	11	18	2	−3	−4	1,115	1,295	1,705	315	341	490
8b	3.8	—	3.7	17	—	17	3	—	2	956	—	946	264	—	248
9	3.1	3.1	2.7	21	15	19	13	6	9	839	849	724	170	177	193
Mean	4.1	4.2	4.0	18	15	17	8	3	5	1,121	1,150	1,078	244	228	240
S.E.	±0.3	±0.5	±0.3	±1.0	±1.0	±1.5	±1	±1	±1	±84	±113	±77	±19	±26	±28

†$P < 0.001$

*CI, cardiac index; PAP, pulmonary artery pressure; PWP, pulmonary wedge pressure; VO_2, oxygen consumption.
†Compares CPAP with PEEP.

(8) J. Thorac. Cardiovasc. Surg. 74:557 – 562, October, 1977.

These findings suggest that, in patients who are able to maintain spontaneous ventilation, CPAP is more effective than the same level of PEEP in improving arterial oxygenation by the lung without adverse effects on cardiac output. Positive end-expiratory pressure hyperinflates the remaining normal lung and diverts blood flow to the abnormal lung, thus the potential benefit from increased mean airway pressure on gas exchange may be negated by the effect of a greater perfusion inequality.

► [The concept of the use of positive-pressure breathing to treat pulmonary edema was introduced in 1938 by Barach and associates (Ann. Intern. Med. 12:454, 1938); during the 1940's and 1950's this was usually accomplished with a fenestrated face mask which had holes of various calibers, creating a graded obstruction to expiration while being supplied with freely flowing oxygen during inspiration. This was essentially positive pressure during expiration. The aim of therapy, whether or not it was crisply formulated at the time, was to reexpand small airways collapsed as a result of interstitial pulmonary edema, and thereby to lessen shunting and improve oxygenation much the same as with present-day devices. It was protocol to dial in progressively smaller holes, thus increasing the mask pressure during expiration until the patient would not tolerate it or until the blood pressure dropped and the pulse rate rose.

Granting that it is a gross oversimplification, acute respiratory failure resembles interstitial pulmonary edema, and its treatment, insofar as it consists of increasing mean airways pressure so as to recruit collapsed airways, is similar in many respects.

Continuous positive airways pressure is a treatment modality within the capabilities of most respiratory therapy units. Insofar as the usual patient with acute respiratory failure or adult respiratory distress syndrome (ARDS) has no problem moving air and in point of fact is usually hyperventilating, CPAP has much to recommend it. If successful, weaning involves only decreasing the pressure in the system and does not require moving from controlled to spontaneous ventilation.

One very attractive option utilizes intermittent mandatory ventilation (IMV) with positive end-expiratory pressure (PEEP) to supplement spontaneous breathing in a pressurized system (CPAP). The most modern of the sophisticated ventilators are equipped to furnish CPAP and IMV together or can be modified to do so (Geodan and Seed: A new versatile breathing system for CPPB, Anesthesia 31:917, 1976).

The continued spontaneous use of the muscles of ventilation keeps them in tone, so to speak, and the characteristics of airways pressures during CPAP are less liable to produce decrease in venous return and hypotension than is continuous PEEP. The physiology of these various interventions is complex, affecting heart, airways, pulmonary vascular resistance and venous return in complex ways. However, if one focuses on end results without getting lost in the intricacies of the physiologic effects, treatment principles can be stated rather simply. The therapeutic aim is to provide an acceptable Pa_{O_2} (60–70 mm Hg) at concentrations of inhaled oxygen less than 60%, and preferably less than 50%, while avoiding serious respiratory alkalosis or hypotension, and to be ever on guard for barotrauma (pneumothorax, pneumomediastinum—always associated with subcutaneous emphysema—and pneumoperitoneum). An important practical point is avoidance of morphine and sympatholytic drugs when possible because these cause loss of venous tone and render the patient much more susceptible to hypotension as a consequence of increased mean intrathoracic pressure. As mentioned several times before, the use of steroids and albumin is controversial and probably falls under the general purview of Loeb's third rule of therapy—when you don't know what to do, do nothing. Pontoppidan, who has contributed so much distinguished work in this area, states, "There is no evidence that treatment with protein-containing solutions results in more rapid recovery from ARF. Crystalloid solutions may be preferable during the capillary leak phase, and protein-containing solutions once capillary integrity is established." (Pontoppidan et al.: Respiratory intensive care, Anesthesiology 47: 96, 1977). Spotting that transition point would be tricky. This review is an excellent one.—Ed.] ◄

► ↓The following article is included in this section because of the remarkable incidence it has recorded of gastrointestinal bleeding in ARDS. The use of cimetidine in this circumstance will almost certainly be studied soon and would seem to be justified *a priori*. – Ed. ◄

Gastrointestinal Hemorrhage in Patients in a Respiratory Intensive Care Unit. There are no data concerning risk factors associated with development of gastrointestinal hemorrhage in patients in the respiratory intensive care unit. In order to identify these factors, Susan K. Harris, Roger C. Bone and William E. Ruth[9] (Univ. of Kansas Med. Center, Kansas City, Kan.) reviewed the charts of 98 patients admitted with primary respiratory diagnosis during 1 year (1974–75). Twenty patients (20%) developed gastrointestinal hemorrhage. They had a mean fall in hemoglobin of 2 gm/100 ml, and required 1.5 units of blood in transfusion per episode of bleeding.

Patients who bled had a mean age of 48 years, compared to 51 years for nonbleeders. Differences between the two groups in steroid therapy and heparin administration were not significant. Rate of bleeding was 9% in the 44 patients with chronic obstructive lung disease and 85% in 13 patients with adult respiratory distress syndrome.

Bleeding patients required longer ventilator support during their illness and had a longer stay in the intensive care unit and in the hospital. Ten patients had more than one episode of bleeding in the same admission. Twelve bleeding patients and 2 nonbleeders were thrombocytopenic. Eight of 14 patients given antacids after onset of bleeding had no further episodes. Only 2 bleeding patients had received antacids prophylactically, compared with 41 of 78 nonbleeders, a highly significant difference.

The mortality was 65% for bleeding patients and 22% for nonbleeders. All 11 autopsies showed multiple diffuse areas of ulceration in the upper gastrointestinal tract.

Diagnosis of the adult respiratory distress syndrome is a significant risk factor for development of gastrointestinal hemorrhage. Patients who bled while in the intensive care unit were more seriously ill than the nonbleeders and had a higher mortality. Prophylactic antacid administration to patients at high risk of bleeding might reduce morbidity and mortality in such patients.

Diagnosis of Causes for Acute Respiratory Distress by Pressure-Volume Curves. Patients often have episodes of deterioration in respiratory status during mechanical ventilation. Determinations of total respiratory compliance have not been generally applied to the evaluation of treatment in this setting. Roger C. Bone[1] (Univ. of Kansas) prospectively evaluated the contribution of pressure-volume relationships in the respiratory system as monitoring measurements in 25 consecutive patients who required continuous mechanical ventilation for 72 hours or longer. Measurements were repeated every 8 hours and whenever increasing hypoxemia or respiratory distress developed. Static and dynamic measurements of pressure and volume were made at tidal volumes of 0.6 to 1.2 L. Pressure-volume curves are illustrated in Figure 15.

---

(9) Chest 72:301–304, September, 1977.
(1) Ibid., 70:740–746, December, 1976.

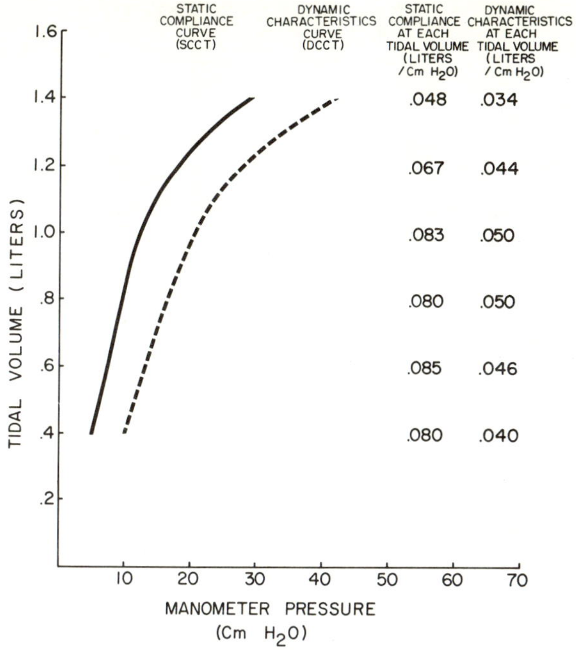

Fig 15.—Pressure-volume curves. Static compliance at each tidal volume is calculated by dividing tidal volume by "plateau" pressure at that tidal volume. Shift to right of compliance curve occurred with pulmonary diseases that decreased total respiratory compliance. Value for dynamic characteristics at each tidal volume is calculated by dividing tidal volume by "peak" pressure at end of inspiration. Shift to right of curve for dynamic characteristics occurred with diseases associated with increased airway resistance, such as bronchoconstriction or retained secretions. (Courtesy of Bone, R. C.: Chest 70:740–746, December, 1976.)

Curve determinations contributed to medical management in 22 of the 25 patients. Thirty-two superimposed respiratory complications occurred in these patients, which resulted in variable changes in the curves for compliance and dynamic characteristics. The curves were most useful when determined at multiple tidal-volume values. No complications resulted from determination of the curves. The changes that occurred with complicating pulmonary diseases are shown in Figure 16. Bronchoconstriction was reflected by a right-shifted curve for dynamic characteristics, with little or no shift in the compliance curve. The curve for dynamic characteristics returned to the left after aspiration of retained secretions in some cases. Curves for static compliance and dynamic characteristics were shifted equally to the right in tension pneumothorax, atelectasis, right main stem bronchial intubation, and pulmonary edema. Right-shifted curves also resulted from widespread bronchopneumonia.

The determination of effective dynamic and static relationships between pressure and volume is a simple, noninvasive means of diagnosing pulmonary disease and the effect of treatment in patients on mechanical ventilation. The equipment needed is the same as that required for continuous mechanical ventilation. The determinations are

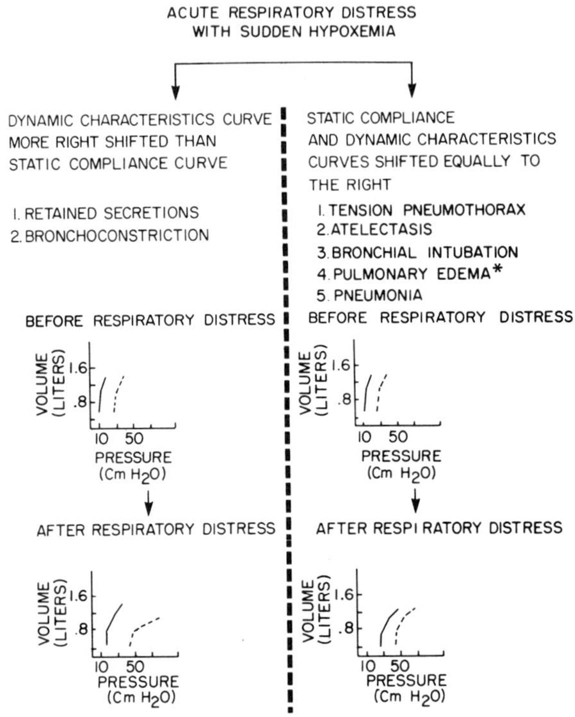

Fig 16.—Causes of acute respiratory distress in patients receiving assisted ventilation. After acute respiratory distress in patients treated with mechanical ventilation, static compliance curves *(solid curves)* and curves for dynamic characteristics *(dashed curves)* compared to same curves plotted prior to respiratory distress will assist in differential diagnosis of cause for acute respiratory distress. Idealized curves obtained before and after respiratory distress categorized by their pattern of abnormality are shown. *Asterisk*, adult respiratory distress syndrome (cardiogenic and noncardiogenic). (Courtesy of Bone, R. C.: Chest 70:740–746, December, 1976.)

now used routinely in all patients having mechanical ventilation.

► [Sophisticated people I have talked to about this have expressed some doubts. This article is included, however, because the basic principles are ones which should be utilized in caring for all patients on controlled ventilation, particularly when the problem is acute respiratory failure with stiff lungs. One should note the peak pressure and the expiratory plateau pressure on the pressure dial. The latter is easier to see when the expiratory retard dial on the MA-1 is turned all the way to the right. Very high peak pressures, out of proportion to the expiratory plateau pressures, suggest that something is wrong with the airways, either bronchospasm or obstruction with secretions. The tidal volume divided by the plateau pressure gives a reasonable index of the stiffness of the lungs and chest cage and, therefore, an index which can be followed to indicate improvement or deterioration. Prolonged (24 hours or more) controlled ventilation with PEEP is almost always associated with further accumulation of interstitial edema (Butler et al.: The hemodynamics of pulmonary edema, Am. Rev. Respir. Dis. [Suppl.] 115: 173, 1977; and Caldini et al.: Effect of continuous positive-pressure ventilation (CPPV) on edema formation in dog lung, J. Appl. Physiol. 39:672, 1975). This may be signaled by a fall in Pa_{O_2} and compliance and may indicate use of a diuretic.—Ed.] ◄

Asthma and Related Disorders

Clinical Significance of Pulmonary Function Tests: The One Best Test for Evaluating the Effects of Bronchodilator Therapy. It has been claimed that body plethysmography is the most sensitive test for evaluating bronchodilators and, that from spirometry, the mid-half flow rate (FEF25–75%) is the most sensitive index. Richard W. Light, Steven A. Conrad and Ronald B. George[2] (Louisiana State Univ. Med. Center, Shreveport) evaluated the 1-second forced expiratory volume (FEV_1), forced vital capacity (FVC), FEV_1/FVC%, FEF25–75%, specific airway conductance (Gaw/V_L) and airway resistance (Raw) for their ability to separate different drug regimens.

Twenty adults with reversible airways disease manifested by a 15% improvement in FEV_1 after administration of 150 μg isoproterenol randomly received fenoterol, 400, 200 or 100 μg, isoproterenol 150 μg, and placebo in a double-blind crossover design. Lung function tests were performed serially at predetermined intervals.

Generally the largest improvement in percentage was in the Gaw/V_L, followed by the FEF25–75% and then the FEV_1, Raw and FVC. The least improvement in percentage was in the FEV_1/FVC%.

Fig 17.—F values for the FEV_1, Gaw/V_L and FEF25–75% at various times after drug administration. Critical values for F where P = 0.01 and P = 0.05 are indicated by the dotted lines. F values are highest for the FEV_1 for the first 240 minutes. (Courtesy of Light, R. W., et al.: Chest 72:512–516, October, 1977.)

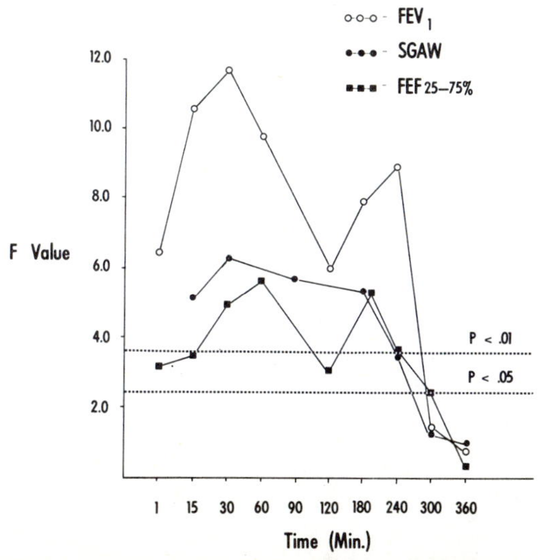

(2) Chest 72:512–516, October, 1977.

With analysis of variance, the F value for the FEV_1 was highest, followed by that for the Raw and FVC. When the drug regimens were compared, the FEV_1 yielded more significant differences than the other parameters. In no drug comparison did plethysmography or the FEF25–75% allow more or different conclusions than did the FEV_1. When the F value for each test was computed at each interval of testing, at no point in time did the Gaw/V_L, Raw or FEF25–75% add to the conclusions available from the FEV_1 and FVC (Fig 17).

The FEV_1 is the best test for evaluating the response to bronchodilators in patients with obstructive airway disease. When combined with the FVC, it permits the maximum number of conclusions. Addition of body plethysmography and the FEF25–75% does not allow further conclusions. With the FEV_1, the highest number of significant differentiations can be made. The FEV_1/FVC% was found to be a poor index for measuring bronchodilatation.

► [During the past several years a number of tests have been developed to detect obstruction or compromise of the small (under 2 mm) airways. Some of these, such as frequency dependence of compliance (1973 YEAR BOOK, p. 104) and closing volumes (ibid., pp. 107–108), seem unlikely to become clinically important. Others, such as the maximum expiratory flow volume curve (MEFV) (1974 YEAR BOOK, pp. 101–103; 1975 YEAR BOOK, pp. 116–119; and 1977 YEAR BOOK, pp. 107–109) and the numbers generated from it and reported on the chart, are liable to be with us from now on, since the pulmonary function consoles now used by most hospitals are based on the MEFVC maneuver. The number of the "numbers" is the cause of some confusion.

This article by Light et al. has attempted to clarify the situation. Its conclusions, while probably valid, need amplification. The problem is that bronchospasm can involve large airways, small airways or even alveolar ducts in any mix. Involvement of larger airways will modify the earlier, effort-dependent portions of the MEFV curve when the lungs are pretty much filled with air and effort makes a difference; these include the percent of FEV in 1 second and the peak expiratory flow rate. Involvement of the smaller airways is thought to produce abnormalities in the more effort-independent portions of the curve when the lungs contain less air and effort makes much less difference; these include the slope of the line drawn between the points representing the instantaneous flow rates after exhalation of 25% and after exhalation of 75% of the vital capacity—FEV 25–75, between 75% and 85% of vital capacity—FEF75–85, and the flow rate of 50% of vital capacity (maximum mid-expiratory flow rate). Involvement of the very, very small airways may produce a constricted FEV with nothing to suggest airways obstruction (Hudgel et al.: Reversible restrictive lung disease simulating asthma, Ann. Intern. Med. 85:328, 1976; and 1977 YEAR BOOK, pp. 122–123) and present with exertional dyspnea and cough without any wheezing (1976 YEAR BOOK, pp. 169–170).

These relationships and the problem facing the pulmonary physiologist are also well discussed by Leifer and Wittig (Differing patterns of pulmonary function response to bronchodilators in asthmatics, Ann. Allergy 38:91, 1977; and Unreliability of maximum mid-expiratory flow rate as sole index of bronchodilator response in chronic asthma, ibid., p. 96). Doctors Sobol and Emirgil (Pulmonary function tests and the diagnosis of bronchial asthma, ibid., 37:340, 1976) caution that the situation is sufficiently complex that the clinician, when he has diagnosed asthma on clinical grounds, should not be too much bothered if the results of the pulmonary function test do not always demonstrate reversible bronchospasm, which may be the most important lesson of all of this.—Ed.] ◄

Asthma: Analysis of Sudden Deaths and Ventilatory Arrests in Hospital. Death may occur suddenly in asthma patients in the hospital, and it is usually difficult to understand why. M. R. Hetzel, T. J. H. Clark and M. A. Branthwaite[3] (Brompton Hosp., London) analyzed

(3) Br. Med. J. 1:808–811, Mar. 26, 1977.

Clinical Features of 9 Patients Who Sustained Respiratory Crises with Ventilatory Arrest

	General ward	High dependency unit
Number of episodes	9*	1
Occurrence between midnight and 0600	7	1
Pulse rate >120/min on admission	0	1
Pulsus paradoxus >20 mm Hg on admission	1	0
Peak expiratory flow rate <100 l/min on admission	4	0
Diurnal variation in peak expiratory flow rate >50%	8†	1
Treated with >10 mg prednisone/day	3	1
Blood gas analysis on admission	2	1
Failed resuscitation	3	0

*One patient had two episodes on two separate occasions.
†One patient with severe nocturnal symptoms but no peak flow chart recovered.

asthma admissions to evaluate accepted criteria of acute attacks as indicators for patients at risk of sudden death. The study was retrospective for 2 years and prospective for a further 6 months. All patients admitted to adult wards with a diagnosis of asthma were studied.

There were 1,345 admissions of 993 patients (540 women), 1,169 for treatment of uncomplicated asthma. Physiologic criteria for uncomplicated asthma were met by 827 patients, 351 of whom were initially treated in a special-care unit.

Only 1 nonfatal ventilatory arrest occurred in the special-care unit. Nine other arrests, 3 of them fatal, occurred on general wards. Accepted clinical criteria of a severe attack were not present in the episodes occurring outside the special unit (table). The risk of sudden death could not be related to severity of the attack, but it did correlate with presence of excessive diurnal variation in the peak expiratory flow rate (PEFR) illustrated in Figure 18. All 9 patients who sustained respi-

Fig 18.—Daily 4-hourly (0600–2200) recordings of peak expiratory flow rate *(PEFR)* in man aged 52. Days are marked at 0000; solid circles indicate readings at 0600. Recurrent >50% morning falls in PEFR precede respiratory crisis at 0400 of 5th day. (Courtesy of Hetzel, M. R., et al.: Br. Med. J. 1:808–811, Mar. 26, 1977.)

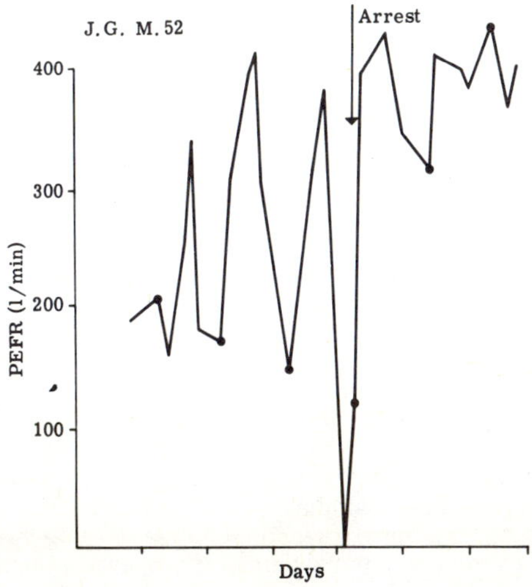

ratory crises exhibited more than 50% swings in PEFR. The 3 deaths occurred 5–8 days after admission. Two autopsies showed extensive mucus plugging of the airways.

Large diurnal swings in PEFR with an early morning fall were observed in all patients who sustained crises. Respiratory crises were common in the first few days of admission. Patients may die suddenly of asthma in the hospital even if the attack is initially judged to be not severe. Patients at risk are not easily recognized, and conventional criteria for diagnosing severe attacks have little value in predicting potentially fatal cases. Wide diurnal variation in the PEFR may be a better clue, and patients who exhibit this finding should receive intensive treatment.

► [This is part of an accumulating body of evidence that the danger period for the hospitalized asthmatic is during sleep, especially in the early morning. It is worth noting that only 4 of the 10 episodes of respiratory crises occurred while the patient was receiving steroids and 9 of these episodes occurred while the patient was on the general ward rather than in the specialized respiratory unit (see the table). Many, including ourselves, feel that patients sick enough with asthma to be in the hospital are sick enough to be receiving steroids. The tendency of physicians and patients alike to underestimate the severity of an attack was also emphasized by MacDonald et al. (Asthma deaths in Cardiff, 1963–74: Fifty-three deaths in hospital, Br. Med. J. 2:721, 1976). Rubinfeld and Pain (How mild is mild asthma? Thorax 32:177, 1977) demonstrated that in some subjects the threshold of symptoms with Mecholyl-induced bronchospasm was associated with advanced derangement of airflow and lung volumes.

Hetzel and associates have made some detailed physiologic observations at 6 A.M. and 2 P.M. in 16 asthmatics with marked diurnal variation in bronchial obstruction (Hetzel et al.: Physiologic patterns in early morning asthma, ibid., p. 418). Some of their mean values expressed as percent of predicted are as follows, the first figures being those measured at 6 A.M. and the second at 2 P.M.: peak expiratory flow rate (PEFR), 35.4% and 68.7%; forced vital capacity (FVC), 64.9% and 90.4%; 1-second FEV (FEV_1), 42.4% and 73%, functional residual capacity (FRC), 132% and 109%; and residual volume (RV), 177% and 128%. Unexpectedly, the arterial oxygen tension and the alveolar-arterial oxygen gradient (see 1977 YEAR BOOK, p. 105) changed very little. Somewhat more than half of their patients showed a good response to salbutamol at 6 A.M., but a large minority did not, while responding well at 2 P.M. There was a notable absence of severe subjective symptoms.

Another study by the same investigators attempted to determine the reason for this diurnal variation (Clark and Hetzel: Diurnal variation of asthma, Br. J. Dis. Chest 71:87, 1977). They found it was not related to being out of bed during the day, such as would be expected to be the case if the important factor were to have been bed-related allergens; lying in bed all day did not eliminate the 2 P.M. improvement. They showed, by studies of patients who changed from day to night working hours, that it was related to sleep; that is to say, the diurnal pattern almost immediately adjusted itself to the patient's wake-sleep pattern – much more promptly, as a matter of fact, than other basic diurnal biorhythms such as body temperature and blood cortisol levels. They also felt it was unrelated to endogenous cortisol and was not modified by exogenous corticosteroid treatment (see below). They concluded that probably a very important contributory factor, if not the most important, was interruption of treatment during sleeping hours. This has obvious therapeutic implications, as discussed below. However, untreated asthmatics also have morning worsening, in our experience.

Margaret Turner-Warwick, in an article she described as "table talk" rather than scientific data, discussed several different patterns of asthmatics based on serial frequent measurements of peak expiratory flow (On observing patterns of air flow obstruction in chronic asthma, ibid., p. 73). First she wisely noted that classification of asthmatics according to causative agent was probably overly simplistic and not very helpful. Patients with atopic (IgE-mediated) asthma may also have attacks provoked by nonimmunologic causes such as "exercise, infection, change in temperature and humidity or emotional upset." Also she noted that whereas "polar cases," such as childhood atopic patients with clearly allergic, intermittent, completely reversible asthma and high levels of IgE, do exist, most cases are not nearly so clear-cut and "extrinsic" and "intrinsic" asthma patients often merge or drift from patterns resembling the former to patterns resembling the latter. Accordingly, classification based on presumed immunopathogenesis is often clinically unrewarding. She proposed a classification based on observed patterns of air flow (an existential classification if you will kindly permit) and drew some interesting although admittedly preliminary therapeutic implications. One clear-cut pattern she perceived was described as "brittle," connoting patients who showed chaotic and unpredictable drops in expiratory flow rate unrelated to time of day or anything else that could be discerned. Characteristically they responded promptly and completely to aerosol bronchodilator, and efforts to stabilize their course with theophylline or corticosteroids did not work. For these she thought that use of an aerosol bronchodilator as required was probably optimal therapy. The second group she termed "morning dippers" with predictable severe morning impairment, the group discussed in this article by Hetzel et al. She noted that measurements made in the afternoon or evening were usually quite good, so that the patient's veracity might be doubted unless early morning values were measured. In these, she felt a long-acting bronchodilator at bedtime, either by mouth or by aerosol or both, had real therapeutic promise. (We have a patient who was unable to go to work several mornings each month until he began to use a long-acting bronchodilator aerosol at bedtime and when he awoke during the middle of the night.) She felt this pattern was not modified by steroids. Her third classification, "irreversible," was less crisp. These patients never achieved a normal PEFR, but some responded partially to bronchodilators and some gradually improved on steroids over a period of weeks. Importantly, in some the FEV showed a clear-cut, gradual, but substantial response to steroids while conventional measurements of bronchial obstruction such as the PEFR or FEV_1 did not. The fourth she termed "drifters," patients who gradually got completely better on steroids while never showing much of a response on bronchodilators. This is an important group, justifying a therapeutic 7- to 10-day trial of steroids.

The question of steroids and diurnal variation is, in our opinion, unresolved. Soutar et al. (Nocturnal and morning asthma: Relationship to plasma corticosteroids and response to cortisol infusion, Thorax 30:436, 1975) showed that infusion of steroids in quantities sufficient to eliminate the diurnal trough of plasma cortisol did not modify the diurnal pattern of airways obstruction. It is of note that therapeutic doses of steroids were *not* studied. Falliers et al. (1973 YEAR BOOK, p. 177) noted elimination of the diurnal variation of PEFR with high doses of steroids. The thrust of their article was that the upper limit of chronic, every-other-day steroid dosage should be that amount which *did not* eliminate the diurnal variation in PEFR on the day *off* steroids. Whereas some effect of steroids can be noted in 2 or 3 hours after injection (1977 YEAR BOOK, p. 117), maximum response is not observed until 6 or 7 days of treatment (1976 YEAR BOOK, discussion on p. 1967). We believe that the effects of pharmacologic doses of corticosteroids in modifying or eliminating diurnal variation in air flow remains an open question.

For completeness sake, mention is made here of the article by Gervais et al. (Twenty-four-hour rhythm in the bronchial hyperreactivity to house dust in asthmatics, J. Allergy Clin. Immunol. 59:207, 1977). As expected, the reactions were more severe in the early morning.

Two good articles discussing severe asthma should be mentioned here. Bondi and Williams (Severe asthma; course and treatment in hospital, N.Y. State J. Med. 77:350, 1977) record experience with 127 patients using the PEFR as a guide to therapy. (The Wright Peak Flow Meter is an inexpensive and reliable device which doctors taking care of asthmatics should have in their bag). The important points of this study are as follows. (1) Hypercapnia was present in 21% of the patients on admission, but only 4 patients (3.2%) required intubation. (Hypercapnia has been regarded by some as sufficient reason for intubation in status asthma. This is clearly not so if you are careful.) Intubation was only necessary "for those whose general condition of fatigue and somnolence suggested impending apnea." (2) Hypercapnia never developed if the PEFR was greater than 130 L/minute. (3) When the PEFR improved with treatment, hypercapnia never developed. (4) Slow gradual improvement of the PEFR mandated prolonged intensive therapy. Only 1 patient died of asthma. (Proper use of the PEFR as a guide to therapy requires that one remember the diurnal variation of bronchospasm and note the time of day at which the observations are made.) Scoggin et al. (Status asthmaticus, a 9-year experience, J.A.M.A. 238:1158, 1977) discuss the major risks attendant on intubation and mechanical ventilation of asthmatics. Nineteen of their 811 patients required mechanical ventilation and 8 of these died. The major complications included pneumothorax, endotracheal tube malfunction, alveolar hypoventilation on the ventilator and pneumonia. See the 1977 YEAR BOOK, page 119, for a similarly grim report concerning mechanical ventilation in asthma.

The use of intravenous isoproterenol in childhood status asthma was mentioned in the 1973 YEAR BOOK, page 176, and an article concerning its use in adults appeared in the 1976 YEAR BOOK, p. 163. The discussion also referred to an article on the use of intravenous salbutamol in this situation (Br. Med. J. 1:53, 1975). Pang et al. report on terbutaline given in children in status by the subcutaneous route, 0.01 – 0.04 mg/kg every 30 minutes until a response was obtained (Terbutaline in the treatment of status asthmaticus, Chest 72:469, 1977). Response was good in 9 of 10, and the failure also failed to respond to intravenous isoproterenol. There were no cardiovascular complications.

While discussing treatment, we would like also to mention the article by Stalcup and Mellins (Mechanical forces producing pulmonary edema in acute asthma, N. Engl. J. Med. 297:592, 1977). It provides evidence that the mean intrapleural pressure in severe asthmatics is much more negative than in normal persons, discuss the reasons why abnormally negative intrapleural pressure produces interstitial pulmonary edema and point out that interstitial pulmonary edema will make everything worse. They are attacking, properly, the time-honored but never established therapeutic practice of hydrating asthmatics in order to "loosen secretions." The amount of fluid an asthmatic should receive is not too much, not too little, but just enough.

Siegler provides useful clinical information in his article, "Reversible Electrocardiographic Changes in Severe Acute Asthma" (Thorax 32:328, 1977). In a group of 63 severe asthmatics, 78% had an abnormally vertical P wave axis (P greater in II and III than in I and negative in AVL), 22% showed P pulmonale as evidence of right atrial hypertrophy (height of P wave in II and III greater than 2.5 mm) and 1 patient had right ventricular hypertrophy. Of greatest interest, 11% had ST-T wave changes looking just like myocardial ischemia. All of these changes went away with resolution of the asthma. – Ed.] ◄

Theophylline Disposition in Patients with Hepatic Cirrhosis. Adverse effects of theophylline such as cardiac arrhythmias and cerebral seizures have been noted when plasma levels exceeded the therapeutic range of 5 – 20 mg/L. Theophylline is eliminated mainly by biotransformation in the liver, and toxicity has sometimes been attributed to reduced drug clearance secondary to impaired liver function. Kenneth M. Piafsky, Daniel S. Sitar, Robert E. Rangno and Richard I. Ogilvie[4] (McGill Univ.) studied the kinetic disposition of theophylline in 9 men with chronic alcoholic hepatic cirrhosis. Mean patient age was 51.6 years. All patients were receiving an adequate diet, and 4 were being treated with spironolactone. None ingested alcohol for at least a week before the study. A single dose of 4.5 or 2.25 mg theophylline ethylenediamine per kg was given intravenously in 15 minutes by infusion pump after an overnight fast. Binding of theophylline to plasma protein was measured using ^{14}C-labeled theophylline.

Rapid initial distribution of theophylline was observed, with variable plasma half-lives (table). Only 3 patients had plasma half-life and clearance values within the normal adult range, and the overall values were significantly different from those in normal subjects. Mean values for central-compartment volume and steady-state volume distribution appeared greater than in normal adults, but the differences were not

(4) N. Engl. J. Med. 296:1495 – 1497, June 30, 1977.

Plasma Theophylline Kinetic Disposition in 9 Cirrhotic Patients

Case No.	$\beta T\frac{1}{2}$	Clearance	V_1	VD_{SS}
	hr	*liters/kg/hr*	*liters/kg*	
1	10.1	0.035	0.448	0.513
2	15.0	0.021	0.144	0.457
3	46.7	0.018	0.781	1.187
4	14.1	0.026	0.095	0.510
5	11.5	0.029	0.157	0.479
6	53.8	0.008	0.163	0.604
7	59.1	0.014	0.146	1.169
8	13.0	0.028	0.282	0.519
9	7.1	0.200	0.753	1.624
Mean	25.6	0.042	0.330	0.785

Abbreviations: $\beta t\frac{1}{2}$, plasma (beta phase) half-life; V_1, volume of central compartment; V_{DSS}, volume of distribution at steady state.

significant. There was no correlation between the steady-state volume distribution and the presence of ascites. Binding of theophylline by plasma proteins was 32.3–40.2% in the 3 patients studied, and 52.6% in 4 normal adults.

Most of an administered dose of theophylline is biotransformed in the liver. The intersubject variability in kinetic disposition of the drug in cirrhotics is consistent with the variable hepatocellular function observed in this disease. Ability to eliminate theophylline cannot readily be predicted from usual laboratory tests of liver function. For the treatment of bronchoconstriction in asthmatics with cirrhosis, the current recommendation for a single loading dose of 6 mg/kg in 20 minutes would be safe, but the usually recommended chronic dose schedules for theophylline may be hazardous in cirrhotic patients. Determinations of plasma theophylline would be useful in designing a chronic dose schedule for a patient with liver disease.

► [Several articles concerning theophylline were summarized in the 1977 YEAR BOOK (pp. 115–117) and in the 1976 YEAR BOOK (p. 167). This article by Piafsky et al. confirms that you have to be careful when giving aminophylline to cirrhotics. Jusko et al. (Intravenous theophylline therapy: Nomogram guidelines, Ann. Intern. Med. 86:400, 1977) provide a useful nomogram which they validated in 72 patients with determination of blood levels. It was based on a loading dose of 5.6 mg aminophylline per kg given in a concentrated solution at a rate not exceeding 50 mg/minute; this was halved or eliminated if the patients had received any theophylline within 12 hours. The maintenance dose was based on 0.9 mg/kg/hour (aminophylline) in normal youngish patients, 0.68 mg/kg/hour in older patients (define that yourself) and 0.45 mg/kg/hour in patients with liver or heart disease. Kordash et al. (Theophylline concentrations in asthmatic patients after administration of aminophylline, J.A.M.A. 238:139, 1977) indicate that asthmatics without manifest heart or liver disease should receive reduced dosage because 34% of their patient population achieved levels greater than 20 μg/ml (generally regarded as the lower limit of the toxic range) on the recommended maintenance dose of 0.9 mg/kg/hour. The elevated levels were all under 40 μg/ml, so probably the intermediate dosage mentioned above would be all right. Levy et al. (Hemodialysis clearance of theophylline, ibid. 237:1466, 1977) demonstrate dialysis removal at a clearance rate of 33 ml/minute. What this means practically is not entirely clear to us, except that one should monitor levels if achieving therapeutic concentrations of the drug in dialyzed patients is thought to be very important (and really, aminophylline probably should not be given unless one intends to achieve therapeutic levels, between 10 and 20 μg/ml). Possibly, although this has not been shown, dialysis might be used to reduce toxic levels. This latter seems unlikely. Weinberger et al. (Inhibition of theophylline clearance by troleandomycin, J. Allergy Clin. Immunol. 59:228, 1977) suggests that this drug-drug interaction might account for some of the beneficial effects of the antibiotic in chronic bronchitis patients taking theophylline and might also carry a toxic risk. Piafsky et al. have shown that phenobarbital does not change theophylline metabolism (Effect of phenobarbital on the disposition of intravenous theophylline, Clin. Pharmacol. Therap. 22:336, 1977).

There is really not much new this year concerning outpatient therapy of bronchospasm. When symptoms are not adequately controlled by sporadic use of a bronchodilator aerosol, most physicians recommend adding oral aminophylline. Dosage of oral aminophylline (the cheapest theophylline by far, and as good as any) was discussed in the 1977 YEAR BOOK (pp. 115–116). Practically, in adults one starts with 200 mg 4 times daily and then increases from there, if necessary, following the results not only with observation of symptoms but hopefully with measurements of the PEFR in the office. If tolerated, addition of an extra dose at night may help the "morning dipper." If larger than usual doses are used and the clinical situation warrants pushing aminophylline, it is wise to check a blood level. People can either take aminophylline or they cannot, principally because of gastrointestinal upset and at times because of cardiac irritability. It may be possible, in some who cannot tolerate aminophylline, to switch to some other theophylline form such as choledyl, but this usually does not work for us. In addition to, or as an alternative to aminophylline, one can add oral terbutaline, a supposedly β_2-specific adrenergic agent, in dosage of 2.5–5 mg 3 times daily. Terbutaline seems to have a substantial advantage over ephedrine in not producing unacceptable central nervous system agitation. Whether or not terbutaline causes fewer cardiac effects, which is purported to be the case, is really not known for certain, or at least one can find articles on either side of the question. Again this has to be individualized. Some people prefer ephedrine.

One easily can be confused by reading the bronchodilator advertisements and literature. The two features of importance in selecting a bronchodilator are duration of action and specificity for the β_2-receptors; the latter is supposed to avoid cardiac excitement, and probably does. These features and the pharmacologic principles underlying them were discussed fairly extensively and referenced in the 1976 YEAR BOOK (pp. 160 and 161). Isoproterenol remains the standard by which others are judged. It is very short acting and accordingly really quite safe for repetitive administration (ibid., pp. 161 and 162). The only longer-acting aerosol now available is Alupent (metaproterenol or Metaprel), benefits from which do persist for several (4–6) hours. This may be particularly important in treatment of the "morning dipper," but the potential for accumulation of the drug with repetitive administration means it should be used no more frequently than every 4–6 hours. Salbutamol will soon be available and is the same sort of drug, widely and successfully used in Europe. The parasympatholytic aerosols (atropine and its esterified analogue, ipratropium) look very good in studies, do have sustained action for 4–6 hours, which is at least as long as Alupent, and some studies indicate that they are particularly useful in bronchospastic chronic bronchitics (Rosenthal et al.: Role of the parasympathetic system in antigen-induced bronchospasm, J. Appl. Physiol. 42:600, 1977; and Baigelman and Chodosh: Bronchodilator action of the anticholinergic drug, ipratropium bromide (Sch 1000), as an aerosol in chronic bronchitis and asthma, Chest 71:324, 1977). They are certain to have a place in treatment, but are not yet available in the United States. Two reviews appeared this past year; one by Webb-Johnson and Andrews (Bronchodilator therapy, N. Engl. J. Med. 297:476, 1977; and ibid., p. 758) and one by Campbell and Soyka (Selective β_2-receptor agonists for the treatment of asthma: Therapeutic breakthrough or advertising ploy?, J. Pediatr. 89: 1020, 1977). Trautlein et al. (Paradoxic bronchospasm after inhalation of isoproterenol, Chest 70:711, 1976) reviewed the literature on this interesting and bothersome phenomenon and demonstrated it in 12 of 41 patients studied.

Inhaled steroid (beclomethasone or Vanceril) remains an important new therapeutic modality. Up until now conventional dosage recommendation has been 100 μg (2 puffs) 4 times daily. Toogood et al. (A graded-dose assessment of the efficacy of beclomethasone dipropionate aerosol for severe chronic asthma, J. Allergy Clin. Immunol. 59:298, 1977) have published a very good study indicating further benefits in some patients by increasing dosage to 400 μg (8 puffs) 4 times daily. Whether or not inhaled steroids should precede oral steroids in the treatment sequence or should be used after oral steroids have been tried successfully (every-other-day dosage if at all possible; see 1973 YEAR BOOK, pp. 177–180), with the aim of trying to decrease or eliminate oral steroid dosage, is dealer's choice. It should be noted that some asthmatics don't like to inhale beclomethasone because it may immediately aggravate bronchospasm. For this reason it works well to have it inhaled following bronchodilator inhalation, which both avoids the immediate bronchospasm and may produce deeper penetration of the drug. – Ed.] ◄

► ↓ The syndrome of pulmonary eosinophilic infiltrates with asthma includes two fairly distinct and serious conditions that are probably seen more frequently than they are diagnosed and that should be recognized and appropriately managed, allergic bronchopulmonary aspergillosis and chronic eosinophilic pneumonia. – Ed. ◄

Asthmatic Pulmonary Eosinophilia: Review of 65 Cases. W. G. Middleton, I. C. Paterson, I. W. B. Grant and A. C. Douglas[5] (Edinburgh) report a study of asthmatic pulmonary eosinophilia, with special reference to the etiologic role of *Aspergillus fumigatus* and the results of corticosteroid therapy. Records of 65 asthmatic patients with documented pulmonary infiltration and peripheral blood eosinophilia of over 0.5×10^9/L were reviewed. There were age peaks at 21–30 and 51–60 years. Thirty-five female and 30 male patients were studied. Fifty-seven patients had an eosinophilia exceeding 10% of the total white blood cell count; in 25 it exceeded 20%. Eosinophils were found in the sputum in 28 of 48 patients in whom it was studied. Fifty-five patients had segmental or lobar opacities at some time. Asthma began before age 10 in 26 patients. In 29 cases the first recorded pulmonary eosinophilia occurred within 2 years of the onset of asthma symptoms. Skin tests were positive to common allergens in 25 of 50 patients tested. An immediate skin reaction to *A. fumigatus* was positive in 30 of 53 cases, and precipitating antibodies were present in 60% of the 48 patients tested. Thirty patients had evidence of allergic aspergillosis.

The prognosis in 62 cases followed for a mean of 6.4 years is given in Table 1 and the factors related to the prognosis in Table 2. Patients without evidence of allergic aspergillosis tended to do better than the

TABLE 1. – Asthmatic Pulmonary Eosinophilia: Relation between Prognosis and Allergic Aspergillosis*

Follow-up grade	*Whole group* (65 patients)	*Aspergillosis-negative subgroup* (22 patients)	*Allergic aspergillosis subgroup* (32 patients)
0 (no symptomatic, functional or radiographic abnormality)	14	8 } 14	3
I (only one of the above)	8	6 }	1
II (two of the above)	15	4	10 } 27
III (all three of the above or death)	25	4	17 }
No follow-up	3	0	1
		$\chi^2 = 14.73$, $P < 0.001$	
Number given long-term daily corticosteroids	34 (52%)	12 (55%)	18 (56%)

*Guidance of allergy to *A. fumigatus* or of *A. fumigatus* in sputum was sought in 54 (22 + 32) of the 65 patients.

(5) Br. J. Dis. Chest 71:115–122, April, 1977.

TABLE 2.—Factors Related to Prognosis in Pulmonary Eosinophilia with Asthma

Follow-up grade	*Sex*	*Mean age at onset of asthma*	*Duration of asthma before first episode of pulmonary eosinophilia* < 2 years	> 10 years	*Allergic* aspergillosis* Absent	Present	*No. requiring long-term corticosteroids*
0 (14 patients)	3M 11F	42 years	13	1	8	3	6 (43%)
III (25 patients)	12M 13F	21 years	6	15	4	17	16 (64%)
			$\chi^2=14.0$ $P<0.001$		$\chi^2=8.0$ $P<0.01$		

*Three patients with grade 0 assessments and 4 with grade III assessments were inadequately investigated for allergic aspergillosis.

others. Opacities recurred during regular daily corticosteroid therapy in 35% of the 34 patients treated. All but 1 of 10 patients not given corticosteroids had further opacities. Most patients had symptoms coincident with the appearance of further opacities. No steroid-treated patient developed invasive pulmonary aspergillosis. All 8 patients who underwent bronchography had evidence of bronchiectasis. Six patients have died, 3 of respiratory failure due to bronchopneumonia. All 3 of these patients had severe, largely irreversible airways obstruction at presentation.

The incidence of pulmonary eosinophilia in asthmatics is difficult to estimate. It appears to be reasonable to try to prevent eosinophilic episodes, especially when allergic aspergillosis is present. This can be achieved by giving prednisolone in a daily dose of at least 10 mg. Treatment should be continued indefinitely.

Studies in Chronic Allergic Bronchopulmonary Aspergillosis: 1. Clinical and Physiologic Findings. J. L. Malo, R. Hawkins and J. Pepys[6] (London) report the findings in 50 asthmatic patients with chronic allergic bronchopulmonary aspergillosis in whom the diagnosis was made a mean of 10.9 years ago (Table 1). Age of the patients

TABLE 1.—Diagnostic Features

	No. of patients
Main diagnostic criteria	
Asthma	50
Previous episode of transient shadow in chest radiograph with blood eosinophilia	50
Immediate positive prick test with an extract of *A. fumigatus*	50
Supporting evidence	
Presence of serum precipitins against *A. fumigatus*	
in the past	44
at time of study	42
History of 'plugs' in sputum	37
Culture of *A. fumigatus* from sputum in the past	23
Suggestive chronic changes in chest radiograph	49

(6) Thorax 32:254–261, June, 1977.

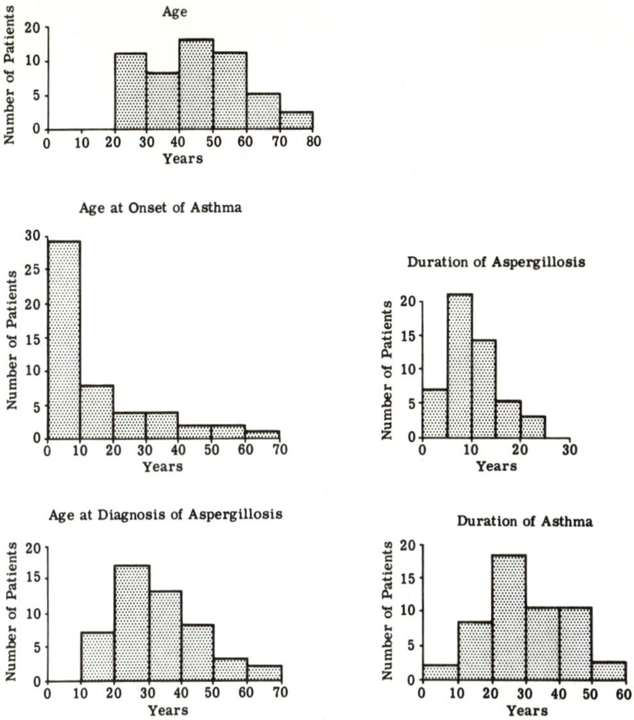

Fig 19.—Histograms of clinical features. (Courtesy of Malo, J. L., et al.: Thorax 52:254–261, June, 1977.)

and duration of asthma and aspergillosis are shown in Figure 19. The mean duration of asthma was 30.4 years. Bronchopulmonary aspergillosis was diagnosed after age 20 in most patients.

The clinical data were obtained from answers to a questionnaire (Table 2). Of the 39 full-time workers, 17 had lost time off work in the past year, and 5 were hospitalized with acute exacerbations of asthma or aspergillosis. Four patients reported absence of asthma and sputum production in the past year, and 39 of the other 46 considered control of their asthma to be good. Twenty-seven patients were being treated with oral steroids with or without beclomethasone dipropionate, 9 with beclomethasone only and 4 with sodium cromoglycate.

Only 12 patients had a normal forced expiratory volume in 1 second (FEV_1) at the time of study, and 12 had severe airways obstruction with an FEV_1 of less than 45% of predicted. In 20 patients, the vital capacity was reduced. In 9 the gas transfer factor was less than 75% of predicted normal. Eighteen patients had a reduced forced vital capacity. Significant improvement (more than 15%) in FEV_1 occurred in only 17 patients after administration of bronchodilator aerosol. The severity of reduction of the gas transfer factor was directly related to patient age and history of aspergillosis. The degree of reversibility was not related to the clinical findings except for the forced vital capacity.

Only 2 patients currently smoked. Patients receiving significant

TABLE 2.—CLINICAL FINDINGS IN 50 PATIENTS*

	None	*2 weeks*	*2–4 weeks*	*> 4 weeks*
Loss of work**	22	4	9	4
	None	*One*	*Two*	
No. of hospital admissions**	45	3	2	
Characteristics of asthma				
	Night	*Day*	*Same*	
Diurnal preponderance	11	13	22	
	Winter (Oct.–Mar.)	*Summer (Apr.–Sep.)*	*Same*	
Seasonal preponderance	21	3	22	
	Present	*Absent*		
Morning tightness	19	27		
	One attack/wk	*Several attacks/wk*	*One attack every day*	*Continuously wheezing*
Severity	29	5	5	7
	Good	*Fair*	*Poor*	
General control	39	4	3	
Sputum production				
	Every day	*Intermittent*		
Frequency	21	25		
	Small	*Up to an eggcupful*	*Up to a teacupful*	
Daily quantity	27	15	4	
	White–grey	*Yellow–green*		
Usual colour	20	26		
	None	*Intermittent*		
'Plugs'	22	24		

*Except for loss of work, where the number of full-time workers is 39, and characteristics of asthma and sputum production, where the number is 46 (4 patients denied asthma and sputum production in the past year).

**From chest symptoms.

doses of oral steroids had significantly reduced lung function compared with those receiving bronchodilator and/or antibiotic therapy only.

Prospective studies of patients selected for treatment at onset of bronchopulmonary aspergillosis may be expected to indicate the overall value of corticoids or other treatment in prevention of permanent pathologic and physiologic impairment.

► [The clinical picture is characterized by a history of intermittent asthma, often beginning in childhood and changing into more or less continuous asthma, prominent sputum production, often sputum plugs, winter worsening and episodes of exacerbation with chest infiltrates at times associated with fever, hemoptysis and chest pain in some combination. As mentioned, the asthmatic component may be stable and not too prominent, responding fairly indifferently to bronchodilator therapy, but serial pulmonary function measurements indicate slow relentless deterioration, particularly in diffusion capacity (gas transfer factor) but also in measurements of obstruction to air flow.

The roentgenographic picture is said to be very suggestive and, in the proper setting, diagnostic (Malo et al.: Studies in chronic allergic bronchopulmonary aspergillosis: 2. Radiologic findings, Thorax 32:363, 1977). Among the 50 patients which the authors followed for an average of 10 years, 267 acute transient pulmonary infiltrates were recorded, an average of 5.3 per patient, 22% of which were asymptomatic. These transient shadows included homogeneous infiltrates without shrinkage, homogeneous shadows with shrinkage, patchy clouding, nodular shadows, bandlike (toothpaste or gloved-finger) shadows 2–3 cm long (presumably representing radiodense secretions in a bronchus or dilated bronchus), parallel linear shadows ("tramlines") representing thickened bronchial walls and 2–3 cm circular nodular shadows. The pattern of proximal bronchiectatic dilatation with normal more peripheral bronchi is thought to be so characteristic that it can be suspected without bronchograms by experienced observers. Permanent shadows included tubular shadows (like "tramline" shadows but more prominent); ring shadows, presumably representing proximal bronchiectatic areas seen on end; shrunken but aerated segments or lobes; loss of vascular shadows; and "long line" shadows. Evidence of overinflation was present more often when the patient was first seen (42%) than when last seen (34%), which the authors attributed to loss of lung substance. Permanent roentgenographic changes were seen in all but 1 case at the end of the period of observation. All lung zones were pretty much equally involved. Two patients appeared to have developed fungus balls. Almost half of the acute infiltrates led to permanent changes.

Although false negatives and false positives may be seen, 70–85% of cases demonstrate precipitins against *A. fumigatus* antigens, the immediate skin test is almost always positive and IgE levels are very high, ranging in some series from 600 to 60,000 ng/ml. A number of conditions are associated with elevated IgE levels in the 1,000- to 3,000-ng/ml range, but these very high levels are quite suggestive of allergic bronchopulmonary aspergillosis, and it seems likely that a normal level would argue strongly against this diagnosis (Malo et al.: Studies in chronic allergic bronchopulmonary aspergillosis: 3. Immunologic findings, ibid., p. 269; and Rosenbert et al.: Ann. Intern. Med. 86:405, 1977).

There is some disagreement among authorities concerning treatment. All agree that symptomatic flares should be treated with corticosteroids, but Middleton et al. suggest that prolonged steroid therapy of at least 10 mg prednisone per day once the diagnosis is made is indicated to prevent progression. Malo et al. do not make that recommendation specifically. Most authors have opted against aerosolized steroid, but Pingleton et al. (Chest 71:782, 1977) say that it works in some.

Hanson et al. (Bronchocentric granulomatosis: A complication of allergic bronchopulmonary aspergillosis, J. Allergy Clin. Immunol. 59:83, 1977) state that this is at least one of the conditions leading to limited invasion of the bronchial wall with fungal forms and a granulomatous reaction. Goodman and Sacca (Pulmonary cavitation, allergic aspergillosis, asthma and bronchocentric granulomatosis, Chest 72:368, 1977) report the case of a young man with a suggestive history including nasal stuffiness (see also Safirstein: Allergic bronchopulmonary aspergillosis with obstruction of the upper respiratory tract, ibid. 70:788, 1976) who presented with hemoptysis, fever, sputum production and a large right upper lobe cavity which on resection resembled bronchocentric granulomatosis pathologically.

There are three acronyms which represent this same process. Of course, ABA is allergic bronchopulmonary aspergillosis. The BEAP syndrome consists of bronchiectasis of the central type, eosinophilia, aspergillosis and recurrent pneumonitis in a patient with chronic asthma, i.e., the same thing. The third, MIP, or mucoid impaction of the bronchus, is the same process with emphasis on bronchial obstruction and atelectasis and less emphasis on asthma and eosinophilia. Repeat four times daily: "ABA! BEAP! MIP!" Feel better?—Ed.] ◄

Peripheral Opacities in Chronic Eosinophilic Pneumonia: Photographic Negative of Pulmonary Edema. Edward A. Gaensler (Boston Univ.) and Charles B. Carrington[7] (Stanford Univ.) reviewed 2,852 radiographs from 591 patients referred with interstitial lung disease since 1950 to determine whether there is a radiographic pattern diagnostic for chronic eosinophilic pneumonia (CEP). Twenty-four patients (4.1%) exhibited a peripheral ground-glass pattern on one or more occasions. In 21 cases (5.7%), CEP was the sole or primary di-

Fig 20.—Initial chest radiographs of 4 patients. All show virtually complete peripheral opacification, giving impression of photographic negative or reversal of pattern usually seen in pulmonary edema. Involvement is symmetric in **A** and **B,** and limited largely to one side in **C** and **D.** (Courtesy of Gaensler, E. A., and Carrington, C. B.: Am. J. Roentgenol. 128:1–13, January, 1977.)

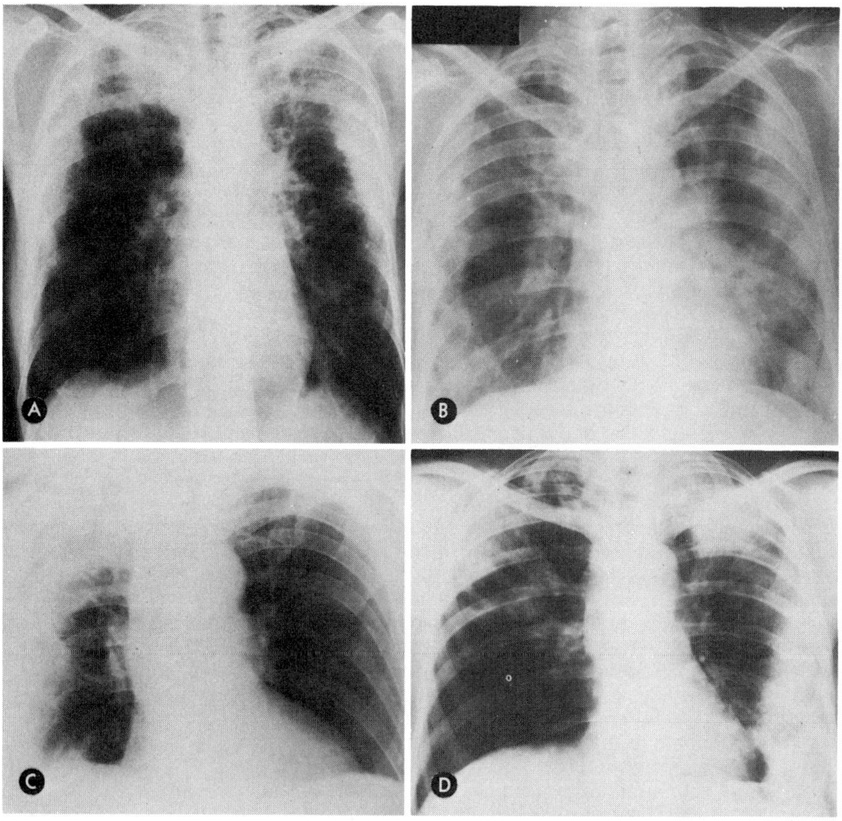

(7) Am. J. Roentgenol. 128:1–13, January, 1977.

agnosis. Sixteen of these patients had typical peripheral shadows and were among those selected by radiographic criteria.

The typical opacities were peripheral, with ill-defined margins and no segmental distribution. They sometimes completely surrounded the lung, suggesting a photographic negative of the opacities seen in pulmonary edema (Fig 20). More often they were limited to the upper or lower lateral portions. The opacities were usually homogeneous, but in 3 cases they contained ill-defined radiolucencies. Occasionally perihilar infiltration was noted. Peculiar peripheral curved lines were seen in 3 patients. The opacities sometimes disappeared and reappeared spontaneously over many years, either in the same sites or in different peripheral sites. Opacities often cleared within 2–3 days with corticosteroid therapy.

Most patients had typical histologic features of CEP in lung tissue and improved within hours of the start of steroid therapy. Most patients were middle-aged housewives. The usual presentation was with dyspnea, cough with mucoid sputum and severe weight loss. Fever was universal, and drenching sweats were frequent. A background atopy was apparent in one third of the cases. Eight patients remained well after long-term therapy. Four had severe relapses after short courses but are now well. Four acquired asthma for the first time in middle age, some years after the last episode of CEP. One patient died of CEP. Functional abnormalities were usually less marked than expected from the radiographs.

The typical radiographic pattern of CEP is virtually diagnostic. Blood eosinophilia is confirmatory, but its absence does not exclude the diagnosis. Lack of appropriate therapy may lead to consolidation, unnecessary surgery or death.

► [Crofton's much used classification of the pulmonary eosinophilic syndromes includes: (1) transient pulmonary eosinophilia or Löffler's syndrome, (2) prolonged pulmonary eosinophilia, (3) tropical eosinophilia (due to microfilariae and responsive to antifilarial chemotherapy), (4) pulmonary eosinophilia with asthma and (5) pulmonary eosinophilia with polyarteritis. We think that a better classification might be: (1) allergic bronchopulmonary aspergillosis complicating asthma, (2) tropical eosinophilia, (3) pulmonary eosinophilia due to known allergens, particularly drugs, (4) pulmonary polyarteritis and its variants, including Wegener's granulomatosis, and (5) idiopathic pulmonary eosinophilia, (a) mild and transient (Löffler's pneumonia), (b) prolonged without asthma and (c) prolonged with asthma. Category 5 is the disease under discussion. This classification assumes that Löffler's pneumonia is a mild variant of chronic eosinophilic pneumonia and that it is the same process whether or not asthma is a concomitant or antecedent condition, both of which assumptions are not established or widely shared.

Angelillo et al. have published another excellent summary of this condition (Chronic eosinophilic pneumonia: A report of four cases and a review of the literature, Am. J. Med. Sci. 273:279, 1977). They feel the "syndrome is sufficiently characteristic that, after appropriate evaluation, therapy can often be initiated . . . without . . . histologic confirmation." The distinctive features of the clinical presentation are peripheral lung shadowing with eosinophilia and serious constitutional symptoms, with or without asthma, and prompt, usually dramatic response to corticosteroid therapy. The physiologic set is principally an alveolitis-like picture (hypoxemia and breathlessness with or without airway obstruction). Most patients are middle-aged or older women. Steroid therapy initially in rather large dosage (30–60 mg prednisone daily) is administered and usually can be rapidly tapered to low (10 mg per day) suppressive therapy. This, however, often has to be prolonged, usually over a year, and the pulmonary infiltrates may recur in exactly the same location when steroids are discontinued. Of the 22 patients in the review of Angelillo et al. for whom data were available, 12 had asthma and 10 did not, and 3 of their own 4 cases were asthmatic.

Two other recent articles have titles which are self-explanatory (Hudgel and Spector: Pulmonary infiltration with eosinophilia: Recurrence in an asthmatic patient treated with beclomethasone dipropionate, Chest 72:359, 1977; and Repo and Nieminen: Pulmonary infiltrates with eosinophilia and urinary symptoms during disodium cromoglycate treatment, Scand. J. Respir. Dis. 57:1, 1976).

For the sake of completeness, extrinsic allergic alveolitis or hypersensitivity pneumonitis should be mentioned. This represents a "group of pulmonary diseases characterized by an inflammatory reaction in the peripheral gas-exchanging portions of the lung . . . in nonatopic individuals after prolonged inhalation of small organic antigens" (Dill et al.: A study of the effects of systemic administration of adrenal glucocorticoids in an experimental model of hypersensitivity pneumonitis, Clin. Allergy 7:83, 1977). It is characterized by dyspnea, dry cough, often systemic symptoms such as fever and malaise, crackling rales, diffuse micronodular infiltrates on x-ray and serum precipitins to the offending antigens (1977 YEAR BOOK, pp. 127–130; and 1975 YEAR BOOK, pp. 171–175). It can be caused by heavy inhalation of *Aspergillus fumigatus* (Yocum et al.: Extrinsic allergic alveolitis after *Aspergillus fumigatus* inhalation: Evidence of a type IV immunologic pathogenesis, Am. J. Med. 61:939, 1976). Schatz et al. (Immunopathogenesis of hypersensitivity pneumonitis, J. Allergy Clin. Immunol. 60:27, 1977) feel that the antigen has to be particulate and not readily digestible by lysosomal enzymes and that the immune response is complex, although always involving cell-mediated immune mechanisms. Olenchock has also written a good review concerning experimental models (Animal models of hypersensitivity pneumonitis: A review, Ann. Allergy 38: 119, 1977). You can get it if your sauna water is contaminated (Metzger et al.: Saunataker's disease: Hypersensitivity pneumonitis due to contaminated water in a home sauna. J.A.M.A. 236:2209, 1976) or you overuse hair spray (Stringer et al.: Hypersensitivity pneumonitis following prolonged inhalation of hair spray, thesaurosis, ibid. 238: 888, 1977). We feel that this is what histoplasmin-sensitive patients get when they are massively exposed to *Histoplasm capsulatum* spores. – Ed.] ◄

Metal Fume Fever in Ferrochrome Workers was studied by John Stoke[8] (Univ. of Rhodesia). The illness is short-lived, occurring some 4–8 hours after exposure to fresh hot metal fumes. It is characterized by shivering, limb pains, a feeling of constriction in the chest, dyspnea, cough and fever. Rales may be heard in the chest, and leukocytosis is usually present. The chest film is usually normal. The condition may progress to a chemical pneumonitis that resembles pneumonia clinically, but does not respond to antibiotics.

During the process of tapping the mix in making chrome alloys, a mixture of dust and fumes in which silicon dioxide and the oxides of chromium and iron are present escapes. Forty of the 70 male workers examined were tapping hands. Half of the tapping hands gave a history of symptoms suggestive of metal fume fever. The 1 other worker with such a history had worked in the furnace area and occasionally helped at tapping. Complications developed in 4 workers known to have had metal fume fever. Another of the 21 subjects acquired bronchial asthma. The mean timed forced expiratory volume (FEV_1) was less than expected in the tapping hands and in 1 control subject, but no significant differences in lung function tests were noted.

The metal fume fever in these workers was probably due to the inhalation of freshly prepared chromium oxide, which was formed during the tapping process. A reduction in the FEV_1-forced vital capacity ratio may represent a defensive reaction in workers who perform tapping in

(8) Cent. Afr. J. Med. 23:25–28, February, 1977.

a hot, dusty environment. Metal fume fever should be considered in any worker who contacts metal fumes, either in a foundry or after welding, and who acquires pyrexia with respiratory symptoms within 8 hours of completing work. A high index of suspicion is necessary, since only after diagnosis can preventive measures be implemented. The condition may well occur in other occupations where metal fumes are produced.

► [The number of occupation-related exposures which can produce pulmonary disease is growing daily and the field is in need of classification and review (see 1977 YEAR BOOK, pp. 127 and 128). In addition to the classic pneumoconioses, there are a large number of conditions related to inhalation of organic molds, of which farmer's lung is the prototype, a large number of conditions related to inhalation of industrial fumes of various sorts, plastics (organic chemicals) and metal fumes. These are often complex, involving more than one substance. The syndromes tend somewhat to sort themselves out according to etiologic agents, but not cleanly so. One can have immediate asthma after exposure; late asthma; pulmonary edema; the syndrome of alveolitis consisting of chest tightness, breathlessness and systemic symptoms including malaise and fever; and more chronically can develop chronic obstructive lung disease, interstitial fibrosis or granulomatosis. Which syndrome develops probably depends in some part on host factors as well as on the agents themselves. It probably makes sense to suspect industrial exposure if it is at all suggested by the circumstances and not get bothered if the condition has not yet been described. This won't help with compensation but may be important to the patient's health. (Health vs. pocketbook is always a closer tradeoff than doctors are prone to believe, however. Bishop Cramner's phrase according distress in mind, body or estate more or less equal weight in the now-departed 1928 *Episcopal Book of Common Prayer* always seemed to us to be closer to the truth than the medical profession's emphasis on optimum health regardless of cost.)

There are several other titles of interest that appeared during the past year (Taylor and Davies: Ferroalloy workers' disease: A report of a recent case against the background of 12 years' experience, Cent. Afr. J. Med. 23:28, 1977; Carlson and Villaveces: Hypersensitivity pneumonitis due to pyrethrum, J.A.M.A. 237:1718, 1977 [pyrethrum is a component of many insecticides]; Brubaker: Pulmonary problems associated with the use of polytetrafluoroethylene, J. Occupational Med. 19:693, 1977; Butcher et al.: Toluene diisocyanate pulmonary disease: Immunopharmacologic and mecholyl challenge studies, J. Allergy Clin. Immunol. 59:223, 1977; Vandervort and Brooks: Polyvinyl chloride film thermal decomposition products as an occupational illness, J. Occupational Med. 19:188, 1977; ibid., p. 192; Fawcett et al.: Asthma due to inhaled chemical agents: Fumes from "multicore" soldering flux and colophony resin, Clin. Allergy 6: 577, 1976; Chester et al.: Phthalic anhydride asthma, ibid. 7:15, 1977; Fawcett, et al.: Asthma due to inhaled chemical agents: Epoxy resin systems containing phthalic acid anhydride, trimellitic acid anhydride and triethylene tetramine, ibid., p. 1; Zeiss et al.: Trimellitic anhydride-induced airway syndromes: Clinical and immunologic studies, J. Allergy Clin. Immunol. 60:96, 1977; Sargent et al.: Respiratory effects of occupational exposure to an epoxy resin system, Arch. Environ. Health 31:236, 1976; and Chan-Yeung and Abboud: Occupational asthma due to California redwood dusts, Am. Rev. Respir. Dis. 114:1027, 1976).—Ed.] ◄

Pulmonary Embolism

Pulmonary Embolectomy, Heparin and Streptokinase: Their Place in Treatment of Acute Massive Pulmonary Embolism. It has been suggested that embolectomy is seldom both technically feasible and clinically appropriate. However, in most reported series, the survival rate quoted for pulmonary embolectomy is considerably higher than actually can be achieved. G. A. H. Miller, R. J. C. Hall and M. Paneth[9] (London) compared embolectomy with medical management by anticoagulants or streptokinase in a relatively large series of 68 patients with isolated active, massive pulmonary embolism; 33 had emergency embolectomy under total bypass since 1964, and 18 patients were primarily treated with heparin and 17 with streptokinase. "Shock" was defined as a systolic arterial pressure of 100 mm Hg or less.

The overall mortality for the entire group was 16%. Results in the 27 patients without shock are given in Table 1 and those in the 41 patients with shock in Table 2. The 20 patients with at least one previous episode of circulatory arrest had a mortality of 45%. Seven of 14 patients in this group who had embolectomy died. Only 2 patients who had not had a circulatory arrest died and neither had embolectomy. The rate of response of medically treated patients is shown in Figure 21. Resolution at 72 hours was significantly more complete in the streptokinase-treated than in the heparin-treated group. Recurrent

TABLE 1.—NONSHOCK: BLOOD PRESSURE $>$ 100 MM HG

Primary treatment	*Embolectomy*	*Streptokinase*	*Heparin*	*Total*
Total number of patients	10	9	8	27
Deaths	1	0	1	2 (7.4%)
"Treatment failure"	–	0	1	
Recurrent embolism	0	0	1	1
Total deaths and failures	1 (10%)	0	3 (37.5%)	

TABLE 2.—SHOCK: BLOOD PRESSURE $<$ 100 MM HG

Primary treatment	*Embolectomy*	*Streptokinase*	*Heparin*	*Total*
Total number of patients	23	8	10	41
Deaths	6	1 (2*)	1	9 (21.9%)
"Treatment failure"	–	1*	4	
Recurrent embolism	0	1*	1†	2
Total deaths and failures	6 (26%)	2 (25%)	5 (50%)	

*This patient failed treatment (hemodynamic deterioration) but died 3 months later of a recurrent embolism. He therefore appears in the failure and recurrent columns and (in brackets) in deaths.

†This patient died of recurrent embolism and also appears in the deaths column.

(9) Am. Heart J. 93:568–574, May, 1977.

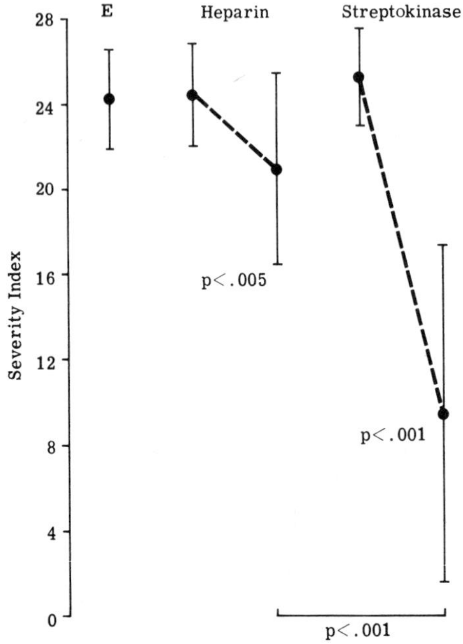

Fig 21.—The response to treatment as assessed by angiographic appearances before and after 72 hours of treatment. Vertical axis shows numerical index of severity obtained from pulmonary arteriograms. Mean values for each group and 1 SD are shown. *Broken lines* join the pretreatment and posttreatment values for the heparin-treated and streptokinase-treated groups. No posttreatment values are available for the patients who were treated by embolectomy but the preoperative index of severity was similar for these and for the medically treated patients. (Courtesy of Miller, G. A. H., et al.: Am. Heart J. 93:568–574, May, 1977.)

massive pulmonary embolism could not be excluded as a cause of 1 of the 5 late deaths that occurred.

Pulmonary embolectomy is necessary in a patient with acute massive embolism who cannot be adequately resuscitated after circulatory arrest or who is deteriorating rapidly despite thrombolytic therapy. Partial bypass may reduce mortality in this group. A patient who has lived 2 hours or longer but is in shock is given streptokinase therapy. Streptokinase is also used in patients with acute massive embolism who are not in shock. With this approach to management, only an occasional patient will require emergency embolectomy.

► [It should be emphasized that the findings of this study are of limited applicability to the United States since streptokinase and urokinase are not now available for treatment of pulmonary embolism and it is not certain that they ever will be. The technique of administering these drugs through a catheter left in the pulmonary artery after angiographic demonstration of massive embolism (defined as obstruction of over 50% of the pulmonary arterial tree) is interesting but, to our knowledge, of no certain advantage over administration by peripheral vein.

The conclusions, based on small numbers, are that patients in refractory shock despite medical management should be operated on and that the mortality is 26% in these authors' hands. They also feel that the actual surgical mortality would have been much lower if patients already having developed severe cerebral ischemia prior to referral to their hospital had been excluded. Note also that of 10 patients in shock treated with heparin, 1 died and 4 others were treatment failures requiring streptokinase or embolectomy. The crux of the argument hinges on how these treatment failures were defined. Kenneth Moser, in his recent excellent review on the state of the art (Pulmonary Embolism: Am. Rev. Respir. Dis. 115:829, 1977), states that overall the mortality experienced with medical management of massive embolization has been less than that reported with embolectomy and that the mortality rate with medical treatment in those who survive long enough to have the diagnosis established is very low "even in those subjects in whom previously accepted criteria for emergency embolectomy are present (systemic hypotension initially unresponsive to therapy and overt right ventricular failure). . . .Perhaps, with available support systems and surgical approaches, emergency embolectomy merits consideration in some institutions, but its effect is likely to be modest indeed." This seems a good interim position to maintain, but the question remains an open one.

In contrast to acute pulmonary embolectomy, the surgical treatment of chronic pulmonary embolism is probably underutilized. This subject was discussed in the 1974 YEAR BOOK (p. 188); the patient was a man with marked obstructive pulmonary artery disease for 10 years who had substantial and persisting improvement after pulmonary embolectomy. Sabiston et al. (Surgical management of chronic pulmonary embolism, Ann. Surg. 185:699, 1977) report their experience with 6 patients who were symptomatic with a syndrome including a history of thrombophlebitis, progressive exertional dyspnea and symptoms and signs of right heart strain for a period of 5 months to 2 years. The diagnosis was made by scan, arteriogram and right heart catheterization. Five were improved by removal of large, arborized clots which adhered firmly to the arterial wall; the sixth was not improved and none died. The authors felt that success depended on a distal pulmonary circulation kept open by flow *via* anastomosis between the pulmonary and bronchial circulations and that this favorable situation could be anticipated by the demonstration of brisk back-bleeding at operation when the clot was removed. They summarized the total of 17 reported cases including their own; 13 patients were improved, 1 was unimproved and 4 died. – Ed.] ◄

Prevention of Pulmonary Embolism by Inferior Vena Cava Filters: Results in 62 Cases are reported by Volker Schlosser, G. Spillner and W. Kaiser[1] (Univ. of Freiburg). Anticoagulation and fibrinolysis are of limited use in the prevention of recurrent pulmonary emboli, and venous thrombectomy does not provide effective prophylaxis. Only surgical interruption of the path of the embolus is effective. Three methods of interrupting blood flow in the inferior vena cava are available (Table 1). Implantation of a screen filter appears to be most advantageous, because it avoids the risks of an extraperitoneal dissection. The umbrella screen filter developed by Mobin-Uddin et al. (1969) is used. The filter is introduced through the jugular vein under local anesthesia and fluoroscopic control, and positioned below the level of the renal veins. When in position, the umbrella is opened and hooked into the caval wall, and unscrewed from the introducing catheter.

TABLE 1. – Operative Prophylaxis of Pulmonary Embolism by Interruption of Inferior Vena Cava

Method	Prevention of embolism	Hemodynamic disturbance	Operative risk
Caval ligation [3]	+++	+++	+++
Caval plication [5]	++	+	+++
Caval clipping [6–9]	++	+	+++
Caval filter [10]	+++	±	±
Caval catheter [11]	++	+	±

(1) World J. Surg. 1:113–116, January, 1977.

TABLE 2.—EARLY COMPLICATIONS OF INFERIOR VENA CAVA FILTER IMPLANTATION FOR PULMONARY EMBOLISM

	World literature up to 1974		Freiburg Experience	
	No. cases	Percent	No. cases	Percent
Total cases	2267	100	62	100
Recurrent pulmonary embolism	77	3.4	1	1.6
Dislocation of filter	33	1.5	2	3.2
Edema of lower extremities	116	5.1	5	9.7
Hemorrhage	7	0.3	0	0

The umbrella screen filter was placed in 62 patients with recurrent and massive pulmonary emboli in 1971–75. Early complications are given in Table 2. Fourteen of the 44 patients seen at 1–2 years reported edema of the lower limbs, and 4 reported having edema for the first time after the operation. No patient had a late recurrence of pulmonary embolism. Thirty patients were on chronic anticoagulation. Eight of 25 patients who had inferior vena cavography 6–24 months postoperatively showed complete blockage of the vena cava with extensive collateral formation and edema of the lower limbs. Eight others had partial blockage of the filter with some collateral circulation but no lower limb swelling. Nine patients showed a patent vena cava without new collateral vessels and no lower limb swelling.

Screen filter implantation is a method of tolerable risk that provides a high degree of protection against recurrent pulmonary embolism. It is much less risky than methods that require extraperitoneal exposure of the vena cava in very ill patients. The procedure is indicated after a single severe pulmonary embolus; after recurrent symptomatic emboli that occur despite correct anticoagulation; and as prophylaxis when fresh pelvic and lower limb thrombosis with free-floating thrombi is demonstrated by phlebography, even in the absence of documented pulmonary emboli. The method is not used for infected thrombi.

► [This article was selected because it summarizes the literature on the umbrella filter and tallies its complications. The total occlusion rate of about 30% is in line with the experience of others. We certainly do not agree with the indications mentioned in this article, which seem far too broad. The Moser review cited in the preceding comment recommends caval interruption "only as a lifesaving maneuver in a closely defined group of patients, namely, those with massive acute embolic obstruction (in whom) an additional embolus during (the first few days of) heparin therapy might be fatal . . . (and) those in whom significant embolization occurs and heparin therapy—even in minidoses—cannot be employed safely." He agrees that the umbrella filter is the procedure of choice for caval interruption when this is necessary.

The review by Doctor Moser (Am. Rev. Respir. Dis. 115:829, 1977), is the one paper about pulmonary embolism you should read if you can read only one. A little of the wealth of information therein can be mentioned briefly. (1) The incidence of venous thrombosis after myocardial infarction is 30–40%. (2) One of the consequences of embolization is loss of surfactant which results in alveolar collapse, loss of the impermeability of the alveolar lining, a hemorrhagic alveolar exudate and "congestive atelectasis." This process may cause chest x-ray infiltrates, pleurisy and hemoptysis but does not represent tissue death and is reversible. Infarction is much more rare, occurring in fewer than 10% of all recognized emboli. (3) The sudden onset of atrial fibrillation in a patient with preexisting cardiac disease should suggest pulmonary embolism. (4) Antiplatelet drugs have not yet been established as helpful. (5) Dopamine is preferred over isoproterenol for hypotension. (6) If thrombolytic therapy, if it becomes available, will have a role, it is likely to be in patients with marked cardiopulmonary compromise due to embolism.

The symptoms and signs of pulmonary embolism are discussed in Moser's review and also in an article by Bell et al. (The clinical features of submassive and massive pulmonary emboli, Am. J. Med. 62:355, 1977) based on the clinical information accumulated during the urokinase cooperative study (see also 1974 YEAR BOOK, pp. 187 and 188). Two thirds of their 754 patients had massive emboli defined as involvement of the equivalent of two lobar arteries or more. The size of the embolus was not related to mortality; massive emboli were slightly more likely to be associated with syncope, shock and diaphoresis; pleuritic chest pain, chills and hemoptysis were more frequently associated with submassive emboli. Patients with massive emboli more frequently had a history of recent surgery and immobilization. Seventy-five percent of women less than age 45 with pulmonary embolism were taking oral contraceptives.

Rostand et al., in "Massive Hemothorax Complicating Heparin Anticoagulation for Pulmonary Embolus (South. Med. J. 70:1128, 1977), comment on the rarity of this complication, only 11 reported cases. Overanticoagulation by laboratory indices was not a feature. Treatment was stopping heparin, tube thoracotomy and, in some, vena cava interruption. Hall et al. report the association of two rare consequences of pulmonary infarction in 1 patient (Pneumothorax complicating asceptic cavitating pulmonary infarction, Chest 72:232, 1977).—Ed.] ◄

Interstitial Lung Disease

Sarcoidosis with Large Nodular Lesions Simulating Pulmonary Metastases: Analysis of 126 Cases of Intrathoracic Sarcoidosis. A rare roentgenologic picture in sarcoidosis is that of large metastasis-like nodular lesions (LNL) with a "snowball" appearance. F. K. Rømer[2] (Aarhus, Denmark) determined the frequency of LNL in a series of 126 new cases of intrathoracic sarcoidosis diagnosed in Denmark in 1970–75 and followed regularly. The 68 female and 58 male patients in the series were aged 14–60 years. The x-rays were evaluated independently by 3 investigators, once blindly.

Eighty-two patients (65%) had only bilateral hilar adenopathy (BHL) at the time of diagnosis. Thirty-seven (29%) had BHL and pulmonary parenchymal lesions, mostly disseminated mottling, stippling and shadowing. Five, (4%) presented with pulmonary involvement without BHL. Two patients (1.6%) exhibited LNL simulating metastases. The appearances in 1 of these patients, a previously healthy man aged 25, who presented with cough, fever, malaise and weight loss over 3 months, are shown in Figure 22. Prednisone therapy was associated with marked regression of the pulmonary changes, and after 9 months

Fig 22.—Lungs 6 weeks after normal chest film was obtained. Multiple, large, round nodules are seen. (Courtesy of Rømer, F. K.: Scand. J. Respir. Dis. 58:11–16, 1977.)

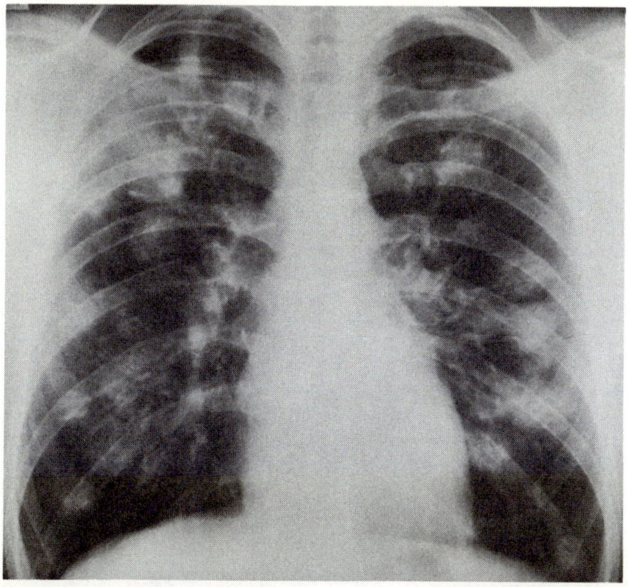

(2) Scand. J. Respir. Dis. 58:11–16, Jan. 1977.

the lungs appeared normal. In the other patient with LNL, the lesions regressed without treatment.

Recent reports from the United States suggest a higher frequency of LNL than was formerly suspected. In some cases the prognosis seems favorable, with lesions disappearing after 1 or 2 years, but the prognosis is unpredictable. All reported cases have been in young patients. Metastasis was suspected in many cases, including 1 of these 2. The method of choice for correct diagnosis in patients presenting with LNL is biopsy, especially of mediastinal lymph nodes. In cases with solitary nodules, thoracotomy and open lung biopsy may be necessary.

► [The observation that sarcoid can look like metastatic cancer, while not new, was new to us when we saw the first case we diagnosed about 2 years ago. We have since seen 5, and the literature this past year indicates that there is growing awareness of this (Dhakhwa et al.: Sarcoidosis presenting as multiple pulmonary nodules, J.A.M.A. 236:2529, 1976; Onal et al.: Nodular pulmonary sarcoidosis, Chest 72:296, 1977). The nodules may have discrete or ill-defined borders and vary in size from quite small to massive. The experience in the literature and our own indicate that at least many of these cases represent early disease, sometimes with other markers of early disease such as hilar nodes and acute arthritis, and tend to fairly prompt spontaneous resolution. The initial diagnostic procedure should probably be transbronchial biopsy, since this is positive in 93% of cases of sarcoid with pulmonary involvement and in 60% of cases in which the only roentgenographic manifestation is hilar adenopathy. These nodules may rarely cavitate (Tellis and Putnam: Cavitation in large multinodular pulmonary disease; a rare manifestation of sarcoidosis, ibid. 71:792, 1977) and even cause pneumothorax (Shiffner and Sharma: Acute pulmonary sarcoidosis with cavitation, West. J. Med. 127:346, 1977). Sharma (Sarcoidosis: Unusual pulmonary manifestations, Postgrad. Med. 61:67, 1977) has presented a nice and brief analysis of 180 personally reviewed cases. Thirteen patients had pleural involvement occurring from the time of diagnosis up to 6 years thereafter. In 4 the fluid showed lymphocytosis, but in 2 it was nearly cell free. In 2, pleural tissue revealed noncaseating granulomas. Seven of his cases had nodular lesions as described above. Two demonstrated peripheral lung shadowing and blood eosinophilia, resembling closely chronic eosinophilic pneumonia except for a lack of serious systemic symptoms. Three had unilateral lymphadenopathy, a feature which usually is taken to argue against sarcoid and for infection, especially tuberculosis. Three had calcified nodes, and 1 demonstrated a unilateral pneumonic infiltrate.

The problem of differentiating sarcoid from tuberculosis when the presenting syndrome is serofibrinous pleurisy with effusion was illustrated by a case reported by Mikhail et al. (Sarcoidosis presenting with a pleural effusion, Tubercle 57:226, 1976. This patient presented with a lymphocytic pleural effusion, and granulomas were found on pleural biopsy. He was started on antituberculous chemotherapy, and 5 months later developed bilateral pulmonary infiltrates which cleared after steroid administration.

Sarcoid of the nose and upper airways was discussed in an article from Dr. Geraint James' group (Neville et al.: Sarcoidosis of the upper respiratory tract and its association with lupus pernio, Thorax 31:660, 1976). Upper respiratory involvement, while seldom a prominent clinical finding, was found in 6% of cases when looked for. Of a total group of 17 with upper airway involvement, 12 had concomitant lupus pernio (a disfiguring violaceous cutaneous tumefaction of the nose, cheeks and ears). The mucous membrane involvement varied from clustered yellow spots to boggy erythematous membranes and, in some, polyp formation. Symptoms were due to obstruction, crusting and bleeding. Bone cysts were seen in 32%, indicating that this is often a part of disseminated and progressive illness. Nasal perforation, both spontaneous and especially after submucous resection, was seen (see also Selroos and Niemisto: Sarcoidosis of the nose, Tubercle 57:226, 1976). – Ed.] ◄

Idiopathic Pulmonary Fibrosis: Clinical, Histologic, Radiographic, Physiologic, Scintigraphic, Cytologic and Biochemical Aspects are discussed by Ronald G. Crystal, Jack D. Fulmer, William

TABLE 1.—CLASSIFICATION OF FIBROTIC LUNG DISORDERS

Known Cause	Unknown Cause
Occupational and environmental* inhalants	Idiopathic pulmonary fibrosis
Drug reactions	Associated with a collagen-vascular disease†
Physical agents	Not associated with any known disorder
Infectious disorders	Associated with pulmonary arteritis‡
Cardiac disease	Sarcoidosis
Pulmonary vascular disease	Ankylosing spondylitis
Neoplastic disease	Congenital; familial
	Eosinophilic granuloma
	Idiopathic pulmonary hemosiderosis
	Alveolar microlithiasis
	Goodpasture's syndrome
	Alveolar proteinosis

*Including those disorders termed "extrinsic allergic alveolitis"; the fibrotic form is called "chronic hypersensitivity pneumonitis."

†Including rheumatoid arthritis, progressive systemic sclerosis, systemic lupus erythematosus, dermatomyositis-polymyositis, Sjögren's syndrome and the mixed connective tissue syndrome; patients with necrobiotic nodules or vasculitis not included.

‡Including periarteritis nodosa; Wegener's granulomatosis; rheumatoid arthritis with necrobiotic nodules; and rheumatoid arthritis, progressive systemic sclerosis and polymyositis-dermatomyositis with arteritis.

C. Roberts, Morton L. Moss, Bruce R. Line and Herbert Y. Reynolds[3] (Natl. Inst. of Health) on the basis of the findings in 29 patients and a comprehensive review of the literature with 195 references. Idiopathic pulmonary fibrosis is now categorized as associated with a collagen-vascular disorder or not associated with any known disorder (Table 1). Clinicians have tended to consider the disease a diagnosis of exclusion;

TABLE 2.—CLINICAL, LABORATORY AND PHYSIOLOGIC FINDINGS IN PATIENTS WITH IDIOPATHIC PULMONARY FIBROSIS

Presenting Symptoms	Percent of Patients	Laboratory	Percent of Patients	Physiologic Studies	Mean Values*
Breathlessness	100	↑ Sedimentation rate	94†	Vital capacity	61.7 ± 2.9‡
Cough	86	+ Antinuclear antibodies	7†		
Systemic§	48†	+ Rheumatoid factor	14†	Total lung capacity	62.9 ± 2.9‡
		+ Cryoimmunoglobulins	41†		
		+ Lupus erythematosus preparations	3†	Residual volume/ total lung capacity	34.4 ± 1.6‖
Physical		Abnormal serum protein electrophoresis			
Tachypnea	46			FEV_1%**	97.6 ± 2.3‡
Clubbing	72	↑ $\alpha 2$ macroglobulins	22		
Chest findings		↑ γ globulins	17	Diffusing capacity††	46.8 ± 3.5‡
Normal	14	Serum immunoglobulins			
Rales	65	↑ IgG	4		
Ronchi or bronchovesicular		↑ IgA	39		
sounds	21	↑ IgM	9		
Cardiac findings		Serum complement (C50) ↓	6†		
Normal	30	Polycythemia	3		
Augmented P_2	70				

*Mean ±SEM.

†Data refer only to the 23 patients with no associated collagen-vascular disorder.

‡Percent predicted.

§Systemic symptoms included flulike illness, fatigue, joint symptoms, fever or weight loss.

‖Percent observed.

**Forced expiratory volume in 1 second/forced vital capacity.

††Single breath, carbon monoxide.

(3) Ann. Intern. Med. 85:769–788, December, 1976.

however, it has clearly defined features that define a characteristic and specific clinical entity.

Of the 29 patients evaluated at this institution, only 20% had an associated disorder. The average age was 51.8 years. The clinical and laboratory features are given in Table 2. The average duration of symptoms before evaluation was 2.9 years. The average patient had a total lung capacity of 62.9% predicted and a diffusing capacity of 46.8% predicted. An increased physiologic dead space, found in 60% of the patients, and a volume-pressure curve shifted downward and to the right are characteristic of the condition.

Histologic observations in the 29 patients showed the anatomical distribution of idiopathic pulmonary fibrosis to be heterogeneous. Increased fibrous tissue in the alveolar septae and inflammatory cells in areas of increased fibrous tissue are characteristic. Many of the "desquamated" cells described are macrophages. Peribronchiolar fibrous tissue or mononuclear inflammatory cells or both were found in 80% of the biopsies. An important distinguishing feature is absence of arteritis, granulomas or evidence of minerals in the lung. The 29 patients showed six radiographic patterns, the dominant patterns being reticular, reticulonodular and ground-glass. There was poor correlation between degree of fibrosis seen on lung biopsy and severity of disease estimated by chest film.

Idiopathic pulmonary fibrosis most likely begins as an alveolitis and gradually develops into alveolar septal fibrosis. It is probably reversible in the alveolitis stage. Thus overall assessment of progression must include methods that monitor the fibrotic process in order to evaluate prognosis and new types of therapy. The two most useful physiologic tools are the volume-pressure curve for staging fibrosis and the exercise study. Nuclear scanning is useful to evaluate lung perfusion, ventilatory function and lung inflammation. Limited bronchoalveolar lavage permits analysis of the cell and protein content of the recovered fluid.

The lung may act as a relatively independent immune organ in this disorder. It is probably not an allergic disorder mediated by IgE. The finding that collagen becomes antigenic to patients with idiopathic pulmonary fibrosis does not answer the question of what triggers the disease. Regardless of the trigger of idiopathic pulmonary fibrosis, several lines of evidence strongly suggest that therapeutic intervention should be directed toward stopping the inflammatory and immune process, rather than toward stopping the fibrotic process.

► [Interstitial fibrosis is a catchall phrase applied to a number of diseases with differing etiologies or associated with different systemic diseases as well as a group for which no etiology or readily understood associated disease process can be established. The pathologic process is variable depending on the stage at which material is available for study and to much less degree on the cause if there is one; in theory it begins with replication and desquamation of the type II alveolar epithelial cell (corner cell, surfactant producing) resulting in a round cell alveolar infiltrate, progresses to involvement of the interstitial areas with lymphocytes, other inflammatory cells, edema and fibroplasia in some mix, and at the most chronic and severe end of the spectrum appears as multiple cystic fibrotic areas most marked at the bases (honeycomb lung). There is also a wide spectrum of x-ray abnormalities depending on the stage of the illness, its severity and occasionally its etiology. The picture may be one of diffuse nodular infiltrates resembling miliary tuberculosis, simple increase in the interstitial markings of the lungs, more marked fibrosis, always with the bases somewhat more involved than the less-dependent areas, and finally basilar cystic and fibrotic changes with marked loss of lung volume. The physiologic picture is characterized by hypoxemia worsened on exercise, usually a normal or low carbon dioxide tension, hyperventilation, a defect in gas transfer across the alveolar-capillary membrane, decreased lung compliance and decreased lung volumes, the so-called alveolar-capillary block syndrome. This name implies thickening of the membrane as the basic defect in the production of gas transfer inhibition, but most feel that this is actually due in larger part to loss of pulmonary capillary cross-sectional area as a result of the fibrotic process. Although it has usually been said that obstruction to air flow is not seen, Fulmer et al. have demonstrated that tests sensitive to obstruction of small (under 2 mm) airways are abnormal in a large proportion of cases (Small airways in idiopathic pulmonary fibrosis, comparison of morphological and physiologic observations, J. Clin. Invest 60:595, 1977). The importance of this new observation, which parallels similar studies in sarcoidosis, is that hypoxemia may be due in part to ventilation-perfusion abnormalities, and this may improve with exercise rather than the converse which is expected with hypoxia due to defective gas transfer.

This process may be due to inhalation of fibrogenic dusts (Suratt et al.: Acute silicosis in tombstone sandblasters, Amer. Rev. Respir. Dis. 115:521, 1977); various drugs, particularly those used to treat cancer (discussed more fully below), but also, prominently, nitrofurantoin; the chronic effects of inhaled noxious agents such as gastric acid or smoke and other atmospheric pollutants including ozone, and NO_2; severe diffuse infections, particularly influenzal pneumonia; and may be associated with a variety of collagen vascular diseases, most prominently scleroderma and rheumatoid arthritis, but also systemic lupus erythematosus and, in a few reported cases, hepatitis B virus infection of the type which is associated with a positive antinuclear antibody. The notion that this is often the result of immune complex injury of the lung is a persistent one with considerable indirect evidence to support it. Doctor Turner-Warwick points out that not only established collagen vascular diseases with associated pulmonary fibrosis but also idiopathic pulmonary fibrosis (cryptogenic fibrosing alveolitis in the British phase) are associated with non-organ-specific autoantibodies in a fairly large proportion of cases (Immune reactions in pulmonary fibrosis, Schweiz. Med. Wochenschr. 107:171, 1977; and Haslam et al.: Antinuclear antibody and lymphocyte responses to nuclear antigens in patients with lung disease, Clin. Exp. Immunol. 20:379, 1975). The autoantibodies demonstrated include not only rheumatoid factor and antinuclear factor, but also anti-smooth muscle antibody and anti-mitochondrial antibody. Surprisingly, evidence for autoimmunity is also seen in fibrotic processes of known etiology such as silicosis and asbestosis. Further, some patients with accelerated silicosis develop connective tissue disorders such as lupus, scleroderma and rheumatoid arthritis, a cause-and-effect confusion which seems pretty impossible to untangle (Ziskind et al.: Silicosis, Amer. Rev. Respir. Dis. 113:643, 1976). The implication is that lung damage induces the autoantibodies which in turn cause wider tissue destruction, but this is simply speculative. Doctor Scadding has reported an association with hemolytic anemia (Fibrosing alveolitis with autoimmune hemolytic anemia: Two case reports, Thorax 32:134, 1977), but again this is only speculation. Not only humoral but cellular immune abnormalities have now been implicated (Kravis et al.: Pathogenic mechanisms in pulmonary fibrosis: Collagen-induced migration inhibition factor production and cytotoxicity mediated by lymphocytes, J. Clin. Invest. 58:1223, 1976).

The earliest stage of fibrosing alveolitis or interstitial fibrosis, in which the most prominent changes are alveoli filled with a mixture of type II alveolar epithelial cells and some macrophages, was initially thought to be a different disease termed "desquamative interstitial pneumonitis," and this is still the position taken by some authorities. It was also thought that lungs characterized by this tissue reaction responded more favorably to corticosteroid therapy than those with predominantly interstitial disease. This may or may not be the case, but some feel that steroid responsiveness cannot be predicted by whether the process is predominantly intra-alveolar or interstitial (Tubbs et al.: Desquamative interstitial pneumonitis: Cellular phase of fibrosing alveolitis, Chest 72:159, 1977). – Ed.] ◄

Severe Radiation Injuries of the Lung are discussed by Bernard

Roswit (VA Hosp., Bronx, N.Y.) and David C. White[4] (Armed Forces Inst. of Pathology, Washington, D. C.). The chief feature of the acute severe exudative syndrome of radiation lung injury is the long latent period for its expression, even after a gross radiation insult to the lung. Not until 2–10 weeks after irradiation is completed will the patient note dyspnea, a cough and low-grade fever. Only 7–10 days later will radiographs show a diffuse haze in the treatment zone, rapidly changing to flocculent patchy infiltrates and then coalescing to define the treatment portals more precisely in a "straight-edge effect."

Profound changes in lung function result from severe damage to the pulmonary parenchyma, bronchial tree and blood vessels. There is no consistent correlation between duration and severity of early radiation pneumonopathy and occurrence of late delayed pulmonary fibrosis. As with the early pneumonopathy, the volume of lung affected by fibrosis is critical to the outward manifestations of the late severe changes.

The early histologic response generally peaks 1–3 months after start of therapy. Much early damage is due to direct injury of the endothelium. Enlargement and a bizarre configuration of proliferating alveolar lining cells occur, and an exudate penetrates into the alveolus. Inspiratory efforts compress the trapped exudate into hyaline membranes. Dissipation or resorption of the exudate is slow, even though it may be limited in extent. The late phase is characterized by progressive vascular sclerosis and progressive interstitial fibrosis. Progressive scarring steadily destroys the respiratory parenchyma. Intercurrent bacterial invasion can produce a necrotizing bronchitis and bronchiolitis resistant to therapy.

For treating both lungs in patients with disseminated metastases, it is unwise to exceed a total of 2,000 rad in 10–13 fractions. In an infant or young child, daily fractions of 140–150 rad and a total of 1,400–1,500 rad represent the limits of lung tolerance. When adjuvant chemicals are used, especially actinomycin D, the total dose of radiation should be reduced by at least 10–15%. The acute exudative reaction is treated with high-dose steroids. Immediate and absolute bed rest is also important. Bronchodilators and oxygen therapy are always helpful.

► [This old subject is one which seems to be foggy in the minds of most internists. It is important; first, because of ever-increasing radiation therapy; second, because of the synergism, probable in most cases and certain in many, between irradiation and cancer chemotherapeutic agents in the production of diffuse interstitial disease (to be discussed below); and third, because the problem, in a patient under treatment for neoplastic disease and worsening pulmonary infiltrates, of differentiation among progression of the underlying process, superimposed infection and drug or irradiation toxicity comes up with increasing regularity on most medical services.

In addition to this article, a second very worthwhile review was published this past year (Gross: Pulmonary effects of radiation therapy, Ann. Intern. Med. 86:81, 1977), the practical major points of which will be summarized here. (1) "The amount of damage produced is less a function of total dose of radiation than the rate . . . delivered, since fractionation permits repair of sublethal dosage to occur between fractions." This fact has led to formulation of a different radiation unit, relative equivalent therapy (RET), which is calculated by a rather complicated formula taking into consideration total dose, number of fractions and interval between fractions (Ellis: Dose, time and frac-

---

(4) Am. J. Roentgenol. 129:127–136, July, 1977.

tionation: A clinical hypothesis; Clin. Radiol. 20:1, 1969). (2) The mean incidence of radiation pneumonitis in several series of breast cancer is 41% and in 11% symptoms occurred. In Hodgkin's disease estimates vary from 6% to 65%. (3) The illness is biphasic; radiation pneumonitis usually begins between 2 and 3 months after completion of treatment. Higher dosage produces earlier injury. Cough, respiratory distress with a sense of limitation of inspiration (doorstop phenomenon) and, in many, fever and constitutional symptoms are seen. Hypoxia is the rule. Severe cases may be promptly fatal but most persist for a week to a month and then gradually subside. The roentgenographic hallmark of radiation pneumonitis is an alveolar infiltrate sharply confined to the radiation port. In a few cases extension beyond the port, as, for instance, to a contralateral lung, is seen. The mechanism of this is not known. (4) The second phase, radiation fibrosis, evolves usually in a period of 6 months or more, in most cases following clinically recognized pneumonitis but occasionally appearing without a recognized antecedent episode of pneumonitis. (5) Pleural effusion infrequently occurs 2–6 months after completion of irradiation, always in association with symptomatic pneumonitis. It is modest to minimal in extent and tends to spontaneous resolution, differentiating it from malignant pleural involvement. (6) Endobronchial neoplastic lesions with potential to obstruct should be treated with prednisone, 20 mg 1 day before and 2 days after irradiation. (7) Pulmonary function tests available at most hospitals, such as simple lung volumes (vital capacity) and diffusion capacity, may become abnormal more promptly than the chest roentgenogram and anticipate the development of radiation pneumonitis, finding of real importance because of therapeutic implications. (8) The roentgenographic picture of radiation fibrosis, the late change, differs from pneumonitis and evolves from it into a series of linear streaks radiating from the area of previous pneumonitis but not confined to it. (9) Not only chemotherapeutic agents but also prior irradiation predispose to radiation pneumonitis and fibrosis. (10) Steroids in dosage of 60–80 mg prednisone daily should be administered to patients in the pneumonitis phase, the earlier the better. Interruption of steroids often is associated with recurrence. Accordingly, treatment should be prolonged and discontinuation carried out carefully with close supervision. Chemotherapeutic regimens containing intermittent steroid may cause confusing waxing and waning of the radiation pneumonitis.

As time goes on, it seems that virtually all cancer chemotherapeutic agents excluding the *Vinca* alkaloids have been observed to cause pulmonary injury. One good review (Green: Pulmonary toxicity of antineoplastic agents, West. J. Med. 127:292, 1977) divides these into those which seem clearly to be on an allergic basis with other extrapulmonary allergic manifestations (L-asparaginase, procarbazine, azothiaprine), those in which the mechanism is unknown, there being no relationship between toxicity and cumulative dose (methotrexate), and those producing direct, dose-related pulmonary toxicity (bleomycin, chlorambucil, cyclophosphamide, busulfan, melphalan). Another good recent review (Sostman et al.: Cytotoxic drug-induced lung disease, Am. J. Med. 62:608, 1977) includes reference to 6-mercaptopurine and azathioprine. Patel et al. review cyclophosphamide in some depth (Cyclophosphamide therapy and interstitial pulmonary fibrosis, Cancer 38:1542, 1976). Crittenden records a case due to BCNU (Pulmonary fibrosis after prolonged therapy with 1,3-Bis-(2-chloroethyl)-1 nitrosourea, Chest 72:372, 1977). Horton et al. (Diffuse interstitial pulmonary fibrosis complicating Hodgkin's disease, Br. J. Dis. Chest ibid., p. 44, 1977) blame a case on the underlying illness which was probably due to nitrogen mustard or procarbazine, both of which the patient received. Farney et al. reported a case which supports this supposition (Diffuse pulmonary disease after therapy with nitrogen mustard, vincristine, procarbazine and prednisone, Am. Rev. Respir. Dis. 115:135, 1977). McInerney and Bullimore implicate adriamycin (Reactivation of radiation pneumonitis by adriamycin, Br. J. Radiol. 50:224, 1976).—Ed.] ◄

Nonmalignant Lymphoid Disorders of the Chest are discussed by David S. Feigin, Stanley S. Siegelman, Elias G. Theros and Francis M. King[5] on the basis of review of the literature and examples collected at the Armed Forces Institute of Pathology. The nonmalignant lymphoid disorders can be divided into those that affect lymph nodes and those that primarily affect extranodal tissues (table).

(5) Am. J. Roentgenol. 129:221–228, August, 1977.

RADIOGRAPHIC CHARACTERISTICS OF LYMPHOID DISORDERS OF THE CHEST

Disorder	Lymph Node Enlargement	Pulmonary Abnormality
Extranodal disorders:		
Lymphocytic interstitial pneumonitis	−	Diffuse interstitial (later ? alveolar) infiltration
Pseudolymphoma	−	Localized infiltration
Lymphomatoid granulomatosis	−	Nodular or alveolar infiltration; cavitation possible
Lymph node disorders:		
Lymphadenitis	+	None or rare
Giant lymph node hyperplasia, and sinus histiocytosis with massive lymphadenopathy	+	None
Angioimmunoblastic lymphadenopathy	+	None or rare
Malignant lymphoma	+/−	Highly variable; infiltration and/or mass

Of the extranodal disorders, lymphocytic (lymphoid) interstitial pneumonitis principally affects middle-aged women and is characterized by coarse shadows or a more confluent alveolar pattern, without hilar or mediastinal adenopathy. There may be disorders of immune globulins or lymphoid infiltrations of other organs. Pulmonary pseudolymphoma is a localized parenchymal infiltrate. It is found primarily in middle-aged patients but with no sex predilection. There is no lymphadenopathy or pleural effusion. Symptoms are usually absent or very mild. Lymphomatoid granulomatosis is a relatively rare parenchymal disease characterized by angiocentric lymphoreticular proliferation and granulomatous change. The condition is considered reactive, but cutaneous, renal and central nervous system lesions are present in many cases. At least half of the patients die of the disease.

Of the lymph node disorders, lymphadenitis is usually caused by a specific inflammatory agent or organism or by one of several other causes, such as systemic lupus erythematosus and infectious mononucleosis. Lymphadenitis, giant lymph node hyperplasia and another form of node enlargement, sinus histiocytosis with massive adenopathy, present with mediastinal adenopathy, usually appearing as bilateral diffuse widening or nodularity. Angioimmunoblastic adenopathy is not universally accepted as distinct from other forms of lymphadenopathy. Some feel that it may be a form of the plasma cell type of giant lymph node hyperplasia. The radiologic appearance is not distinct from adenopathy of any other cause. The prognosis is extremely variable. With the exception of lymphadenitis, which is usually of viral origin, the exact nature of these nonmalignant lymphoid disorders is unclear. Malignant change is not known to occur in lymphocytic interstitial pneumonitis. Some feel that lymphomatoid granulomatosis can evolve into a malignant neoplasm. None of these disorders has a distinctive radiographic appearance. Diagnosis requires pulmonary biopsy or node biopsy and a complete hematologic workup. When the histologic appearance suggests a nonmalignant lymphoid disorder, aggressive combination cytotoxic drug therapy is usually not appropriate treatment.

► [Helman et al. have reported lymphoid interstitial pneumonitis (LIP) associated with chronic active hepatitis (Lymphoid interstitial pneumonia with associated chronic active hepatitis and renal tubular acidosis, Am. Rev. Respir. Dis. 115:161, 1977). The article is a nice one to note because it references the literature concerning the association of the broad category of interstitial fibrosis and chronic active hepatitis. The association of LIP with a wide variety of "immunologic" diseases is discussed in the 1977 YEAR BOOK (pp. 132 and 133) and the 1975 YEAR BOOK (p. 175). Weisbrot reported a confusing case with features of Sjögren's syndrome, lung biopsies interpreted during life as LIP, a downhill course with the appearance of cavitation and, at postmortem, the histologic features of lymphomatoid granulomatosis (Lymphomatoid granulomatosis of the lung, associated with a long history of benign lymphoepithelial lesions of the salivary glands and lymphoid interstitial pneumonitis, Am. J. Clin. Pathol. 66:792, 1976). Yockey et al. (Lymphomatoid granulomatosis presenting as fever of unknown origin, J.A.M.A. 237:2633, 1977) report a fatal case in a young man with "an unremitting illness consisting initially of fever, lymphadenopathy, hepatosplenomegaly and central nervous system dysfunction. Abnormal chest roentgenogram findings did not develop until 6 months after the patient became ill." The clinical features which set lymphomatoid granulomatosis apart from Wegener's granulomatosis are a greater incidence of necrotizing skin lesions, often misdiagnosed as suppurative panniculitis, massive central nervous system involvement in almost a quarter and a tendency in many to evolve into malignant lymphoma (1975 YEAR BOOK, p. 176).

Angioimmunoblastic lymphadenopathy was described in this article by Feigin et al. as very rarely having pulmonary involvement. Asher et al. (Immunoblastic lymphadenopathy presenting as pulmonary interstitial fibrosis, J.A.M.A. 237:2411, 1977) reported what they believe to be the first case with substantial lung parenchymal involvement.

Obviously sorting out these disorders, if they can be sorted out, and working through the therapeutic implications will be lively pursuits during the next several years. – Ed.] ◄

Pleural Diseases

Cirrhotic Pleural Effusion in the Absence of Ascites. Pleural effusions occur in about 5% of cirrhotic patients with ascites and occasionally they may develop in such patients without detectable ascites. James A. Singer, Marshall M. Kaplan and Ruth L. Katz[6] (Boston) report data on a woman who presented with a transudative pleural effusion in the absence of ascites or other stigmas of chronic liver disease. Cirrhosis with secondary hydrothorax was diagnosed eventually, but ascites was not demonstrated until just before death when hypertonic saline was administered.

Woman, 61, was admitted for progressive shortness of breath, present for 6 months, and ankle swelling for 1 month. She had had hepatitis 25 years before. The entire right side of the chest was dull, with absent breath sounds. The abdomen was distended but without shifting dullness and the liver was palpable 2 cm below the right costal margin. A large right pleural effusion was present with a mediastinal shift to the left. The serum glutamic-pyruvic transaminase was 71 IU and the alkaline phosphatase was 4 Bodansky units. Clear sterile fluid was obtained from a chest tube. Two peritoneal taps yielded no fluid. Lethargy and asterixis were noted on hospital day 3; the mental status cleared on treatment for hepatic encephalopathy. A liver biopsy specimen showed postnecrotic cirrhosis. The pleural effusion cleared over several weeks on salt restriction and diuretic therapy but reaccumulated 3–4 months later. Symptomatic hyponatremia developed despite cessation of diuretics, and small

Fig 23.—Hole (1 mm) in tendinous portion of right hemidiaphragm. (Courtesy of Singer, J. A., et al.: Gastroenterology 73:575–577, September, 1977.)

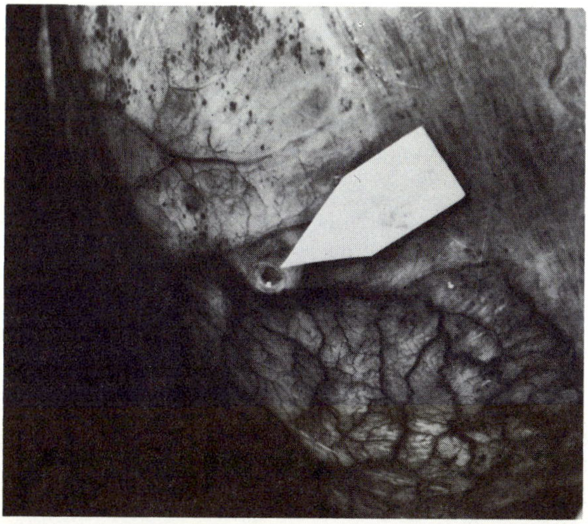

(6) Gastroenterology 73:575–577, September, 1977.

doses of hypertonic saline were given that lead to detectable ascites for the first time. The patient died after a relatively rapid downhill course.

Autopsy showed about 200 ml ascitic fluid that flowed through a 1-mm hole in the tendinous part of the right hemidiaphragm when the body was tilted (Fig 23). The right thorax contained 2,500 ml of clear fluid and the right lung was collapsed. The diaphragm contained a defect lined by a single layer of mesothelial cells continuous with the peritoneal and pleural lining cells; inflammation was absent.

The small diaphragmatic defect explains the occurrence of pleural effusion in the absence of detectable ascites in this case. The flow of ascitic fluid into the pleural space equalled the rate of ascites production. Similar diaphragmatic defects have been described at autopsy in 10 patients with cirrhotic hydrothorax. Probably rupture of diaphragmatic blebs, formed from evagination of peritoneum through a congenital diaphragmatic weakness, is responsible for the hydrothorax in these cases. The absence of ascites should not prevent the inclusion of cirrhosis in the differential diagnosis of an otherwise unexplained pleural effusion.

► [This is an old observation, although new to us. The mechanism in this case was clearly direct transmission via a diaphragmatic defect. The unusual feature of the case was the absence of ascites. It was proposed that the negative pressure in the thorax relative to the abdomen in this instance caused the fluid to be sucked into the chest as rapidly as it was formed. Stanley et al. (Hypoxia and hydrothoraces in a case of liver cirrhosis: Correlation of physiologic, radiographic, scintigraphic and pathologic findings, Thorax 32:457, 1977) demonstrated direct peritoneal to pleural communication by inducing pneumoperitoneum during life. They make the point that thoracentesis is indicated only for diagnosis and that repeated removal of fluid from the chest may prevent the diaphragmatic defect from healing. Johnston and Loo (Hepatic hydrothorax: Studies to determine the source of the fluid and report of 13 cases, Ann. Intern. Med. 61:385, 1964) studied 5 cases with labeled albumin and concluded that the mechanism of formation was via transdiaphragmatic lymphatics rather than an actual anatomical defect. Lieberman et al. (Pathogenesis and treatment of hydrothorax complicating cirrhosis with ascites, ibid. 64:341, 1966), using similar techniques and also pneumoperitoneum, provided evidence for actual diaphragmatic defects; so it seems reasonable to assume that both mechanisms may obtain. They stated that repeated attempts might be necessary to position air over the liver but once it was there it went to the chest. They emphasized that repeated thoracenteses were useless and often debilitating as fluid usually rapidly reaccumulated and that the only effective therapy was diuresis and salt limitation to decrease the formation of ascites. They said that at times the defect might seal and then rupture, making the pleural fluid transiently bloody when the ascites was not. In most series quoted, the incidence of hydrothorax in cirrhosis is about 5–8% although in some it is lower. Two-thirds are on the right side, the remainder being more or less equally divided between bilateral and left-sided effusions. Our interest in this subject was stimulated by a case with spontaneous peritonitis in a cirrhotic with a simultaneous infected right-sided pleural effusion, the organism being the same in the pleural fluid and the ascites. – Ed.] ◄

Pleural Effusion: Diagnostic Dilemma. Whatever its cause, pleural effusion requires investigation because it may represent serious or fatal disease. Often the cause is elusive. Donald D. Storey, David E. Dines and Douglas T. Coles[7] (Mayo Clinic), in order to determine the cause of pleural effusion, reviewed the clinical and laboratory data of 72 male and 61 female patients who had had 204 thoracenteses during 1973–74. The cause was determined in 108 patients and was indeter-

(7) J.A.M.A. 236:2183–2186, Nov. 8, 1976.

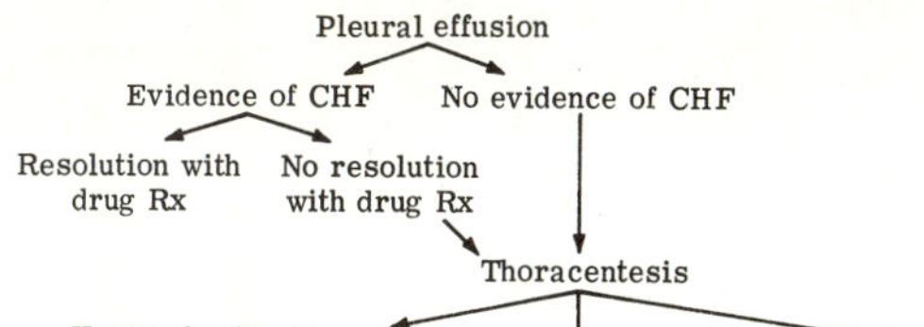

Primary diagnosis	Hemorrhagic, serous or serosanguineous	Chylous	Purulent
1. Cancer	Pr + Cy	Pr, Cy, F	Pr, Cy, RC
2. Lymphoma	Pr	Pr, F	Pr, RC
3. Miscellaneous	Pr + Cy + O	Pr, Cy, F, O	Pr, Cy, RC, O
4. Unknown	Pr, Cy, AC, FC	Pr, Cy, AC, FC, F	Pr, Cy, AC, FC, RC

Fig 24.—Algorithm for evaluation of pleural effusion; *CHF*, congestive heart failure; *Pr*, protein determination; *Cy*, cytology; *F*, triglyceride and cholesterol determinations; *RC*, routine culture; *O*, other tests (including those known to have high correlation with specific diagnosis, such as glucose with rheumatoid effusion or amylase with pancreatic disease); *AC*, acid-fast bacillus culture; *FC*, fungal culture. (Courtesy of Storey, D. D., et al.: J.A.M.A. 236:2183–2186, Nov. 8, 1976; copyright 1976, American Medical Association.)

minate in the other 25. There were 164 diagnostic thoracenteses; various tests on the fluid were done in these.

The result was positive for cancer in 15% of the 136 cytologic examinations. Five of 19 patients with primary bronchogenic carcinoma, 13 of 25 with clinical metastatic lung cancer and 2 of 20 with lymphoma had positive cytologic findings.

Of 105 patients studied, 35 had a pleural fluid protein level below 3 gm/100 ml; 16 of the 35 had congestive heart failure, and 6 had hypoproteinemia. Of 70 with a protein level above 3 gm/100 ml, 30 had malignant neoplasms and 14 had lymphoma.

Four positive aerobic cultures and 1 positive anaerobic culture were obtained in 143 routine bacterial cultures.

Transthoracic needle biopsy of the pleura in 28 cases revealed 8 specimens positive for malignant neoplasms; 2 of these patients had normal cytologic findings. Cell counts on 46 effusions revealed 17 with over 50% lymphocytes, 13 of these were secondary to neoplasm.

None of 7 amylase determinations was diagnostic of pancreatitis. Cholesterol and triglyceride values, obtained in 5 cases, confirmed chylous effusion in only 1 case. Pleural fluid complement tests in 5 cases were not contributory. Eight of 107 effusions had a glucose content below 50 mg/100 ml; 3 of these were associated with bronchogenic carcinoma. Six effusions had a glucose content of over 150 mg/100 ml; 2 were associated with lymphoma.

Laboratory study of pleural fluid has a low yield of positive results for cancer. Routine culture is not indicated unless tuberculosis is strongly suspected. Certain tests are indicated only in specific situations. Only protein measurement and cytologic examination should be ordered routinely at diagnostic thoracentesis. A logical and cost-effective approach to evaluation of pleural effusions is shown in Figure 24.

► [This conservative and reasoned approach based on a large series of cases is welcome indeed. The recent series of excellent studies on what can be done with pleural fluid led our housestaff to follow them all in each case, which clearly is not indicated (1976 YEAR BOOK, p. 180; 1974 YEAR BOOK, p. 196; and 1973 YEAR BOOK, p. 189).—Ed.] ◄

Internal Pancreatic Fistulas: Pancreatic Ascites and Pleural Effusions. John L. Cameron, Richard S. Kieffer, William J. Anderson and George D. Zuidema[8] (Johns Hopkins Hosp.) report their experience with 34 patients with a diagnosis of internal pancreatic fistulas during 1966–75. There were 29 male and 5 female patients; the average age at presentation was 40 years. Thirteen patients were from a Veterans Administration hospital.

Twenty-two patients had a fistula into the peritoneal cavity and presented with ascites. Seven had fistulas tracking up into the mediastinum and into a pleural cavity and presented with massive pleural effusion. Five patients presented with both ascites and pleural effusions. Only 2 patients presented with acute pancreatitis; 12 others had a history of attacks of acute pancreatitis (Table 1). The diagnosis was easily made by determination of the amylase and albumin levels in ascites or pleural fluid.

Patients were generally treated nonoperatively for up to several weeks. Those with ascites underwent multiple paracenteses and those with pleural effusions, multiple thoracenteses; if the fistula remained unclosed, operation was performed (Table 2). Many patients underwent pancreatography in an attempt to define the anatomy of the internal fistula; 1 patient underwent retrograde transduodenal pancreatography before surgery (Fig 25). Seventeen patients ultimately came to surgery. Thirteen were found to have pseudocysts and 4 to have direct duct leaks with no pseudocyst. Nine patients underwent resection of the involved pancreas. Two patients had pseudocyst drainage into the duodenum by way of a large sphincteroplasty; 1 had recurrence of ascites and then underwent a cystogastrostomy. A third patient with a duct leak had no definitive procedure.

The overall mortality of 18% in these 34 patients with internal pancreatic fistulas is significant. The mortality generally represents the debilitated state that many patients were in but, with careful manage-

TABLE 1.—ACUTE PANCREATITIS

Pancreatic Fistula	# Patients	Current	Previous History	None
Ascites	22	1	9	12
Pleural Effusion	7	1	2	4
Both	5		1	4

TABLE 2.—TREATMENT

	Medical				Surgical			
Pancreatic Fistula	# Patients	Success	Failure	Death	# Patients	Success	Failure	Death
Ascites	17	7	6	4	10	8	0	2
Pleural effusion	3	2	1		5	4	1	
Both	5	3	2		2	2		

(8) Ann. Surg. 184:587–593, November, 1976.

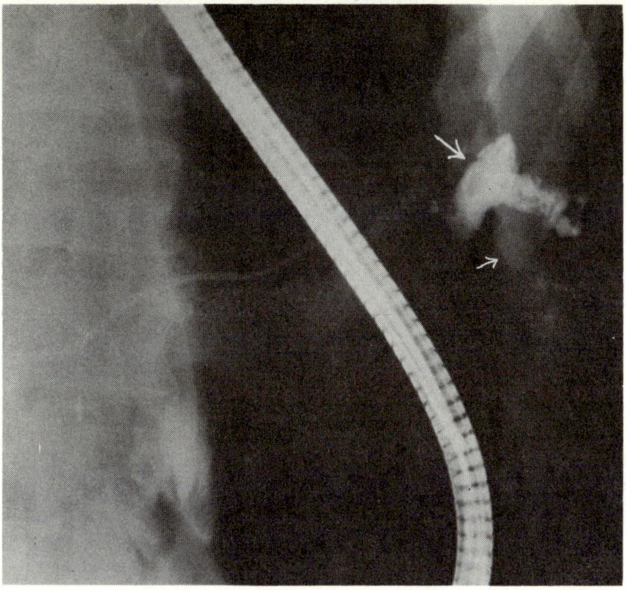

Fig 25.—Retrograde transduodenal pancreatogram demonstrating a normal proximal duct, a distal pseudocyst *(large arrow)* and extravasation into the free peritoneal cavity *(small arrow)*. (Courtesy of Cameron, J. L., et al.: Ann. Surg. 184:587–593, November, 1976.)

ment and use of intravenous hyperalimentation, most patients should be treated successfully. The long-term outlook is much better than that of patients with the entities with which pancreatic ascites and pleural effusions usually are confused, cirrhotic ascites and lung cancer.

► [This is the largest series collected from one institution and the only one from which firm diagnostic and therapeutic guidelines can be derived. The use of elective retrograde cannulation of the pancreatic duct is impressive. The frequency with which these syndromes appear in the absence of a clinical history of pancreatitis remains surprising. The fact that the fluid amylase level is always very high whereas the serum amylase level can be normal or minimally elevated bears emphasis. Although not mentioned in this article, this syndrome can result from blunt abdominal trauma such as can be sustained in automobile accidents (personal case).

The literature concerning the occurrence of the adult respiratory distress syndrome in acute pancreatitis is summarized in part by McKenna et al. (The pleuropulmonary complications of pancreatitis, Chest 71:197, 1977). Although the etiology of this problem must be multifactorial, an experimental study in dogs by Reinitz et al. (Pulmonary sequelae of experimental pancreatitis, J. Surg. Res. 22:566, 1977) makes a strong point for the concept that serum lecithinase A, which is elevated in pancreatitis, alters lung surfactant, with resulting alveolar atelectasis and vascular congestion. Murphey et al. (The "negative chest radiograph" in acute pancreatitis, Br. J. Radiol. 50:264, 1977) make the point that the initial chest x-ray is often normal in patients who go on to develop substantial respiratory distress and that arterial hypoxemia may be a more sensitive indicator of pancreatitis-induced diffuse lung disease than is the x-ray.

There are some other articles of interest concerning the pleura. Askin et al. (Reactive eosinophilic pleuritis, a lesion to be distinguished from pulmonary eosinophilic granuloma, Arch. Pathol. Lab. Med. 101:187, 1977) found lesions suggestive of eosinophilic granuloma in the pleural specimens of 37% of 57 patients treated for spontaneous pneumothorax with pleurectomy, none of whom had evidence of parenchymal eosinophilic granuloma. Since this latter condition is frequently complicated by pneumothorax, this potential source of confusion seems worthwhile to know. Rubin et al.

briefly review the subject of chylothorax (Chylothorax: therapeutic alternatives, Am. Surg. 43:292, 1977) and its successful medical and surgical management in 8 and 6 patients, respectively. The article "Granulomatous pleuritis secondary to blastomycosis," by Nelson and Light (Chest 71:433, 1977), is mentioned in the section Infections, in this YEAR BOOK. The important feature is that the clinical syndrome resembled tuberculosis clinically and histologically. Sokolowski et al. have briefly reviewed the association of pneumothorax with underlying pulmonary disease (Spontaneous pneumothorax as a manifestation of pulmonary disease, J. Med. Soc. N. J. 74:127, 1977). – Ed.] ◄

Tuberculosis and Other Infections

Transmission of Tubercle Bacilli: The Effects of Chemotherapy are discussed by A. Rouillon, S. Perdrizet and R. Parrot[9] (Paris) Patients in whom tubercle bacilli are detectable by direct examination of the sputum smear are the main sources of transmission of the bacillus. In addition, persons infected by smear-positive patients break down more often with the disease. A Canadian study demonstrated the relation of certain factors to prevalence of infection among contacts (table).

In the individual patient, use of antibacterial drugs completely alters the natural history of the disease. Patients are cured, their period of infectivity is considerably reduced and chronicity disappears. The impact of chemotherapy is reflected in a twofold to threefold increase in rate of decline of risk of infection, a decline that had begun before introduction of the drugs. Patients given the right drug combination lose their infectivity in a few weeks, probably most often within 2 weeks. Obviously, treatment must be continued much longer on a regular basis to insure maintenance of conversion and absence of relapse.

Direct sputum examination is important when tuberculosis is suspected, and as wide as possible a circle of contacts of positive patients should be examined. The best form of isolation is achieved by regular chemotherapy. Bacteriologic supervision and radiographic review can be considerably reduced in the course of treatment. A rapid return to work is desirable as soon as general and functional symptoms have resolved, as long as drugs are taken regularly. Indefinite supervision of

PREVALENCE (PERCENTAGE) OF ACTIVE TUBERCULOSIS IN INFECTED CONTACTS OF THE PATIENT ACCORDING TO BACTERIOLOGIC STATUS OF THE INFECTIOUS PATIENT, CLOSENESS OF THE CONTACT AND AGE OF THE CONTACTS

Age group (years)	*Degree of contact*	*Bacteriological status of infected patient**			*Total*
		Microscopy+	*Culture+*	*Culture–*	
0–14	Close	*37.7 (11.0)*	*18.2 (9.1)*	*9.7 (0)*	*33.0 (9.6)*
	Occasional	*23.8 (6.6)*	*18.2 (0)*	–2	*21.8 (5.6)*
15–29	Close	*10.6 (4.5)*	*1.2 (0)*	–2	*7.2 (2.9)*
	Occasional	*6.2 (3.9)*	*3.2 (1.1)*	–2	*5.2 (3.1)*
30 or more	Close	*4.6 (3.7)*	*0.8 (0.4)*	–2	*2.9 (2.3)*
	Occasional	*1.9 (1.3)*	*2.1 (1.5)*	–2	*1.7 (1.2)*
Total	Close	*15.0 (5.9)*	*3.3 (1.5)*	*1.2 (0)*	*10.5 (4.1)*
	Occasional	*5.6 (2.6)*	*3.1 (1.3)*	–2	*4.5 (2.1)*

*Numbers in parentheses represent percent of cases with bacteriologic confirmation.

(9) Tubercle 57:275–299, December, 1976.

patients can be abandoned 2 years after satisfactory treatment is completed.

Wider and more systematic use of chemoprophylaxis, as in subjects with "minimal fibrotic lesions" or those merely tuberculin-positive, will depend on results of studies to define the groups capable of benefiting from this approach and to determine the level of risk of tuberculosis to which these subjects are actually exposed, as well as on comparisons between risk of disease and risks from chemoprophylaxis.

► [This scholarly and extensive review, which really cannot be summarized too well, gathers together evidence, some of it from European sources, to support the recent radical changes in attitudes toward the infectiousness of patients, identification of the people at risk to develop tuberculosis and where people ought to be treated. It is written in a personal, almost polemic style and is fun to read. Some of the major points will be repeated here. (1) The person by all odds most likely to infect others is the untreated patient with a positive smear on direct microscopy. Patients who are culture positive but have negative results on direct microscopic examination of the sputum are almost no risk at all, and patients who remain positive by microscopy but have been on treatment for 2 weeks or so are likewise noninfectious to all intents and purposes. As illustrated in the table, the microscopy-positive patient infects almost 40% of close contacts under age 14, an enormous risk. The average undiscovered active patient infects 5–10 persons a year. (2) The closeness of the contact to an index case influences not only the risk of infection but also the incidence of active disease. In other words, the closer the contact and larger the inoculum the more likely it is that active disease rather than just infection will occur. (3) A positive smear connotes 5,000–10,000 bacilli per ml sputum. A bout of coughing produces up to 3,500 infectious particles, most of which remain suspended in the air; 5 minutes of talking does the same; and a sneeze disperses one million particles. (4) Most microscopy-positive patients have rapidly evolving disease; practically, this means that one can go from a negative x-ray to a far-advanced x-ray between 2 yearly routine chest films. (5) Although estimates vary widely, infection carries about a 5% risk for evolution into active disease during the first 2 years and a 10% lifetime risk. If one looks only at those patients between the ages of 15 and 30, this is much higher, in one study 15%. (6) High degrees of tuberculin reactivity may indicate a larger than usual initial infection and risk of development of active disease, at least in younger individuals. (7) Prior to chemotherapy, 50% of microscopy-positive tuberculosis patients died, a quarter of the cases were arrested and a quarter became chronic active cases. (8) Chemotherapy virtually eliminates the risk of relapse, which is as high as 20% in the patient who had disease arrested prior to the chemotherapy era or who was treated and arrested with inadequate chemotherapy. (9) Drugs decrease infectiousness not only by an effect on the organism but also by suppressing the vehicle of transmission, that is to say, cough.

A similar article with less extensive but still interesting data was published by Sbarbaro (Tuberculosis: The new challenge to the practicing clinician, Chest [Suppl.] 68: 436, 1975). He summarizes USPHS data indicating that only 8% of new active cases each year come from the 93% of the population which is uninfected (tuberculin negative) at the outset. Ninety-two percent of active cases will come from the 7% of the population which is infected, either tuberculin positive only, tuberculin positive with apparently quiescent small lesions or individuals with a history of active disease who have in the past received either no chemotherapy or inadequate chemotherapy.

These facts have altered the approach both to case finding and to treatment in ways which are not as widely recognized as they might be. It is necessary to really be very thorough about contacts, tuberculin testing them all as much as possible, getting chest x-rays of those who are positive, treating contacts who have positive tuberculin tests and retesting after a 2-month interval those with negative tests. Although an initial brief period of hospitalization for new active cases is convenient and on balance advisable in most, it is quite acceptable, from the point of view of contagion, to treat a reliable new patient entirely at home. If efforts are made to control cough (coughing into tissues) and to keep children out of the room for 2 weeks or so, the risk is truly minimal compared to that which preceded diagnosis. After 2 or 3 weeks of treatment have been accomplished, patients who feel well can go back to work with no risk to co-workers.

The single most important duty of the physician is to make sure that appropriate chemotherapy is prescribed and, more importantly, taken.—Ed.] ◄

Clinical and Roentgenographic Spectrum of Pulmonary Tuberculosis in the Adult. Because patients with tuberculosis are no longer managed predominantly by physicians with special interest in the disease or in special hospitals, physicians today have much less experience with the disease than in the past. M. Anees Khan, Daniel M. Kovnat, Bruce Bachus, Michael E. Whitcomb, Jerome S. Brody and Gordon L. Snider[1] reviewed newly diagnosed cases seen in a 12-month period at Boston City Hospital and the Boston VA Hospital to determine how often adults with tuberculosis present with atypical roentgenographic manifestations. Data on all patients aged 16 or more with a diagnosis of pulmonary tuberculosis made in a 1-year period were reviewed.

Of 225 patients with pulmonary tuberculosis, 88 had new active cases; 30 of these cases (34%) were considered unusual. There were 76 men and 12 women in the series. More than a third of the patients were less than age 40 years, and 23% were more than age 60. Thirty-six patients had a history of alcohol abuse, 6 had bronchogenic carcinoma and 3 had diabetes. Symptoms were more frequent in usual than in unusual cases. More women than men had the unusual type. The unusual cases are summarized in Table 1, and the clinical features of 12 patients with primary tuberculosis are given in Table 2. Six patients had parenchymal infiltrates isolated to the lower or middle lobe. Four had miliary infiltration of the lungs. Eight patients had discrete tuberculomas, which were multiple in 3 of them.

Pulmonary tuberculosis in the adult often does not present as an upper lobe infiltrate. One third of the patients in this study had unusual roentgenographic manifestations. At least 14% had primary dis-

TABLE 1.—UNUSUAL PULMONARY TUBERCULOSIS

Category		Number	Per Cent of Total
I. Primary tuberculosis		12	13.5
i. Isolated pleural effusion	5		
ii. Pleural effusion with infiltrate in lower lobe	1		
iii. Pleural effusion with ipsilateral hilar adenopathy and infiltrate	1		
iv. Isolated unilateral hilar adenopathy	1		
v. Unilateral hilar adenopathy with infiltrate	3		
vi. Bilateral hilar adenopathy	1		
II. Tuberculosis in lower lung field		6	6.8
i. Lower lobe	4		
ii. Middle lobe	2		
III. Miliary tuberculosis		4	4.5
IV. Tuberculoma		8	9.1
i. Solitary (coin lesion)	5		
ii. Multiple (2 to 4 nodules)	3		
Total		30	34

(1) Am. J. Med. 62:31–38, January, 1977.

TABLE 2.—ADULT PRIMARY TUBERCULOSIS

Case No.	Age (yr), Race and Sex	Symptoms	Location of Pulmonary Lesion	Hilar Adenopathy	Pleural Effusion	Source of Bacteriologic Confirmation
1	28,B,M	Fever, pulmonary and constitutional symptoms for 1 mo	...	+	—	Sputum culture
2	24,B,M	Pulmonary and constitutional symptoms for 3 mo	Infiltrate in lower lobe of left lung	+	—	Sputum smear and culture
3	27,B,F	Fever, pulmonary and constitutional symptoms for 4 mo	Infiltrate in lower lobe of right lung	+	—	Sputum smear and culture
4	25,W,F	Pulmonary symptoms for 1 mo	Infiltrate in upper lobe of right lung	+	—	Sputum smear and culture
5	38,W,M*	Pulmonary and constitutional symptoms for 2 mo	Infiltrate in lower lobe of right lung	+	R	Pleural biopsy
6	31,W,M†	Fever for 6 wk	...	—	L	Pleural biopsy and sputum culture
7	30,W,M	Fever and pulmonary symptoms for 2 wk	...	—	L	Pleural biopsy
8	19,B,F‡	Fever and pulmonary symptoms for 4 days	...	—	R	Pleural biospy
9	29,W,M†	Fever, pulmonary and constitutional symptoms for 1 wk	...	—	R	Pleural biopsy
10	67,B,M	Fever and constitutional symptoms for 2 mo	...	—	L	Pleural fluid and pleural biopsy
11	64,W,M	Pulmonary and constitutional symptoms for 6 wk	Infiltrate in lower lobe of right lung	—	R	Sputum smear and culture
12	37,B,M	Pulmonary and constitutional symptoms for 2 mo	Diffuse nodular	Bilateral	—	1. Sputum smear and culture 2. Mediastinal node biopsy

*Right hilar lymphadenopathy was noted on chest roentgenogram taken 20 days before admission.
†5 TU skin test turned positive 2 weeks later.
‡Infiltrate developed in superior segment of lower lobe of right lung on 3d hospital day.

ease. When the cause remains unclear, tissue must be obtained for histologic study and culture. The flexible fiberoptic bronchoscope has been useful in diagnosing endobronchial disease and in obtaining secretions and tissue in difficult cases. The need for prompt, accurate diagnosis and recognition of the total spectrum of roentgenologic manifestations of tuberculosis persists.

► [These forms of tuberculosis are by no means new or different and have probably existed in this proportion in the patient population studied more or less forever. What is new or different, as compared to 40 years ago when much of the material traditionally taught about the clinical features of tuberculosis was generated, or even 20 years ago, is that universal or even frequent infection in childhood or the early adolescent years no longer takes place, so that one is seeing initial infections in later life—often, as in this group of patients, in people with some compromise of their overall health. When tuberculosis infection is acquired in persons with some degree of immune compromise such as children (if you are willing to grant that childhood constitutes a period of somewhat decreased cellular immunity), sequestered races such as Indians or at times blacks, or in this instance alcoholics, a lower lobe infiltrate and hilar adenopathy often result, many times associated with pleural effusion (although pleural effusion can occur later than the early postprimary period during the course of tuberculous infection, see 1973 YEAR BOOK, p. 146). When infection is acquired by vigorous adolescents or young adults of European extraction, the site of the initial infection and the hilar node component are minimal and often not seen at all and the first apparent consequence of the infection is progression of a metastatic infectious focus in the apical posterior aspect of the lungs. This is the so-called adult type or reinfection type of tuberculosis, but it still represents a direct and fairly prompt (within a year usually) consequence of the initial infection in the lower or mid-lung fields.

The production of what looks like an atelectatic pneumonitis of the dependent portions of the lung, particularly the middle lobe, by rupture of an adjacent node and bronchogenic spread of infectious material from it is a well-established mechanism with which doctors dealing with tuberculosis have long been familiar (see 1975 YEAR BOOK, p. 201). Since one of the patients in this article by Khan et al. had concomitant cancer, it perhaps bears repeating that cancer and other destructive lung diseases such as lung abscess can erode a previously quiescent focus and reactivate tuberculosis either in that location or distal to it by bronchogenic spread (see 1977 YEAR BOOK, comment on p. 175). – Ed.] ◄

Short-Course Chemotherapy in Pulmonary Tuberculosis was evaluated in a controlled trial by the British Thoracic and Tuberculosis Association.[2] Treatment of 696 patients with pulmonary tuberculosis with rifampicin plus isoniazid for 6 – 18 months, supplemented for 2 months by ethambutol or streptomycin, resulted in bacteriologic quiescence in all cases but 1 at 18 months. In this report, the findings are extended to 33 months from the start of chemotherapy.

Patients aged 15 – 70 years with culture-proved pulmonary disease were included in the study if they were not known to be pregnant or to have impaired renal, hepatic or visual function. Patients with no cavity larger than 2 cm in diameter were treated for 6 or 12 months and those with larger cavities for 9 or 18 months. Rifampicin, 600 mg/day or 450 mg for patients weighing under 50 kg, isoniazid, 300 mg/day, and ethambutol, 25 mg/kg/day, were given orally. Streptomycin, 0.75 gm, was given intramuscularly 6 days a week. The oral drugs were taken all together in a single daily dose on an empty stomach.

The 665 evaluable patients have completed 33 months in the study. No relapses occurred in patients given 9 months of chemotherapy, and the relapse rate in those treated for 12 months was 1%. The same regimen given for 6 months resulted in a relapse rate of 5% in the subsequent 27 months. Adverse reactions occurred with streptomycin but not with ethambutol.

It is concluded that treatment with rifampicin plus isoniazid for 9 months, supplemented by ethambutol, 25 mg/kg, for the first 2 months, is now acceptable as standard chemotherapy for pulmonary tuberculosis in Britain. This regimen is well tolerated by patients, is totally effective in sputum conversion and has not been followed by relapse.

► [This is the last of a large series of studies which appear definitively to have established that 9 months' treatment with isoniazid plus rifampin (the editors doubt the contribution of 2 months of ethambutol, but it cannot hurt, and those were the conditions of the study) produces results equal to but not better than those obtained with 18 – 24 months' treatment with a double- or multiple-drug regimen containing isoniazid but not rifampin. It is of interest that 9 rather than 6 months is the optimum period. The question invariably arises, "Why do anything else if this works so well?" and indeed one gathers that in England this is now the official position.

We still feel that there are some good reasons to individualize. In the patient in whom compliance really seems certain and who has less than far-advanced disease and a drug-sensitive infection, equally good results can be obtained by administration of isoniazid and ethambutol for 18 months or 2 years. In more far-advanced disease, equally good results can be obtained by regimens containing INH and streptomycin. Rifampin still appears to many to increase the risk of hepatotoxicity from isoniazid, and there are studies which give some basic scientific rationale to the notion that this should be the case (rifampin is an inducer of the hepatic microsomal system which metabolizes isoniazid, and it is a toxic product of isoniazid metabolism which is thought to be the important factor in the production of hepatitis (Black et al.: Isoniazid-associated hepatitis in 114 patients, Gastroenterology 69:289, 1975; and Mitchell and

(2) Lancet 2:1102 – 1104, Nov. 20, 1976.

Jollows: Metabolic activation of drugs to toxic substances, ibid. 68:392, 1975). However, firm data that isoniazid plus rifampin is more toxic than INH alone are very hard to develop and this remains opinion. Further, rifampin in combination with other drugs to which the infection has not been exposed has entirely changed the outlook of INH-resistant relapse cases. It will be argued that if you treat properly you do not get relapses, but in a practical sense you do, most often due to patient failure to comply. See Zaki et al. (Tuberculosis patients; reactivation, N.Y. State J. Med. 77:1441, 1977) for a discussion of factors leading to reactivation and a review of the literature. Failure to comply with a regimen containing both major agents, or taking these drugs intermittently, is quite liable to produce acquired microbial resistance to both, creating the unfortunate and difficult to treat situation of tuberculosis resistant to both of the really effective agents.

It remains our preference, even in the face of the above very good evidence, to reserve administration of isoniazid and rifampin together for those cases in which the ability or willingness of the patient to comply with therapy seems uncertain and in which the most rigid type of control, preferably in a hospital, can be maintained. Another acceptable approach to the patient in whom noncompliance seems likely but who cannot be hospitalized is intermittent (less than daily) chemotherapy under rigid clinic supervision (Trial of two intermittent short-course regimens (78 doses) in the initial treatment of pulmonary tuberculosis, Tubercle 58:1, 1977; and Controlled trial of 6-month and 9-month regimens of daily and intermittent streptomycin plus isoniazid plus pyrazinamide for pulmonary tuberculosis in Hong Kong, Am. Rev. Respir. Dis. 115:727, 1977). Unfortunately the number of patients who cannot or will not take drugs on a regular basis always exceeds the estimate of the physician. The use of INH-containing regimens without rifampin in the relatively well, compliant patient with the intention to treat for 2 years or so may be an old-fashioned or stubborn opinion, but the results remain excellent, the uncertainty of increased toxicity with INH plus rifampin, if this does work out to be the case, is avoided and, perhaps most importantly, one does not risk losing the effectiveness of both agents if the patient proves to be irregular and unreliable in his drug administration habits. See the 1977 YEAR BOOK (p. 171) for more discussion on chemotherapy.

Some other tuberculosis titles are of interest. Strumpf et al. (The reliability of gastric smears by auramine-rhodamine staining technique for the diagnosis of tuberculosis, Am. Rev. Respir. Dis. 114:971, 1976) have shown that sputum staining with this fluorescent technique is reliable, with a sensitivity of 78% and false positive smears in 11%. In this experience, if the sputum smears were positive the chances were only 1 in 10 that the cultures would be negative; if the sputum smears were negative the chances were only 1 in 5 that the cultures would be positive. Gastric smears were in general not nearly so reliable, with many false positives and false negative results. It is implied, although not stated, that the auramine-rhodamine technique is superior to the traditional acid-fast techniques.

Bassi et al. quantitated the appearance of antirifampin antibodies (Antibodies against rifampin in patients with tuberculosis after discontinuation of daily treatment, ibid., p. 1189) and found them most frequent and in highest titer 3 weeks after discontinuation, suggesting that this would be a particularly bad time to start up the drug again. The relative safety of daily administration of rifampin is likely to be due to maintaining a situation of antigen excess. Riska et al. (Acute renal failure subsequent to the administration of rifampicin, Scand. J. Respir. Dis. 57:183, 1976) summarize the literature concerning this syndrome (see also Bansal et al.: Prolonged renal failure after rifampin, Am. Rev. Respir. Dis. 116:137, 1977). Grennan and Sturrock record a severe immune complex-type illness complicating rifampin treatment (Polyarthritis, hepatitis and anti-native DNA antibodies after treatment with ethambutol and rifampicin, Tubercle 57:259, 1976). – Ed.] ◄

Osteomyelitis, Pericarditis, Mediastinitis and Vasculitis due to *Mycobacterium chelonei*. Luis Jauregui, Augustin Arbulu and Francis Wilson[3] (Wayne State Univ.) report a fatal case of osteomyelitis, costochondritis, mediastinitis, pericarditis and vasculitis, due to *M. chelonei* ssp *abscessus* infection after coronary bypass surgery.

(3) Am. Rev. Respir. Dis. 115:699–703, April, 1977.

Man, 55, with angina for 5 years, was admitted after 2 weeks of crescendo angina with ECG evidence of anteroseptal ischemia and left ventricular hypertrophy. Nitrate and propranolol therapy did not lead to improvement and catheterization and angiography showed a complete block of the left anterior descending, posterior branch of the left circumflex and right coronary arteries. A triple revascularization procedure was carried out but the sternotomy incision became swollen and painful shortly after discharge and separated. A Ziehl-Neelsen stain of the purulent exudate showed clumps of acid-fast organisms. Antituberculosis therapy was initiated, but painful erythema developed over the lower sternal scar and growth of *M. chelonei* ssp *abscessus* was subsequently reported. Intravenous erythromycin was given and the appearance of the wound improved, but complete resection of the sternum and costal cartilages was necessary. Vancomycin was begun postoperatively. Chest pain developed and bleeding from a presumed infected perforation of a saphenous vein graft was observed. The patient died of exsanguination.

Autopsy showed massive acute hemorrhage of the anterior chest wall and mediastinum from a vein graft to the left circumflex coronary artery, where thrombosis and necrosis of the vessel wall were noted. Acid-fast organisms were present at this area. Microabscesses and extensive granulomatous involvement of the mediastinum, pericardium, pleural surfaces and epicardium were observed. The sternal bone and muscle obtained at surgery were similarly affected. *Mycobacterium chelonei* was grown from vein grafts, pericardium, pleura and blood in the anterior aspect of the chest. Cultures of the lungs and bronchi were negative.

Mycobacterium chelonei was only recently clearly separated from other group IV organisms. Once the organism has penetrated the skin barrier, it is capable of extensive tissue destruction. The organism was apparently introduced into the surgical wound in the present case. The organism is resistant to virtually all standard antituberculosis drugs, but combination therapy may prove to be of value. Local measures are indicated for cutaneous infections and abscesses. Sternal infections are managed by early incision and drainage and antimicrobial therapy.

► [This article references the literature concerning *M. chelonei* and cardiac surgery, including infection of prosthetic valves and infections of sternotomy wounds. This case appears to have been much worse than any previously recorded. As indicated in this article, antibiotic treatment of this and other atypical mycobacteria (or mycobacteria other than *M. tuberculosis*) is more or less up in the air, and when one is faced with such a case there is no way of avoiding going to the literature, finding out what drugs have shown promise and, depending on the gravity of the situation, treating accordingly. Fortunately, many such infections resolve with no treatment or with simple surgical débridement and do not require drug therapy. In any event, in most atypical infections excluding *Mycobacterium kansasii,* one has to look elsewhere than the drugs generally used to treat tuberculosis. For instance, minocycline, a lipid-soluble tetracycline, is good against *Mycobacterium marinum* (Loria: Arch. Dermatol. 112:517, 1976), the aminoglycosides, particularly amikacin, and also erythromycin show promise for *Myobacterium intracellularis,* and amikacin may be good against *Myobacterium fortuitum* (Sanders: Antimicrob. Agents Chemother. 12:295, 1977). This is anecdotal and incomplete information; one hopes that it will be all pulled together soon. – Ed.] ◄

Pulmonary and Articular Sporotrichosis. *Sporotrichum schenckii* is known to cause lymphocutaneous infection after direct trauma and also produces lung disease that resembles tuberculosis and other chronic granulomatous lung diseases roentgenographically and clinically. Charles J. Brook, K. P. Ravikrishnan and John G. Weg[4] review a

(4) Am. Rev. Respir. Dis. 116:141–143, July, 1977.

case documenting active sporotrichosis that simultaneously involved a knee and the lung and possibly represented late systemic spread from chronic pulmonary sporotrichosis.

Man, 46, had had swelling and pain in the right knee for 6 months that started several days after a nonpenetrating injury and he reported a chronic cough and weight loss of 50 lb in the past year. Bilateral apical infiltrates and a positive tuberculin test had been treated with isoniazid and ethambutol 7 years before, despite negative sputum smears and cultures. The patient had abused ethanol periodically for over 10 years. The right knee was swollen and tender and the fingers were clubbed. An increase in the upper lobe infiltrates was noted and a film of the right knee showed effusion and new periosteal bone formation in the distal femur. A synovial biopsy specimen showed multiple caseating granulomas. Bronchoscopy showed inflammation and edema in the apical segmental bronchus of the right upper lobe. *Sporotrichum schenckii* was cultured from synovium, sputum and bronchial washings. A bronchial biopsy specimen showed only chronic inflammation. Joint aspirations were carried out and a total of 1,776 mg amphotericin B was given before the serum creatinine increased. Knee findings were improved at hospital discharge. After 10 months there was no recurrence of the knee symptoms, but the chronic cough persisted.

The lung has been proposed as a portal of entry for *S. schenckii* in cases of articular sporotrichosis not preceded by penetrating trauma or skin lesions. The present case is thought to represent hematogenous spread of *S. schenckii* from a chronic pulmonary infection to the knee. It supports the hypothesis that the lung serves as a portal of entry in noncutaneous systemic sporotrichosis.

► [Another article of interest is by Nelson and Light (Granulomatous pleuritis secondary to blastomycosis, Chest 71:433, 1977), who report a case that looked just like serofibrinous tuberculous pleurisy with effusion but cultured out blastomycosis. Goodwin et al. (Chronic pulmonary histoplasmosis, Medicine 55:413, 1976) make a strong case that chronic cavitary pulmonary histoplasmosis is always superimposed on chronic obstructive pulmonary disease and that the cavities represent superinfected preexisting emphysematous air spaces. They also took issue with the generally accepted practice of treating all active pulmonary histoplasmosis with amphotericin. —Ed.] ◄

Carcinoma

► ↓ Lung cancer is a terrible illness in both men and women. Surgical removal remains the only real hope. Yet the overall results are quire disappointing (approximately 15% 5-year survival in all diagnosed cases is an optimistic figure). Activity to improve the situation continues in several areas: (1) early diagnosis, (2) selection of patients for surgery and (3) radiotherapy and chemotherapy. – Ed. ◄

Preliminary Report of the Lung Cancer Detection Program in New York. Myron Melamed, Betty Flehinger, Daniel Miller, Raymond Osborne, Muhammad Zaman, Carolyn McGinnis and Nael Martini[5] report the results obtained to date at Memorial Sloan-Kettering Cancer Center in a program undertaken in 1971 by the National Cancer Institute to determine whether periodic sputum cytology as a supplement to chest x-ray screening could reduce significantly the mortality from lung cancer in a high-risk population. Cigarette-smoking men over age 45 were encouraged to enroll in the program and, to date, 6,612 have done so. Annual posteroanterior and lateral chest films are obtained and about half the subjects also have sputum cytology every 4 months. Cough specimens of sputum are obtained with a saline-propylene glycol aerosol solution. When cancer cells are found on cytologic study and the chest film is normal, specific diagnostic procedures are initiated to find the source of the cancer cells. Occult lung cancers are managed by lobectomy with mediastinal node dissection.

Cytologic and radiologic studies have been done in 3,225 subjects, whereas 3,387 have been screened by radiology only. Fifteen cases of late lung cancer in pathologic stages II and III were detected at initial examination, as were 11 early (stages 0 and I) cases. Three early cancers were found in the group having radiologic screening only. In the group screened by both methods, 4 early cancers were detected by x-ray examination and 4 by cytologic study. In addition, 3 larynx cancers were detected by cytology.

The early cancers found by x-ray were peripheral and most were

TABLE 1. – CONFIRMED CASES OF LUNG CANCER ACCORDING TO METHOD OF DETECTION

	No. in Group "A"	(Per thous.)	No. in Group "B"	(Per thous.)
Total no. subjects	3225		3387	
No. cases lung cancer	15	(4.6)	11	(3.4)
Detected by:				
X-ray	9	(2.8)	11	(3.4)
Cytology	5	(1.5)		
X-ray and cytology	1	(0.3)		

(5) Cancer 39:369–382, February, 1977.

TABLE 2.—PATHOLOGIC STAGE OF CONFIRMED LUNG CANCERS*

	Group "A" detected by Cytology	Group "A" detected by X-ray	Group "A" detected by Both	Group "B" detected by X-ray
Stage 0	4			
Stage 1		4		3
Stage 2				2
Stage 3	1	5	1	6

*AJC postsurgical stage, determined at surgery and by examination of the pathologic specimen. Stage 0 is used here to mean carcinoma in situ in the bronchus or invading into the bronchial wall but not extending outside the bronchus.

TABLE 3.—HISTOLOGY AND ORIGIN OF CONFIRMED LUNG CANCERS

	Cytology detection		X-ray detection	
	Epid ca	Bronchiolar & ad ca	Epid ca	Bronchiolar & ad ca
Lobar or segment broncus	4	—	3	2
Sub-segmental bronchus	1	—		1
Peripheral	1*	—	6*	9

*One case detected simultaneously by x-ray and cytology.

bronchiolar or adenocarcinoma. Those detected by cytology were central epidermoid carcinomas of major bronchi. No early lesions were detected by both techniques. The findings are summarized in Tables 1, 2 and 3. All early lesions were resectable and are not potentially cured. Eight patients had lobectomy. Only 7 of the 15 late cancers were resectable.

A combination of chest films and sputum cytology can be an effective means of detecting early lung cancer. Regular repeat examinations are now being carried out to determine whether a substantial percentage of the new lung cancers that develop after initial negative screening studies can be detected in an early stage.

► [This article is another interim report from one of several institutions cooperating to determine whether or not high-risk (smoking male) patients might benefit from thrice-yearly sputum cytologic examination (see also 1977 YEAR BOOK, pp. 159–161; Fontana, A.: Early diagnosis of lung cancer, Am. Rev. Respir. Dis. 116:399, 1977; and Nasiell et al.: Clinically occult lung cancer with positive sputum cytology and primarily negative radiologic findings, Scand. J. Respir. Dis. 58:134, 1977). Although whether or not such a screening mechanism will prove productive enough to justify the cost remains to be seen, several important points have been learned. (1) the frequency of multiple primary pulmonary tumors remains impressive; as high as 25% of cases is a defensible figure. These are both synchronous and sequential. Accordingly, it is a virtue to elect as conservative a resection as possible since another may well be required in the future. (2) As many as 10–15% of positive cytologies in patients with negative roentgenograms originate from the pharynx and larynx (the frequency with which cancer of the upper airways and lung occur together is well known). (3) As many as 50% of the group with positive cytologies and negative chest roentgenograms will actually have invasive bronchial carcinoma extending deeper than the submucosa rather than carcinoma in situ when examined pathologically; in other words, highly productive, truly early diagnosis in the sense that this is possible with routine Papanicolaou smears of the cervix in women will never be the case. (4) Exploratory thoracotomy without secure tumor localization is not advisable as the tumors most often cannot be found by palpation at operation. Localization by fiberoptic bronchoscopy is possible in most instances. New in vivo mucosal staining techniques to highlight mucosa involved with cancer are being developed which will hopefully make this easier. When one has only a positive cytology to go by, it should be recovered from the same lobar orifice on two or more repeated bronchoscopies before surgery is recommended. This sort of searching for the source of positive cells is a tricky, expensive, fairly prolonged endoscopic procedure best done under general anesthesia and requiring a great deal of expertise. (5) Most of the cases of positive sputum with negative x-rays are fairly proximal squamous cell lesions. Tumors discovered on screening x-ray with negative cytologies tend to be peripheral adenocarcinomas. (6) Submission of sputum cytology for persistent respiratory symptoms of any sort is very probably an underutilized procedure by most doctors. By the use of heated hypertonic aerosol inhalations (20% propylene glycol, 15% saline is one good preparation) and very inexpensive commercially available equipment, good specimens can be obtained from persons not producing sputum. The sputum is coughed directly into fixative jars. (7) Although it is not absolutely certain (see 1977 YEAR BOOK, pp. 159–161 for a more pessimistic statement), present and past evidence indicates that patients with cases diagnosed on the basis of a positive sputum cytology have a much better prognosis than patients diagnosed in other ways; some series claim a two-thirds or greater 5-year survival (Martinik et al.: Radiologically occult lung cancer: Report of 26 cases, Surg. Clin. North Am. 54:811, 1974; and Woolner et al.: In situ and early invasive bronchogenic carcinoma: Report of 28 cases with postoperative survival data, J. Thorac. Cardiovasc. Surg. 60:275, 1970). (8) Cytology is a quite accurate means to determine all types (see Mittman and Bruderman: Lung cancer: To operate or not?, Am. Rev. Respir. Dis. 116:477, 1977).—Ed.] ◄

Multiorgan Scans for Staging Lung Cancer: Correlation with Clinical Evaluation. Joe W. Ramsdell, Richard M. Peters, Andrew T. Taylor, Jr., Naomi P. Alazraki and Gennaro M. Tisi[6] prospectively studied 100 consecutive patients with findings suggestive of resectable bronchogenic carcinoma to determine if routine multiorgan scans would detect metastases not suggested by the history, physical findings or serum chemistries. Scans were compared with clinical evaluations in 52 patients found to have operable carcinoma. Scans of the liv-

FINAL DIAGNOSES OF FALSE POSITIVE SCANS IN PATIENTS WITH NO ABNORMALITIES ON CLINICAL EVALUATION

Diagnosis		*No.*
Liver		3
No metastasis after greater than 18 months	2	
No metastasis at open biopsy	1	
Brain		0
Bone		19
Osteoarthritis	9	
Trauma	1	
No metastasis after greater than 12 months	1	
No metastasis at autopsy	2	
Nonmalignant primary disease	6	
Total		22

(6) J. Thorac. Cardiovasc. Surg. 73:653–659, May, 1977.

er, brain and skeletal system were obtained within 2 weeks of clinical evaluation. Liver-spleen scans were made with ^{99m}Tc-sulfur colloid and brain scans with ^{99m}Tc-labeled pertechnetate; perchlorate was used to block choroid plexus uptake. Total body scans were performed after the administration of ^{99m}Tc-labeled pyrophosphate or polyphosphate.

A total of 153 scans were obtained in the 52 patients with proved bronchogenic carcinoma. Fourteen scans confirmed abnormalities found on clinical evaluation. The two approaches were discordant in 16.3% of the scans. Eight scans (5.2%) were negative with clinical abnormalities present, and 2 were false negative scans. Seventeen scans (11.1%) were positive in the absence of clinical findings that suggested metastases, but 16 were false positive scans. The results are summarized in the table. None of 23 patients with nonmalignant disease had positive liver or bone scans. Only 1 of 131 scans done in patients without clinical evidence of metastasis was true positive.

These data indicate that the routine use of multiorgan scans in the initial staging of potentially resectable bronchogenic carcinoma is not justified when the history, physical findings and serum chemistries give no evidence of metastases. If a diligent clinical evaluation and liver function tests are negative and the patient has adequate cardiopulmonary reserve to tolerate pulmonary resection, the extent of intrathoracic spread should be determined by bronchoscopy and mediastinal exploration. If, after these studies, the tumor is considered resectable, operation is indicated.

► [For several years it was almost routine at our hospital, and probably many others, to obtain scans of liver, brain and bone prior to undertaking thoracotomy for bronchogenic carcinoma, and this was certainly not discouraged by nuclear medicine sections (recall Pogo's comment that nuclear physics might be new but wasn't very clear) despite skepticism on the part of most of us. This study by Ramsdell et al. is important ammunition for those who oppose in principle unbridled use of expensive technologic procedures. It is perhaps useful to present a little more of the data than is contained here. The basis on which liver abnormality was evaluated clinically was not defined, but it was implied that abnormalities on liver function tests, in particular the alkaline phosphatase, were the most important factors. Of 51 patients with lung cancer, liver scans were negative in 46 (mottled defects such as commonly seen in cirrhosis were not counted as positive). Six of the 46 patients had elevated alkaline phosphatase values; 2 of these had liver metastases confirmed, 1 had no metastases at autopsy and 3 could not be followed. Five of the 51 scans were positive; metastases were present in only 2 of these patients, both with elevated alkaline phosphatase levels. The other 3 were shown to be false positives. A study presented in the 1975 YEAR BOOK, page 166, also found that all cases of hepatic metastases were associated with an elevated alkaline phosphatase. The conclusion of Ramsdell et al., "liver scanning adds nothing to the staging of bronchogenic carcinoma in patients who have no evidence of hepatic dysfunction," seems valid and important.

Brain scans have been on the way out in patients with no signs or symptoms of neurologic disease and this study confirms that opinion. Bone scans have been the most bothersome of all, however. The proliferation of those little skeletons seemed at one point unstoppable. Therefore, the data presented in the table are most welcome.

A short report by Williams et al. (Br. Med. J. 1:1004, 1977) presents the opposite opinion. Of 100 scans, 37 were true positive for metastatic disease and in 7 x-rays were normal and the patients symptom free. They agreed that most patients with positive scans had symptoms.—Ed.] ◄

Major Pulmonary Resection for Bronchogenic Carcinoma in the Elderly. Marvin M. Kirsh, Harold Rotman, Edward Bove, Louis

TABLE 1.—FIVE-YEAR SURVIVAL ACCORDING TO METASTASES AND CELL TYPE AMONG 55 ELDERLY PATIENTS OPERATED ON FOR BRONCHOGENIC CARCINOMA

	All Cell Types		Squamous Cell Carcinoma		Adenocarcinoma	
Metastases	No. Treated	Survivors	No. Treated	Survivors	No. Treated	Survivors
None	35	13	18	7	15	5
Hilar only	9	2	5	2	4	0
Mediastinal (with radiation therapy)	11	2	7	2	3	0

Argenta, Vincent Cimmino, Jeanne Tashian, Pauline Ferguson and Herbert Sloan[7] (Univ. of Michigan) reviewed the results of major pulmonary resection in 58 patients aged 70 years or more, who underwent lobectomy or pneumonectomy for bronchogenic carcinoma since 1959. Seventeen other patients were denied surgery because of poor general condition or insufficient cardiopulmonary reserve. Lobectomy was done where technically feasible. The perihilar and hilar nodes were removed en bloc with the primary lesion whenever possible. Three patients did not have curative resections, 2 because of the proximal extent of tumor and 1 because of inadequate pulmonary reserve.

All 17 unoperated patients received radiotherapy, but none lived 5 years; the average survival was 7.7 months. Survival in the operated group is shown in Table 1. Thirteen of 35 patients without hilar or mediastinal metastases were alive without disease at 5 years, as were 2 of 11 patients with mediastinal metastases, who received postoperative irradiation. None of 6 patients who had pneumonectomy lived 5 years without disease. Survival is related to age in Table 2. Most patients who lived for 2 years survived for a reasonably long time, with satisfactory quality of survival. The overall postoperative mortality for patients who had resection was 14%; 1 of 6 patients who had pneumonectomy and 7 of the 49 who had lobectomy died postoperatively.

Age itself does not adversely influence long-term survival after pulmonary resection for bronchogenic carcinoma. The 5-year survival of 30% in patients who had a major resection has encouraged the authors to continue this program in elderly patients. The decision on operating should be based on the patient's cardiovascular status and pulmonary reserve. The question of what constitutes inadequate cardiovascular or

TABLE 2.—FIVE-YEAR SURVIVAL ACCORDING TO AGE AMONG 55 ELDERLY PATIENTS OPERATED ON FOR BRONCHOGENIC CARCINOMA

	Overall		Squamous Cell Carcinoma		Adenocarcinoma	
Age	No. Treated	Survivors	No. Treated	Survivors	No. Treated	Survivors
70–75	43	13	24	8	17	4
76–79	7	2	3	2	3	0
80	5	2	3	0	2	1

(7) Ann. Thorac. Surg. 22:369–373, October, 1976.

pulmonary reserve for a proposed pulmonary resection remains to be answered. Patients with small peripheral lesions and cardiopulmonary reserve inadequate for lobectomy may tolerate a lesser procedure, such as wedge resection or segmentectomy.

► [The influence of age, associated disease in other organ systems and pulmonary function in assessing operability remains an area of judgment more than data. The above experience certainly suggests that age of itself should not constitute a contraindication to surgery with intent to cure. This surgical group again recorded survival of patients who had squamous cell carcinomas with mediastinal implants treated with postoperative irradiation (2 of the 5-year survivors). Their pulmonary function criteria for exclusion included resting hypercapnia, hypoxemia under 50 mm Hg at rest or after exercise, a vital capacity under 2 L and a 1-second vital capacity under 1.2 L. They advised the use of lung scans in borderline cases to see whether the lung to be resected was good lung (well perfused) or bad lung (underperfused or nonperfused).

Lung scanning has never been established as a very useful technique in the evaluation of neoplasia, although all of us have seen instances in which scan provided very important information. Stinson and Goodwin (Pulmonary vein obstruction by bronchogenic carcinoma, South. Med. J. 69:1482, 1976) demonstrate cases in which virtual absence of perfusion was shown to be caused by inconspicuous hilar implants. A similar experience was recorded by Grant et al. (Radioisotope perfusion and ventilation studies in bronchial hilar neoplasia, Australas. Radiol. 20:122, 1976). – Ed.] ◄

Selective Mediastinoscopy. Jerry L. Acosta and Felice Manfredi[8] (Indiana Univ.) sought definite criteria for selecting patients for mediastinoscopy that would reduce the number of negative studies while maintaining an acceptably low incidence of unnecessary thoracotomy. Patients hospitalized with suspected lung carcinoma who had (1) central neoplasms, (2) enlarged mediastinal nodes, (3) a history of hoarseness or documented paresis of the recurrent nerve or (4) hilar extension were selected for mediastinoscopy (group A). Patients exhibiting none of these criteria (group B) underwent exploratory thoracotomy without mediastinoscopy. No patient with distant metastasis, direct involvement of the chest wall or phrenic nerve paralysis or with incomplete staging was included in the study.

Fifty-four patients were evaluated completely. Criteria for selecting the 34 group A patients are given in the table. With exclusion of 7 pa-

Criteria for Selection and Results of Mediastinoscopy in Group A

Criteria for Selection	Results: Positive for Neoplasm	Negative for Neoplasm
Mediastinal nodes	6	1
Mediastinal nodes and laryngeal nerve	4	0
Perihilar mass and laryngeal nerve	4	0
Perihilar mass	3	4
Perihilar mass and mediastinal nodes	5	0
Hilar extension (linear stranding)*	0	7
Total	22	12

*These 7 patients were subsequently included in group B.

(8) Chest 71:150–154, February, 1977.

tients with linear stranding as the only suggestive radiologic finding who were placed in group B, positive mediastinal nodes were found in 22 (81%)) of 27 patients. All 8 patients with recurrent nerve involvement had lymphatic metastases at mediastinoscopy. Only 2 of 5 patients with negative mediastinoscopic findings had resectable masses. No evidence of lymphatic metastases was found at thoracotomy in 23 group B patients. Four of 27 group B patients had unresectable disease. The incidence of negative mediastinoscopic findings for neoplasm in this series was 19% and that of unnecessary thoracotomy, 15%.

Mediastinoscopy for staging lung cancer should be done on a selective basis in patients with tracheobronchial lymphadenopathy demonstrated on chest films or tomograms, or both; those with central lesions; and those with paresis of the recurrent laryngeal nerve, either suspected clinically or demonstrated at bronchoscopy. With this approach, few patients have unnecessary mediastinoscopy, and an acceptable level of productive exploratory thoracotomy is maintained.

► [The role of mediastinoscopy and mediastinotomy in the assessment of local metastases was discussed at some length in the 1977 YEAR BOOK (pp. 157–159). The question as to whether these procedures should be selective or form a part of routine preoperative evaluation remains open and largely a matter of the surgeon's choice. This article by Acosta and Manfredi advocates a selective point of view. Fleming (Mediastinal biopsy: Selective or routine, Am. Surg. 43:74, 1977) also reserves the procedure for patients in whom (1) x-ray evidence of mediastinal or carinal widening is seen, (2) the trachea or carina is suspicious on bronchoscopy, (3) small cell anaplastic carcinoma is strongly suspected or established, (4) tissue diagnosis is required in clinically nonresectable disease and (5) undiagnosed bilateral hilar node disease is present; the procedure was done in only 23 of 138 cancer patients. Other reports favor its use routinely or almost routinely in preoperative evaluation of almost all cases of carcinoma (Gardner and Lomas: Mediastinoscopy, Med. J. Aust. 2:437, 1976; Weissberg: Mediastinoscopy and anterior mediastinotomy in patients with lung cancer, Isr. J. Med. Sci. 13:866, 1977; Hansen and Marshio: Mediastinoscopy in bronchogenic carcinoma: A routine or a selective preoperative procedure, Dan. Med. Bull. 24:30, 1977). The following impressions have been gained by the editor from all of these sources. (1) Most agree that mediastinoscopy is indicated with x-ray (including tomographic) evidence suggesting mediastinal involvement, with centrally located tumors and with clinical evidence of involvement of mediastinal structures such as recurrent laryngeal paralysis. (2) It is indicated in the rare peripheral oat cell lesion without evidence of spread; the vast majority of oat cell carcinomas present with evidence of spread, however. (3) Most surgeons are not subjecting small (under 2 cm) peripheral cancers of other than oat cell type to preoperative mediastinoscopy in the absence of tomographic evidence of mediastinal involvement. Some patients will be subjected to needless thoracotomies following this policy, however, since the x-ray will have been normal in up to 25% of cases with mediastinal implants discovered at operation. (4) Lesions originating on the left side, especially the left upper lobe, may be associated with metastases behind the aortic arch which are not accessible to the mediastinoscope; some surgeons approach these, after negative mediastinoscopy or at the same time, with a left parasternal mediastinotomy. (5) When all comers are subjected to mediastinoscopy, 35–45% will have positive findings, and those who are negative will prove to have resectable lesions in 80–90% of cases. (6) Disagreement remains on the issue as to whether or not ipsilateral solitary mediastinal deposits from a squamous cell carcinoma constitute resectable lesions when treated with postoperative radiation. Recent authors have suggested that this may be the case only when the metastasis has not reached the surface of the node, that is to say, is entirely intranodal.

Scalene node biopsy, the forerunner of mediastinoscopy, has fallen into disuse on most services. Brosseau et al. (The continuing importance of scalene node biopsy in lung cancer patients, Wis. Med. J. 76:97, 1977) reported that in their hospital over 90% of palpable supraclavicular nodes in lung cancer patients were positive, and the scalene fat pad (bilateral exploration) was positive in 22% of cancer patients without palpable nodes. As would be expected, oat cell cancers were most frequently associated with positive findings, adenocarcinoma next and squamous cell least. They felt that it remained a useful procedure because it could be done without general anesthesia.

Mediastinoscopy can be surprising. Our surgeons harvested one unsuspected parathyroid adenoma that way. The indication for the procedure was a round mass on x-ray adjacent to the top of the aorta and shown by angiography not to be vascular. In retrospect, calcium values had been intermittently elevated. – Ed.] ◄

Prophylactic Cranial Irradiation in Small Cell Carcinoma of the Lung: Randomized Study. Don V. Jackson, Jr., Frederick Richards II, M. Robert Cooper, Carolyn Ferree, Hyman B. Muss, Douglas R. White and Charles L. Spurr[9] (Bowman Gray School of Medicine) studied the ability of prophylactic cranial irradiation, added to irradiation of the primary tumor and multiagent chemotherapy, to prevent central nervous system (CNS) metastasis from small cell carcinoma of the lung. Twenty-nine patients with untreated small cell carcinoma and no evidence of brain metastasis were entered into the study during 1974 – 76. The diagnosis was confirmed by tissue biopsy in 22 patients.

There were two treatment groups: (1) prophylactic cranial irradiation, 3,000 rad to the whole brain at the outset of therapy, 14 patients, and (2) no prophylactic cranial irradiation, 15 patients. Both groups received, from day 1, the same extracranial irradiation (3,000 rad to the primary lung tumor and mediastinum and 3,000 rad to the supraclavicular regions) and chemotherapy with CAV – cyclophosphamide, Adriamycin (doxorubicin hydrochloride) and vincristine sulfate – for 3 months alternating with CM – lomustine (CCNU).

Objective responses were observed in 26 (90%) of the patients (table). Complete responses occurred in 20% of group 2 patients and 43% of group 1 patients, for an overall complete response rate of 31%. The median duration of remission was 4.9 months. All but 7 patients have relapsed. The median survival of the entire group was 9.3 months, with no difference in the two groups.

Response and Survival

	Non-PCI*	PCI*	All
Complete response, No.(%)	3/15(20)	6/14(43)	9/29(31)
Partial response, No.(%)	11/15(73)	6/14(43)	17/29(59)
Time of response†	0.7(0.4-1.7)	1.1(0.4-1.8)	1.1(0.4-1.8)
Duration of remission†	4.5(1-24+)	4.7(2-25+)	4.9((1-25+)
Survival†	7.2(1-26+)	9.8(2-26+)	9.3(1-26+)
Local disease	>10.0‡	8.7	10.0
Extrathoracic disease	4.5	6.0	5.5
Ambulatory	7.9	9.0	9.0
Nonambulatory	3.0§	5.0	4.0
Partial response	6.1	10.2	8.4
Complete response	>25‖	9.0	10.0

*PCI indicates prophylactic cranial irradiation.
†Response and survival data are expressed in median number *(No.)* of months (range).
‡Includes 5 living patients: 3+, 8+, 25+ and 26+ months.
§Includes only 3 patients: 1, 3 and 5 months.
‖Includes 3 living patients: 22+, 25+ and 26+ months.

(9) J.A.M.A. 237:2730 – 2733, June 20, 1977.

Symptomatic CNS metastasis occurred in 4 group 2 patients; 3 of these showed a marked change in mental status. Two patients responded briefly to steroids and cranial irradiation, but their CNS disease was ultimately fatal.

Cranial irradiation was well tolerated. There were no major limiting drug toxicities.

Prophylactic cranial irradiation prevented development of brain metastasis with its attendant neurologic complications, with minimal toxicity. It appears that prophylactic cranial irradiation should be an integral part of the initial therapy of patients with small cell carcinoma of the lung.

► [There is wide agreement now that roughly one third of patients with oat cell cancer will develop cerebral metastases which are extremely symptomatic, often fatal, usually multiple and, once established, respond only partially and variably to radiotherapy and that prophylactic irradiation at the time of diagnosis will reduce the incidence to 5%. In disease which is widespread at the outset, prophylactic brain irradiation does nothing to prolong life and its use is probably optional. In this group the overall benefits of combined radiotherapy-chemotherapy remain marginal. It is in the small subset with limited disease (confined to the thorax and supraclavicular area, not involving the pleura, not spread to other organs and able to be encompassed by one radiotherapy portal) that chemotherapy-radiotherapy holds real promise. Although the data are not published, it now appears that 20–30% of these patients will survive 2 years (as opposed to 2% of the widespread group) and will show no clinical evidence of disease. How many may survive much longer than that is an open question, but the experience with histiocytic lymphoma would lead one to hope that some will be actual cures. In this particular group, prophylactic brain irradiation would seem to be most important, as the chemotherapeutic agents by and large are excluded from the central nervous system. – Ed.] ◄

Combination Chemotherapy of Advanced Lung Cancer: Randomized Trial. Previous single-agent studies have shown cyclophosphamide to be effective in small cell carcinoma of the lung and mechlorethamine to be effective in the treatment of epidermoid carcinoma. Heine H. Hansen, Oleg S. Selawry, Richard Simon (Natl. Inst. of Health), David T. Carr (Mayo Clinic), C. E. van Wyk, R. D. Tucker and Rossall Sealy[1] (Univ. of Capetown) conducted a controlled trial that compared two- and three-drug combination chemotherapy in 206 patients with advanced bronchogenic carcinoma. Small cell carcinoma and adenocarcinoma were the most common types. All patients had

TABLE 1. – Objective Response Rate to Two-Drug Treatment as Related to Cell Type

	Cyclophosphamide or mechlorethamine + methotrexate					CCNU + hydroxyurea			Vincristine + procarbazine		
Cell type	No. patients	Measurable or evaluable	% response	Median duration response (days)	Range (days)	No. patients	Measurable or evaluable	% response	No. patients	Measurable or evaluable	% response
Epidermoid	25	20	10	135	85–185	11	8	0	2	1	0
Small cell	29	24	38	153	36–423	13	7	0	3	2	0
Adenocarcinoma	28	17	6	115	115	10	8	0	3	1	0
Large cell carcinoma	17	14	7	437	437	8	8	0	4	2	0
Total	99	75	16	160	36–437	42	31	0	12	6	0

(1) Cancer 38:2201–2207, December, 1976.

TABLE 2.—OBJECTIVE RESPONSE RATE TO THREE-DRUG TREATMENT AS RELATED TO CELL TYPE

	Cyclophosphamide or mechlorethamine + methotrexate + CCNU					Vincristine + procarbazine + hydroxyurea				
Cell type	No. patients	Measurable or evaluable	% response	Median duration response (days)	Range	No. patients	Measurable or evaluable	% response	Median duration response (days)	Range
Epidermoid	29	17	6	334	334	3	2	0	0	0
Small cell	33	30	56	176	89–330	15	13	15	58	21–95
Adenocarcinoma	28	21	38	112	68–611	15	14	7	233	233
Large cell undifferentiated	17	10	10	108	108	6	4	0	0	0
TOTAL	107	78	35	160	68–611	39	33	9	95	21–233

tumor involvement beyond surgical control, extending beyond one hemithorax, and ipsilateral scalene node involvement. Each drug combination consisted of agents with different modes of action, including those sensitive and nonsensitive to cell cycle stages. Cyclophosphamide, mechlorethamine, methotrexate, CCNU, hydroxyurea, vincristine and procarbazine were the drugs used.

Adenocarcinoma responded significantly better to three-drug treatment than to the two-drug combinations. Three-drug therapy also resulted in longer survival in small cell carcinoma, but the difference was not significant. Response rates are given in Tables 1 and 2. Small cell carcinoma and adenocarcinoma were the most sensitive tumor types; patients with these types had a total objective response rate of 48.2% and 23.6%, respectively. Over half of the small cell carcinomas responded to three-drug therapy. All responses but one occurred during treatment with the first drug combination. The main dose-limiting toxicity was hematologic, consisting of leukopenia and thrombocytopenia. No major difference between the two treatments was apparent.

Small cell carcinoma and adenocarcinoma of the lung may benefit most from combined chemotherapy. There is a need for more effective antineoplastic modalities of treatment for advanced epidermoid carcinoma and large cell anaplastic carcinoma of the lung. On-going studies are evaluating the effect of combination chemotherapy, plus radiotherapy and surgery, in patients with less advanced disease.

► [In contrast to limited oat cell carcinomas, the effectiveness of chemotherapy and radiotherapy in adenocarcinoma, large cell undifferentiated carcinoma and squamous cell carcinoma is much less well established. (This article indicates that patients with adenocarcinomas do somewhat better, but this is not a usual experience.) There seems to be an emerging consensus that "high-dose" methotrexate in combination with other drugs shows promise in squamous cell lesions (Selawry et al.: Methotrexate compared with placebo in lung cancer, Cancer 40:1, 1977; and Straus: Combination chemotherapy in advanced lung cancer with increased survival, ibid. 38:2232, 1976). There is evidence that the level of radiation dose is an important determinant of survival (Petrovich: Clinical report on the treatment of locally advanced lung cancer, Cancer 40:72, 1977).

Although most nononcologists view treatment of disseminated oat cell cancer and all nonresectable non-oat cell cancers as pretty much bootless exercises, all of us have seen occasional patients with all cell types who do beautifully with radiation or radiation and chemotherapy and live happily for long periods. It is the memory of those uncommon great results which keeps us sending everyone to the oncologist. It is now becoming common practice in oncologic papers to have the patients separated into "responders" and "nonresponders." Presumably whether or not a patient is a responder can be determined within the first 2 or 3 months. (About 1 in 5 patients with squamous cell cancers is a responder at present.) We would regard it as desirable if it becomes common oncologic practice to go for cure only in the responders and to treat the remainder with support and palliation after nonresponse has been determined.

Another area which is likely to be productive eventually is adjuvant therapy (either chemotherapy, immunotherapy or both) at the time of putatively curative resection; but this will remain experimental for several years. The topic was recently reviewed by Legha et al. (Adjuvant chemotherapy in lung cancer: Review and prospects, ibid. 39: 1415, 1977). – Ed.] ◄

Acromegaly Caused by Pulmonary Carcinoid Tumors. Occasionally, carcinoid and pituitary adenomas are two aspects of a widespread pluriglandular syndrome involving also tumors of other endocrine glands. Also a carcinoid tumor could be responsible for acromegaly directly be secreting a growth hormone-like substance or indirectly by secreting a growth hormone releasing factor. P. H. Sönksen, A. B. Ayres, M. Braimbridge, B. Corrin, D. R. Davies, G. M. Jeremiah, S. W. Oaten, C. Lowy and T. E. T. West[2] (St. Thomas' Hosp. Med. School, London) encountered a patient with acromegaly and a bronchial carcinoid in whom the last mechanism seems to be the most likely explanation.

Woman, 60, referred with a diagnosis of acromegaly, had classic clinical features of acromegaly, bilateral carpal tunnel syndrome and a history of recurrent attacks of right-sided pneumonia for 19 years.

The pituitary fossa was enlarged, and the fasting plasma GH level was 156 – 260 mU/L, which was not suppressed during an oral glucose tolerance test. Glucose tolerance was normal. A chest x-ray showed a mass involving the right lower lobe bronchus with distal lung collapse. Bronchoscopy revealed an adenoma, shown by biopsy to be a carcinoid tumor. Urine levels of vanilylmandelic and 5-hydroxyindole acetic acids were normal.

The collapsed right lower lobe and middle lobe were removed. Plasma GH measurements were 7 and 6 mU/L postoperatively. The patient has been well since operation.

The tumor was very cellular and argyrophilic. The tumor cells were small, with the pattern of a bronchial carcinoid tumor. They contained numerous dense-core granules. The tumor contained 5-hydroxytryptamine, 3.46 μg/gm, dopamine, 5.03 μg/gm, and noradrenaline, 0.166 μg/gm. No growth hormone was detected.

Another patient, a woman aged 53, had clinical features of acromegaly and a carcinoid tumor obstructing a segmental bronchus. The acromegaly apparently improved after operation.

In some instances, the pluriglandular syndrome may not represent spontaneous tumor development in a number of endocrine glands, but rather tumor development as a result of chronic stimulation by releasing factors produced by a carcinoid tumor. Small bronchial carcinoids grow slowly and may stimulate tumor development in an endocrine gland. Every effort should be made to detect these since the syndrome may remit if the carcinoid is completely removed.

► [Other articles on ectopic hormone production that are of interest are by Luey and Scobie (Watery diarrhea (WDHA) syndrome associated with carcinoma of the lung,

(2) Clin. Endocrinol. (Oxf.) 5:503 – 513, September, 1976.

Aust. N.Z.J. Med. 6:490, 1976) (see also Said and Faloona: Evaluated plasma and tissue levels of vasoactive polypeptide in the watery diarrhea syndrome due to pancreatic, bronchogenic and other tumors, N. Engl. J. Med. 293:155, 1975), Coscia et al. (Ectopic production of antidiuretic hormone (ADH), adrenocorticotropic hormone (ACTH) and β-melanocyte-stimulating hormone (β-MSH) by an oat cell carcinoma of the lung, Am. J. Med. 62:303, 1977), Padfield et al. (Plasma arginine vasopressin in the syndrome of antidiuretic hormone excess associated with bronchogenic carcinoma, ibid. 61:825, 1976), Yokoyama et al. (Amylase-producing lung cancer, Cancer 40:766, 1977) and Otsuki et al. (Amylase in the lung, ibid. 39:1656, 1977). This last article indicates that salivary-type amylase is produced in normal lung, that left atrial blood amylase is always higher than right atrial blood amylase and that nonneoplastic lung disease such as pneumonia or tuberculosis may be associated with hyperamylasemia.

Some other cancer subjects which merit brief mention: The frequency and variety of the thoracic manifestations of renal carcinoma were the subject of several articles. Latour and Shulman (Thoracic manifestations of renal cell carcinoma, Radiology 121:43, 1976) note that 30–45% of patients with renal carcinoma metastases have no symptoms referable to the kidney, that thoracic metastases occur in over 50% and that their manifestations are quite variable, including multiple nodules, single masses, pleural effusion, destructive lesions of the chest wall, bilateral hilar adenopathy resembling sarcoid, and tumor in the atrium and pulmonary arteries (see also Wright: Enlarged hilar and mediastinal nodes (and especially lower right hilar node enlargement) as a sign of metastasis of a renal tumor, Clin. Radiol. 28:431, 1977). Daughtry et al. emphasize pulmonary emboli (Pulmonary embolism presenting as the initial manifestation of renal cell carcinoma, Ann. Thorac. Surg. 24:178, 1977). Donaldson et al. discuss the long latent period which may be seen (Metastatic renal cell carcinoma 24 years after nephrectomy, J.A.M.A. 236:950, 1976).

Gonzalez-Vitale and Garcia-Bunuel, in an article entitled "Pulmonary Tumor Emboli and Cor Pulmonale in Primary Carcinoma of the Lung (Cancer 38:2105, 1976), reported tumor emboli in 10% of autopsied lung cancer patients, most frequently those with adenocarcinoma. The authors comment that unexplained breathlessness, evidence of pulmonary hypertension, and cor pulmonale may be due to this mechanism.

Several articles address the subject of detection of pulmonary metastases and what to do when they are found (Didolkar et al.: Accuracy of roentgenograms of the chest in metastases to the lungs, Surg. Gynecol. Obstet. 144:903, 1977; Neifeld: Suspected pulmonary metastases: Correlation of chest x-ray, whole lung tomograms and operative findings, Cancer 39:383, 1977; Muhm: Detection of pulmonary nodules by computed tomography, Am. J. Roentgenol. 128:267, 1977; and Vidne et al.: Surgical treatment of solitary pulmonary metastasis, Cancer 38:2561, 1976). Tomography is better than plain films; computerized axial tomographic scans are better than tomography; solitary metastases should in most instances be removed if the primary tumor has been eliminated, because the prognosis is at least as good as in primary lung cancer; and in selected situations resection of more than one metastasis has been associated with lasting benefit.

Three articles discuss pneumothorax due to both primary and metastatic pulmonary cancer (Yeung and Bonnet: Bronchogenic carcinoma presenting as spontaneous pneumothorax, ibid. 39:2286, 1977; Brufman et al.: Spontaneous pneumothorax complicating lung metastases from carcinoma of the breast, Radiol. Clin. (Basel) 46:38, 1977; and Yusuf et al.: Spontaneous pneumothorax as a presenting feature of primary lung carcinoma, Conn. Med. 42:210, 1977).

In the 1976 YEAR BOOK, page 201, note was taken of a theoretically attractive notion, the use of anticoagulant therapy to enhance chemotherapy in lung cancer (Elias et al.: Heparin and chemotherapy in the management of inoperable lung carcinoma, Cancer 36:129, 1975). This has not been restudied by the Veterans Administration Lung Cancer Study Group (Rohwedder and Sagastume: Heparin and polychemotherapy for treatment of lung cancer, Cancer Treat. Rep. 61:1399, 1977), who found no benefit and "severe infection and troublesome occult bleeding . . . unacceptably frequent." (We thank Doctor Rohwedder of Ann Arbor, Michigan, for taking the trouble to bring this information to our attention.) – Ed.] ◄

Miscellaneous

Pulmonary Hemorrhage in Fiberoptic Transbronchial Biopsy. According to Donald C. Zavala[3] (Univ. of Iowa), transbronchial forceps biopsy of the lung through a flexible fiberoptic bronchoscope has been widely used in the past 2 years, with a diagnostic yield of 58–79%. The incidence of bleeding averaged 9% in a collected series of 438 patients (table).

This technique, although relatively safe, is definitely more hazardous than routine fiberoptic endoscopy and bronchial brushing. The chief potential danger is bleeding, with hypoxemia and cardiac arrest resulting. Pneumothorax usually poses no real threat. Pulmonary hypertension is a relative contraindication. Also, patients on mechanical ventilation must be approached cautiously. Absolute contraindications are lack of patient cooperation; presence of an uncorrected bleeding dithathesis, severe hypoxemia or a resting Pa_{CO_2} above 44 mm Hg; an acute asthmatic attack; serious arrhythmia; and recent myocardial infarction.

The most important premedication is atropine, 0.8–1.0 mg intramuscularly, given 30 minutes before the biopsy. All biopsies should be done through an oral endotracheal tube. Fluroscopy with image intensification is necessary to position the biopsy forceps on a peripheral

MATERIALS, METHODS AND COMPLICATIONS OF TRANSBRONCHIAL FORCEPS BIOPSY IN A COLLECTED SERIES OF 438 PATIENTS*

Study	No. of Patients	Route of Introduction	Fluoroscopy	Pneumothorax	Hemorrhage	Deaths
Levin et al	33	Transnasal	Yes	0	4 (mild)	0
Schoenbaum et al	18	Transnasal	Yes	0	0	0
Scheinhorn et al	21	Transnasal	No	0	0	0
Koerner et al	26	Transnasal	Yes	1	1 (mild)	0
Joyner and Scheinhorn	37	Transnasal	No	1	3 (1 mild and 2 with 200 ml)	0
Ellis	107	Transnasal	Yes	1	9 (8 mild and 1 with 100 ml)	0
Flick et al	1	Transnasal	Yes	0	1 (massive)	1
Hanson et al	164	Oral endotracheal tube	Yes	7	15 (12 with 25-100 ml and 3 with >100 ml)	0
Unpublished data †	31	Oral endotracheal tube	Yes	6	8 (25-100 ml)	0
Total	438	...	...	16	41	1
Percent		...	...	4	9	0.2

*All procedures were done with use of fiberoptic bronchoscope (Olympus 5B2) and forceps (Olympus BF-5B2)

†Cunningham, Zavala, Corry et al., University of Iowa.

(3) Chest 70:584–588, November, 1976.

density. A cardiac monitor should always be used. Prophylactic supplemental oxygen is given by nasal cannula and/or endotracheal-tube swivel adapter to all patients. Platelets should be infused when indicated just before biopsy.

Patients on immunosuppressive and cytotoxic therapy and those who are azotemic are at high risk for bleeding. Mild bleeding can be managed by suctioning through the bronchoscope, local instillation of epinephrine and oxygen therapy. A new procedure consists of wedging the bronchoscope tip into a selected distal bronchus before, during and after biopsy to confine bleeding to a segmental bronchus until clotting occurs. This method has been used in 55 cases, with encouraging results. Tamponade with the bronchoscope tip was effective in all 6 patients who bled, preventing blood from flooding the airway. If this method can be followed closely, transbronchial forceps biopsy with the flexible fiberoptic instrument is an excellent diagnostic technique with minimal risks of hemorrhage, hypoxemia and cardiac arrest.

► [In this experience, 1 patient died of severe hemorrhage, a mortality of about 0.2%. Another compilation of 5,450 transbronchial lung biopsy procedures, from which exact data were available in 2,628 (Herf et al.: Deaths and complications associated with transbronchial lung biopsy, Am. Rev. Respir. Dis. 115:708, 1977), recorded pneumothorax in 5.5%, hemorrhage exceeding 50 ml in 1.3% and death in 0.2%. Hemorrhage accounted for 9 deaths, and in 8 of these cases abnormal coagulation studies were known to be present, usually thrombocytopenia. However, 1 patient had entirely normal coagulation studies and the responsible physician indicated that even in retrospect there was nothing to indicate that the patient would bleed. One patient died from a tension pneumothorax which developed slowly after the biopsy, indicating the necessity for continued observation. Presumably this was a preventable death. One of the most attractive applications of transbronchial lung biopsy is in the immunocompromised host in whom a pulmonary infiltrate may be due to underlying malignancy, to therapy with immunosuppressive or oncolytic agents or to intercurrent infection. Feldman et al. (Transbronchial lung biopsy in the compromised host, J.A.M.A. 238:1377, 1977) recorded the results in 38 such patients: 10 were diagnostic of infection, 13 of nonspecific interstitial pneumonitis and 6 of tumor and 9 were nondiagnostic. The infections included 6 cases of *Pneumocystis carinii,* 2 cases of fungal pneumonia (mucormycosis and cryptococcosis), 1 case of tuberculosis and 1 of cytomegalovirus infection. Obviously 9 of these 10 diagnoses had therapeutic implications. Also, the finding of interstitial pneumonitis in a patient on immunosuppressive or oncolytic therapy would often indicate discontinuation of the drugs. Overall the results have to be regarded as excellent. Fossieck et al. (Fiberoptic bronchoscopy and culture of bacteria from the lower respiratory tract, Chest 72:5, 1977) confirm what has been generally assumed, that it is useless to submit fiberoptic bronchoscopy specimens for routine bacteriologic culture. Kane et al. (Diagnosis of asbestosis by transbronchial biopsy, a method to facilitate demonstration of ferruginous bodies, Am. Rev. Respir. Dis. 115:689, 1977) digest the biopsy material with sodium hypochlorite and concentrate it with Millipore filtration, which greatly increases the ability to recover ferruginous bodies, a useful thing to know. Weber et al. (Lung biopsy in *Pneumocystis carinii* pneumonia: A histopathologic study of typical and atypical features, Am. J. Clin. Pathol. 67:11, 1977) indicate that 47% of biopsy specimens shown to contain *Pneumocystis* by silver staining had no histologic features generally regarded as suggestive of *Pneumocystis.* The atypical features included interstitial fibrosis, epithelioid granulomas, focal multinucleated giant cells, dense interstitial infiltrate, infiltration of alveolar macrophages and calcification. The message is that meticulous examination of special stains, usually the methenamine silver stain, is essential to the pathologic diagnosis of this treatable condition. There are, incidentally, no typical x-ray findings either. – Ed.]

Pulmonary Hypertension in the CREST Syndrome Variant of Progressive Systemic Sclerosis (Scleroderma). Although the

TABLE 1.—CLINICAL DATA*

Patient	Age	Sex	Duration of Raynaud's Phenomenon at Time of Study	Calcinosis	Sclerodactyly	Telangiectasia	Esophageal Dysfunction	Pulmonary Fibrosis (Roentgenogram)	Pulmonary Diffusing Capacity Percent of Predicted	Electrocardiogram	Follow-Up from Time of Study	Associated Diseases
	yrs		*yrs*								*months*	
1	60	F	19	+	+	+	+	0	38	RVH	11∤	Hashimoto's thyroiditis
2	41	F	9	0	+	+	0	0	—	RVH	14∤	Hypothyroidism (? Hashimoto's thyroiditis)
3	56	F	24	0	+	+	0	0	50	RVH	38∤	? Sjögren's syndrome
4	69	F	3	0	+	+	+	0	—	RVH	1∤	? Sjögren's syndrome
5	64	F	40	+	+	+	+	0	52	RVH	5∤	
6	66	F	30	+	+	+	0	0	—	Sick sinus	20	Sjögren's syndrome
7	28	F	18	0	+	+	+	0	42	RVH	4∤	Sjögren's syndrome
8	48	F	9	0	+	+	0	0	37	RVH	6	
9	61	M	3	+	+	+	+	0	—	LBBB	34	Calcified mitral annulus
10	46	M	23	+	+	+	+	0	—	RVH/LVH	37	Rheumatic heart disease

*+, present; 0, absent; –, not available; ∤, expired; RHV, right ventricular hypertrophy; LVH, left ventricular hypertrophy; LBBB, left bundle-branch block.

CRST (calcinosis, Raynaud's phenomenon, sclerodactyly, telangiectasia) syndrome tends to pursue a slowly progressive course, it is associated in many instances with serious internal disturbances, including esophageal (E) dysfunction. Rosemarie Salerni, Gerald P. Rodnan, Donald F. Leon and James A. Shaver[4] (Univ. of Pittsburgh) observed 10 patients with the CREST syndrome and severe pulmonary hypertension without pulmonary fibrosis among more than 120 patients seen with the CREST syndrome in the past 2 decades. Two patients had associated mitral valve disease; 1 had severe annulus calcification producing mitral obstruction and incompetence and 1, rheumatic heart disease with mitral stenosis and mild aortic regurgitation.

All patients but the 2 with mitral valve disease were women; all were aged 28–66 years at the time of hemodynamic evaluation (Table 1). Raynaud's phenomenon had been present for 3–40 years. Calcinosis was evident clinically in 4 patients. Six patients had x-ray evidence of esophageal dysfunction without symptoms, except for reflux in 1 patient. Exertional dyspnea had been present for 6–24 months. All patients had clinical evidence of pulmonary hypertension; 5 with the most severe pulmonary hypertension showed tricuspid regurgitation. Four patients had congestive heart failure at the time of study; 8 had ECG evidence of right ventricular hypertrophy. Four deaths were directly attributable to pulmonary hypertension and a fifth patient died suddenly 5 days after a cholecystectomy. The hemodynamic findings are summarized in Table 2. Autopsy of 3 patients who died of pulmonary hypertension showed intimal proliferation with myxomatous change in small- and medium-sized pulmonary arteries that resembled the changes seen in the digital arteries of patients with scleroderma and the interlobular renal arteries of those with "scleroderma kidney."

The CREST syndrome is not entirely benign, but may be complicated after a long clinical course by progressive pulmonary vascular obliteration, pulmonary hypertension and death in the absence of significant pulmonary fibrosis. The CREST syndrome appears to be a subset of the connective tissue disease progressive systemic sclerosis with predominantly vascular manifestations.

TABLE 2.—HEMODYNAMIC DATA*

Patient	Pressures					C.O.	C.I.	Pulmonary Resistance	
	$\bar{m}$RA	RV	PA	$\bar{m}$	$\bar{m}$ Wedge or LA			Total	Vascular
	mm Hg			*mm Hg*		*litres/min*	*litres/min/m²*	*dynes · sec ·cm⁻⁵*	
1	14	100/0 (15)	98/37	63	6	1.89	1.16	2667	2413
2	7	80/0 (7)	80/25	40	8	5.29	3.19	605	484
3	4	60/0 (8)	65/20	35	8	4.85	2.89	577	445
4	14	100/0 (15)	100/40	65	...	3.21	1.95	1620	...
5	10	94/0 (12)	87/36	43	5	1.50	1.19	2293	2027
6	5	60/0 (6)	60/16	32	15	...	...	...	...
7	8	... ...	75/35	50	6	...	...	...	...
8	12	... ...	60/30	...	8	...	...	...	...
†9	7	70/0 (7)	72/25	40	16	6.66	3.41	480	288
‡10	5	55/4 (7)	55/24	36	18	3.52	1.89	818	409

*$\bar{m}$, mean pressure; RA, right atrium; RV, right ventricle; number in parentheses, end-diastolic pressure; PA, pulmonary artery; LA, left atrium; CO, cardiac output; CI, cardiac index.

†Mitral annulus calcification.

‡Rheumatic heart disease with mitral stenosis and mild aortic insufficiency.

(4) Ann. Intern. Med. 86:394–399, April, 1977.

► [Kay and Banik (Unexplained pulmonary hypertension with pulmonary arteritis in rheumatoid disease, Br. J. Dis. Chest 71:53, 1977) report a case of medial hypertrophy and intimal fibrosis of muscular pulmonary arteries in a young woman with rheumatoid arthritis of fairly prolonged duration. There were no changes suggestive of interstitial fibrosis to which the arterial changes might have been secondary. Although the authors did not state that the diseases were associated, they did review similar cases from the literature. Sanderson et al. (A case of pulmonary veno-occlusive disease responding to treatment with azathioprine, Thorax 32:140, 1977) report a case which almost certainly was immune complex in origin since it was associated with alopecia, digital vasculitis ulcers, Raynaud's phenomenon, polyarthritis and muscle weakness. The remarkable thing was an excellent response to azathioprine. They noted that fine pulmonary rales and orthopnea are common in this condition whereas they are rare in pulmonary arterial hypertension. Dye et al. (Sclerosing mediastinitis with occlusion of pulmonary veins, J. Thorac. Cardiovasc. Surg. 74:137, 1977) review the entity of sclerosing mediastinitis, often due to infections such as histoplasmosis, tuberculosis, other fungal infections and syphillis, but also associated with processes of unknown etiology including retroperitoneal fibrosis. Sclerosing mediastinitis can cause compromise not only of the pulmonary veins, so as to produce pulmonary hypertension, but of the pulmonary arteries, bronchi, the vena cava and the esophagus. – Ed.] ◄

Management of Flail Chest: Comparison of Ventilatory and Nonventilatory Treatment. The treatment of flail chest injuries continues to be difficult. Intubation and internal pneumatic stabilization with volume-cycled ventilators have supplanted external stabilization of the flail segment as the treatment of choice, but the mortality remains high. Steven R. Shackford, David E. Smith, Christopher K. Zarins, Charles L. Rice and Richard W. Virgilio[5] (Naval Regional Med. Center, San Diego) have treated selected patients without mechanical ventilation in the past year. Mechanical ventilation has been reserved for patients with clinical respiratory distress. The Bennett MA-1 volume-cycled respirator was used. Using criteria of a Pa_{O_2} below 60 mm Hg or a P_{CO_2} above 60 mm Hg, patients were classed as appropriately

TABLE 1.—COMPARISON OF TREATMENT GROUPS

	Group I	Group II	Group III
	"Appropriately" Ventilated	"Inappropriately" Ventilated	Nonventilated
Number of patients	16	15	11
Age (yr)	49	35	45
Admission PO_2	43*	68	65
Admission PCO_2	35	34	32
Associated injuries	1.44	1.27	0.64
Number of fractured ribs	4.6	5.3	4.2
Hemopneumothorax	8/16	6/15	2/11
Ventilator time (days)	18.6	12.9	0.3*
Complications	2.8	1.9	0.3*
Treatment-associated complications	12/16	9/15	4/11
Deaths	5*	1	0

*$P < 0.01$.

(5) Am. J. Surg. 132:759–762, December, 1976.

TABLE 2.—REVIEW OF 10-YEAR EXPERIENCE WITH FLAIL CHEST

Author	Year	Patients	Deaths	Mortality (%)
Reid and Baird [1]	1965	33	12	36
Perry and Galway [2]	1965	74	26	35
Ransdell [3]	1965	86	43	50
Garzon et al [4]	1966	19	9	47
Duff et al [5]	1968	71	16	22
Sankaran and Wilson [6]	1970	100	24	24
Diethelm and Battle [7]	1971	75	9	12
Relihan and Litwin [8]	1973	85	30	35
Total		543	169	31

ventilated (group I), inappropriately ventilated (group II) or nonventilated (group III).

The 40 men and 2 women had a mean age of 43 years. Thirty were injured in automobile accidents. Twelve patients had a chest injury only. Sixteen had hemothorax or pneumothorax. Twenty-four of 27 patients admitted before October, 1973, were intubated and ventilated. Nine were in group I and 15 in group II. Of the 15 patients admitted later, 7 were in group I and 5 were treated by chest physiotherapy and analgesia only (group III). Three were ventilated at operation for associated injuries and were extubated before stabilization of the flail segment. The mortality was 14%. Two patients died of adult respiratory distress syndrome. Thirty patients had complications, including pneumonia in 18, atelectasis in 10 and tracheolaryngeal injury in 10. The treatment groups are compared in Table 1. The complication rate in group II was significantly greater than in group III.

Mechanical ventilation has failed to improve survival in flail chest injury (Table 2). Ventilation, when indicated, should be used to correct abnormalities in gas exchange rather than to overcome chest wall instability. Hypoxemia in these cases results from ventilation-perfusion abnormalities secondary to splinting of the chest wall and pulmonary contusion. Initial hypoxemia is a good indicator of the need for ventilation, but other factors must be considered. If respiratory support is necessary, it should be discontinued when normal gas exchange has been restored.

► [The term "appropriately ventilated" indicated patients with respiratory failure as defined by blood gases and "inappropriately ventilated" indicated those in whom the only indication for ventilation was the chest injury itself. The major thrust was that one should be conservative and use ventilators only when blood gas data are sufficiently abnormal to warrant this. Baker reports a similarly conservative approach with good results (The treatment of flail chest injury, Aust. N.Z.J. Surg. 47:170, 1977). Artificial ventilation was restricted to patients in whom hypoxemia could not be corrected with administration of oxygen, patients with high and unstable Pa_{CO_2} concentrations and unconscious patients. The emphasis was on relief of pain and splinting and attention to secretions. The results with this conservative approach were appreciably better than in the period in which artificial ventilation was used routinely. Ginsbert and Kostin (New approaches to the management of flail chest, Can. Med. Assoc. J. 116:613, 1977) likewise advocate conservatism as regards ventilator therapy but also favor early surgical fixation of the unstabilized chest with wires and such devices as soon as the general condition permits. – Ed.] ◄

PART THREE

THE BLOOD AND BLOOD-FORMING ORGANS

MARTIN J. CLINE, M.D.

Bone Marrow Failure Syndromes

Recovery from Aplastic Anemia after Treatment with Cyclophosphamide. The prognosis for survival in severe aplastic anemia remains poor. Immune processes may be involved in the pathogenesis of aplastic anemia in some patients. At least 4 recoveries have been reported in cytotoxic drug-treated patients given bone marrow transplants, despite failure of engraftment or graft rejection. Daniel T. Baran, Paul F. Griner and Martin R. Klemperer[1] (Univ. of Rochester) report a successful recovery from aplastic anemia in a patient given cytotoxic therapy without attempted bone marrow transplantation.

Man, 22, had received chloramphenicol for an intestinal infection 6 months before and had also taken clindamycin for acne. Petechiae and retinal hemorrhages were present, with a hematocrit of 14%, a white blood cell count of 1,700 and a platelet count of 7,000. Bone marrow aspiration and biopsy showed marked hypocellularity. Oxymetholone and prednisone were given, the latter without benefit. Eighteen units of platelets and 10 of packed red blood cells were given in a 7-week period. Fever and a large anal fissure were then noted, and blood cultures were positive for *Pseudomonas aeruginosa.* Infusions of donor platelets were no longer effective, and epistaxes and rectal bleeding occurred. No HLA-compatible sibling or unrelated bone marrow donor was identified.

The patient was given cyclophosphamide, 30 mg/kg daily, intravenously, for 4 days. Resistance to platelets subsided within 1 week, but multiple abscesses and hectic fever ensued. The white blood cells increased spontaneously about a month after treatment, and the abscesses resolved. The reticulocytes peaked at 10%, and bone marrow studies showed active myeloid and erythroid cell lines. Bone marrow cellularity was nearly normal several months later, but megakaryocytes remained reduced in number. Currently the patient is active and asymptomatic.

This patient's course suggests but does not prove a causal relationship between cyclophosphamide therapy and improvement. This treatment must be considered experimental and must be restricted to patients with severe aplasia. Additional case reports and further experimental observations should clarify the pathogenesis of aplastic anemia and the possible role of immunosuppressive therapy in selected patients.

► [I have observed a patient with severe aplastic anemia reconstitute her own bone marrow after failure of attempted bone marrow transplantation with high-dose cyclophosphamide conditioning (Territo, M. C.: Br. J. Haematol. 36:306, 1977). My conclusions were (1) that the hematopoietic stem cell can be very resistant to cytotoxic drugs and (2) that my ability to predict the outcome of severe aplasia is distinctly fallible. Doctor Baran and his colleagues, observing another patient in rather similar circumstances, suggest that immunologic mechanisms may operate in aplasia and that immunosuppressive-cytotoxic drugs may be effective therapy. Clearly all the facts are not in.

(1) N. Engl. J. Med. 295:1522–1523, Dec. 30, 1976.

Swiss and French investigators have claimed good results in the treatment of aplastic anemia with antithymocyte globulin (ATG). Certainly cyclophosphamide and ATG are potentially dangerous in a patient already prone to bleeding and infections. Cyclophosphamide can produce further myelosuppression as well as hemorrhagic cystitis. Antithymocyte globulin can produce immunosuppression, serum sickness and acute hypersensitivity reactions. My own view is that such agents should only be used in controlled trials in a few centers with excellent support facilities for bone marrow failure. – Ed.] ◄

Suppression of Erythroid Colony Formation by Lymphocytes from Patients with Aplastic Anemia. Lymphocytes from patients with congenital hypoplastic anemia can inhibit erythroid colony formation by normal human marrow in vitro. Ronald Hoffman, Esmail D. Zanjani, John D. Lutton, Ralph Zalusky and Louis R. Wasserman[2] (City Univ. of New York) used this assay technique to evaluate the peripheral blood lymphocytes from 7 patients with severe aplastic anemia. Eighteen normal subjects donated peripheral blood. Three patients given multiple transfusions for other diseases and 2 with acquired pure red blood cell aplasia were studied also. The in vitro plasma clot culture technique was used to measure growth of erythroid colonies from the marrow.

Addition of serum from 5 patients with aplastic anemia failed to suppress the number of colonies formed and resulted in an increase of 18–47% over normal controls. The increase probably was due to the elevated serum erythropoietin levels present in the anemic patients. In no case was any inhibition by serum of aplastic patients seen. Serum from patients with pure red blood cell aplasia markedly depressed ery-

EFFECT OF PERIPHERAL BLOOD LYMPHOCYTES FROM DONORS WITH NORMAL BONE MARROW AND PATIENTS WITH APLASTIC ANEMIA ON EYRTHROID COLONY FORMATION BY NORMAL HUMAN BONE MARROW CELLS IN RESPONSE TO 2 IU ERYTHROPOIETIN IN VITRO*

SUBJECTS	ERYTHROID COLONIES/6 × 10⁵ BONE-MARROW CELLS AT LYMPHOCYTE CONCENTRATION INDICATED †				
	0.5 × 10⁵ cells	*1 × 10⁵ cells*	*2 × 10⁵ cells*	*4 × 10⁵ cells*	*6 × 10⁵ cells*
Normal donors	246±14	296±21	317±31	374±16	287±22
Transfused patients	293±12	272±42	‡	363±54	297±18
Case 1	255±10	205±30	44±5	22±6	12±4
Case 2	374±28	497±60	291±30	282±87	‡
Case 3	15±5	20±3	‡	48±4	12±3
Case 4	72±14	84±18	78±12	50±16	‡
Case 5	293±47	286±32	218±21	197±34	203±48
Case 6	250±26	275±32	279±18	80±14	20±4
Case 7	110±13	95±21	27±3	‡	‡

*No erythroid colonies were formed by normal marrow at lymphocyte concentration of $0.5-6\times10^5$ cells in absence of erythropoietin. In presence of 2 IU erythropoietin, however, 206 ± 14 were formed. This value represents mean ± 1 SEM of all marrow specimens (23) used in these studies.

†Each value represents mean ± 1 SEM for mean for either of duplicate cultures (Cases 4 and 7) or for duplicate cultures in all studies.

‡Not determined.

(2) N. Engl. J. Med. 296:10–13, Jan. 6, 1977.

throid colony formation. These serums also contained elevated erythropoietin activity.

Lymphocyte effects on erythroid colony formation are shown in the table. Lymphocytes from the transfused control subjects behaved like those of the normal donors, but the peripheral blood lymphocytes of most aplastic patients inhibited erythroid colony formation by normal human bone marrow. Persistence of such lymphocytes could explain the difficulty seen with marrow engraftment of HLA-compatible cells. Autologous marrow reconstitution has occurred in patients with severe aplastic anemia after treatment with antilymphocyte globulin and HLA-semi-incompatible marrow transplants. Suppressor lymphocytes are being increasingly implicated in the pathogenesis of disease in man, and the present findings suggest that acquired aplastic anemia may be an additional disorder whose pathogenesis might be attributed to lymphocyte autoaggression.

► [A number of recent reports describe lymphocyte suppression of hematopoiesis in aplastic anemia, Diamond-Blackfan syndrome, and red blood cell agenesis (Hoffman et al.: Science 193:899, 1976; Ascensao et al.: Lancet 1:669, 1976; and Litwin and Zanjani: Nature 266:57, 1977). I am skeptical about the significance of these observations. Controls for the effects of sensitization by transfusions and for technical artifacts generally have been inadequate. Most cases of bone marrow failure probably are not caused by immunologic autoaggression and one must be cautious in extrapolating these in vitro studies to the treatment of the aplastic patient with cytotoxic immunosuppression. — Ed.] ◄

Diamond-Blackfan Syndrome: Lymphocyte-Mediated Suppression of Erythropoiesis. Congenital hypoplastic anemia (CHA), or Diamond-Blackfan syndrome, is a disorder of childhood characterized by progressive anemia and sparing of the white blood cells and platelets. Erythroid precursors in the bone marrow are virtually absent. Erythropoietin production appears to be adequate, and a serum inhibitor of erythropoiesis is not present. Ronald Hoffman, Esmail D. Zanjani, Jose Vila, Ralph Zalusky, John D. Lutton and Louis R. Wasserman[3] (Mt. Sinai School of Medicine, New York) report evidence that peripheral blood lymphocytes from patients with CHA inhibit red blood cell production by normal bone marrow cells, an indication that CHA may have an immunologic basis.

Lymphocytes were obtained from 6 patients with clinically established CHA, 24 normal subjects, 5 subjects given multiple transfusions and 3 adults with acquired pure red blood cell aplasia. Lymphocytes from all patients with CHA suppressed the formation of erythroid colonies by marrow cells in the presence of erythropoietin. Prior repeated freeze-thawing of the cells removed their ability to suppress erythroid colony formation. Serums from the study patients did not exhibit erythropoietic-inhibitory activity, and the addition of CHA serum increased the number of colonies formed. Serums from patients with pure red blood cell aplasia inhibited erythroid colony formation, but their lymphocytes did not suppress colony formation. No inhibition of colony formation was seen with lymphocytes from multiply transfused patients.

---

(3) Science 193:899–900, Sept. 3, 1976.

A component of peripheral blood lymphocytes from patients with CHA may be the primary agent in the production of anemia in this disorder. It is not clear whether the suppressive lymphocytes reside in the bone marrow or arrive there as part of the recirculating lymphocyte pool. Steroid therapy does not lead to the preferential selection of a population of lymphocytes capable of inhibiting erythropoiesis. The ameliorative effects of steroids may be mediated through an effect on the erythroid precursor cell. Possibly CHA is an additional disorder characterized by lymphocyte autoaggression.

► [Taken at their face value, the data in this report clearly suggest that lymphocytes suppress erythropoiesis in patients with Diamond-Blackfan syndrome. Again, I am skeptical about this simplistic explanation. It seems inconsistent with the clinical features of the disorder. We are only beginning to appreciate the complex interactions between T lymphoid cells and erythroid progenitors (Wiktor-Jedrezejczak et al.: Science 196:313, 1977). Various recent experimental observations suggest that T lymphocytes or their products may modulate the responsiveness of early erythroid progenitors to erythropoietin. More information may allow us to put the observations of Hoffman and his colleagues into perspective. – Ed.] ◄

Marrow Transplantation for Treatment of Aplastic Anemia: Analysis of Factors Associated with Graft Rejection. Treatment with transplantation of bone marrow from HL-A-identical siblings has introduced optimism into the problem of severe aplastic anemia, but marrow graft rejection is associated with a high initial mortality of marrow transplantation. Rainer Storb, Ross L. Prentice and E. Don-

Fig 1. – Conditioning regimens, marrow infusions, platelet support, hematologic events and methotrexate administration in patient who showed initially successful marrow engraftment followed by marrow rejection and subsequent successful marrow engraftment. *MTX*, methotrexate; *Cy*, cyclophosphamide (50 mg/kg); *Pz*, procarbazine (12.5 mg/kg); *ATG*, antithymocyte globulin (12 mg IgG/kg); and *WBC*, white blood cells. (Courtesy of Storb, R., et al.: N. Engl. J. Med. 296:61–66, Jan. 13, 1977.)

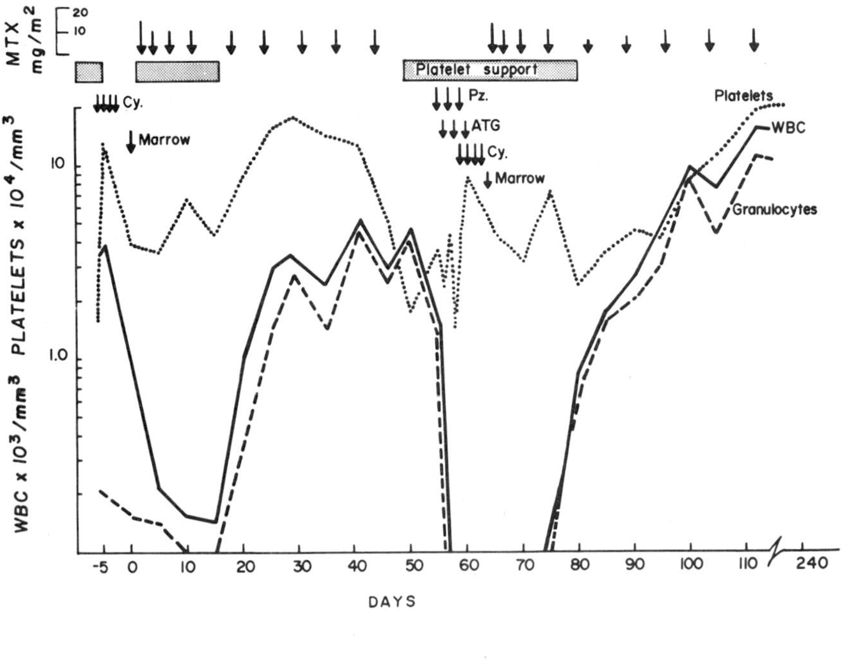

nall Thomas[4] (Seattle) analyzed the factors associated with marrow graft rejection in 21 of 73 patients treated for severe aplastic anemia in 1970–75. Five other patients died 1–8 days after marrow transplantation before success of the procedure could be evaluated. All patients received methotrexate within 100 days of transplantation.

An example of initially successful marrow engraftment followed by marrow rejection is shown in Figure 1. Graft rejection was associated with the extent of previous blood or platelet support, the number of marrow cells infused and the relative response index in mixed leukocyte culture. A low marrow cell dose was associated with a higher rate of graft rejection. Nineteen of the 21 patients in whom the graft was rejected died. The only other factors that correlated strongly with graft rejection were fewer than 3×10^8 marrow cells per kg and a positive relative response index in mixed leukocyte culture. The transplant year was not a significant factor when the marrow cell dose and relative response index were taken into account.

This study clearly established strong associations between the fate of the marrow graft and two prognostic factors, the results of mixed leukocyte culture testing before transplantation and the number of marrow cells injected. It seems important to obtain the greatest possible amount of donor marrow by harvesting cells from the anterior and posterior iliac crests and sternum. Also, alternate sources of hematopoietic stem cells must be investigated. It may suffice to select a group of patients with little risk of graft rejection who could be conditioned with cyclophosphamide alone and another group with a high risk of rejection in whom a more powerful conditioning regimen is indicated. One such regimen consists of procarbazine, antithymocyte globulin and total body irradiation.

► [Severe aplastic anemia is defined by an empty bone marrow, neutrophils < 500/cu mm and platelets < 20,000/cu mm. Approximately 40% of patients with severe aplastic anemia are alive and show hematologic improvement 2 years after marrow grafting. In contrast, less than 10% of such patients treated by conventional methods are alive (see the following article). Clearly, therefore, transplantation offers greater hope, at least in the patient less than age 30 years. It is distressing, therefore, that often the bone marrow graft fails after an initial period of proliferation. The reasons for failure of engraftment are unclear although Doctor Storb and his colleagues believe they have identified some prognostic factors. Unfortunately, the UCLA Bone Marrow Transplant Team has not found the relative response index to be a useful predictor of the success of engraftment. Preliminary data suggest that more aggressive immunosuppression can increase the percentage of "takes" of marrow transplants; however, the more aggressive programs may be associated with an increased incidence of lethal infections and interstitial pneumonitis, thus offsetting the beneficial effects of better graft survival. Our pressing need is for reliable tests for identifying the patient at high risk of graft failure and for nonlethal conditioning programs that will prepare such a patient for engraftment.—Ed.] ◄

Bone Marrow Transplantation in Severe Aplastic Anemia was evaluated by the UCLA Bone Marrow Transplant Team[5] (Univ. of California, Los Angeles). The outlook for patients with severe aplastic anemia is grave. Transplantation of normal bone marrow may be beneficial to patients with no or defective hematopoiesis. The course of 21 patients seen in 1972–75 with severe aplastic anemia was analyzed.

(4) N. Engl. J. Med. 296:61–66, Jan. 13, 1977.
(5) Lancet 2:921–923, Oct. 30, 1976.

Transplantation was done when an HLA-identical sibling was available and the clinical and hematologic data indicated a poor prognosis. When a matched sibling was not available, patients were managed by conventional means. All patients received comparable blood product and antibiotic therapy. Patients had a granulocyte count of 500/μl or less and two or more bone marrow biopsy specimens that showed moderate to severe aplasia or a bone marrow aspirate with 70% or more nonmyeloid cells, or some combination of these findings. Most patients received a trial of oxymetholone for 1–3 months. Transplant patients received donor buffy coat-rich plasma in conjunction with cyclophosphamide, followed by donor bone marrow and then posttransplantation methotrexate administration. Two patients received total body irradiation in preparation for marrow transplantation.

Twelve of the 21 patients received bone marrow transplants and 9 were managed conservatively. All 9 conventionally managed patients died, 4 from infection and 5 from hemorrhage. The median survival from diagnosis was 82 days. The study patients received transplants a median of 37 days after diagnosis. A mean dose of 3.9×10^8 nucleated bone marrow cells per kg was given. The procedure was well tolerated. Seven patients are alive; the actuarial survival at 1 year was 53%. Five patients have returned to full activity. Four patients rejected their grafts and 3 died, but 1 is alive after retransplantation from a second HLA-identical sibling. Graft-vs.-host disease developed in 4 of 8 patients at risk. Eight transplants were between ABO-identical pairs and 5 were mismatched; ABO compatibility had no effect on engraftment, graft rejection, graft-vs.-host disease or survival.

Bone marrow transplantation is useful in selected patients with severe aplastic anemia. The long-term fate of patients given bone marrow transplants is unknown, but the survival of transplant recipients has been better than that of patients managed conventionally.

► [It is important to be familiar with the criteria for *severe* aplastic anemia because the severe form of the disease has a mortality in excess of 80%. This study once again demonstrates the poor prognosis of severe disease and the usefulness of bone marrow transplantation in selected patients. About 40% of transplant recipients will be alive and hematologically reconstituted at 2 years. Major causes of failure are still graft rejection, graft-vs.-host disease and interstitial pneumonitis (Camitta et al.: Blood 48: 63, 1976).—Ed.] ◄

Disorders of Hemoglobin

Radioimmunoassay for Abnormal Hemoglobins. The common method of preliminary identification of hemoglobin variants is based on electrophoretic differences, but many different abnormal hemoglobins have similar or identical mobilities that necessitate structural analyses for conclusive identification. Fred A. Garver, Marilyn B. Baker, C. Sidney Jones, Marsha Gravely, Gultekin Altay and Titus H. J. Huisman[6] (Med. College of Georgia) have developed a radioimmunoassay system with monospecific antiserums capable of recognizing and quantifying hemoglobin variants in red blood cell hemolysates. Included in the study are the abnormal hemoglobins S, C, D and E, as well as G, Philadelphia. Blood samples for isolation of hemoglobin variants were obtained from patients whose abnormal hemoglobins had been characterized structurally.

Antiserums to the variants were prepared in rabbits with complete adjuvant. Antiserum to hemoglobin E was produced in chickens. Antibody preparations were made monospecific for the variants by absorption with hemoglobin A conjugated to AH-Sepharose activated with glutaraldehyde. The extent of binding of absorbed antiserums with the corresponding ^{125}I-labeled variant hemoglobin was measured. Standard radioimmunoassay inhibition assays were done to insure the specificity of the antiserum for each mutant. Red blood cell hemolysates containing hemoglobin S or C from newborn infants could be distinguished from those lacking these variant hemoglobins. In studies of cross-reactivity, only the homologous antigen was effective in inhibiting the antigen-antibody reaction, thus emphasizing the dominant role of a single amino acid side chain in an antigenic determinant in combining with antibody. All the variants eliciting monospecific antibody contained substitutions exposed to the exterior of the macromolecular surface.

► [The authors describe a sensitive and specific means of identifying and quantifying a number of human hemoglobin variants. Absorption of antiserum prepared against human hemoglobin A with a variety of variant hemoglobins should help clarify the structural basis of the immunogenicity and antigenicity of human hemoglobin. — Ed.]

Prenatal Diagnosis of Hemoglobinopathies: Review of 15 Cases. Blanche P. Alter, C. Bernadette Modell, Denys Fairweather, John C. Hobbins, Maurice J. Mahoney, Fredric D. Frigoletto, Anita S. Sherman and David G. Nathan[7] attempted prenatal diagnosis for sickle cell disease or thalassemia in 15 cases in an 18-month period in 1974–75. Adequate fetal cell samples were obtained in 12 cases, in 7 by fetoscopy and in 5 by placental aspiration. In another case, premature labor resulted from repeated placental aspirations. Homozygosity

(6) Science 196:1334–1336, June 17, 1977.
(7) N. Engl. J. Med. 295:1437–1443, Dec. 23, 1976.

SUMMARY OF PRENATAL DIAGNOSIS FOR HEMOGLOBINOPATHIES

FINDING	FETOSCOPY	ASPIRATION	TOTALS
		no. of cases	
All cases	7	8	15
Fetal loss	0	1	1
Inadequate samples	0	3*	3
Evaluable cases	7	5	12
% fetal cells	70 (4 - 100)	37 (1 - 100)	64
Homozygosity:			
Established	2	0	2
Incorrectly diagnosed	1	0	1
Missed (infant born)	1	0	1
Ruled out, with confirmation at birth	3	4†	7

*Sample produced in case of fetal loss was inadequate.

†In 1 additional case, in which β-thalassemia trait was diagnosed in utero, the family chose abortion, but the fetal sample was not available for confirmation.

was diagnosed correctly in 2 cases and ruled out in 8 cases. Homozygous disease was not detected in 1 case, and 1 uncertain case of β-thalassemia trait was terminated.

The series included 11 cases studied for β-thalassemia and 4 studied for sickle cell disease. Globin synthesis was assessed by incubation of samples with ^{3}H-leucine and hemoglobin chain separation on carboxymethylcellulose columns. Seven predictions that infants would not have homozygous disease were confirmed. One prediction of sickle trait proved to be sickle cell disease. The findings are summarized in the table. Transfusion of the mother in an effort to reduce her reticulocyte count and thus decrease the maternal reticulocyte contribution to the mixed sample was attempted 8 times and became an established part of the procedure. There was no sampling failure or fetal death in the fetoscopy series, but one diagnostic error and a recommendation for a repeat procedure were made despite adequate samples.

Prenatal diagnosis of antenatal defects and selective abortion of homozygotes offer an opportunity to prospective affected parents to have children without fear. Prenatal diagnosis of hemoglobinopathies, although useful and often successful, remains experimental. Better methods are needed to separate fetal and maternal cells from one another. The greatest biochemical hazard appears to be misinterpretation of peaks in the beta region of the chromatographic system.

► [A perfect prenatal test for thalassemia or sickle cell disease would correctly identify all homozygotes and all heterozygotes and cause no fetal mortality. This objective has not been achieved in the present study. The investigators failed to identify sickle cell disease in 1 of 4 fetuses at risk and may have induced premature labor with fetal loss by repeated placental aspirations. Nevertheless, the studies of Y. W. Kan et al. (see the following article) and this group represent important advances in the technology of antenatal diagnosis of the serious hemoglobinopathies. The technology is sufficiently complex that it presently should be restricted to a few centers. – Ed.] ◄

Prenatal Diagnosis of β-Thalassemia and Sickle Cell Anemia: Experience with 24 Cases. Yuet Wai Kan, Mitchell S. Golbus, Richard F. Trecartin, Roy A. Filly (Univ. of California, San Francisco),

Carlo Valenti (Rome), Mario Furbetta and Antonio Cao[8] (Univ. of Cagliari) attempted prenatal diagnosis of β-thalassemia and sickle cell anemia by fetal blood sampling and analysis of globin-chain synthesis in fetal reticulocytes in 24 at-risk pregnancies since 1974. Twenty-two pregnancies were at risk for β-thalassemia and 2 for sickle cell anemia; 6 were first pregnancies. Fetal blood was sampled from the placenta by aspiration at 18–23 weeks' gestation after ultrasonic location of the placenta, and amniotic fluid was also withdrawn. Placental samples containing fetal blood were incubated with ^{3}H-leucine before globin-chain separation on carboxymethyl-cellulose columns. Similar studies were performed on the cord blood of the aborted fetuses.

Adequate fetal blood was obtained in 22 of the 24 patients. Three complications occurred, including 1 case of amnionitis and 2 abortions associated with excessive fetal bleeding. A fetal bleed of about 25 ml occurred in these 2 cases and a bleed of less than 10 ml was detected in 8 other cases. Sickle cell anemia was diagnosed in both patients at risk and the diagnoses confirmed after abortion. Six fetuses with β-γ ratios of 0.068–0.094 have been born and are normal. Four fetuses with ratios of 0.037–0.057 were found after birth to have β-thalassemia trait. Four fetuses with ratios of zero were considered homozygous and the pregnancies were terminated; the diagnosis was confirmed in these cases. Three pregnancies are continuing uneventfully.

Prenatal diagnosis of β-thalassemia and sickle cell anemia by fetal blood sampling and analysis of globin-chain synthesis in fetal red blood cells is feasible. Enrichment of fetal red blood cells by differential agglutination with anti-i serum permits the successful study of samples containing as little as 7% fetal red blood cells. The biochemical analysis of fetal blood has proved to be extremely reliable. The overall risk needs to be determined and if too high, safer methods that do not require fetal blood must be devised.

► [Once again, this study demonstrates the feasibility of antenatal diagnosis of serious hemoglobinopathies. It also emphasizes the risks associated with blood sampling. – Ed.] ◄

Lead Poisoning: Association with Hemolytic Anemia, Basophilic Stippling, Erythrocyte Pyrimidine 5′-Nucleotidase Deficiency and Intraerythrocytic Accumulation of Pyrimidines. Hereditary hemolytic anemia occurs in association with a severe genetic deficiency of pyrimidine-specific 5′-nucleotidase in erythrocytes. The syndrome is associated with marked basophilic stippling on the stained blood film and with large intraerythrocytic accumulations of nucleotides. The pyrimidine 5′-nucleotidase of normal red blood cells is inhibited markedly in vitro by low concentrations of lead and certain other heavy metals. William N. Valentine, Donald E. Paglia, Kay Fink and Glenn Madokoro[9] (Univ. of California, Los Angeles) postulated that severe lead-induced nucleotidase deficiency should lead to hemolytic anemia, increased basophilic stippling and accumulation of pyrimidine necleotides in erythrocytes in a manner analogous to the

(8) Lancet 1:269–271, Feb. 5, 1977.
(9) J. Clin. Invest. 58:926–932, October, 1976.

genetic deficiency. A patient in whom the hypothesis could be evaluated is described.

Man, 26, a spray painter, presented with epigastric and back pains for 2 days, with anorexia and vomiting. He had worked as a spray painter for 8 years. A "lead line" was noted on the gingiva and orthostatic hypotension was documented. Moderately severe anemia with reticulocytosis of up to 24% was observed. The red blood cells on the stained blood film were anisocytocic, hypochromic and polychromatic and many were stippled. The marrow was mildly hypercellular, with abundant stainable iron. X-rays showed a mild deformity of the duodenal bulb and probable paralytic ileus. Blood and urine lead levels were elevated markedly, as were the urinary aminolevulinic acid, coproporphyrin and uroporphyrin levels. Abdominal pain subsided, but the hematologic changes persisted. Orthostatic hypotension was corrected by intravenous saline. Lead intoxication was traced to paint used by the patient for the past 9 months. Both parents and 2 siblings of the patient had normal hemograms and the parents had normal blood lead levels.

Cytidine was present in 12% of red blood cell nucleotides in the blood of this patient. Nucleotidase activity was about 25% of that in normal red blood cells and 15% or less of that expected in comparable reticulocyte-rich blood. The findings indicate that the hemolytic anemia and increased basophilic stippling characteristic of certain cases of lead intoxication may share a common etiology with the genetically determined disorder.

► [The suggestion that lead poisoning may inhibit erythrocyte pyrimidine 5′-nucleotidase came from the observation of the intense basophilic stippling associated with hereditary deficiency of this enzyme (Valentine, W. N., et al.: J. Clin. Invest. 54:866, 1974). Both conditions are associated with intraerythrocytic accumulations of nucleotides. These nucleotides are believed to retard breakdown of RNA within the developing red blood cell, with resulting undegraded or partially degraded ribosomes which give rise to the basophilic stippling seen on conventional stained smears. — Ed.] ◄

Disorders of the Erythrocyte and of Erythropoiesis

Cerebral Blood Flow in Polycythemia. The pathogenesis of cerebrovascular accidents in patients with polycythemia vera is not clear. D. J. Thomas, G. H. du Boulay, John Marshall, T. C. Pearson, R. W. Ross Russell, L. Symon, G. Wetherley-Mein and E. Zilkha[1] (London) determined the effect of reducing an elevated hematocrit on cerebral blood flow (CBF) in 16 patients with definite polycythemia, having a mean age of 60.1. The diagnosis was based on a red blood cell volume exceeding the expected normal mean by more than 25% in men and 30% in women. Thirteen patients had primary polycythemia, 2 had a renal origin and 1 had hypoxic lung disease; 7 patients had cerebral symptoms, 4 had had a mild completed stroke. Control patients were hospitalized for a disk syndrome. Cerebral blood flow was measured by the intravenous xenon-133 clearance method.

The mean CBF of all polycythemic patients was 37.9 ml/100 gm/minute, significantly below the control mean of 69.1 ml. The 7 patients with cerebral symptoms had a mean CBF of 34.3 ml compared with 40.7 ml for those without. The CBF level was inversely related to the hematocrit level. Venesection resulted in a 73% increase in CBF in 15 patients. The mean CBF returned to normal in patients without cerebral symptoms and increased 60% in those with symptoms. Whole blood viscosity was reduced substantially at all shear rates. Lethargy resolved in all 9 patients with this symptom. Both patients with lower extremity ischemia lost their rest pain. A patient with vertebrobasilar attacks became symptom free and 1 with multi-infarct dementia improved. Only 2 of 19 CBF values with a hematocrit above 0.50 were normal, whereas 3 of 21 with a hematocrit below 0.46 were low.

Cerebral blood flow is reduced in polycythemic patients whose hematocrit is in the range 0.53 – 0.62. The reductions in CBF may be corrected by venesection. Prevention of cerebrovascular complications is as important as the relief of current symptoms. Because a low CBF may predispose to the development of cerebral infarction, the hematocrit should be reduced and maintained at levels lower than those generally accepted.

► [The message seems clear. Keep the hematocrit below 50% in polycythemic patients if normal cerebral blood flow is an important parameter. – Ed.] ◄

Polycythemia Vera: Hormonal Modulation of Erythropoiesis In Vitro. Some clinical observations cast doubt on the concept of complete autonomy of erythropoiesis in polycythemia vera. Recent bone marrow culture studies have provided evidence for erythropoietin re-

---

(1) Lancet 2:161 – 163, July 23, 1977.

sponsiveness of red blood cell progenitors in vitro. David W. Golde, Noelle Bersch and Martin J. Cline[2] (Univ. of California, Los Angeles) cultured bone marrow from 5 patients with polycythemia vera to characterize the interaction of erythropoietin with red blood cell progenitors in this disease. In 4 patients the disease was newly diagnosed and untreated; the fifth had had only phlebotomy. All had splenomegaly, a red blood cell mass over 36 ml/kg and a hemoglobin-oxygen saturation of 92% or greater.

A mean 10-fold higher erythroid cloning efficiency was found with polycythemic marrow than with normal marrow without added erythropoietin. With erythropoietin concentrations of 0.01–1 units/ml, about sevenfold more colony formation was generated in the patients' cultures. Cloning efficiency was substantially greater than normal in 4 of the 5 patients. Dexamethasone consistently increased erythroid colony formation in the patients' cultures as well as in normal subjects' cultures.

These findings provide evidence for functional erythropoietin and glucocorticoid receptor mechanisms on erythroid precursors in polycythemia vera. The results are consistent with a concept of this disease as a disorder of hematopoietic stem cells in which peripheral erythrocytosis is caused by an expanded erythroid progenitor compartment that maintains responsiveness to hormonal modulation. It remains uncertain whether effective erythropoiesis can occur in vivo in the complete absence of erythropoietin stimulation. The role of serum myelostimulatory factors remains to be clarified, as do possible defects in negative regulation.

► [Evidence from a variety of sources suggests that erythropoiesis in polycythemia vera is not autonomous. The red blood cell precursors in this disease appear to retain responsiveness to erythropoietin and to other hormones that modulate red blood cell proliferation. They do not appear to be unusually sensitive to erythropoietin. Strong evidence supports the notion that the disease originates in an aberration in a single hematopoietic stem cell, i.e., is clonal in nature and affects lymphocytes, granulocytes and platelet-producing cells (Adamson et al.: N. Engl. J. Med. 295:913, 1976). – Ed.] ◄

Ferrokinetics and Erythropoiesis in Man: Evaluation of Ferrokinetic Measurements. Standard measures of iron kinetics may be only qualitative reflections of the degree and effectiveness of erythropoiesis. C. Ricketts, I. Cavill, J. A. F. Napier and A. Jacobs[3] (Welsh Natl. School of Medicine, Cardiff) compared the plasma iron clearance half-time ($T^{1/2}$), plasma iron turnover (PIT) and percentage red blood cell utilization of ^{59}Fe (RCU) with the total bone marrow iron turnover (MIT) and effective red blood cell iron turnover determined by the method of Ricketts et al. (1975). Ferrokinetic studies were done in 10 normal subjects and in 51 patients with a variety of hematologic disorders, including 9 with megaloblastic anemia, 14 with iron deficiency anemia, 12 with refractory hypoplastic anemia and 6 with hemochromatosis. Transferrin-bound ^{59}Fe was injected intravenously.

A linear relationship between $T^{1/2}$ and MIT was not observed. The $T^{1/2}$ was prolonged in cases in which the MIT was most markedly re-

(2) Blood 49:399–405, March, 1977.
(3) Br. J. Haematol. 35:41–47, January, 1977.

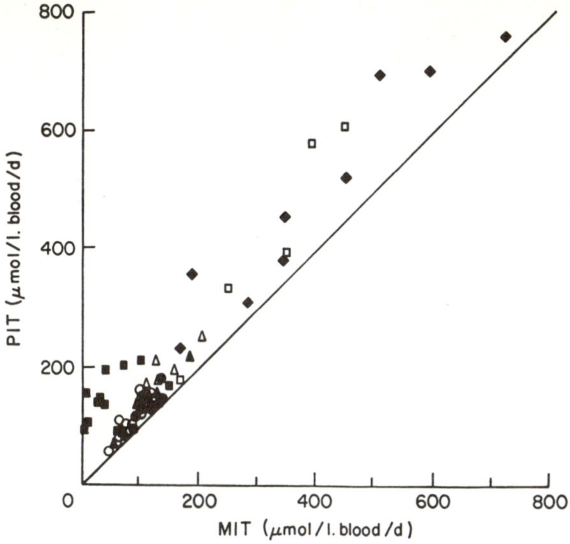

Fig 2.—Relationship between MIT and PIT in normal subjects *(solid circles)* and patients with iron deficiency anemia *(open circles)*, refractory hypoplastic anemia *(solid squares)*, megaloblastic anemia *(diamonds)*, hemochromatosis *(open triangles)*, hemolytic anemia *(open squares)* and rheumatoid arthritis *(solid triangles)*. (Courtesy of Ricketts, C., et al.: Br. J. Haematol. 35:41–47, January, 1977.)

duced and usually was short when the MIT was greatly increased. However, a short $T^{1/2}$ was also found where the MIT was normal or even reduced. There was a significant correlation between PIT and MIT (Fig 2), although PIT was consistently greater than MIT. When the MIT fell below normal levels, there was no proportional reduction in PIT. In patients with refractory hypoplastic anemia, PIT overestimated MIT by as much as 20-fold. Red blood cell utilization was not closely related with red blood cell iron turnover. Red blood cell iron turnover and effective red blood cell iron turnover were significantly correlated, but erythrocyte iron turnover was consistently greater than red blood cell iron turnover.

These findings cast doubt on the validity of $T^{1/2}$ and PIT as measures of erythropoiesis. Red blood cell utilization and red blood cell iron turnover are also inadequate estimates of effective erythropoiesis in many circumstances. The traditional measurements offer poor insight into the nature of a patient's hematologic disease.

► [These investigators reexamine traditional and more sophisticated recent analyses of ferrokinetics in clinical disorders of erythropoiesis. They once again point out how misleading the measurements of plasma iron clearance and red blood cell iron utilization can be in estimating effective erythropoiesis when the marrow is diseased.—Ed.]

Continuous Subcutaneous Administration of Deferoxamine in Patients with Iron Overload. Methods of removing iron in diseases associated with marked dyserythropoiesis have been largely unsuccessful and patients with thalassemia major and other transfusion-dependent iron-overload states usually have died of the toxic manifestations of chronic iron overload. Long-term trials of iron-chelating agents have given disappointing results but continuous intravenous administration of deferoxamine has been found to enhance urinary iron excretion markedly. Richard D. Propper, Barry Cooper, Robert R. Rufo, Arthur W. Nienhuis, W. French Anderson, H. Franklin Bunn, Amnon Rosenthal and David G. Nathan[4] studied the effect of the route of deferoxamine administration on urinary iron excretion in 26 patients aged 3–68 with severe iron overload. Seventeen had severe homozygous β-thalassemia. Most patients received ascorbic acid for at least 2 weeks before subcutaneous deferoxamine therapy was begun. A dose beyond which only minimal additional iron excretion occurred was selected for chronic treatment.

All patients excreted notable amounts of iron and were continually in net negative iron balance. More iron was excreted with a continuous subcutaneous infusion than with intramuscular injection in all 7 patients who received identical doses of deferoxamine. On a milligram-for-milligram basis, subcutaneous administration was 84% as effective as intravenous administration. Thalassemic patients with high serum ferritin values tended to excrete more iron than those with lower ferritin values. No substantial change in daily urinary iron excretion occurred in the 5 patients treated for 6–11 months. Oral ascorbic acid supplementation more than doubled urinary iron excretion. Toxicity has been confined to symptoms at the injection site.

No tachyphylaxis has been observed with the treatment of severely iron-overloaded patients. Ascorbic acid supplementation markedly enhances urinary iron excretion in deferoxamine-treated patients. No systemic toxicity has accompanied chronic subcutaneous deferoxamine administration. Preliminary evidence suggests that this approach may improve or at least stabilize cardiac function and rhythm. The method is practical and can promote sustained urinary iron excretion for at least a year. Further clinical trials certainly are warranted.

► [This article and the following one confirm the usefulness of deferoxamine in iron mobilization when the compound is administered appropriately. — Ed.] ◄

Subcutaneous Infusion and Intramuscular Injection of Desferrioxamine in Patients with Transfusional Iron Overload. Iron overload with cardiac toxicity is the chief cause of death in patients with thalassemia major and other severe refractory anemias who are treated by regular blood transfusions. Multiple endocrine involvement and hepatic cirrhosis are other serious results of excessive iron accumulation. Recent studies have raised the possibility of treatment of transfused patients by the continuous subcutaneous infusion of desferrioxamine (DF) with the use of a portable constant-infusion pump.

M. A. M. Hussain, D. M. Flynn, N. Green, S. Hussein and A. V. Hoffbrand[5] (London) compared iron excretion after continuous delivery of DF over 24 hours and a single intramuscular injection of a similar dose. Eleven patients with β-thalassemia major and 1 with congenital sideroblastic anemia were studied. A dose of 750 mg DF was given by intramuscular injections 4–5 days before and 1–2 days after blood

(4) N. Engl. J. Med. 297:418–423, Aug. 25, 1977.
(5) Lancet 2:1278–1280, Dec. 11, 1976.

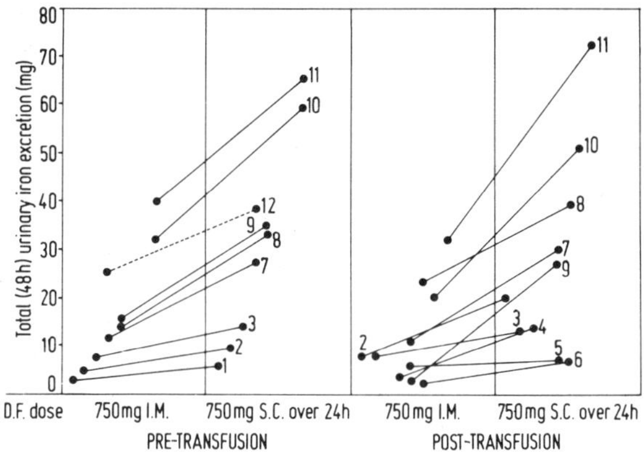

Fig 3.—Total urinary iron excretion after intramuscular *(I.M.)* and subcutaneous *(S.C.)* DF in patients studied before and after transfusion. (Courtesy of Hussain, M. A. M., et al.: Lancet 2:1278–1280, Dec. 11, 1976.)

transfusion, or by continuous subcutaneous infusion into the abdominal wall over 24 hours, at a rate of 0.67–1.83 ml/hour in physiologic saline. Six patients received infusion therapy.

Iron excretion after the two types of DF administration is compared in Figure 3. Subcutaneous infusion increased iron excretion by a mean of 101% in 9 patients. In all cases iron excretion was greater after infusion than after intramuscular injection, the mean difference being 128%. In both pretransfusion and posttransfusion studies, the increase in iron excretion with subcutaneous infusion was highly significant. The number of units transfused was correlated with total urinary iron excretion. Posttransfusion iron excretion was related more closely to serum ferritin levels and to the number of units transfused. Iron excretion was increased by a mean of 429% in 6 patients who had 1,500 mg DF infused subcutaneously, compared with an intramuscular dose of 750 mg in the same patients.

It is thought that DF acts by chelating iron from a continuously renewable labile iron pool inside cells. A slow-release parenteral preparation of DF may prove more convenient than use of a portable pump. Continuous administration of DF may be valuable in preventing and treating iron overload in anemic patients given regular blood transfusions. The effects of ascorbic acid and oral iron chelators in conjunction with continuous DF remain to be evaluated.

► [Propper and his colleagues (N. Engl. J. Med. 294:1421, 1976) demonstrated that a given dose of desferrioxamine (deferoxamine) was more effective at mobilizing iron when the dose was given by continuous intravenous infusion than by the intramuscular route. Now this article by the group from the Royal Free Hospital, London, and the preceding article by Propper et al. have established that chronic subcutaneous infusion is also effective at enhancing iron excretion. The amounts of iron excreted are in the range where the technique is likely to be therapeutically effective if carried out for a sufficient period. The approach is cumbersome, however, and the disadvantages of use of a continuous-infusion pump are obvious. Interestingly, none of the reports have noted complications of long-term treatment with this chelating agent derived from microbial sources. Surely some complications must exist.—Ed.] ◄

Molecular Lesion of Hereditary Spherocytosis (HS): Continuing Enigma is discussed by William N. Valentine[6] (Univ. of California, Los Angeles). The assumption that a genetic abnormality of the red blood cell membrane underlies HS has pervaded studies of its pathophysiology, but the ultimate molecular lesion remains unknown. Several abnormal properties have been found in HS red blood cells, including abnormal permeability to sodium and instability of HS membrane lipid under conditions of glucose deprivation. No specific abnormalities in membrane lipid structure have been demonstrated.

The failure of lipid-free proteins from HS membranes to increase in sedimentation on treatment with divalent cations has been attributed to an inability to form properly aggregates or microfilaments. The postulate that a protein kinase-mediated phosphorylation affects the state and function of microfilamentous, perhaps contractile membrane proteins is attractive. The protein kinase system in intact membranes is potentially one of great complexity, and it remains unclear whether one or more protein kinases play significant roles.

It is difficult to determine definitely whether differences between HS and normal membranes are due to a fundamental disturbance in the protein kinase system or are merely secondary to disturbed membrane relationships not fundamental to the system itself. Parallels between membrane phosphorylation and sphering and its attendant osmotic phenomena, whether induced by heating or by reagents that bind sulfhydryl groups, must be interpreted with great caution. The possibility of proteolytic attack on enzyme subunits in the membrane is always present and is difficult to evaluate. The specificity of observed decreases in membrane phosphorylating capacity in HS is challenged by a report of analogous, even more severe aberrations in cases of hemoglobin SS disease and by the reported occurrence of similar aberrations in hereditary stomatocytosis.

► [This is a brief but thorough and well-balanced overview of more than 4 decades of research into the nature of the primary defect in the hereditary spherocytosis erythrocyte. As Doctor Valentine points out, many of the studies have not been controlled adequately or have failed to distinguish between a primary and a secondary abnormality. The definition of the basic defect has remained elusive. — Ed.] ◄

(6) Blood 49:241–245, February, 1977.

Hematologic Malignancies

Target Cell in Chronic Myeloid Leukemia and Its Relationship to Acute Lymphoid Leukemia are discussed by George Janossy, Marion Roberts and Melvyn F. Greaves[7] (Univ. College, London). The findings that the Philadelphia (Ph′) chromosome is observed in granulocytic, erythroid, monocytic and megakaryocytic lines in chronic myeloid leukemia (CML) whereas phytohemagglutinin-stimulated lymphocytes are Ph′-negative have been interpreted as indicating that the potential diversity of two stem cell derivatives may be relatively restricted, one stem cell line giving rise to lymphocytes and the other to myeloid cells. Chronic myeloid leukemia is presumed to arise in a single myeloid stem cell which differentiates preferentially into granulocytes. Chronic myeloid leukemia, however, often progresses to an acute phase, with blast cells resembling those of acute lymphoblastic leukemia (ALL) in a minority of cases. Also, Ph′-positive ALL cases have been observed with no preceding chronic phase, and rare patients may convert from ALL into classic Ph′-positive CML.

Of 40 patients studied during an acute blast crisis of Ph′-positive leukemia, 18 had lymphoid leukemic cells at certain stages of the disease. In 15 cases, lymphoid leukemic blasts reacted with anti-ALL serum. This was a clinically heterogeneous group. Myeloid blast crisis developed in 22 patients. With one possible exception, cells from these patients did not react with anti-ALL serum.

Probably Ph′-positive blast crisis and the common Ph′-negative variety of ALL involve the same or closely related target cells. These target cells express the same membrane antigen irrespective of the precise etiology of the disease. The ALL antigen would then be a normal stem cell antigen or a determinant that is only expressed when the stem cell is "transformed." It appears that the target cell in some CML patients is the pluripotential stem cell. The character of blastic crisis phase cells is likely to be influenced by the target cell in which the original Ph′ defect arose. In blast crisis cases with a myeloid character and a long initial CML course, the Ph′ defect perhaps occurred in a relatively mature myeloid stem cell.

► [This group of sophisticated immunologists has attempted to develop antiserums to antigens specific to ALL cells or antigens specific to AML cells. They have failed to make a specific anti-AML antiserum. Their antiserum to ALL cells (of the null cell variety) probably reacts with antigens common to ALL and to normal prothymocytes. Utilizing this antiserum, they have constructed an elaborate hypothesis which basically concludes that some chronic myelocytic leukemias and some acute lymphoblastic leukemias originate in a common target cell that is possibly a pluripotent stem cell or close relative. The clinical implications of this hypothesis are summarized in the following article. – Ed.] ◄

(7) Lancet 2:1058–1061, Nov. 13, 1976.

Blast Crisis of Chronic Myeloid Leukemia (CML): II. Cell Surface Marker Analysis of Lymphoid and Myeloid Cases. The terminal stage of CML may take several forms. The most frequent is blastic transformation, which is highly variable at both the clinical and the morphological levels. The blast crisis has a lymphoid appearance in a minority of cases, and in a minority the blastic change appears to occur in extramedullary sites such as lymph nodes. G. Janossy, M. F. Greaves, T. Revesz, T. A. Lister, Marion Roberts, Jill Durrant, Barbara Kirk, D. Catovsky and M. E. J. Beard[8] analyzed the cell membrane characteristics of leukemic blasts in the acute blast crisis of CML. In addition to markers for thymocytes, T lymphocytes and B lymphocytes, rabbit antiserums to acute lymphoid leukemia (ALL) were used. Binding of antiserums to cell surface structures was studied by indirect immunofluorescence.

Fourteen cases were studied. In none of 4 lymphoid cases that presented in blast crisis did the blast cells show definite evidence of differentiation. Leukemic blast cells in all cases were negative in sheep erythrocyte rosette and surface Ig tests. In 6 of 8 lymphoid cases, blast cell populations reacted strongly with anti-ALL serum. Large proportions of lymphoid and myeloid blast cells were deficient in cholera toxin receptors. More than 90% of cholera toxin-positive cells belonged to the myeloid differentiation series. In 1 patient the blast cells were anti-ALL negative at presentation, but central nervous system leukemia subsequently developed with anti-ALL-positive blast cells in the cerebrospinal fluid.

There was good correlation between surface marker analyses and morphological data in this study. The findings suggest that the blastic phase of CML may involve different cellular derivatives of a pluripotential stem cell in which the primary malignant-genetic changes reside. The blast crisis of CML can be heterogeneous with respect to cellular expression and, in a significant proportion of patients, involves a cell indistinguishable by membrane markers and morphological criteria from that seen in the common form of ALL. The Philadelphia chromosome may be the only distinguishing cellular feature in these cases. The ALL antigen(s) can be expressed in diseases of differing etiology that involve a common target cell.

► [Cell surface membrane markers have helped in characterizing the origin of non-myeloid leukemias. A B cell origin is defined by the presence of one or more markers, including surface membrane immunoglobulin (smIg), receptors for complement bound to antibody-coated erythrocytes (EAC) and, in some cases, so-called Ia-like antigens (Humphreys, R. E., et al.: J. Exp. Med. 144:98, 1976). A T cell lineage is often defined by rosette formation with sheep erythrocytes (E rosettes) and T-specific antigens. On the other hand, the presence of receptors for cholera toxin probably correlates with granulocytic differentiation. The most frequent type of acute lymphoblastic leukemia lacks any of these markers and is often called non-B, non-T cell, or null cell leukemia. Greaves and his colleagues (Clin. Immunol. Immunopathol. 4:67, 1975) raised an antiserum in rabbits which they originally believed was specific for null leukemic lymphoblasts. It is now clear that this antiserum also reacts with primitive progenitors of normal lymphocytes (prothymocytes). Nevertheless, the antiserum is a useful reagent for identification of lymphoid origin of malignancy.

The present study confirms a number of previous observations. In a minority of

(8) Br. J. Haematol. 34:179–192, October, 1976.

cases of blastogenic transformation of CML, the emergent acute leukemic clone is lymphoid in origin. The cell surface markers are of use in analyzing the biology of malignant transformation, but in most cases morphology suffices to identify the lymphoid characteristics. It is likely that it is these lymphoblastic transformants that are most apt to show a therapeutic response to corticosteroids and vincristine (Canellos, G. P., et al.: Blood 38:671, 1971), whereas the more common transformation to an acute myeloid leukemia is generally unresponsive to therapy. Another clinically useful point is that occasional patients may present with "lymphoid" blast crisis. In such patients the origin of disease may be unclear until an analysis for the Ph^1 chromosome is performed. – Ed.] ◄

Terminal Deoxynucleotidyl Transferase Levels and Membrane Phenotypes in Diagnosis of Acute Leukemia were investigated by A. V. Hoffbrand, K. Ganeshaguru, G. Janossy, M. F. Greaves, D. Catovsky and R. K. Woodruff[9] (London). Terminal deoxynucleotidyl transferase (TDT) polymerizes a single-stranded deoxynucleotidyl sequence onto a primer without need of a template. Its level tends to be elevated in the cells of patients with acute lymphoblastic leukemia (ALL) but not in the cells of those with acute myeloblastic leukemia (AML). The TDT values were compared with immunologic phenotypes in 112 patients, including 40 with untreated ALL, 17 with untreated AML, 30 with Ph^1-positive chronic granulocytic leukemia (CGL), 17 with unclassified acute leukemia, 10 control subjects with nonleukemic hematologic disorders and hypercellular marrows and 10 hematologically normal adults.

The mean TDT activity in normal marrow samples was 0.13 unit/10^8 cells and that in hyperplastic, nonleukemic marrow samples, 0.67 units. Only values above 1.4 units were considered abnormal. The mean value in patients with active untreated ALL was 59 units/10^8 cells; 1 patient had a normal value. The enzyme level was normal in all but 1 of 8 patients with ALL in remission. All but 1 of the patients with AML had normal TDT levels in the marrow. In the group with CGL in blast transformation, TDT values clearly separated anti-ALL-serum-positive and serum-negative transformation. Results were variable in the group with unclassified acute leukemia.

The assay of TDT in peripheral blood or marrow of patients with acute leukemia is of value in differentiating lymphoid from myeloid leukemia. The correlation between TDT levels, membrane phenotypes and response to therapy in acute leukemias, especially acute undifferentiated leukemia, is under study.

► [The observation that in most cases of null cell ALL there are elevated levels of terminal transferase suggests that the cases are of prothymocyte or pre-T cell origin but have not developed surface phenotypic markers of T cells. – Ed.] ◄

Characteristics of Blast Crisis in Chronic Granulocytic Leukemia. Blast crisis is the major cause of death in chronic granulocytic leukemia (CGL) but the reasons for its occurrence are unknown. Susan Rosenthal, George P. Canellos, Vincent T. DeVita, Jr., and Harvey R. Gralnick[1] (Natl. Inst. of Health) analyzed the blastic phase of CGL in 44 male and 29 female patients followed during 1968–75 who received combination chemotherapy. Sixty-seven patients had marrow biopsies

(9) Lancet 2:520–523, Sept. 10, 1977.
(1) Blood 49:705–714, May, 1977.

Clinical Presentation of Blast Crisis

	Lymphoblastic (n = 21)		Myeloblastic (n = 46)		Total* (n = 73)	
	N	(%)	N	(%)	N	(%)
Fever	14	(67)	26	(57)	44	(60)
Musculoskeletal pain	9	(43)	26	(57)	39	(53)
Abdominal enlargement/pain	7	(33)	18	(39)	28	(38)
Malaise	10	(48)	34	(74)	48	(66)
Dyspnea, cough	10	(48)	15	(33)	28	(38)
Nausea, vomiting	10	(48)	23	(50)	34	(47)
Weight loss	4	(19)	15	(33)	21	(29)
Hemorrhage	3	(14)	9	(20)	13	(18)
Infection	1	(5)	5	(11)	6	(8)
Ankle edema	1	(5)	5	(11)	6	(8)
Hepatomegaly	7	(33)	29	(63)	38	(52)
Splenomegaly	14	(93)†	30	(88)†	47	(85)†
Adenopathy	1	(5)	2	(4)	4	(5)
Accelerated phase ‡	8	(38)	22	(48)	32	(44)

*Includes 6 patients for whom blast crisis bone marrow specimens were unavailable.
†Percent of those who had not been splenectomized.
‡A minimum of a 1-month period prior to blast crisis characterized by rising white blood cell count, anemia, thrombocytopenia, refractoriness to previous therapy or significant hypermetabolic symptoms.

or aspirations at the time of blast crisis. Marrow samples were obtained within 2 weeks before the initiation of blast crisis chemotherapy. The patients had a mean age at onset of the blast crisis of 43. Most were treated primarily with busulfan or dibromomannitol during the chronic phase. Most blast crises were treated with vincristine-prednisone or with cytosine arabinoside-6-thioguanine chemotherapy.

At onset of blast crisis, 21 patients had blast cells in the marrow that were indistinguishable from the lymphoblasts of acute lymphocytic leukemia (ALL), whereas 38 had cells indistinguishable from the myeloblasts of acute myelocytic leukemia (AML). Seven patients had an erythroblastic transformation. One patient had a unique blast type; its morphology was most consistent with a histocytic cell line. The clinical features present at the time of blast crisis are summarized in the table. Percentage of blasts in marrow equaled or exceeded the percentage in the peripheral blood in about two thirds of cases. More myeloblastic than lymphoblastic patients had various peripheral blood abnormalities. Marrow hypercellularity was the rule, except in patients with extensive marrow fibrosis. The lymphoblastic patients almost all had reduced or absent megakaryocytes. About a third of patients had extramedullary leukemia. Six patients died of complications of blast crisis chemotherapy; 2 patients had second malignancies.

Death in blast crisis is caused primarily by infection and hemorrhage. Similar outcomes are seen in AML and ALL. Blast crisis in a patient with previously diagnosed CGL should be defined as 30% or more blast forms in either peripheral blood or bone marrow. Patients who have either an extramedullary myeloblastic tumor or a major new aneuploid cell line in the marrow are at a very high risk of imminent blastic transformation. Many patients with marked leukocytosis and progressive granulocytic immaturity, accompanied by transfusion-dependent anemia and thrombocytopenia, have fewer than 30% blasts but require intensive treatment. They may be considered to be in an accelerated phase of CGL but not necessarily in blast crisis.

► [This is a good summary of the hematologic and clinical manifestations of blast crisis in CGL. The varied cell lines of the blast cells include myeloid, erythroid, monocytic and lymphoid. This observation supports the recent concept that the clonal evolution of CGL may involve any of the primitive hematopoietic stem cells (see the three preceding articles). – Ed.] ◄

Mediastinal Irradiation for Chronic Lymphocytic Leukemia. Arthur Sawitsky, Kanti R. Rai, Isamettin Aral, Richard T. Silver, Arvin S. Glicksman, Robert W. Carey, Salvatore Scialla, C. J. Cornell, Jr., Barbara Seligman and Lorne Shapiro[2] (New Hyde Park, N.Y.) evaluated mediastinal irradiation in 31 patients with chronic lymphocytic leukemia who manifested active or progressive disease. Megavoltage irradiation was used in all cases.

Complete remission was not achieved in any patient, but 52% of the patients had partial remission or clinical improvement. All responses were short. Patients with stage I or II disease had a response rate of 73% and those with stage III or IV disease, a rate of 37%. The response rate was 77% for patients given a total dose of more than 3,000 rad and 45% for those given lower doses. Severe life-threatening toxicity was found in 11 patients. More severe toxicity occurred in patients with stage IV disease (thrombocytopenia). Two of 5 patients not previously treated had life-threatening toxicity. Seven patients (22.5%) had treatment-associated deaths. None of these patients had previously received radiotherapy. Two patients had radiation pneumonitis, and 1 of them died. Two patients died in complete bone marrow aplasia. Six patients had thrombocytopenia, 4 had anemia, 4 had leukopenia and 5 had a life-threatening infection. The severity of reactions and death were not correlated with the total dose of radiation or the dose per week.

The high incidence of severe toxicity and treatment-associated deaths in patients with chronic lymphocytic leukemia who are given mediastinal irradiation suggests caution should be exercised in selecting such patients for this type of treatment. This is particularly true for patients who are anemic or thrombocytopenic and those who have had previous chemotherapy.

► [The present study was based on an earlier report by Richards et al. (Am. J. Med. 57: 862, 1974) that thymic irradiation produced a partial or total response in 21 of 22 patients with chronic lymphocytic leukemia. The presently reported collaborative investigation by Doctor Sawitsky and his colleagues fails to confirm the optimistic earlier results. Mediastinal irradiation appears to be sufficiently hazardous for this group of patients that its use should be strictly curtailed. – Ed.] ◄

Splenectomy in Chronic Lymphocytic Leukemia. The favorable effects of splenectomy in selected cases of chronic lymphocytic leukemia (CLL) have long been known but the procedure does not seem to have been generally adopted in the treatment of patients with predominant splenomegaly, possibly because its long-term consequences are not entirely known. B. Egelund Christensen, M. Mørk Hansen and Aa.

(2) Am. J. Med. 61:892–896, December, 1976.

Videbaek[3] (Copenhagen) reviewed the effects of splenectomy in 42 patients having operations in the past 20 years. Seven of the 22 men and 20 women were over age 70. The spleen weighed over 1,000 gm in most patients. The main indication for splenectomy was anemia, but in 9 patients it was thrombocytopenia and in 14, hypercatabolism. In addition, data on 37 nonsplenectomized patients with CLL and appreciable splenomegaly who were treated in 1954–63 were also reviewed.

A marked increase in hemoglobin level was found 3 months after splenectomy, with constant levels at least during the 1st postoperative year. Platelet counts showed a prompt increase and the lymphocyte count usually increased. The need for corticosteroids was reduced after splenectomy. The basal metabolic rate usually declined after splenectomy in the 7 patients studied. Fewer patients had elevated serum uric acid levels after splenectomy. No systematic changes in serum γ-globulin or protein levels were recorded after splenectomy. No change in the tendency to infection was evident. No patient died in direct connection with splenectomy but 1 died 7½ weeks postoperatively of pulmonary embolism and bronchopneumonia. Eleven patients had definite infections postoperatively, but these were usually easy to control.

Spontaneous remission of marked splenomegaly was not observed in the control group. The effect of irradiation was modest and only 2 patients obtained a sustained effect on spleen size from irradiation of the spleen. Prednisone therapy decreased spleen size and produced a partial remission in 2 patients. The median survival time was 30 months, compared with 54 months for the splenectomized group.

Splenectomy should be done at an early stage in cases of CLL complicated by splenomegaly, at least before the spleen weight greatly exceeds 1,000 gm. Splenectomy appears to be superior to other methods of treatment in selected cases and should be done far more often and earlier than has been recommended.

► [This report summarizes a large experience with splenectomy in patients with CLL. It confirms one's impression that splenectomy may be beneficial, and occasionally dramatically successful, in alleviating severe hemolytic anemia or thrombocytopenia in affected patients. In contrast, splenic irradiation is rarely helpful. Usually splenectomy is an act of desperation performed relatively late in the disease when other measures have failed. The authors argue that the operation should be performed early rather than late in patients with prominent splenomegaly. They do acknowledge, however, that if splenectomy is to have a rational place in the treatment of CLL, chronologically and in relation to other treatment modalities, then a prospective, randomized study must be performed. – Ed.] ◄

Immunoglobulin Synthesis in Hairy Cell Leukemia. The weight of evidence suggests that hairy cell leukemia is a B-lymphocyte malignancy, but some studies have indicated that the hairy cell is derived from the monocytic line. David W. Golde, Ronald H. Stevens, Shirley G. Quan and Andrew Saxon[4] (Univ. of California, Los Angeles) performed in vitro studies with leukemic cells from 2 patients with hairy cell leukemia. One (patient A) was a man aged 60 with a history of monoclonal gammopathy for 17 years before presenting with spleno-

(3) Scand. J. Haematol. 18:279–287, April, 1977.
(4) Br. J. Haematol. 35:359–365, March, 1977.

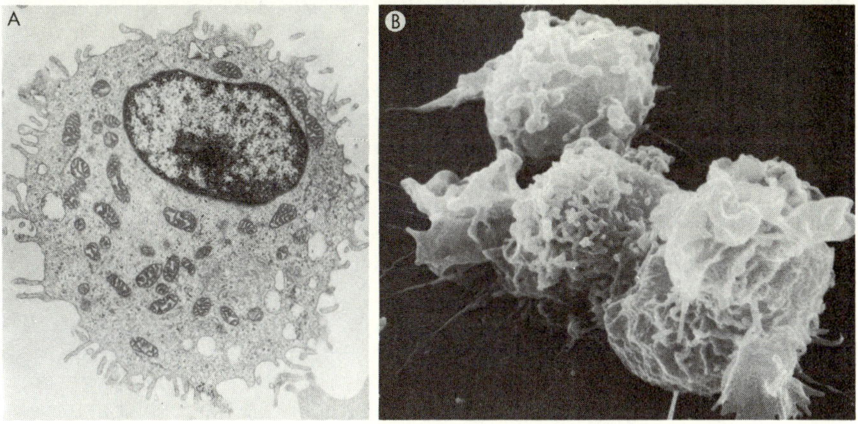

Fig 4.—In patient B, transmission electron micrograph (**A**) of peripheral blood leukocyte shows numerous small microvilli, many mitochondria and extensive rough endoplasmic reticulum in cytoplasm; reduced from ×16,800. **B,** scanning electron micrograph shows ruffles and microvilli; reduced from ×4,480. (Courtesy of Golde, D. W., et al.: Br. J. Haematol. 35:359–365, March, 1977.)

megaly and circulating hairy cells. The other (patient B) was an asymptomatic man aged 50, found to have splenomegaly on routine examination. Elective splenectomy was performed in this case.

The neoplastic cells from both patients stained prominently for tartrate-resistant acid phosphatase and contained a "dot" of α-naphthyl butyrase activity in the Golgi area that was fluoride resistant. The cells were ultrastructurally consistent with lymphocytes (Figs 4 and 5).

Fig 5.—In patient A, scanning electron micrograph (**A**) shows microvilli; reduced from ×10,000. **B,** immunofluorescence shows capping of membrane IgM, with the use of class-specific goat anti-human IgM; reduced from ×360. (Courtesy of Golde, D. W., et al.: Br. J. Haematol. 35:359–365, March 1977.)

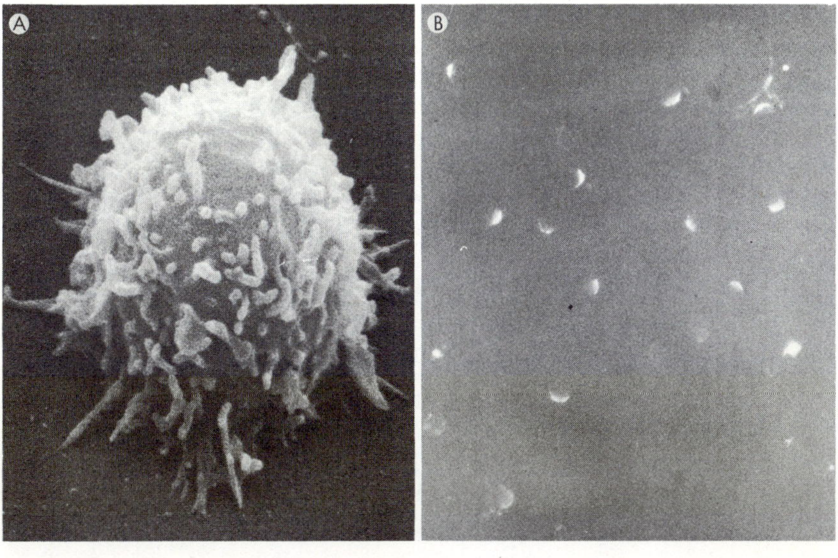

Fresh cells from both patients stained prominently for membrane immunoglobulin, and cytoplasmic fluorescence was easily detected in patient A. These cells stained for surface IgM and IgD, whereas IgM was found cytoplasmically. Patient B's peripheral blood and spleen cells stained for IgG only. Established cell cultures grew as typical B cell lymphoblastoid lines. The cell line derived from patient B contained, in addition to 17% weakly IgG cytoplasmic staining cells, a few cells that reacted with IgM or IgA with the appearance of mature plasma cells. Fresh peripheral blood cells from patient A synthesized only immunoglobulin of the IgM class in vitro, whereas patient B's cells synthesized only IgG.

The hairy leukemic cells from these 2 patients are dissimilar, existing at different levels of maturity along the continuum of B cell development with regard to immunoglobulin production and secretion. The findings unequivocally demonstrate the B-lymphocyte nature of the hairy cells in these patients. There is also good evidence for a clonal origin of the leukemia.

► [This study and a number of other recent reports strongly suggest that hairy cell leukemia (leukemia reticuloendotheliosis) is lymphoid in origin rather than monocytic, as originally believed. It would be reasonable to conclude from this report that the disease is a monoclonal B lymphocyte disorder; however, the situation appears to be more complex than this. These same investigators have recently described another case of hairy cell leukemia of T lymphocyte origin (Golde et al.: Ann. Intern. Med., in press, 1978). Both the B and T cell variants have the distinctive tartrate-resistant acid phosphatase in the hairy cells. The physiologic significance of this specific isozyme in a subpopulation of lymphoid cells is presently uncertain. It is likely that hairy cell leukemia encompasses several neoplastic disorders with common clinical features. – Ed.]

Hairy Cell Leukemia: B Lymphocyte and Phagocytic Properties. Hairy cell leukemia is considered to be a rare type of chronic leukemia in which a high proportion of the abnormal cells have a characteristic ribosome-lamella complex rarely seen in other human tumors. Peter D. Utsinger, William J. Yount, C. Randall Fuller, Marshall J. Logue and Eugene P. Orringer[5] (Univ. of North Carolina) studied the neoplastic cells of 3 men with hairy cell leukemia. All had splenomegaly, fever and no adenopathy. Two were pancytopenic.

Peripheral blood smears from all 3 patients showed large mononuclear cells with slender, hairlike cytoplasmic projections. Tartrate-resistant acid phosphatase isoenzyme was demonstrated in the cells. Over 75% of mononuclear cells were hairy cells in each case. A large proportion of the hairy cells stained strongly for IgM and IgD in all 3 cases. There was minimal or no staining with antiserums to IgA and IgG. Trypsinization studies gave further evidence that the immunoglobulin present on the cell surfaces was produced by the cells. Minimal incorporation of tritiated thymidine by the mononuclear cell populations after stimulation by phytohemagglutinin was observed, and DNA analyses excluded abnormal thymidine transport. A similar impairment in blastic transformation was found when the mononuclear cells were reconstituted with allogeneic monocytes. Dilution of T lymphocytes by the proliferating neoplastic cells was not responsible for the impaired phytohemagglutinin response.

(5) Blood 49:19–27, January, 1977.

These patients exemplified the key clinical features of hairy cell leukemia. Strong evidence for B cell characteristics of the neoplastic cells was obtained. In some patients with hairy cell leukemia a malignant proliferation of monocyte-histiocyte-like cells is documented, whereas in others there is a proliferation of B lymphocyte-like cells. Alternatively, hairy cell leukemia may involve malignant proliferation of a hypothetical subpopulation of B lymphocytes with phagocytic potential. The prognosis of hairy cell leukemia is generally very good, which suggests the cell type involved may represent a malignancy of a more differentiated, minor subpopulation of B lymphocytes.

► [Since the early descriptions of hairy cell leukemia (Bouroncle et al.: Blood 13:609, 1958), uncertainty has existed about the line of origin of these neoplastic cells. Because of their phagocytic activity, an origin in the monocyte-macrophage system has been considered. More recently, clear examples of B cell and T cell hairy cell leukemia have been described (Golde, D. W., et al.: N. Engl. J. Med. 296:92, 1977). Some of these show moderate phagocytic activity.

The occurrence of hairy cell leukemia is probably more common than previously has been appreciated. Most large hematologic practices have a few patients with this disorder masquerading as atypical chronic lymphocytic leukemia. The usual atypical features are prominent splenomegaly without commensurate lymphadenopathy and a bone marrow that is packed with cells and difficult to aspirate. The correct diagnosis usually is established by staining for tartrate-resistant acid phosphatase and identification of isozyme 5 of acid phosphatase. The distinction between hairy cell leukemia and chronic lymphocytic leukemia is important because of the differences in prognosis and management. Splenectomy is often effective therapy in hairy cell leukemia (Catovsky et al.: Br. J. Haematol. 26:9, 1974). – Ed.] ◄

Acute Nonlymphocytic Leukemia: A Delayed Complication of Hodgkin's Disease Therapy – Analysis of 109 Cases. Acute nonlymphocytic leukemia has been seen after successful treatment of Hodgkin's disease, and there is concern that it is caused by the multimodal therapy that has been responsible for the dramatic increase in survival of patients with Hodgkin's disease.

E. C. Cadman, R. L. Capizzi and J. R. Bertino[6] (Yale Univ.) present a critical analysis of 4 cases seen at the Yale-New Haven Medical Center and 105 cases reported in the world literature through early 1976. Cases in which leukemia was diagnosed within 6 months of diagnosis of Hodgkin's disease were considered to be simultaneous occurrences. Both clinical features and treatment were evaluable in 69 cases. There were 36 female patients with a median age of 26 years and 28 male patients with a median age of 37 years; age was not given for 13 patients. The clinical stage and histology of Hodgkin's disease were similar to those usually noted. Eleven patients were in complete remission of Hodgkin's disease.

Cytopenia was a characteristic finding and was present a median of 3 months before the diagnosis of leukemia. Abnormal red blood cell precursors were noted in 14 of 31 patients having marrow examination. All 17 cytogenetic studies of bone marrow gave abnormal results.

The leukemia was refractory to treatment. Only 5 of 77 patients (6.5%) had remission on antileukemic therapy. The median survival after diagnosis of leukemia was 1 month, but 3 patients with partial remission survived for 5–13 months, and 1 patient with a complete

(6) Cancer 40:1280–1296, September, 1977.

remission lived 18 months. Four patients received only aggressive combination chemotherapy before development of acute nonlymphocytic leukemia. Fourteen received chemotherapy followed by radiotherapy; the median interval to diagnosis of leukemia was 5 years. Onset of leukemia after diagnosis of Hodgkin's disease was significantly sooner in patients given radiotherapy alone than in those given radiotherapy followed by chemotherapy. Eleven patients received only MOPP (nitrogen mustard, vincristine, prednisone and procarbazine) before or after total nodal irradiation. Aggressively treated patients had an interval to diagnosis of leukemia about half that of less aggressively treated patients.

The incidence of reported acute nonlymphocytic leukemia in patients with Hodgkin's disease is increasing at present. The leukemia appears to be a distinct clinicopathologic entity, characterized by pancytopenia, megablastoid marrow, nucleated red cells in the peripheral blood, random chromosomal aberrations in the bone marrow and refractoriness to antileukemic therapy with a very short survival.

► [It now looks as if the incidence of acute leukemia in aggressively treated patients with Hodgkin's disease will exceed 1–2%. The leukemias are almost always refractory to treatment.—Ed.] ◄

Prolonged Maintained Remissions of Adult Acute Nonlymphocytic Leukemia. Complete remissions can now be obtained with intensive induction chemotherapy in most adults with acute nonlymphocytic leukemia (ANLL) but the median duration of remission has rarely exceeded a year. Bruce A. Peterson and Clara D. Bloomfield[7] (Univ. of Minnesota) describe a simple outpatient maintenance regimen that has resulted in a median duration of complete remission of 16.5 months. Twenty-four of 40 adults with ANLL achieved complete remission and were placed on maintenance therapy with 6-thioguanine and cytosine arabinoside. The median patient age was 44.5; 1 patient was over age 70. Maintenance therapy consisted of 2 mg 6-thioguanine per kg orally on 4 successive days, followed by 1.5 mg cytosine arabinoside per kg intramuscularly on the 5th day.

The median duration of complete remission was 16.5 months, with a range of 3–56+ months; 9 patients (38%) remain in complete remission. Eight patients have been in complete remission for over 2 years and 5 for 3 years. The 6 patients over age 60 have a median duration of complete remission of 18 months. Patients whose remissions lasted less than a year had higher initial leukocyte and myeloblast counts than the others. Patients received a median of 90% of their full calculated dose of cytosine arabinoside and 68% of their dose of 6-thioguanine. Over half the patients had hepatic enzyme or bilirubin abnormalities. Maintenance therapy rarely was changed because of leukopenia or thrombocytopenia. Six of 14 patients given reinduction chemotherapy for relapse achieved a second complete remission. The current median survival of the 24 patients is 22.5 months. Eleven patients remain alive, 9 in their original complete remission and 2 in a second

(7) Lancet 2:158–160, July 23, 1977.

remission. One patient died after 17 months in remission with no autopsy evidence of leukemia.

Over half the patients in this series achieved complete remission. Home treatment with a simple weekly cycle of cytosine arabinoside and 6-thioguanine is effective maintenance chemotherapy in adults with ANLL. The regimen is well tolerated and easily administered on an outpatient basis.

► [This program sounds simple enough. Hopefully other studies will confirm its efficacy.—Ed.] ◄

One Hundred Patients with Acute Leukemia Treated by Chemotherapy, Total Body Irradiation and Allogeneic Marrow Transplantation. E. Donnall Thomas, C. Dean Buckner, Meera Banaji, Reginald A. Clift, Alexander Fefer, Nancy Flournoy, Brian W. Goodell, Robert O. Hickman, Kenneth G. Lerner, Paul E. Neiman, George E. Sale, Jean E. Sanders, Jack Singer, Mary Stevens, Rainer Storb and Paul L. Weiden[8] (Univ. of Washington, Seattle) performed bone marrow transplantation in 54 patients with acute myelogenous leukemia (AML) and 46 with acute lymphoblastic leukemia (ALL). The 100 patients were considered to be in the end stages of disease after combination chemotherapy. Grafts from HLA-identical siblings were given after total body irradiation. Cyclophosphamide was given to 43 patients, additional chemotherapy to 31 and BCNU as well as cyclophosphamide to 19. Seven patients received other chemotherapy regimens before total body irradiation. The median dose of bone marrow cells infused was 2.8×10^8/kg.

Six patients died 3–17 days after bone marrow infusion without evidence of engraftment, whereas 94 had engraftment documented. Seventeen patients are alive. No deaths have occurred at 2–4½ years, but 4 of the 17 living patients have had a relapse of leukemia. Survival was similar in the groups with ALL and AML. Three of the 13 living, disease-free patients have chronic graft-vs.-host disease that significantly compromises their activity. The condition of patients at the time of transplantation affected their survival. No significant differences related to the preparative regimen were observed. Half the patients in the series acquired moderate to severe graft-vs.-host disease. Interstitial pneumonia was the primary cause of 34 deaths. Thirty-one patients had a relapse of leukemia; relapse was not definitely related to graft-vs.-host disease.

Bone marrow transplantation should now be undertaken earlier in the management of patients with acute leukemia who have an HLA-matched sibling bone marrow donor. Protocols comparing the therapeutic efficacy of bone marrow transplantation with chemotherapy in patients without matched siblings should help determine the true value of bone marrow transplantation in the treatment of leukemia.

► [In this study, 13 of 100 patients receiving bone marrow transplantation for end-stage leukemia are alive and apparently free of disease 2–4½ years later. This 13% figure is roughly comparable to that achieved in other large transplantation series. Although the figure seems discouragingly low, it is clearly superior to that observed in a

(8) Blood 49:511–533, April, 1977.

comparable group of patients managed by conventional (i.e., nontransplantation) methods (Gale et al.: Lancet 2:1197, 1977).

A major cause of treatment failure in this series was recurrent leukemia despite high-dose cyclophosphamide and lethal total body irradiation (TBI). This observation had led to trials of either more intensive antileukemic "conditioning" programs (e.g., Sarna et al.: Ann. Intern. Med. 86:155, 1977) or to the use of cyclophosphamide plus TBI very early in the treatment of leukemia before drug resistance has emerged. The latter approach apparently has failed in acute lymphoblastic leukemia but may be useful in acute myeloid leukemia.

Interstitial pneumonitis is another cause of transplant failure. Cytomegalovirus infection has been implicated as a major cause of this syndrome. Trials of prophylaxis against cytomegalovirus are now in progress. – Ed.] ◄

Lymphoma and Myeloma

Monoclonality of Human B Cell Lymphomas. Restrictions on differentiated lymphoid cells in their potential for immunoglobulin expression are somewhat more relaxed than was previously believed. In Ig-producing lymphoid tumors, leukemic cells produce immunoglobulin of different heavy chain classes; however, Ig products of the same clone all contain a single light chain of either κ or λ type. Ronald Levy, Roger Warnke, Ronald F. Dorfman and Joseph Haimovich[9] performed immunofluorescent staining studies of lymphoma cells in tissue sections to investigate the clonality of human lymphomas in situ. Human lymphoma tissues were examined in frozen sections for Ig-bearing cells by a technique that involved double-label immunofluorescence with mixed anti-κ and anti-λ antibodies. F(ab′) 2 fragments of purified antibodies were used to avoid binding via Fc receptors.

A human B lymphoblastoid cell line stained exclusively for κ, whereas a T lymphoblastoid line stained for neither. Blood cells from a patient with acute lymphoblastic leukemia were uniformly negative for immunoglobulin. Thirteen of 14 patients with chronic lymphocytic leukemia (CLL) showed a monoclonal staining pattern; 8 were κ and 5, λ. One case was negative for Ig. Cells from 3 patients with lymphosarcoma cell leukemia and from 1 with hairy cell leukemia gave monoclonal Ig staining. Exclusive κ staining was observed in a node from a patient with well-differentiated lymphocytic lymphoma. Cells staining only for λ were found in a case of hairy cell leukemia. A polyclonal staining pattern was found in 2 cases of Hodgkin's disease and 1 of angioimmunoblastic lymphadenopathy.

About 10 – 20% of lymphoma patients have what appear to be two different histologic types of lymphoma that occur simultaneously in different sites. The B cell lymphomas are composed of monoclonal populations of Ig-bearing cells, whereas normal or reactive lymphoid follicles contain a mosaic of Ig-bearing cells derived from multiple clones. Nodules of lymphoma are often surrounded by normal polyclonal B cell populations. This approach should provide a sensitive and reliable tool for investigating the immunobiology of human lymphoma.

► [Some lymphoproliferative disorders are characterized by the production, but rarely the secretion, of immunoglobulin. These include CLL, lymphosarcoma cell leukemia, well-differentiated lymphocytic lymphoma, hairy cell leukemia, nodular poorly differentiated lymphocytic lymphoma and some cases of histiocytic lymphoma. All these tumors appear to be monoclonal in origin, i.e., to arise from a single cell. This concept is based, as in the present report, on the occurrence of a single type of immunoglobulin light chain. Interestingly, all the CLL cells from a single patient have the same type of light chain on their surface but may have two types of immunoglobulins – IgM and

(9) J. Exp. Med. 145:1014 – 1028, April, 1977.

IgD. The heavy chains of these two immunoglobulins will then have identical variable regions and different constant regions.

The polyclonal staining observed in 2 patients with Hodgkin's disease suggests that this is not a monoclonal B cell neoplasm. – Ed.] ◄

Treatment Results of 54 American Patients with Burkitt's Lymphoma Are Similar to the African Experience. Burkitt's lymphoma in Africa may be curable by chemotherapy alone, but results are reportedly less favorable in nonendemic regions. John L. Ziegler[1] (Natl. Inst. of Health) reviewed the results of two sequential trials with combined treatment protocols incorporating treatment approaches from clinical trials in Africa in 54 Americans with Burkitt's lymphoma. Both regimens included cyclophosphamide, vincristine and methotrexate, both intrathecal and intravenous, and one also included prednisolone.

Four patients died during induction therapy. Of the other 50 patients, 48 achieved complete remissions. Twenty-two patients relapsed a median of 3 months after the start of therapy. The overall 2-year actuarial survival was 54%. Patients under age 12 and those with a minimal tumor burden had better survivals than older patients and those with advanced abdominal tumors. No survival differences were apparent between patients treated with the two protocols. Hematologic toxicity from both regimens was predictable and manageable. Toxicity from whole abdominal irradiation was troublesome in nearly all cases. Cerebrospinal fluid relapse was noted in 11 patients, 6 of whom had meningeal involvement and 4, widespread bone marrow relapse. Only 2 of 26 patients who remained in complete remission at 6 months or longer after induction therapy received maintenance chemotherapy. The quality of life for 24 patients with remissions who are not receiving maintenance chemotherapy is excellent.

It is not possible at present to conclude that combination chemotherapy has a distinct advantage over cyclophosphamide alone in Burkitt's lymphoma. Early surgical removal of tumor bulk and large doses of chemotherapy with marrow autografting may prove useful in older patients and those with advanced disease. The use of maintenance chemotherapy with intensification courses during the time of relapse risk remains to be evaluated. Further study of the immunologic aspects of Burkitt's lymphoma may reveal an immunotherapeutic approach that can be rationally targeted at the appropriate lesion.

► [This study concludes that complete response rates, relapse frequency and survival in American patients with Burkitt's lymphoma are similar to the results in African patients. In Africa a 95% complete response rate and a 60% relapse rate is observed (Ziegler: Cancer 30:1534, 1972).

Whole abdominal irradiation is not well tolerated and its therapeutic utility has not been well established by the available data.

This study does identify subgroups of patients who are likely to respond to aggressive combination chemotherapy. – Ed.] ◄

Survival of Patients with Localized Histiocytic Lymphoma. J. D. Bitran, J. Kinzie, D. L. Sweet, D. Variakojis, M. L. Griem, H. M. Golomb, J. B. Miller, Nina Oetzel and J. E. Ultmann[2] (Univ. of Chica-

(1) N. Engl. J. Med. 297:75–80, July 14, 1977.

(2) Cancer 39:342–346, January, 1977.

go) attempted to determine w'.ether pathologic staging is of clinical importance for treatment decisions in patients with diffuse histiocytic lymphoma (DHL) and whether their survival is affected by the procedure. Review was made of the data on 65 patients with DHL who had pathologic staging in 1969–75. All patients were initially untreated. Ten were over age 65 years, and 2 were poor risks for staging laparotomy. Staging laparotomy and biopsy of any suspicious extrathoracic, supradiaphragmatic nodes were done in 28 cases in which stage IV disease could not otherwise be established. Open bone biopsy, multiple liver biopsies and splenectomy were carried out. Twenty patients received radiotherapy as primary treatment.

Of 42 sites of nodal involvement with disease, 29 were in the head, neck and thorax. All but 1 of 20 patients had complete responses to radiotherapy; none had a partial response. Radiotherapy was given to patients classed as having pathologic stage I, IE, II and IIE disease. The cumulative survival at 5 years was 71%. Three patients (15%) died of the disease and 1 of radiation pneumonitis and superimposed bacterial pneumonia. All relapses occurred within 4 months after the completion of radiotherapy. Relapses and deaths occurred in patients having stage II disease with more than 4 sites of involvement. Relapses were outside the initial radiotherapy ports in 2 of 3 cases.

The relatively high relapse-free survival rate of 78% in this series can be ascribed to the use of accurate pathologic staging to define patients with potentially curable disease. Failure to assess the stage of disease accurately does not, however, explain all relapses in DHL. Localized DHL may be treated with involved- or extended-field radiation. Patients with fewer than 3 sites of involvement have been cured by radiotherapy. When relapse occurs in DHL, chemotherapy should be instituted. A regimen of cyclophosphamide, vincristine, methotrexate with leukovorin rescue, and cytosine arabinoside is recommended.

► [In this series, survival rate and relapse-free survival at 4 years were, respectively, 71% and 78% in patients with limited disease. These excellent results favor radiation therapy as the single modality of treatment if pathologic staging is accurate and disease is stage I or stage II with ≤3 sites involved. Unfortunately the series is not large enough to evaluate how extensive the radiation therapy should be. Johnson et al. have also suggested that localized diffuse histiocytic lymphoma should be treated with involved- or extended-field radiotherapy (Br. J. Cancer 31 (Suppl. 2):237, 1975). – Ed.] ◄

Combination Chemotherapy of Advanced Non-Hodgkin's Lymphoma with Bleomycin, Adriamycin, Cyclophosphamide, Vincristine and Prednisone (BACOP). Combination chemotherapy is superior to single-agent therapy in the treatment of advanced non-Hodgkin's lymphoma (NHL). Arthur T. Skarin, David S. Rosenthal, William C. Moloney and Emil Frei, III[3] (Boston) evaluated BACOP chemotherapy in 73 patients with advanced NHL seen in 1973–75. Response and survival data were available in 63 cases. The treatment regimen is outlined in Figure 6. A 7-week, remission-induction period was followed by a consolidation phase for a total of 28 weeks of treatment. Patients with a complete remission or a stable partial remission were maintained on 2 mg cyclophosphamide per kg daily until relapse.

(3) Blood 49:759–770, May, 1977.

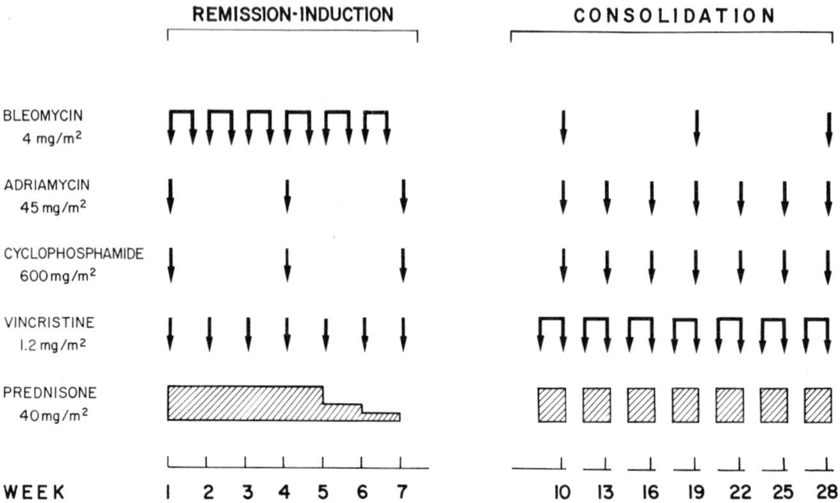

Fig 6.—Diagram of BACOP schema for advanced NHL. Maintenance therapy consisted of cyclophosphamide, 2 mg/kg/day orally. (Courtesy of Skarin, A. T., et al.: Blood 49:759–770, May, 1977.)

The objective response rate in 44 patients with diffuse histology was 86%, with 66% achieving a complete remission. In nodular lymphomas the complete remission rate was 89%. The median time to complete remission was 6 weeks. Partial responses occurred in 1 patient with nodular histology and in 9 with diffuse histology. Five of 6 patients with diffuse histology who had no response had diffuse histiocytic lymphoma. A projected 75% of patients with nodular lymphoma remained in complete remission at 14 months, with a median follow-up of 17 months. The projected median duration of complete remission in patients with diffuse histology was 14 months. The median survival of patients with nodular histology will exceed 25 months, and that of patients with diffuse histology is 14 months, with projected survival beyond 20 months in 42% of patients.

Toxicity included 1 case of heart failure attributed to Adriamycin, 10 cases of reversible peripheral neuropathy and 2 cases of cyclophosphamide-induced hemorrhagic cystitis. Pulmonary infiltrates attributed to bleomycin toxicity occurred in 8 patients. Two patients had fatal bacterial infection during periods of drug-induced pancytopenia. Eleven of 37 complete remitters relapsed. Eleven patients acquired lymphoma of the central nervous system.

Therapy with BACOP has resulted in a higher rate of complete remission and longer survival than a previous three-drug regimen, COP, particularly in patients with diffuse histology. Interposition of methotrexate may overcome the problem of high proliferative thrust between treatment courses. Central nervous system involvement may be controlled by intermittent methotrexate and the use of dexamethasone instead of prednisone. Inadequate cytoreduction may be overcome by increasing the doses of cyclophosphamide and Adriamycin and by adding methotrexate-citrovorum factor. Fatal complications should be reduced by deleting continuous prednisone and frequent doses of bleomycin.

► [The combination BACOP is superior to COP (cyclophosphamide-Oncovin-prednisone) in remission-induction in advanced non-Hodgkin's lymphoma of diffuse histology and it is marginally superior in lymphoma of nodular histology. Not all groups have achieved the extremely high complete remission rates in diffuse lymphoma with BACOP reported in this study (see Schein et al.: Proc. Am. Assoc. Cancer Res. 16:248, 1975). I am not convinced that BACOP is superior to CHOP (cyclophosphamide-Adriamycin-Oncovin-prednisone) in this patient group. I find CHOP easier to use with less toxicity. Bleomycin is simply too toxic – 11% of patients in this series had significant toxic manifestations.

Central nervous system involvement in advanced lymphoma is emerging as an important problem. Possible therapeutic approaches include high-dose methotrexate with citrovorum rescue or central nervous system irradiation combined with intrathecal therapy. The investigators in this group have recently modified BACOP by reducing the rate of bleomycin administration, decreasing the total duration of prednisone therapy and inserting high-dose methotrexate with rescue. – Ed.] ◄

Combination Chemotherapy ("CHOP-Bleo") in Advanced (Non-Hodgkin's) Malignant Lymphoma. Combination chemotherapy of the non-Hodgkin's lymphomas has been shown to be superior to single-drug therapy, and new agents have recently become available. Victorio Rodriguez, Fernando Cabanillas, Michael A. Burgess, Eugene M. McKelvey, Manuel Valdivieso, Gerald P. Bodey and Emil J Freireich[4] (M. D. Anderson Hosp. and Tumor Inst.) combined cyclophosphamide, Adriamycin, vincristine and prednisone (CHOP) with bleomycin in the treatment of 25 men and 22 women seen in 1973 – 75

TABLE 1. – CHOP-BLEO REGIMEN

Drugs	Dosage and Schedule
Cyclophosphamide*	750 mg/sq m/day, day 1, i.v.
Hydroxyldaunorubicin (Adriamycin)*	50 mg/sq m/day, day 1, i.v.
Oncovin (vincristine)	2 mg/day, days 1 and 5, i.v.
Prednisone	100 mg/day, days 1–5, p.o.
Bleomycin†	15 units/day, days 1+5, i.v.

*Starting dose to be reduced by 20% for patients with prior extensive radiotherapy or hypocellular bone marrow (<20%).
†Dose to be reduced to 4 units/sq m on days 1 and 5 for patients older than age 60.

TABLE 2. – RESPONSE TO CHOP-BLEO

Type	No.	Complete Response	Partial Response	Failure
DH*	26	18 (69)†	5 (19)	3 (12)
NPDL	13	8 (62)	5 (38)	—
DPDL	3	2 (67)	1 (33)	—
NM	3	2 (67)	1 (33)	—
UNDIFF	2	1 (50)	—	1 (50)
Total	47	31 (66)	12 (26)	4 (8)

*Abbreviations: DH, diffuse histiocytic; NPDL, nodular poorly differentiated, lymphocytic; DPDL, diffuse poorly differentiated, lymphocytic; NM, nodular mixed; UNDIFF, undifferentiated.
†Numbers in parentheses indicate percentages.

(4) Blood 49:325 – 333, March, 1977.

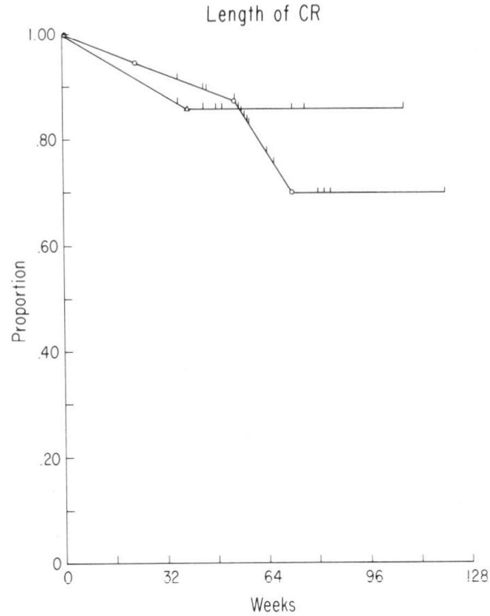

Fig 7.—Duration of complete remission *(CR)* in patients with diffuse histiocytic malignant lymphoma *(circles)* and nodular poorly differentiated lymphocytic lymphoma *(triangles)*. Total remission occurred in 18 and 8, respectively, and relapse in 3 and 1, respectively. (Courtesy of Rodriguez, V., et al.: Blood 49:325–333, March, 1977.)

with advanced malignant lymphoma. Median patient age was 56 years. Most had stage IV disease.

The regimen is outlined in Table 1. Courses were given at 2- to 3-week intervals until a response occurred or were stopped if progression occurred after two courses. Prophylactic Ara-C was injected intrathecally after complete remission. Maintenance therapy was given every 3–4 weeks at the highest tolerated doses for up to 1 year.

The overall response rate was 92%; 66% of the patients had a complete response (Table 2). The durations of the complete responses are shown in Figure 7. Thirteen patients have died. The estimated median survival is more than 3 years. Myelosuppression occurred in all patients, but was transient. Only 6 patients had severe infections; in 2 the infection was fatal. No hemorrhagic problems from thrombocytopenia occurred. Two episodes of congestive heart failure may have been related to Adriamycin therapy. About a third of the patients had mild peripheral neuropathy that was reversible. No pulmonary toxicity from bleomycin was clinically evident.

A significant number of patients with advanced malignant lymphoma remitted completely with the combination CHOP-bleo chemotherapy in this series. Combination chemotherapy has a definite place, not only in the palliation of advanced lymphoma, but also in the permanent control of these diseases in some patients. The addition of combination chemotherapy to radiotherapy for early-stage disease, or perhaps the use of chemotherapy alone in stages I and II, deserves consideration.

► [Many of the patients in this series had histologic varieties of malignant lymphoma that are associated with a poor prognosis. In this study the rate of complete remission was 69% in patients with diffuse histiocytic lymphoma, and only 3 of 18 patients have relapsed. The rate of complete remission was 62% in patients with nodular poorly differentiated lymphocytic lymphoma, and only 1 of 8 has relapsed.

It is clear that CHOP-bleo is an effective combination for the treatment of advanced non-Hodgkin's lymphoma. It is not yet certain that this protocol of drugs is superior to the four-drug combination of Adriamycin, vincristine, prednisone and cyclophosphamide (CHOP) that produces complete remission rates of about 68% and 76%, respectively, in patients with diffuse histiocytic and nodular poorly differentiated lymphocytic lymphoma (McKelvey et al.: Cancer 38:1484, 1976).

The investigators in the present study treated the central nervous system prophylactically because of their recognition of the frequently reported relapses in this site in recent years. It is a logical approach, although the value of such prophylaxis is still uncertain. – Ed.] ◄

Initial Treatment of Stage IIIA Hodgkin's Disease: Comparison of Radiotherapy with Combined Chemotherapy was carried out in the British National Lymphoma Investigation.[5] The optimal primary treatment for stage III Hodgkin's disease remains controversial. A prospective comparison of radiotherapy and chemotherapy was begun in 1970 and continued to 1975. A total of 117 patients with stage IIIA disease were allocated to supervoltage or megacurie radiotherapy after splenectomy or to combination chemotherapy. A tumor dose of 4,000 rad was delivered in 4 weeks to affected node regions by the conventional mantle and inverted-Y techniques, and 3,500 rad to node regions apparently free from disease. Chemotherapy was with mustine, vincristine, procarbazine and prednisone (MOPP). Repeated courses were given to complete remission, and 3 consolidation courses followed; at least 6 courses of therapy were given.

Among 81 patients who had staging laparotomy, 40 of 42 treated by total node irradiation achieved complete remission; 9 have relapsed, and 3 of these have died of Hodgkin's disease. Two patients had partial responses but remain alive. Of 39 patients given MOPP therapy, 29 had complete remissions; 11 have relapsed, and 1 of these has died of Hodgkin's disease. Three of 10 patients with partial responses have died of the disease. The recurrence-free survival curve was better for patients given radiotherapy, but overall survival curves did not differ significantly. In 36 patients who did not have staging laparotomy, the 2-year recurrence-free survival rates were 71% for total node irradiation and 53% for MOPP therapy. The respective overall 2-year survival rates were 76% and 86%. The differences were not significant.

Total node irradiation is the optimal initial treatment for patients with stage IIIA Hodgkin's disease whose staging includes laparotomy.

► [This British National Lymphoma Investigation compared total nodal irradiation (TNI) with MOPP chemotherapy in patients with stage IIIA Hodgkin's disease and concluded that irradiation was superior. In follow-up studies of up to 4 years, approximately 20% of patients treated with TNI have relapsed and another 5% never achieved complete remission. Thus, the overall "failure" rate is at least 25% with TNI. The investigators conclude, with good reason, ". . . there is room for improvement." Consequently, they and other investigators (Rosenberg, S. A., and Kaplan, H. S., Cancer 35:55, 1975) are examining the use of multiagent chemotherapy in combination with total nodal irradiation in stage IIIA Hodgkin's disease. The results are not yet conclusive but suggest a prolonged disease-free survival with the combination. – Ed.] ◄

---

(5) Lancet 2:991–995, Nov. 6, 1976.

Fulminant Sepsis after Successful Treatment of Hodgkin's Disease. Treatment of Hodgkin's disease has become increasingly aggressive in recent years. Sigmund Weitzman and Alan C. Aisenberg[6] describe 3 patients staged by splenectomy and treated by total nodal irradiation and combination chemotherapy at Massachusetts General Hospital who acquired fulminant sepsis with encapsulated bacteria when Hodgkin's disease was in remission. No similar episodes of sepsis were seen in patients with less aggressively managed Hodgkin's disease.

The 3 patients were among the 160 patients under age 65 who were treated for Hodgkin's disease in 1969–74. Laparotomy and splenectomy were done in 118. Patients whose disease was in stage I or IIA were treated by extended-field irradiation and those with disease in stage IIB, by irradiation to all nodal areas. A dose of 3,600–3,900 rad of 2-Mev therapy was delivered in 3½–4 weeks. Combination (MOPP) chemotherapy was used in stages III and IV. Fourteen splenectomized patients received both total nodal irradiation and MOPP chemotherapy.

All 3 patients were young. Two had nodular sclerosis Hodgkin's disease and 1, mixed cellularity disease. Septicemia occurred 0, 4 and 14 months after completion of the last phase of treatment. *Hemophilus influenzae* was responsible in 2 cases and pneumococcus type 18 in 1. Two patients died within hours after admission with adrenal hemorrhage, after 12–33 months of clinical remission of Hodgkin's disease. No autopsy evidence of residual lymphoma was found in these cases.

Splenectomy was probably partly responsible for septicemia in these cases, but the extent of its contribution is not clear. Caution is needed when both total nodal irradiation and combination chemotherapy are used in the primary treatment of splenectomized patients with Hodgkin's disease.

► [It is generally believed that splenectomy in young children predisposes them to certain bacterial infections, particularly those caused by the pneumococcus and *Hemophilus influenzae* (Erakalis et al.: N. Engl. J. Med. 276:1225, 1967). Infection in such children may be fulminant with a high mortality. In contrast, the evidence is weak that the asplenic state predisposes immunologically intact adults to bacterial infection. In this article, Weitzman and Aisenberg raise the possibility that splenectomy combined with aggressive chemotherapy and radiotherapy may increase susceptibility to lethal infection in patients with Hodgkin's disease in clinical remission. The suggestion may have merit, and such patients should be followed carefully when any febrile illness develops.

A recent report (Ammann et al.: ibid. 297:898, 1977) suggests that immunization of sickle cell anemia patients and splenectomized patients with polyvalent pneumococcal polysaccharide may protect against systemic *Streptococcus (Diplococcus) pneumoniae.*—Ed.] ◄

Eleven-Year Follow-up on 64 Subjects with M Components is reported by Uno Axelsson[7] (Karlstad, Sweden). In a survey of 6,995 persons in Sweden, M components of Ig were found in 64 subjects. Thirty-seven of the subjects evaluated in 1964 were alive at follow-up, and plasma samples from 31 subjects were evaluated. One subject had clear signs of myelomatosis, and 1 had lymphatic leukemia. Twenty-seven

(6) Am. J. Med. 62:47–50, January, 1977.
(7) Acta Med. Scand. 201:173–175, 1977.

subjects had died after 11 years. The lymphatic leukemia had changed to myelomatosis after 6 years. One patient died of malignant lymphoma after 9 years. No clustering of diseases was apparent in the 37 surviving patients. The overall observation time was 487 years. No further myelomas or lymphomas were detected at follow-up. One M component had disappeared and been replaced by an oligoclonal gammopathy.

Malignant disease of immunocytes was associated with an M component only three times in this series. Two myelomas and 1 lymphoma were observed. In no other case did a trace component increase in parallel with progression of disease.

► [It is reassuring that, even in the long term, most benign monoclonal gammopathies do indeed represent benign conditions. – Ed.] ◄

Leukocyte Transfusion and Leukocyte Disorders

Randomized Clinical Trial of Granulocyte Transfusions for Infection in Acute Leukemia. Infection is one of the major causes of morbidity and death in patients with granulocytopenia, and many antibiotics are less effective in the presence of granulocytopenia. Jane B. Alavi, Richard K. Root, Isaac Djerassi, Audrey E. Evans, Stephen J. Gluckman, Rob Roy MacGregor, DuPont Guerry, Alan D. Schreiber, John M. Shaw, Penelope Koch and Richard A. Cooper[8] (Philadelphia) evaluated the clinical efficacy of granulocyte transfusions prepared by filtration leukapheresis in leukemic patients with granulocytopenia and infection. Patients with acute leukemia or the blastic phase of chronic myelogenous leukemia with a granulocyte count below 250/cu mm were included in the study if infection was documented or strongly suspected. Most donors were unrelated to the recipients. All patients received broad-spectrum antibiotics initially. About 5×10^{10} granulocytes were given daily to each transfused patient. Hydrocortisone was given if febrile reactions to any transfusions occurred.

Thirteen patients were given transfusions and 19 were assigned to a control group. The groups were similar in age and diagnoses. Twelve surviving study patients received 176 granulocyte transfusions, for an average of 7 per febrile episode. No fatal or severe anaphylactic reactions followed the transfusions. Forty febrile episodes occurred in control patients and 22 in transfused patients. Infection was proved in 40% and 55% of the episodes, respectively. Survival was better for patients with fever of unknown origin than for those with proved or probable infections. When bone marrow recovery was observed, with a granulocyte count above 500/cu mm at day 21, 89% of control patients

Fig 8.—Survival curve for independent episodes of proved or probable infection in patients who did not have bone marrow recovery. (Courtesy of Alavi, J. B., et al.: N. Engl. J. Med. 296:706–711, Mar. 31, 1977.)

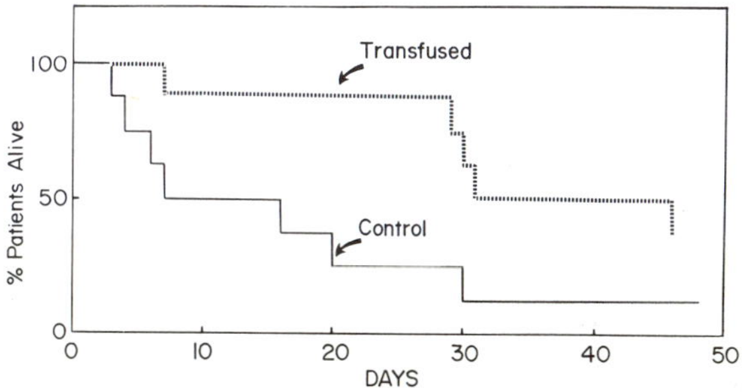

(8) N. Engl. J. Med. 296:706–711, Mar. 31, 1977.

and 83% of study patients survived to day 21, compared with 20% and 75%, respectively, when the count failed to rise. Survival after independent episodes of infection in patients without bone marrow recovery is shown in Figure 8. There was no difference in the proportions of episodes followed by superinfection in the two patient groups.

Filtration-leukapheresis granulocytes were given without serious complications in this study and appeared to offer a survival advantage to infected, persistently granulocytopenic patients with acute leukemia. Some patients with prolonged neutropenia apparently can be supported for several weeks during severe infection until their own bone marrows recover. Procurement methods need to be refined and standardized to eliminate variability in cell function and to minimize reactions in recipients.

► [The two major techniques for procuring granulocytes are by filtration and by differential centrifugation. Both methods yield cells that perform at 70–100% of control levels in in vitro tests of phagocytic function. In most studies the cells obtained by filtration did not circulate very well and frequently caused febrile transfusion reactions. Nevertheless, this study, as well as several other recent reports, indicates that these transfused granulocytes reduce the incidence of lethal infection in severely granulocytopenic patients. Granulocyte transfusion must now be considered an important adjunct during the induction of remission in acute myeloid leukemia when infection unresponsive to antibiotics is present. – Ed.] ◄

Successful Granulocyte Transfusion Therapy for Gram-Negative Septicemia: Prospectively Randomized Controlled Study. Recently there have been several reports of the successful clinical use of transfusions of normal circulating granulocytes. Roger H. Herzig, Geoffrey P. Herzig, Robert G. Graw, Jr., Malcolm I. Bull and Karyl K. Ray[9] (Natl. Inst. of Health) report a prospective trial of granulocyte transfusions in granulocytopenic patients with documented gram-negative septicemia. Patients with hematologic neoplasia, aplastic anemia and solid tumors who had granulocytopenia from primary bone marrow involvement or from treatment and who had culture-proved gram-negative septicemia were eligible for study after the institution of triple-antibiotic therapy. The circulating granulocytes were below 1,000/μl. Transfusions were continued daily until the granulocyte count exceeded this level or after at least 5 days with negative blood cultures and 3 days without fever. Granulocytes were obtained by continuous-flow centrifugation or filtration leukapheresis and were irradiated before transfusion.

Fifteen patients received 197 transfusions for 16 episodes of sepsis. Reactions were frequent after transfusions of leukapheresis cells, but were lessened by slow infusion rates and by acetaminophen, diphenhydramine or corticosteroids. All survivors had complete resolution of sepsis. Bone marrow function was recovered in 10 of 30 episodes. All 8 patients not given granulocyte transfusions died with persistent gram-negative septicemia, whereas 8 of 12 transfused patients survived the bout of sepsis. The duration of granulocytopenia after the initial positive blood culture was important in determining survival from sepsis. Fungus infections did not contribute to mortality to any great extent.

---

(9) N. Engl. J. Med. 296:701–705, Mar. 31, 1977.

Patients who recover bone marrow function nearly always survive episodes of granulocytopenic gram-negative sepsis, whether treated with antibiotics alone or with granulocyte transfusions as well. Patients with prolonged, severe granulocytopenia appear to benefit most from granulocyte transfusions. Daily compatible granulocyte transfusions, combined with appropriate antibiotics, improve survival from gram-negative septicemia in patients with persistent neutropenia.

► [This article makes the point that granulocyte transfusions are effective in many clinical situations in which granulocytopenia is the common denominator. Their use is not restricted to patients with acute leukemia. – Ed.] ◄

Correction of Leukocyte Function in Chediak-Higashi Syndrome by Ascorbate. Patients with the Chediak-Higashi syndrome have frequent, severe pyogenic infections secondary to abnormal polymorphonuclear leukocyte function. The impaired bactericidal activity of the leukocytes appears related to delayed delivery of lysosomal contents into phagosomes. The defect may arise from abnormal microtubular assembly in polymorphonuclear leukocytes. Treatment of such leukocytes with agents that increase cyclic 3′5′-guanosine monophosphate (GMP) levels will improve microtubular function. Laurence A. Boxer, August M. Watanabe, Manfred Rister, Henry R. Besch, Jr., John Allen and Robert L. Baehner[1] (Indianapolis) studied the effects of

Fig 9. – In vivo effect of ascorbic acid on bactericidal capacity of mixed leukocytes in Chediak-Higashi *(C-H)* syndrome. Phagocytes, 1×10^7, were incubated with equivalent amount of *Staphylococcus aureus* 502A. Recorded values are mean ±SEM of three separate experiments. Differences in values at various intervals were statistically significant at the 0.001 level between untreated patient and control. (Courtesy of Boxer, L. A., et al.: N. Engl. J. Med. 295:1041–1045, Nov. 4, 1976.)

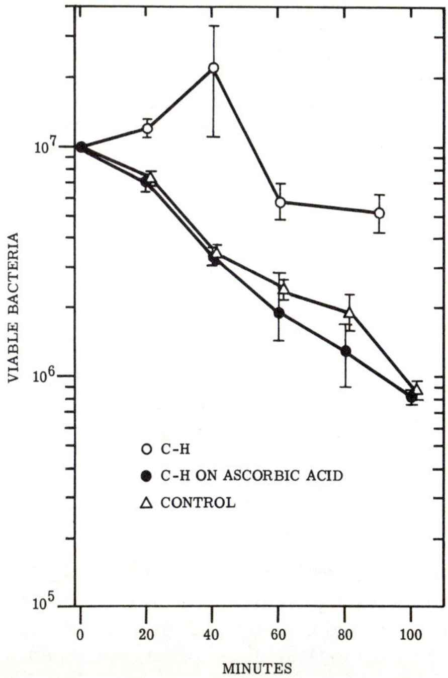

(1) N. Engl. J. Med. 295:1041–1045, Nov. 4, 1976.

ascorbic acid, which increases cyclic GMP levels in monocytes in vitro, on cyclic nucleotide levels and polymorphonuclear leukocyte function.

Girl, aged 11 months, with Chediak-Higashi syndrome, had been placed on 200 mg ascorbic acid daily for 2 months at age 9 months. The abnormal leukocyte morphology persisted, but the absolute leukocyte count increased. The vitamin was discontinued twice for 1-month intervals. The serum lysozyme level was 50 mg/ml. The polymorphonuclear leukocyte ascorbate level was 4.09 $\mu g/10^8$ cells (control, 4.65 μg). Polymorphonuclear chemotaxis was impaired before, and significantly improved after, oral ascorbic acid therapy. Abnormal β-glucuronidase release on exposure of leukocytes to opsonized zymosan was observed, and it was corrected by ascorbic acid therapy. Treatment eliminated the delay in bacterial killing by neutrophils in this case; the overall rate of bacterial killing was comparable to that of control leukocytes (Fig 9). Cyclic adenosine monophosphate (AMP) levels in polymorphonuclear leukocytes were markedly above normal, and they were substantially reduced by ascorbic acid in vitro. Levels of both cyclic AMP and cyclic GMP were reduced during ascorbic acid therapy.

Ascorbic acid reduces cyclic AMP levels in leukocytes from patients with the Chediak-Higashi syndrome, and leukocyte function returns to normal without dramatic changes in granular morphology. Whatever the mechanism of the beneficial effects of ascorbic acid in leukocytes from these patients, it appears the functional defect in the polymorphonuclear leukocytes is corrected by the vitamin.

► [The Chediak-Higashi syndrome (CHS) is a rare disorder whose importance rests on its biologic uniqueness rather than its frequency. The clinical disorder is characterized by frequent infections from early childhood, granulocytopenia, abnormal hair and skin pigmentation and a tendency to develop widespread tissue infiltration. Morphologically, the distinctive feature is giant granules (lysosomes) in leukocytes. Lysosomes are membrane-bound cytoplasmic inclusions containing hydrolytic enzymes. Similar lysosome anomalies widely distributed throughout various tissues occur in CHS, and comparable disorders are known in a variety of animal species, including Hereford cattle, mink and mice. The defect in the ability of CHS leukocytes to kill bacteria is thought to result from an abnormality of the disruption of the giant granules into the phagocytic vacuole containing the ingested bacteria. Maneuvers that raise intracellular cyclic AMP in normal neutrophils appear to produce a similar, but perhaps not identical, defect in degranulation. It is speculated that cyclic GMP may have an opposing effect in the phagocytic process. Ascorbic acid may modulate the intracellular concentrations of cyclic nucleotides in phagocytic leukocytes, and this is suggested as the mechanism of the beneficial effect of the vitamin in this child with CHS. – Ed.] ◄

Acquired Granulocyte Abnormality during Drug Allergic Reactions: Possible Role of Complement Activation. The active locomotion of polymorphonuclear neutrophils toward increasing concentrations of various substances, including soluble bacterial products and complement components, is crucial in localizing infections in that it attracts and accumulates phagocytes at sites of infections. Timothy K. Bowers, Philip R. Craddock and Harry S. Jacob[2] (Univ. of Minnesota) report studies in a patient with an allergic drug reaction and transient hypocomplementemia, whose granulocyte chemotactic function was markedly impaired in vitro and probably also in vivo.

Man, 21, presented with tenderness and swelling in the neck, sore throat and fever that did not respond to oral clindamycin therapy. Intravenous cephalothin was followed by an urticarial eruption, and oxacillin gave no benefit.

(2) Blood 49:3–8, January, 1977.

Cellulitis without abscess formation was evident. After antibiotics were stopped and prednisone given, the fever resolved along with the rash. Total hemolytic complement (CH 50) was undetectable initially and then became normal.

Initially the chemotactic response of the patient's granulocytes was markedly impaired, migrating about one-third as well as normal leukocytes with complement chemotactic factors. They were almost incapable of responding toward *Escherichia coli* chemotactic factor. Responses were much improved after 5 days of steroid therapy, when the serum complement had returned to normal, and were normal 10 days after the cessation of steroid therapy. The chemotactic potency of the patient's serum was markedly increased over that of normal serum. The complement-induced chemotaxes of normal granulocytes incubated with patient serum was markedly impaired. Granulocytes from infected patients given cephalothin or other penicillin-related antibiotics without allergic reactions had normal chemotactic responses.

A defect in chemotaxis was verified in this case. The patient's serum contained a specific inhibitor of complement-induced chemotaxis during the period of impaired chemotaxis. The allergic reaction to cephalothin presumably led to immune complex activation of complement and to complement-induced granulocyte paralysis. The chemotactic defect in patients with exacerbations of systemic lupus erythematosus and hypocomplementemia is a manifestation of this phenomenon, as is the correlation of chemotactic response and complement levels in patients with rheumatoid arthritis.

► [Components of the complement system act as chemoattractants for phagocytic leukocytes. Components C5a, C3a and the trimolecular complex of C5-6-7 are particularly active in orienting the movement of neutrophils. This is probably one of the principal mechanisms by which phagocytic cells are attracted to an inflammatory focus. The chemotactically active products of certain bacteria serve as additional attracting mechanisms.

In clinical situations in which there is activation of all or part of the complement cascade in the bloodstream, the neutrophils appear to be temporarily insensitive to chemotactic stimuli. For example, persons exposed to bacterial endotoxin have neutrophils that are transiently indifferent to such stimuli. A similar situation is described in this report by Bowers and his colleagues in a patient with an allergic reaction. The result of chemotactic insensitivity may be failure of granulocyte localization at the nidus of inflammation and failure of abscess formation. When complement activation is abrupt and profound, the neutrophils may temporarily agglutinate and be sequestered in the lungs, producing a transient neutropenia. — Ed.] ◄

Serum Myeloperoxidase and Lactoferrin in Neutropenia. Results of studies correlating plasma lysozyme and neutrophil turnover rate in neutropenic patients have varied. Tor Olofsson, Inge Olsson, Per Venge and Börje Elgefors[3] describe radioimmunosorbent assays for determining the serum contents of the neutrophil proteins myeloperoxidase (MPO) and lactoferrin. Serial studies were performed in 2 cases of cyclic neutropenia, 1 case of persistent neutropenia without cycling and 1 of drug-induced agranulocytosis. Radioimmunosorbent assays utilizing ^{125}I-labeled MPO and ^{125}I-labeled lactoferrin were carried out.

Normal levels of MPO and lactoferrin were 252×10^{-5} gm/L and

(3) Scand. J. Haematol. 18:73–80, January, 1977.

385×10^{-6} gm/L, respectively. The MPO level was normal in the patients with cyclic neutropenia, even during profound neutropenia, but the serum lactoferrin level fluctuated with the neutrophil cycle. In persistent profound neutropenia the serum lactoferrin was persistently extremely low, but levels of MPO were normal. Lactoferrin was extremely low in the patient with drug-induced agranulocytosis and increased with the neutrophil count during regeneration. Although MPO showed an initial increase followed by some fluctuations, all values were in the normal range. Analysis of all data showed a good correlation between serum lactoferrin and neutrophil counts, but no correlation between serum MPO levels and neutrophil counts.

Serum MPO appears to derive primarily from MPO-rich granulopoietic precursor cells of the bone marrow, whereas serum lactoferrin seems to derive from leakage of more mature granulopoietic cells of the blood and marrow. Studies of neutrophil proteins in serum may aid in the evaluation of neutropenic patients.

► [There are no good simple tests available that reliably correlate with or measure neutrophil production rates. Isotopic labeling techniques are too cumbersome for routine clinical use, and measurements of serum lysozyme show a poor correlation with neutrophil kinetics. In assessing the etiology of a neutropenic disorder, one is usually left with crude morphological estimates of marrow cellularity and myeloid maturation. The use of lactoferrin techniques shows considerable promise for analyzing neutropenic states. Lactoferrin is an iron-binding protein that appears to be restricted in its distribution to the secondary granules of the neutrophil. Consequently, it is a unique marker of neutrophilic granulocytes beginning at roughly the promyelocyte-myelocyte stage of development. It seems reasonable that lactoferrin concentration in blood might correlate with neutrophil turnover rates. Myeloperoxidase and lysozyme, on the other hand, are more widely distributed in blood cells and are not unique markers of the neutrophilic series. The next logical step in these studies is to do detailed neutrophil kinetic studies in a variety of clinical conditions and correlate these with lactoferrin levels. – Ed.] ◄

Endomyocardiopathy with Eosinophilia. Graham O. Solley, Jorge E. Maldonado, Gerald J. Gleich, Emilio R. Giuliani, H. Clark Hoagland, Robert V. Pierre and Arnold L. Brown, Jr.[4] describe 5 patients seen in 1967 – 74 who exhibited striking eosinophilia, cardiomyopathy, hepatosplenomegaly and either a rapidly fatal or a prolonged debilitating illness.

Young man, 17, exhibited chest pains and malaise, and was found to be anemic and have marked eosinophilia. Blood and cortisone were given, but arterial occlusion affected both the lower limbs a month later, and surgery revealed complete aortic obstruction by a saddle embolus, as well as splenomegaly. The arterial supply improved only temporarily after embolectomy, and fibrinous material was removed by bilateral common femoral arteriotomies. Eosinophilia persisted on treatment with prednisone and oral anticoagulation, but good progress was made.

About 2 years after the original presentation, vomiting, diarrhea and weight loss occurred, but improved on treatment with prednisone and diphenhydramine. Tachycardia and pansystolic murmurs were noted, and the liver was enlarged. *Staphlyococcus aureus* was cultured from the blood. The patient deteriorated despite intensive therapy and died a month later.

Autopsy showed a massive mural thrombus that virtually filled the left ventricular cavity. The right ventricular endocardium was markedly thickened,

(4) Mayo Clin. Proc. 51:697 – 708, November, 1976.

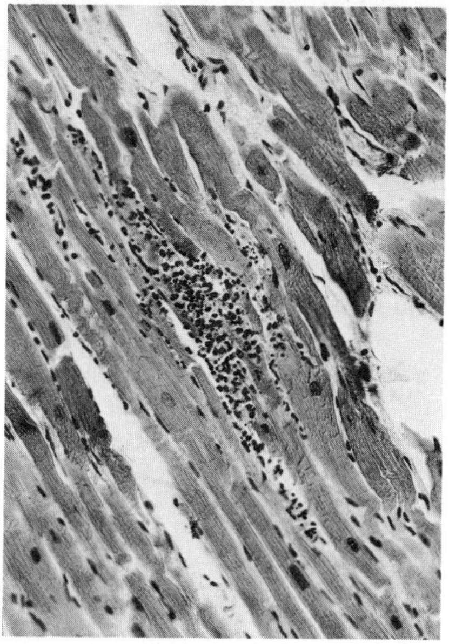

Fig 10.—Myocardium showing focal collection of cells, mainly eosinophils, plus muscle cell damage and infiltration into interstitium. Hematoxylin-eosin; reduced from ×205. (Courtesy of Solley, G. O., et al.: Mayo Clin. Proc. 51:697–708, November, 1976.)

and both ventricles were focally scarred. The kidneys had many small infarcts, and the glomeruli showed marked recent proliferative changes. Eosinophilic hyperplasia was seen in the bone marrow. The spleen was greatly enlarged, had a recent infarct and was markedly infiltrated by mature eosinophils.

A male preponderance (4:1) was evident in this series; the mean age was 32 years. Three patients died within 4–5 years of the first symptoms. Significant eosinophilia usually preceded definite cardiac impairment. The eosinophilia regressed in only 1 case. Large, electron-dense cytoplasmic inclusions were seen in the eosinophils. All patients had mitral insufficiency, tricuspid insufficiency and congestive heart failure. All 3 autopsies showed mural thrombi in the left ventricle. Endocardial scar tissue was infiltrated by lymphocytes, and in 1 case there were focal collections of eosinophils in the myocardium (Fig 10). The glomeruli showed early membranous changes in 2 cases and focal proliferation in 1. Treatment has been generally disappointing, but the illness appears to have become inactive in 1 case.

None of these patients appeared to have a leukemic process. Extreme persistent eosinophilia may herald a rapidly fatal illness and calls for thorough cardiac evaluation if such diseases as polyarteritis nodosa, Hodgkin's disease or benign conditions such as bronchial asthma are not evident.

► [Eosinophilic endocarditis was first described by Löffler in the *Swiss Journal of Medicine* in 1936. The major features are peripheral blood eosinophilia, cardiac failure and peripheral embolic phenomena. Men 30–50 years of age predominate in most series. At autopsy, fibrosis usually involves the walls of the heart rather than the valves, and mural thrombi are common. The etiology of this disorder is unknown and response to treatment is poor. Most patients die within 3 months to 6 years of onset of manifestations. The disorder is probably not a true eosinophilic leukemia, which occurs very rarely. Eosinophilic leukemia is probably a variant of chronic myelogenous leukemia, and patients with eosinophilia, diffuse organ infiltration and the Ph^1 chromosome have been described (Gruenwald et al.: Am. J. Med. 39:1003, 1965).

One wonders whether the eosinophil produces the cardiac lesions in Löffler's carditis or is a secondary manifestation of some other process. If the eosinophil is a primary protagonist, then it is logical to consider manipulations aimed at reducing the total numbers of eosinophils. – Ed.] ◄

Purine Nucleoside Phosphorylase Deficiency Associated with Selective Cellular Immunodeficiency. A causal relationship between deficiency of adenosine deaminase and severe combined immunodeficiency disease has been proved. J. W. Stoop, B. J. M. Zegers, G. F. M. Hendrickx, L. H. Siegenbeek van Heukelom, G. E. J. Staal, P. K. de Bree, S. K. Wadman and R. E. Ballieux[5] (Utrecht, The Netherlands) studied a child with severely defective T cell immunity, normal B cell immunity and no measurable nucleoside phosphorylase activity in the red blood cells and lymphocytes. Two older girls in the family had had the same immune defect and had died.

Girl, aged 15 months, the fourth child of unrelated parents, had 2 older female siblings who had had severely defective T cell immunity. One had died of lymphosarcoma and the other of a severe graft-vs.-host reaction after a blood transfusion. The child had been clinically well, but presented with otitis and a throat infection, both of which responded well to specific therapy. No tonsillar tissue was visible and lymph nodes were not palpable. A slight spastic tetraparesis and slightly retarded motor development were evident. X-ray study at age 3 months had shown no thymus shadow.

Adenosine deaminase activity was present in the patient's red blood cells and lymphocytes but purine nucleoside phosphorylase activity was absent. The serum and urine contained high levels of inosine and guanosine, and hypouricemia and hypouricuria were noted. The marrow was megaloblastic and the blood hypochromic and microcytic. The percentage of E-rosetting cells was low. Despite a low number of circulating Ig-bearing B lymphocytes, the serum Ig levels were normal at age 1 year. At age 15 months the serum IgM was high, as was the IgD level.

The patient's parents and brother had intermediate nucleoside phosphorylase values. The selective cellular immunodeficiency was inherited as an autosomal recessive trait in this family. The T cell function was presumably normal at birth, although elimination of precursor substances became less adequate after birth or the supply of an essential metabolic product became inadequate. It is not clear why T cell immunity is impaired and B cell immunity at least partially intact. The cause of the spastic tetraparesis is unknown. Fetal thymus was transplanted several times in the eldest sister but had only a short-term effect on T cell immunity. The most obvious therapeutic approach would be enzyme substitution or correction of the consequences of the metabolic defect.

► [The pathogenetic mechanisms of the T cell abnormality in this case are obscure; nevertheless, one must wonder whether infusion of normal red blood cells containing normal levels of purine nucleoside phosphorylase would be beneficial. A similar approach has been reported to be successful in adenosine deaminase deficiency and severe combined immunodeficiency disease (Polmar, S. H.: Lancet 2:743, 1975). – Ed.]

(5) N. Engl. J. Med. 296:651–655, Mar. 24, 1977.

Platelets and Hemostasis

Spectrum of von Willebrand's Disease: Study of 100 Cases is reported by T. Barbui, F. Baudo, N. Ciavarella, G. Mariani, Anna Capitanio, P. M. Mannucci, F. Pareti and Z. M. Ruggeri.[6] Von Willebrand's disease (VWD) was diagnosed on the basis of reduced levels of procoagulant factor VIII (VIII_{AHF}), low platelet retention to glass bead columns, prolonged bleeding time and a lifelong bleeding diathesis. All laboratory findings were abnormal in 61 cases.

Seventeen patients from 14 different families (group I) had no family history and a severe clinical form of the disease, with spontaneous joint and muscle bleeding. Levels of VIII_{AHF} and ristocetin co-factor (VIII_{VWF}) were very low, and platelet retention and bleeding time were markedly abnormal in all cases. Factor VIII-related antigen (VIII_{AGN}) was undetectable in 6 patients and extremely low in 11.

Eighty-three patients from 33 families (group 2) had a moderately severe clinical course, with mucosal and postoperative bleeding. Autosomal dominant transmission was apparent in most of these families. Eleven patients had normal platelet retention, and 15 had a normal bleeding time. The VIII_{AHF} level was normal in 2 cases and VIII_{AGN} in 13 cases. Plasma VIII_{VWF} was reduced in all patients and undetectable in 41. Correlation between VIII_{VWF} and the bleeding time was poor (Fig

Fig 11.—Relationship between VIII_{VWF} and bleeding time in group 2 patients. *Triangles,* patients with decreased ristocetin-induced platelet aggregation (RIPA) in platelet-rich plasma; *squares,* those with normal RIPA; *circles,* those with increased RIPA. (Courtesy of Barbui, T., et al.: Br. J. Haematol. 35:101–112, January, 1977.)

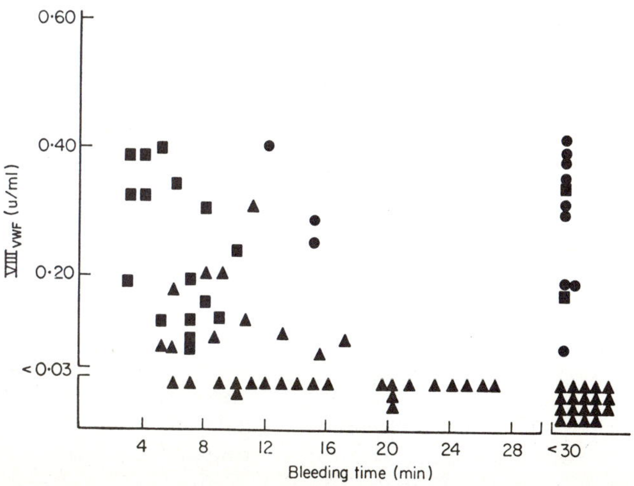

(6) Br. J. Haematol. 35:101–112, January, 1977.

11). A strong correlation was found between VIII_{VWF} and ristocetin-induced platelet aggregation.

It appears that VIII_{VWF} is the most useful single parameter for diagnosing VWD. Autosomal recessive inheritance appears likely in group 1 cases. The features of group 2 patients are more similar to those of classic VWD. Decreased plasma levels of VIII_{VWF} and VIII_{AGN} are not the only factors involved in the pathogenesis of the bleeding time abnormality. It cannot be ruled out, however, that these factors play a key role in primary hemostasis in the endothelial cells of the vessel wall.

► [Von Willebrand's disease (VWD) is one of the most common congenital bleeding disorders. The classic criteria for VWD are (1) a prolonged bleeding time, (2) reduced platelet retention on glass beads, (3) reduced concentrations of factor VIII procoagulant activity, (4) with a parallel reduction in factor VIII-related antigen, (5) impaired ristocetin aggregation of platelets and (6) reduction of a plasma factor associated with factor VIII (VIII_{VWF}) which is needed for aggregation of normal platelets by ristocetin. Although some patients demonstrate all these abnormalities, it has become clear that the spectrum of disease is more complex than was appreciated earlier. This study by Barbui et al. examined a large number of patients with VWD. Only 61% had abnormalities of all laboratory tests. Seventeen patients had severe clinical disease without a positive family history. It appeared that VIII_{VWF} was the best single parameter in diagnosing VWD, since it was abnormal in all patients and its decrease in the plasma was consistently accompanied by hemorrhagic manifestations. – Ed.] ◄

Platelet Membrane Defects in Glanzmann's Thrombasthenia: Evidence for Decreased Amounts of Two Major Glycoproteins. Glanzmann's thrombasthenia, an inherited platelet disorder, is characterized by a prolonged bleeding time, abnormal clot retraction, a normal platelet count and absence of platelet aggregation. Along with enzymatic differences, the molecular basis of the disorder appears to be an altered membrane surface. A decrease in concentration of glycoprotein IIb has been documented in thrombasthenic platelets. David R. Phillips and Patricia Poh Agin[7] (Memphis, Tenn.) labeled the membrane polypeptides of normal and thrombasthenic platelets by two techniques to identify other possible surface defects in thrombasthenic platelets. Platelets were obtained from 6 normal donors and 5 patients with Glanzmann's thrombasthenia. The patients were from two different families. The platelets were labeled by lactoperoxidase-catalyzed iodination and galactose oxidase oxidation, followed by reduction with tritiated sodium borohydride, and labeling patterns were determined after separation of the polypeptides by two-dimensional polyacrylamide gel electrophoresis. Platelet samples were incubated with β-mercaptoethanol before the second dimension was run.

Comparison of the labeled polypeptides of normal and thrombasthenic samples after reduction indicated strikingly decreased labeling of two major glycoproteins in thrombasthenic platelets, IIb and III (apparent molecular weight, 114,000). The relative percentages of radioactivity incorporated by these polypeptides were about 60% and 80% less, respectively, than control values. With either Coomassie Blue or periodic acid-Schiff reagent, glycoprotein III stained much less intensely in thrombasthenic than in normal samples, indicating that

(7) J. Clin. Invest. 60:535–545, September, 1977.

the labeling deficit was due to a decreased concentration of the molecule rather than steric inaccessibility on the membrane surface. Analysis of normal plasma membranes by affinity chromatography showed that glycoprotein IIb has receptors for lectin from *Lens culinaris,* the common lentil, whereas glycoprotein III does not.

A characteristic feature of Glanzmann's thrombasthenia is a reduced concentration of two discrete glycoproteins in the platelet plasma membrane. The inability of thrombasthenic platelets to retract clots is undoubtedly linked to their inability to aggregate. Probably one or both of the deficient glycoproteins is involved in platelet aggregation. However, the receptor involved in aggregation may be a low molecular weight component that is not detected by present techniques.

► [This article provides some of the experimental detail for the analysis provided in the following article. – Ed.] ◄

Thromboxane Synthesis and Platelet Release Reaction in Bernard-Soulier Syndrome, Thrombasthenia Glanzmann and Hermansky-Pudlak Syndrome. The unstable prostaglandin endoperoxide PGG_2, a precursor of prostaglandins E_2 and $F_{2\alpha}$ as well as the thromboxanes, causes rapid, irreversible aggregation of human platelets. C. Malmsten, H. Kindahl, B. Samuelsson (Stockholm), S. Levy-Toledano, G. Tobelem and J. P. Caen[8] (Paris) investigated aggregation, release of adenosine diphosphate (ADP) and ^{14}C-serotonin and synthesis of thromboxane B_2 (TXB_2) in healthy subjects and patients with various platelet disorders.

Both TXB_2 synthesis and ADP-^{14}C-serotonin release and platelet aggregation were essentially normal in a patient with Bernard-Soulier syndrome when platelets were incubated with collagen, ADP, arachidonic acid or PGG_2. In a patient with Hermansky-Pudlak syndrome, aggregation was normal with ADP, but aggregation with collagen and PGG_2 was markedly reduced. Release of ADP and ^{14}C-serotonin was reduced more than 50% with all inducers investigated in this disorder, whereas TXB_2 synthesis was normal with arachidonic acid and PGG_2 but reduced with collagen. In 3 patients with Glanzmann's thrombasthenia, almost no aggregation was noted with any of the compounds. Platelet TXB_2 formation from arachidonic acid or PGG_2 was normal, whereas ADP and collagen both induced significantly less TXB_2 formation than in normal platelets.

These findings provide further evidence for the hypothesis that the Bernard-Soulier syndrome and Glanzmann's thrombasthenia are primarily associated with glycoprotein abnormalities at the receptor level. A hypothetical model for the relationship between the two proposed glycoprotein receptor complexes and thromboxane synthesis is illustrated in Figure 12. Defective arachidonic acid synthesis may be responsible for impaired storage capacity within the dense bodies of the platelets in the Hermansky-Pudlak syndrome. The decreased TXB_2 formation with collagen may be due to lack of secondary stimulation of TXB_2 synthesis by released ADP, or it may be due to abnormal synthe-

(8) Br. J. Haematol. 35:511–520, April, 1977.

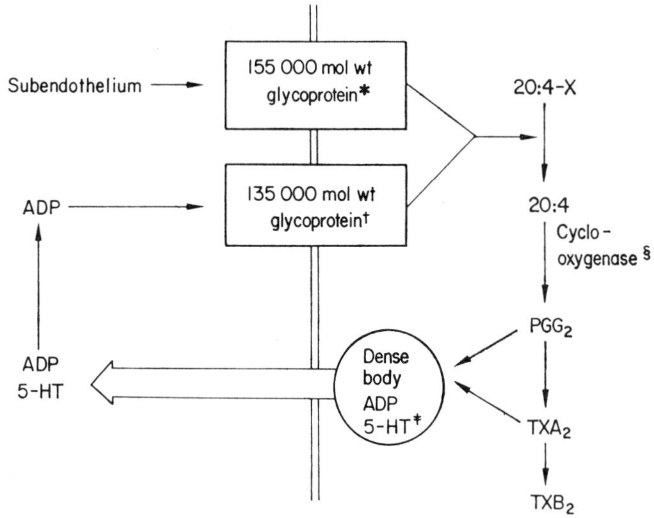

Fig 12.—Hypothetical scheme for the platelet release reaction induced by subendothelium or ADP. Meaning of symbols: *, missing or reduced in Bernard-Soulier syndrome; †, missing or reduced in Glanzmann's thrombasthenia; ‡, reduced in Hermansky-Pudlak syndrome; §, missing in platelet cyclo-oxygenase deficiency. *HT,* hydroxytryptamine; *20:4-X,* arachidonic acid in a phospholipid pool. (Courtesy of Malmsten, C., et al.: Br. J. Haematol. 35:511–520, April, 1977.)

sis of arachidonic acid and other lipids in platelets. Further studies of receptor complexes in platelets from normal donors and those with hemostatic defects and of the relationship between the membrane glycoproteins and the liberation of arachidonic acid for the synthesis of prostaglandin endoperoxides and thromboxanes may help elucidate the mechanism of initiation of the platelet release reaction.

► [Bernard-Soulier syndrome (BS) Hermansky-Pudlak syndrome and Glanzmann's thrombasthenia (GT) are all rare congenital disorders of platelet function that have provided insights into normal platelet physiology. In contrast to cyclo-oxygenase deficiency, none of these disorders is associated with abnormal thromboxane synthesis from arachadonic acid. It has recently been reported that BS and GT are each associated with a specific abnormality in glycoproteins of the platelet membrane (see the preceding article). The BS abnormality is a 155,000 molecular weight glycoprotein and may be a receptor for macromolecular elements of the subendothelium. The GT abnormality is a 135,000 dalton glycoprotein that is associated with the mechanism for ADP-induced aggregation. In contrast, the Hermansky-Pudlak syndrome appears to be a platelet "storage pool" disease with a primary defect in the number of very dense granules containing ADP and 5-hydroxytryptamine.

This article nicely summarizes current observations in a useful working hypothesis.—Ed.] ◄

Red Cell and Platelet Fragmentation in Idiopathic Autoimmune Thrombocytopenic Purpura. It generally is assumed that patients with thrombocytopenic purpura have antibodies to platelets, but it is not known whether autoimmune mechanisms are operative against other cells or tissues in these cases. Dorothea Zucker-Franklin and Simon Karpatkin[9] (New York Univ. Med. Center) investigated the abnormal small particle spike found in the platelet-rich plasma of pa-

(9) N. Engl. J. Med. 297:517–523, Sept. 8, 1977.

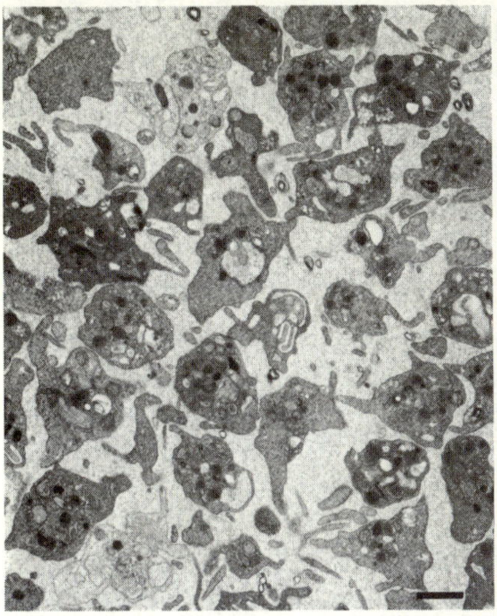

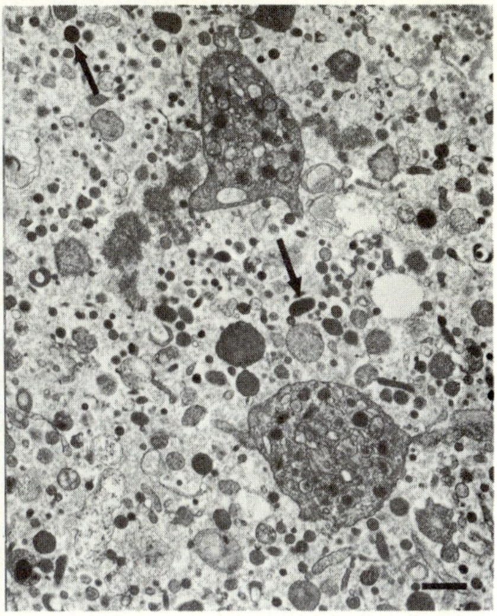

Fig 13 (left).—Survey electron micrograph of platelet fraction III from normal subject. Platelets are deformed due to centrifugation at 27,000 × g, but they are not surrounded by debris.

Fig 14 (right).—Survey electron micrograph of platelet fraction III from a patient. Platelets are much larger than those in Figure 13 and are surrounded by cellular debris and red blood cell fragments *(arrows)*.

(Courtesy of Zucker-Franklin, D., and Karpatkin, S.: N. Engl. J. Med. 297:517–523, Sept. 8, 1977.)

tients with severe idiopathic autoimmune thrombocytopenic purpura. Study was made of the platelets of 17 patients with idiopathic autoimmune thrombocytopenic purpura, 12 normal subjects and 2 normal asplenic subjects. The platelets were fractionated by differential centrifugation and the isolated fractions subjected to electron microscopy and planimetry. Two of the 17 study patients were in remission at the time of study.

Both erythrocytes and platelet fragments were found in the sediment of plasma that had been centrifugated at 27,000×g of the 15 patients with severe disease (Figs 13 and 14), but not in the plasma sediment of normal subjects, asplenic subjects or 3 patients with thrombocytopenia of nonimmunologic origin. Weak complement sensitization of red blood cells was noted in 7 of 12 study patients. Coating of red blood cells with IgG or IgM was not detected in the patients. Erythrophagocytosis was absent, but phagocytosis of intact platelets as well as platelet fragments and other cellular debris were frequently observed.

These observations support Evans' original suggestion that autoimmune thrombocytopenia and hemolytic anemia represent a spectrum of diseases and indicate that a spectrum of cell sensitization may be operative in each patient with severe idiopathic autoimmune thrombocytopenic purpura.

► [Sequestration of platelets in reticuloendothelial organs and the association of radioactively labeled platelets with splenic macrophages in vitro have suggested that antibody-coated platelets may be phagocytized. This study demonstrates that peripheral blood monocytes of patients with idiopathic autoimmune thrombocytopenic purpura can phagocytize platelets in toto.—Ed.] ◄

Thrombotic Thrombocytopenic Purpura-like Syndrome Associated with Infective Endocarditis: Possible Immune Complex Disorder. The diagnosis of infective endocarditis is often elusive. Arnold S. Bayer, Argyrios N. Theofilopoulos, Robert Eisenberg, Sidney G. Friedman and Lucien B. Guze[1] report data on 2 patients with endocarditis whose chief presenting feature was a thrombotic thrombocytopenic purpura (TTP)-like syndrome. The patients were a man aged 24 who presented with a 2-week history of fever, confusion and easy bruising and a woman aged 33 who presented with a 5-day history of confusion, bizarre behavior and fever.

The first patient had high levels of circulating immune complexes at the time endocarditis was diagnosed and the TTP-like syndrome was present. The platelet count and serum complement level returned to normal with successful antimicrobial therapy of the *Streptococcus viridans* bacteremia, in parallel with marked reductions in levels of circulating immune complexes. Complexes became undetectable with continued antibiotic therapy. The second patient had moderately elevated levels of circulating complexes when *Staphylococcus aureus* endocarditis and the TTP-like syndrome were apparent. Platelets and serum complement levels returned to normal with the eradication of bacteremia. Levels of circulating immune complexes became normal with successful antimicrobial therapy and later became undetectable, but subsequently complexes reappeared in association with biopsy-proved interstitial nephritis that occurred during methicillin therapy.

The complete TTP syndrome is rarely seen in association with endocarditis. The entire syndrome is rapidly reversed by antimicrobial therapy of the bacteremia. Both the present patients had hypocomplementemic renal failure. Antimicrobial therapy would have no benefit in true TTP and therapy for true TTP would be both ineffective and hazardous in ineffective endocarditis. Thus distinction of the two syndromes is of paramount importance. The syndrome in the present patients appeared to result from immune complex-mediated vasculitis. Whether TTP has a similar pathogenesis remains to be determined.

► [The pathogenesis of TTP is usually unknown. The 2 patients described in this report provide an interesting insight into one potential pathogenetic mechanism. – Ed.]

Plasmapheresis in Treatment of Thrombotic Thrombocytopenic Purpura. Various treatment methods have been tried in thrombotic thrombocytopenic purpura. R. M. Bukowski, John W. King and James S. Hewlett[2] (Cleveland Clinic) treated 15 patients with exchange transfusions in the past 16 years, with complete, lasting remission in 9 instances. The possibility that these remissions may be related to removal of soluble toxic material led to use of plasmapheresis in this syndrome. Two patients so treated are described.

Man, 32, had had a recent acute inferior myocardial infarction and treatment with warfarin and quinidine. Easy bleeding was noted 6 days before admission and warfarin was discontinued. Fever and chills developed 2 days later. The hemoglobin was 8 gm/dl and the platelet count 15,000/cu mm. A blood smear showed marked red cell fragmentation and multiple nucleated red

(1) J.A.M.A. 238:408 – 410, Aug. 1, 1977.
(2) Blood 50:413 – 417, September, 1977.

cells. No improvement followed administration of whole blood, platelets and hydrocortisone, and the patient was transferred to this hospital.

On admission, he was unconscious and minimally responsive to deep pain and had a temperature of 102 F. A gingival biopsy showed fibrin thrombi in submucosal vessels. The reticulocytes were 8.3%; the platelet count was 4,000/cu mm. The prothrombin time was 13 seconds (control, 11).

Dexamethasone was given, and serial plasmapheresis was carried out with an Aminco cell separator. Ten plasmaphereses were performed with 3 – 6 units of plasma replaced by fresh frozen plasma at each procedure. The patient became awake and responded to commands. After six plasmaphereses, the neurologic status was normal. The blood smear was normal after nine plasmaphereses. The patient was well 7 months after onset of illness and has required no further treatment.

The other patient was a woman aged 21 who, in the 28th week of pregnancy, experienced leg swelling and confusion and aborted. Normal hematologic values and neurologic status followed two exchange transfusions with whole blood. A month later, thrombotic thrombocytopenic purpura recurred, and 10 plasmaphereses were performed. She was well when last seen 5 months after the last plasmapheresis.

About 60% of patients with thrombotic thrombocytopenic purpura may achieve remission with exchange transfusions. The present 2 patients appeared to respond to plasmapheresis. Plasmapheresis appears to be a simpler treatment method than exchange transfusion and does not require large amounts of fresh whole blood. Since this syndrome is complex, possibly plasmapheresis may not be effective in all instances.

► [It has recently been speculated that some cases of thrombotic thrombocytopenic purpura involve soluble immune complexes. The preceding article may present an example of this phenomenon (see also Bukowski et al.: Semin. Hematol. 13:219, 1976). Plasmapheresis has been applied with occasional success to other disorders involving immune complexes, including Goodpasture's syndrome (Lackwood et al.: Br. Med. J. 2:252, 1975) and systemic lupus erythematosus (Jones et al.: Lancet 1:709, 1976). As we begin to understand the pathogenetic mechanisms involved in thrombotic thrombocytopenic purpura we are evolving a series of logical countermeasures: prevent initial endothelial damage, inhibit platelet adhesion and aggregation by pharmacologic approaches and prevent secondary activation of coagulation in the occasional cases in which this is a problem. – Ed.] ◄

Blood Clotting: Role of the Prostaglandins is discussed by Jean L. Marx.[3] Recent findings indicate that the balance between activities of a new prostaglandin and a thromboxane may determine whether or not a clot will form. The findings are of potentially great clinical import because heart attacks and strokes are often caused by abnormal clot formation. The endoperoxides are key intermediates in the synthesis of several prostaglandins and the thromboxanes. Much or all of the effect of endoperoxides in causing platelets to clump may be attributable to their serving as a source of the thromboxane called TXA_2. The synthesizing enzyme, thromboxane synthetase, has been identified in the microsomes of platelets. An enzyme that generates prostaglandin I_2 (PGI_2) in human blood vessels has been located in the innermost lining of the vessels. Many believe that destruction of the inner lining of arteries is an initial step in the formation of atherosclerotic

(3) Science 196:1072 – 1075, June 3, 1977.

plaques; platelets are present in plaques and may promote formation of the lesions.

The effects of TXA_2 on the contraction of arterial smooth muscle could contribute to blockage of an artery through constricting it, whereas the opposed effect of PGI_2 may help protect against restriction of blood flow. Human platelets aggregating with thrombin have been found to release TXA_2. Coronary arteries appear to release a substance that relaxes arterial smooth muscle. Probably arachidonic acid must be converted continuously to an unstable prostaglandin that causes the relaxation. Discovery of the role of TXA_2 and PGI_2 in clotting may make it possible to design more effective strategies for preventing heart attacks. Stable analogues of PGI_2 are being synthesized and the development of specific inhibitors of the enzyme that synthesizes TXA_2 represents another approach. The fact that most prostaglandins act on more than one system makes it difficult to design an agent acting only on the desired target and having no unwanted side effects.

► [The discovery last year of a new prostaglandin that appears to prevent the formation of blood clots has introduced a new field of investigation of these potent regulatory chemicals. This article is a nice summary of the current concepts of the role of prostaglandins in blood clotting. – Ed.] ◄

Laboratory Diagnosis of the Carrier State for Classic Hemophilia was investigated by Oscar D. Ratnoff and Paul K. Jones[4] (Case Western Reserve Univ.). Female relatives of patients with classic hemophilia often wish to learn whether they are carriers of the disorder. In most obligate carriers, the concentration of antihemophilic factor (AHF)-like antigens is disproportionately higher than the titer of procoagulant AHF, thus providing a basis for diagnosing the carrier state. Previously the distinction between normal women and carriers has been based on linear regression analysis of procoagulant AHF values, but discriminant analysis provides a sharper distinction and avoids the artificial assumption that the concentration of AHF-like antigen is linearly related to the titer of procoagulant AHF.

Of 87 obligate carriers, 82 (94%) could be identified as carriers by logarithmic discriminant analysis, because the titer of procoagulant AHF was disproportionately lower than the concentration of AHF-like antigens relative to normal women. Women who were mothers of isolated subjects with hemophilia appeared to be carriers in at least 85% of instances, suggesting that the frequency of cases due to new mutations is low. The validity of the technique used was supported by the frequency with which the carrier state was recognized in daughters of hemophiliacs who had no sons. Corrected for the known error of the method, 48% of 75 such daughters appeared to be carriers, not significantly different from their anticipated chance of 50%.

Methodologic improvements may increase the certainty with which carriers can be detected in the laboratory but it is doubtful that it will be possible to identify all carriers without a major change in technology. Although women with positive tests can assume that they are carriers, those with negative tests must interpret the result with caution. The technique is useful only in close relatives of hemophiliacs.

(4) Ann. Intern. Med. 86:521–528, May, 1977.

► [This method of detection of the carrier state of hemophilia A derives from the observation of Shanberge and Gore (J. Lab. Clin. Med. 50:954, 1957) that hemophiliac plasma contains an AHF-like substance that can be detected by heterologous antiserum, i.e., AHF-like antigen. Subsequent studies have shown that AHF-antigen is normal or even elevated in hemophiliac plasma. This, of course, contrasts with the situation in von Willebrand's disease where procoagulant activity and antigen concentration are proportionately diminished. The present study takes advantage of the fact that the concentration of AHF-like antigens is normal or elevated in obligate carriers whereas procoagulant activity is disproportionately lower. – Ed.] ◄

Hemophilia B: Characterization of Genetic Variants and Detection of Carriers. Carol K. Kasper, Bjarne Østerud, Judy Y. Minami, William Shonick and Samuel I. Rapaport[5] used various laboratory tests to determine plasma factor IX clotting activity, bovine thromboplastin time and plasma factor IX antigen in order to evaluate the genetic heterogeneity of hemophilia B in 92 male patients from 71 kindreds. Factor IX activity was also measured in 51 definite carriers from these kindreds, and the role of measurement of factor IX antigen in carrier detection was examined in 49 carriers. The normal group included 50 healthy males and 48 females who were not pregnant or using contraceptive hormones. Prothrombin times were also measured in 50 patients with severe hemophilia A.

Eighty patients in 60 kindreds had severe or moderately severe hemophilia B on the basis of a factor IX clotting activity of less than 4%; 12 patients in 11 kindreds had mild hemophilia B on the basis of a clotting activity of 4–22%. Thirty-six patients from 26 kindreds had immunologic evidence of factor IX antigen in excess of factor IX clotting activity. Of 24 patients from 15 kindreds with a bovine thromboplastin time over 2 SD above the normal mean, one group from 5

CLASSIFICATION OF PATIENTS WITH HEMOPHILIA B ACCORDING TO LABORATORY TEST RESULTS

Group No.	No. of Kindreds	No. of Patients	Range of Factor IX Activity (%)	Bovine Thromboplastin Time*	Mean (and Range) of Antigen Level (%): Human Inhibitor Neutralization	Rabbit Antibody Electroimmunoassay
I	5	7	<1–1.4	Greatly prolonged	105 (80–145)	111 (56–135)
II	10	17	<1–3	Slightly prolonged	56 (18–100)	71 (27–145)
III	7	8	<1–3	Normal	38 (11–83)	52 (20–90)
IV	38	48	<1–3	Normal	<10†	<10‡
V	4	4	7–22	Normal	43 (31–50)	77 (67–92)
VI	7	8	4–12	Normal	<10 (<10–16)	<10 (<10–23)

*Values for bovine thromboplastin times are not given in seconds because two lots of thromboplastin were used which gave mean values for normal males of 40.9 and 57.4 seconds. Normal bovine thromboplastin times are defined as times within 2 SD of the normal mean for the thromboplastin used; slightly prolonged times were within +5 SD of the normal mean; greatly prolonged times exceeded +9 SD of the normal mean.

†Three patients had levels >10% (11%, 14% and 27%, respectively); they had <10% antigen by electroimmunoassay.

‡Two patients had levels >10% (17% and 27%, respectively); they had <10% antigen by inhibitor neutralization test.

(5) Blood 50:351–366, September, 1977.

kindreds had markedly prolonged times of over 80 seconds. With use of all the data, patients were divided into six groups (table). No patient without evidence of abnormal factor IX had a prolonged bovine thromboplastin time. Human brain thromboplastin times did not distinguish the patients with excess factor IX antigen. Factors II, V, VII and X were all lower in patients with hemophilia B than in normal males.

Female carriers of severe hemophilia B had a normal distribution of factor IX activity. Factor IX antigen exceeded factor IX clotting activity in most definite carriers from kindreds in which affected males had excess factor IX antigen.

Most of the patients with severe hemophilia B had no measurable evidence of an abnormal factor IX molecule, either by antigen assays or by clotting assays with bovine thromboplastin. Immunoassays will provide no help in carrier detection in most hemophilia B kindreds, but they may aid in detection of carriers in kindreds in which affected males possess excess factor IX antigen. Measurement of bovine thromboplastin time may help detect an occasional carrier with low-normal factor IX clotting activity from a kindred with hemophilia B_M, a variant of hemophilia with prolonged prothrombin time with bovine thromboplastin, but will not help in recognizing carriers with high-normal factor IX clotting activity.

As in hemophilia A, measurement of cord blood factor IX activity can establish the diagnosis of hemophilia B at birth.

► [About one third of these 92 patients with hemophilia B had evidence of an abnormal factor IX molecule. In those kindreds in which affected males had antigen in excess of procoagulant activity, some but not all carriers also had excess factor IX antigen. The situation in hemophilia B in regard to detection of carriers is therefore not so well characterized as in hemophilia A (see preceding article). – Ed.] ◄

Factor IX Levels in Patients with Hemophilia B (Christmas Disease) Following Transfusion with Concentrates of Factor IX or Fresh Frozen Plasma (FFP). Fresh frozen plasma provided the basis of replacement therapy for hemophilia B until concentrates of factor IX became available, but some concentrates appear to carry a high risk of hepatitis B, and thromboembolism has also been described. N. Peter Zauber and Jack Levin[6] (Johns Hopkins Univ.) studied rela-

TABLE 1.—Initial Response to Different Types of Concentrates of Factor IX

Source of Factor IX concentrate	Number of transfusion episodes	Number of patients	Increase of Factor IX per U/kg (mean)
Proplex[R] (Hyland, USA)	17	11	1.10%
Konyne[R] (Cutter, USA)	52	18	0.98%
British	56	31	0.65%
PPSB (French)	31	16	1.14%
Swedish	11	8	0.57%

(6) Medicine (Baltimore) 56:213–224, May, 1977.

TABLE 2.—HALF-LIVES ($T^{1/2}$) OF FACTOR IX AFTER TRANSFUSION

	Source of Factor IX	Number of transfusion episodes	Number of patients	$T^{1/2}$ (mean)
$T^{1/2}$ of the Second Component	Concentrate	89	60	27.5 hr
	FFP	12	6	25.9 hr
$T^{1/2}$ of the First Component	Concentrate	33	18	4.5 hr
	FFP	10	4	2.7 hr
Direct $T^{1/2}$	Concentrate	14	10	6.4 ± 1.0 hr
	FFP	4	3	3.5 ± 0.6 hr

tionships between the dose and initial posttransfusion factor IX levels, the biologic half-life of transfused factor IX and the necessary frequency of transfusion in 171 separate transfusion episodes involving 86 patients with factor IX deficiency, seen in 1964–76. Detailed analysis of 20 previously described patients who received factor IX in 32 transfusion episodes was possible; responses in 11 of the authors' patients who received factor IX in 26 episodes and 11 who received FFP in 12 episodes were analyzed also.

The mean initial response in 32 previously reported transfusion episodes was a rise in the factor IX level of 0.82% per unit/kg. The mean initial response to concentrate therapy in 26 determinations in the authors' patients was 1.01% per unit/kg. The response to FFP therapy in 12 episodes was only 0.5% per unit/kg. The responses to factor IX are summarized in Table 1 and factor IX half-lives are given in Table 2. The mean direct half-life calculated for 7 previous transfusion episodes was 6.2 hours and for 7 episodes involving concentrate, 6.6 hours. The mean direct half-life after 4 episodes with FFP was only 3.5 hours. Patients who bled had a significantly shorter half-life than those who did not bleed. There was no difference in mean direct half-life after concentrate therapy whether or not previous treatment had been administered.

An increase in factor IX of 1% (0.01 unit)/unit administered per kg follows the transfusion of American concentrates. The initial frequency of transfusion therapy should be based on a direct half-life of only 6–8 hours. Wide patient-to-patient variation may exist, regardless of the method of administration, and factor IX levels should be measured during the treatment of any significant hemorrhagic episode. This will show that the desired levels have been achieved, detect the presence of a circulating anticoagulant and avoid excessive overtreatment with a valuable, expensive biologic resource.

► [Hemophilia B occurs with approximately one-fourth the frequency of hemophilia A. Its overall prevalence in the United States is approximately 2–3 per 100,000 population. It therefore represents a significant disease problem. The present study was undertaken with the objective of acquiring data regarding the use of factor IX concentrates. After infusion of concentrates, average recoveries of 25–50% of predicted values have been observed, suggesting an initial space of distribution of 2.5 times the plasma volume. Thrombotic episodes and alterations in coagulation have been associated with factor IX concentrates, especially in the presence of liver disease. This article stresses the need for monitoring factor IX levels during replacement therapy. – Ed.]

Syndrome of Acquired Factor X Deficiency and Systemic Amyloidosis: In Vivo Studies of the Metabolic Fate of Factor X. An acquired form of factor X deficiency has been described in association with systemic amyloidosis. The condition appears to be characterized by enhanced destruction rather than reduced synthesis of factor X. Patients have usually died rapidly of bleeding or amyloid infiltration of vital organs. Bruce Furie, Edith Greene and Barbara C. Furie[7] (Tufts Univ.) evaluated a therapeutic strategy with use of bovine factor X as replacement therapy in a man with the syndrome. The patient, aged 49, had had a myocardial infarction and a bleeding duodenal ulcer before presenting with calf pain and recent mucosal bleeding and muscle weakness. Study elsewhere had shown an isolated factor X deficiency. Intermittent episodes of hypotension and bradycardia secondary to heart block occurred and the patient gradually deteriorated and, despite melphalan and prednisone therapy, died with severe anasarca, liver failure and hyperkalemia.

Infusion of human or bovine ^{131}I-labeled factor X established a triphasic plasma clearance pattern. About 85% of the factor disappeared with a half-time of less than 30 seconds, whereas subsequent phases had half-times of 90 minutes and 9 hours, respectively. Factor X in plasma did not appear to be rapidly modified or degraded. Relatively minor amounts were cleared into the urine. A diffuse distribution of activity over the body surface was observed, with concentration in the hepatic and splenic regions.

Factor X deficiency associated with systemic amyloidosis is due to binding of factor X to body tissue, probably within the circulatory system. Highly organized amyloid deposits in the subendothelium and perhaps the endothelium may have a high affinity and specificity for factor X. Bovine factor X does not appear to be useful for treating this coagulopathy. A detailed in vitro study of the interaction of factor X with affected tissue or purified amyloid protein should provide understanding of the relationship of factor X structure with the ultrastructure of amyloid.

► [One important lesson from this interesting study in pathophysiology is that bovine factor X does not appear to be a useful component for the rational treatment of this coagulopathy. – Ed.] ◄

Aspirin Hepatotoxicity and Disseminated Intravascular Coagulation in a patient with juvenile rheumatoid arthritis is described by J. A. Sbarbaro and R. M. Bennett[8] (Univ. of Chicago). This association has been described only once before.

Girl, 17, who previously had been healthy, acquired ankle and knee stiffness after an uncomplicated delivery, followed by fever, diffuse myalgias and polyarthritis. A diffuse macular rash and marked tenderness and swelling of many joints were noted on admission. Microcytic hypochromic anemia and diffuse hypergammaglobulinemia were documented. The sedimentation rate was 174 mm/hour. The serum glutamic-oxaloacetic transaminase was 35 IU. A

(7) N. Engl. J. Med. 297:81–85, July 14, 1977.
(8) Ann. Intern. Med. 86:183–185, February, 1977.

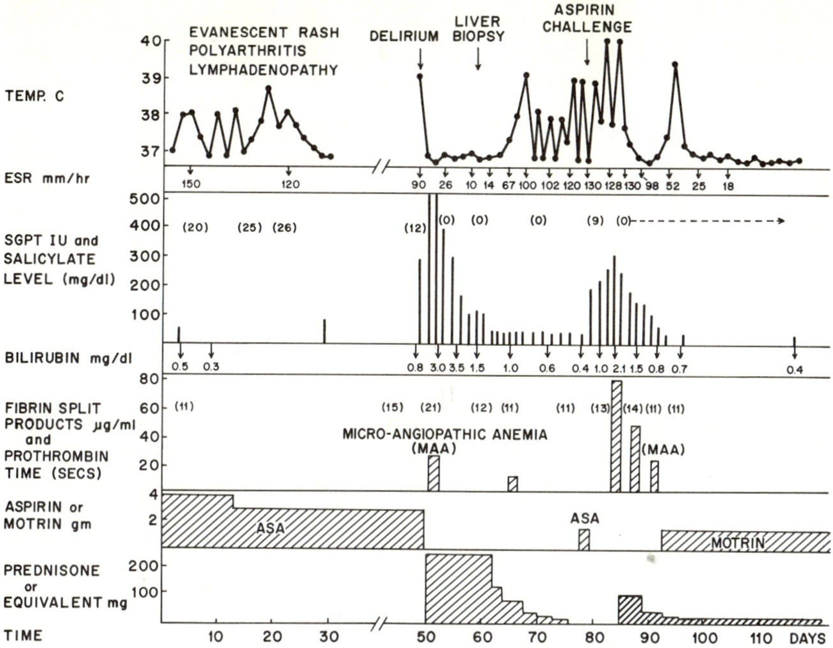

Fig 15. – Clinical course of patient. Figures in parentheses are salicylate levels *(upper)* and prothrombin times *(lower)*. (Courtesy of Sbarbaro, J. A., and Bennett, R. M.: Ann. Intern. Med. 86:183–185, February, 1977.)

bone marrow aspirate showed diffuse hypercellularity. Adult-onset Still's disease was diagnosed. The patient responded only partially to 3.6 gm aspirin daily and continued to have fever, arthritis and severe weakness, as well as draining axillary nodes. The plasma salicylate level was 12 mg/dl. The blood smear showed marked microangiopathic changes, and fibrin split products were 20 µg/ml. Solu-Medrol therapy was given with antibiotics, and the arthritis and constitutional symptoms improved markedly within 48 hours (Fig 15). All cultures were negative, and the antibiotics were withdrawn after 8 days.

A liver biopsy showed vacuolation of hepatocytes and scattered foci of inflammatory cells in areas of focal necrosis. A muscle biopsy showed focal basophilic degeneration without active vasculitis. A challenge with aspirin after steroid therapy was discontinued led to signs of microangiopathic anemia and a fibrin split-products value of 80 µg/dl. The abnormalities resolved when aspirin was stopped and steroid therapy reinstituted. Flares of acute synovitis ensued during an 8-month follow-up, but no hepatic dysfunction or coagulation disorder was evident.

Hepatic injury appears to contribute to the development of disseminated intravascular coagulation in this syndrome. The clinical manifestations depend on the degree of compensation afforded by the liver and bone marrow. A fall in platelets and fibrinogen to normal levels in a patient with active inflammatory disease may represent the start of compensated disseminated intravascular coagulation. Therapy with the nonsteroidal anti-inflammatory agent ibuprofen did not result in a recrudescence of the hepatic and coagulation disorders in the present case.

► [There is evidence that the clearance of procoagulant serum factors from the circulation is impaired in liver disease (Coleman, R. W., et al.: Am. J. Med. 52:679, 1972). The authors suggest that hepatic injury due to aspirin (see Athreya, B. H., et al.: Arthritis Rheum. 18:347, 1975) might have contributed to the coagulopathy in this patient. – Ed.]

Estrogen-Containing Oral Contraceptive Agents: Basis for Their Thrombogenicity. Some estrogens cause venous thromboembolism in man, but the mechanism of this effect is obscure. Protection from thrombosis may be obtained with heparin through increasing the reaction rate between activated factor X (Xa) and antithrombin III, but it is not clear that a reduction in Xa inhibitory activity diminishes protection against thrombosis. Stanford Wessler, Sanford N. Gitel, Livia S. Wan and Bernard S. Pasternack[9] (New York Univ.) assayed antithrombin III and Xa inhibitory activity in 105 women who were attending a family planning clinic (57 were receiving oral contraceptives) and in 7 patients with congenital deficiencies of antithrombin III.

No substantial differences in antithrombin III levels were found between the contraceptive users and nonusers, but Xa inhibitory activity was significantly reduced in the contraceptive users. Patient age and type of contraceptive agent were not related to Xa inhibitory activity, and the reduction was not time dependent. Five of the 7 patients with deficient antithrombin III had clinical episodes of venous thrombosis or pulmonary embolism. Their antithrombin III levels were 46–52% of normal, and Xa inhibitory activities were 34–57% of normal. Small amounts of heparin increased Xa inhibitory activity when added to plasma from control subjects or from women who were using contraceptives, but the quantity of antithrombin III remained constant. Heparin increased Xa inhibitory activity when added to plasma congenitally deficient in antithrombin III, but not to the same extent as in women with low Xa inhibitory activity who were taking oral contraceptives.

Mean Xa inhibitory activity is significantly reduced in women who are taking oral contraceptives. It is reasonable to suggest that the increased tendency to thrombosis in patients with antithrombin III deficiency is due to a reduced amount of antithrombin III in their plasma. When Xa inhibitory activity is below 60%, an increased tendency to thrombosis may be present. Such a subject may be at an increased risk for thrombosis if exposed to surgery, trauma or other events that can initiate the thrombotic process. If this is confirmed, low-dose heparin might be given prophylactically to women on oral contraception who require emergency surgery or are subjected to trauma.

► [The thesis that decreased Xa inhibitory activity may be in part responsible for the increased venous thrombosis associated with oral contraceptives is interesting. In a preliminary report by Sagar et al. (Fifth International Society for Thrombosis and Haemostasis, Paris, 1975), 37 young women undergoing minor abdominal surgery were followed postoperatively by ^{125}I-labeled fibrinogen extremity scanning. Deep venous thrombosis diagnosed by scans developed in 6 of 22 women (27%) taking oral contraceptives, and all 6 had preoperative Xa inhibitory activities at or below 50% of normal by an assay similar to that used in the present study. Deep venous thrombosis did not

(9) J.A.M.A. 236:2179–2182, Nov. 8, 1976.

develop in the other 16 women taking oral contraceptives or the 15 matched controls. These findings are in keeping with earlier data that have demonstrated a threefold to sixfold increased incidence in postoperative venous thromboembolism in women receiving estrogen-containing contraceptives at the time of surgery, compared to their controls (Vessey et al.: Br. Med. J. 3:123, 1970). — Ed.] ◄

Noninvasive Screening for Venous Thromboembolic Disease. Venous thromboembolism is a frequent occurrence and 8% of all hospital deaths are due primarily to a major pulmonary embolus, usually clinically unsuspected. Y. B. Gordon, E. D. Cooke, Sally A. Bowcock, Susan M. Ratky, M. F. Pilcher and T. Chard[1] (London) found that a combination of two noninvasive techniques, thermographic scanning of the lower limbs and estimation of serum levels of fibrin-fibrinogen degradation fragment E (FgE), is a safe and practical means of monitoring medical patients in whom the diagnosis is suspected. Ninety-three patients with a presumptive diagnosis of venous thromboembolism, 81 of them inpatients, were studied. The 63 women and 31 men were aged 25–81. All patients had bilateral ascending phlebography, thermography and estimation of serum FgE levels. Those with clinical evidence of pulmonary embolism had perfusion lung scanning with ^{99m}Tc-albumin. A typical abnormal thermograph is shown in Figure 16.

Thirty-four patients had evidence of deep venous thrombosis (DVT)

Fig 16. — Ascending phlebography of the right thigh and bilateral gray-tone thermography of both thighs. The phlebograph shows recent thrombus in the superficial femoral vein. The thermograph shows an increase in the temperature of the medial aspect of the right thigh, whereas the normal thigh has an overall gray tone. (Courtesy of Gordon, Y. B., et al.: Br. J. Haematol. 35:505–510, April, 1977.)

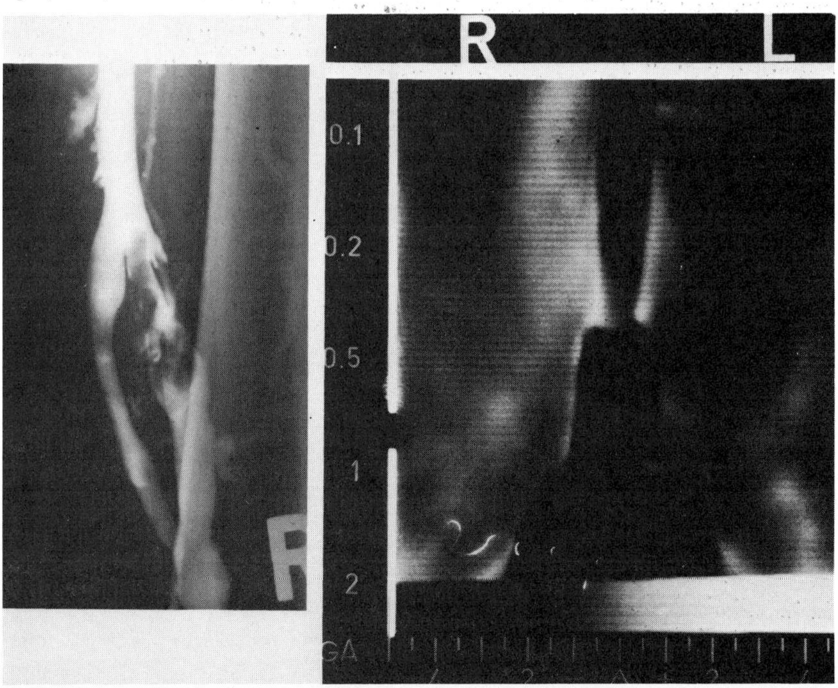

(1) Br. J. Haematol. 35:505–510, April, 1977.

on phlebography; 19 had DVT extending above the knee. A comparison with thermography showed one false positive result and one false negative result. Serum FgE levels were higher in the patients with DVT; a level of 400 μg/L distinguished clearly between the normal and abnormal groups. No patient with symptoms confined to the legs and without DVT had a level above 300 μg/L. All 8 patients with clinical and lung scan evidence of pulmonary embolism had serum FgE levels exceeding 800 μg/L.

The unreliability of diagnosing DVT clinically is paralleled by the difficulty of diagnosing pulmonary embolism clinically. Elevated FgE levels are associated with thrombus extending to the knee or above and a much increased risk of embolism. Negative results of both thermography and FgE determination exclude venous thromboembolism and avoid both invasive procedures and the haphazard administration of potentially hazardous anticoagulant therapy. Thermography reveals the local lesion in the lower limbs and serum FgE levels indicate the likelihood of an embolic episode. Positive results make further investigation and treatment mandatory, especially when extensive DVT is diagnosed. The combined technique is easy to apply and the results are available quickly.

► [At present, clinical suspicion of thromboembolism is generally followed by an invasive procedure such as venography or by ^{125}I-fibrinogen scanning. The authors suggest that the combination of thermography and the measurement of the concentration of fibrinogen degradation fragment E also serves as effective screening for venous thromboembolic disease.

Bilateral ascending venography remains the definitive diagnostic procedure, although it has certain limitations. It is inconvenient, moderately technically demanding, has minor radiation hazards and is not easily repeated. The ^{125}I-fibrinogen uptake is positive only when the thrombus is evolving and continues to deposit fibrin. Thrombi above the midthigh are not reliably detected by the fibrinogen method. – Ed.] ◄

Miscellaneous

Clinical Course and Survival after Elective Splenectomy in 19 Patients with Primary Myelofibrosis. The advantages of splenectomy in myelofibrosis do not always outweigh the mortality and complications. H. Mulder, J. Steenbergen and C. Haanen[2] (Univ. of Nijmegen) report a follow-up study of 11 men and 8 women with primary myelofibrosis and myeloid metaplasia (MMM) who underwent elective splenectomy as soon as the diagnosis was confirmed. All patients had increased fibrous tissue, collagen and reticulin in the bone marrow; proved extramedullary hemopoiesis in the spleen; leukoerythroblastosis in the peripheral blood; and splenic enlargement. Mean patient age at diagnosis was 56 years; mean follow-up after splenectomy was 19.1 months. Bone marrow cellularity was reduced preoperatively in 15 cases. Iron kinetic studies, performed in 9 patients, showed increased plasma iron turnover rate and reduced red blood cell iron incorporation in all 9. All 6 patients studied for red blood cell survival had reduced survival and increased splenic sequestration.

The mean time between admission and operation in 17 cases was 2.4 months. The duration of symptoms and splenic size were slightly correlated. Nine patients had complications during or directly connected with splenectomy. Three had intra-abdominal bleeding with hemorrhagic shock and required reoperation. One patient died of portal vein thrombosis. One required ligation of the inferior cava for rupture. Three patients had Australia antigen-positive hepatitis. The number of immature white blood cells in the peripheral blood declined in 13 patients after splenectomy. Normoblasts disappeared completely in 7 cases. Four patients had an increase in immature white blood cells and 8 an increase in nucleated red blood cells in the peripheral blood. The quality of life improved in all surviving patients. Two patients died of causes unrelated to the disease. The corrected median survival after splenectomy was 55 months.

These results warrant a further trial of elective splenectomy in an early stage of primary myelofibrosis and myeloid metaplasia. Splenectomy appears not to have reduced life expectancy in the present series, and the quality of life was improved in all surviving patients.

► [The decision regarding splenectomy in myeloid metaplasia is usually extremely difficult. When surgery is delayed until disease is advanced, the operation is hazardous and there is a high incidence of serious morbidity or mortality. In advanced disease the spleen is huge and often bound to the surrounding peritoneum by vascular adhesions. These factors combine to make the surgery technically difficult and inadvisable for the novice surgeon.

This article examines the results of splenectomy in relatively early disease. Even in this situation the incidence of operative complications was impressive, but mortality

(2) Br. J. Haematol. 35:419–427, March, 1977.

was low (1 death among 19 patients). The authors state that both the hematologic status and the quality of life improved in 17 of 19 patients. It should be noted, however, that the period of follow-up was relatively short for a chronic disease (a mean of 19 months). I shall maintain a "wait and see" attitude until all the facts are in before advising early splenectomy. – Ed.] ◄

Continuous-Flow Plasmapheresis in Management of Severe Rhesus Disease. J. Graham-Pole, W. Barr and M. L. N. Willoughby[3] (Univ. of Glasgow) used continuous-flow plasmapheresis in 8 patients with exceptionally severe rhesus isoimmunization and determined whether circulating maternal anti-D antibody can be removed faster than it reaccumulates and whether a decrease in fetal hemolysis results. All patients but 1 had amniotic fluid spectrophotometry before treatment. Maternal antibody was estimated by both the indirect antiglobulin assay and the anti-D immunoglobulin concentration. Volumes of 2.5 – 7 L plasma were exchanged for reconstituted freeze-dried plasma or plasma protein fraction with use of an Aminco Cell Separator. Fresh frozen plasma was given after plasma protein fraction to replace clotting factors. Heparin was used as anticoagulant. Plasmapheresis was begun at 16 – 27 weeks' gestation and continued until planned intrauterine transfusion, delivery or the rhesus disease became uncontrolled again. Totals of 24 – 237 L plasma were exchanged over periods of 7 – 16 weeks.

The anti-D level after each run was about half the pretreatment level. Most patients had high initial antibody levels, which were prevented from rising. The value after the final plasmapheresis many weeks later was lower in 7 of the 8 patients and in 5 it was below 4 mg/L (15 IU/ml), below which level fetal death is unlikely in the natural disease. The fall in individual levels was statistically significant. In 3 patients the disease was controlled but the fetus died as a direct result of intrauterine transfusion; 2 other infants survived after delivery, whereas 1 died of respiratory distress syndrome and 2 died after worsening rhesus disease. The only maternal side effect was hypocalcemic symptoms from the citrate in freeze-dried plasma. Immunoglobulin levels remained normal throughout intensive plasmapheresis.

Intensive plasmapheresis can prevent a rise in anti-D antibody levels as pregnancy progresses in patients with exceptionally severe rhesus disease. The fetus can be saved through plasmapheresis alone. Fetal hemolysis may be reduced by this treatment. Only highly motivated patients should be selected for this treatment. The chief contribution of intensive plasmapheresis may be to tide the fetus over to 30 weeks' gestation or later, when intrauterine transfusion is less hazardous.

► [This is an innovative approach to severe anti-Rh hemolytic disease. The observations suggest that our preconceptions about the effectiveness of plasmapheresis in sustained reductions of antibody titer may be wrong. We have generally thought that plasmapheresis is ineffective in dealing with IgG antibody which is distributed both in the vascular space and extracellular fluid volume and whose synthetic rate is high. The present study suggests this may not be true for anti-D antibody. It would seem, however, that the technique requires perfection before it is applied more widely. The reported fetal survival of 25% does not balance the potential risks of bleeding and hepatitis. – Ed.] ◄

(3) Br. Med. J. 1:1185 – 1188, May 7, 1977.

Systemic Capillary Leak Syndrome and Monoclonal IgG Gammopathy: Studies in a Sixth Patient and Review of the Literature. John P. Atkinson, Thomas A. Waldmann, Sidney F. Stein, Jeffrey A. Gelfand, Walter J. MacDonald, Louis W. Heck, Edwin L. Cohen, Allen P. Kaplan and Michael M. Frank[4] report data on a patient with recurrent episodes of increased systemic capillary permeability resulting in angioedema and an associated monoclonal IgG gammopathy and present a review of 5 previous cases.

Man, 38, had had an attack of hemoconcentration and shock due to loss of intravascular fluid about 3 years before, followed by further attacks of varying severity, progressive in frequency to once every 4 days. Typically a peculiar nervous or irritable feeling was followed by abdominal fullness and discomfort that progressed to explosive watery bowel movements, weakness and myalgias of the extremities and diffuse interstitial edema. The attacks reached their height in 12–24 hours and lasted 1–3 days, ending with polyuria and a sense of well-being. One in 10 attacks was severe, with a hematocrit over 65, marked tachycardia and hypotension. Fluid reentered the intravascular space when normal capillary integrity returned. Seven older siblings had had no similar illness. Hemoconcentration and mild prerenal azotemia were consistently present during attacks. The right kidney exhibited multiple cysts and mild interstitial nephritis at laparotomy. An IgG paraprotein and intermittent elevation of serum transaminases were the only abnormalities present between episodes.

The course was not altered by treatment with epsilonaminocaproic acid, thorazine and promethazine, acetylsalicylic acid, diphenhydramine or dexchlorpheniramine, prednisone, 9-α-fluorohydrocortisone and salt-loading, atropine or plasma transfusions. Normal endocrine function was demonstrated. Abnormalities in bradykinin generation did not change in relationship to the attacks. The patient died with tracheal obstruction due to airway edema; death was related directly to a severe attack about 4 years after onset of the syndrome. Autopsy showed cardiomegaly and subendocardial hemorrhage related to resuscitative efforts, stellate periportal hepatic fibrosis, chronic cholecystitis and cholelithiasis and a microscopic, nonbeta islet cell tumor of the pancreas.

The only persistent abnormality in the patient's serum was a monoclonal IgG paraprotein with λ light chains of subclass 2. Injections of serum and plasma into the patient's skin did not produce a reaction. No vasoactive material was detected. Up to half the total circulating albumin passed to the extravascular spaces during edematous periods.

Five similar cases have been reported in the literature. There was an IgG paraprotein in at least 4 and possibly all. In most cases the disease appears to run a course such that a lethal attack will eventually occur. Treatment was unsuccessful and attempts to prevent episodes with a wide variety of agents have failed.

► [This is an extremely thorough description of an extraordinarily interesting syndrome whose pathogenesis remains totally obscure. – Ed.] ◄

Intravascular Hemolysis, Thrombocytopenia, Leukopenia and Circulating Immune Complexes after Jejunal-Ileal Bypass Surgery. Immune complex-induced arthritis has been described at varying intervals after jejunocolonic and jejunoileal bypass surgery for

(4) Medicine (Baltimore) 56:225–239, May, 1977.

the treatment of obesity. J. L. Moake, W. V. Kageler, P. L. Cimo, R. W. Blakely, R. D. Rossen and W. Haesse[5] (Univ. of Texas, Houston) report data on a patient with a jejunoileal anastomosis who had hemolysis, thrombocytopenia and neutropenia, associated with the presence of circulating immune complexes and reduced serum titers of complement components.

Man, 25, had a jejunoileal bypass operation for obesity and had a weight decline from 195 to 100 kg in the next 2 years, with mild diarrhea. He became weak and passed tea-colored urine 2 years postoperatively. The hemoglobin had fallen to 7–8 gm/100 ml and the platelets to 9,000/cu mm. Splenomegaly was noted. Schistocytes and spherocytes were present on blood films and reticulocytes were 8%. The serum hemoglobin was 7.4 mg/dl and hemopexin was reduced to 7 mg/dl. Hemoglobin and hemosiderin were present in the urine. The bone marrow showed erythroid and megakaryocytic hyperplasia and normal iron stores. Hemoglobin electrophoresis was normal. Serum IgM was increased to 315 mg/dl. Fever and transient leukopenia developed and prednisone therapy was given. The blood elements returned to near normal over 2 weeks and the urine became clear. Prednisone was withdrawn over 6 weeks. The patient has been asymptomatic with normal blood counts during 30 months of follow-up.

Antiserums to C4-C3 agglutinated this patient's red blood cells. The serum induced 23% complement-dependent lysis of aminoethylisothiouronium bromide-treated normal platelets (abnormal, lysis exceeding 5%). Increased ^{125}I-C1q binding activity was present in the patient's serum. Serum levels of C4 and C3 were reduced and later returned to normal.

► [Wands and his colleagues (N. Engl. J. Med. 294:121, 1976) have suggested that in patients with intestinal bypass shunts, bacterial antigens from overgrown blind loops enter the blood, form immune complexes with circulating antibodies and may induce manifestations of immune complex disease such as acute arthritis. The authors of this article postulate that a similar immune complex mechanism might have accounted for complement activation and blood cell destruction in the patient whom they describe. —Ed.] ◄

(5) Ann. Intern. Med. 86:576–578, May, 1977.

PART FOUR

THE HEART AND BLOOD VESSELS

EUGENE BRAUNWALD, M.D.

Ischemic Heart Disease

Risk Factors

HDL Cholesterol and Other Lipids in Coronary Heart Disease: Cooperative Lipoprotein Phenotyping Study. William P. Castelli, Joseph T. Doyle, Tavia Gordon, Curtis G. Hames, Marthana C. Hjortland, Stephen B. Hulley, Abraham Kagan and William J. Zukel[1] analyzed data from the Cooperative Lipoprotein Phenotyping Study of subjects drawn from epidemiologic studies of five diverse populations. The groups included male Civil Service employees in Albany, New York, a general population of blacks and whites in Georgia, a general population in Framingham, Massachusetts, and populations of men of Japanese ancestry living in Honolulu and in San Francisco. Fasting lipid levels were related to coronary heart disease (CHD) prevalence in these groups. Two thirds of patients with CHD had definite myocardial infarction and about half had angina pectoris.

Mean high-density lipoprotein (HDL) cholesterol levels were consistently lower in persons with CHD. This finding obtained for both angina and myocardial infarction. Differences in total and low-density lipoprotein (LDL) cholesterol were also apparent but were less uniform than those in HDL cholesterol. The prevalence of CHD in subjects with extremely low HDL cholesterol levels was about twice that of subjects with intermediate levels. Correlations between HDL cholesterol and other fractions were of a low order of magnitude. No association between triglyceride and CHD was evident. At each level of HDL cholesterol there was a highly regular increase in CHD prevalence with increasing LDL cholesterol levels. Both triglyceride and LDL cholesterol were significantly associated with CHD prevalence when the other was held constant.

The data indicate a direct relation between fasting plasma triglyceride concentration and the prevalence of CHD. The value of partitioning total cholesterol in assessing CHD risk is unequivocal. A lipid profile based on HDL and LDL cholesterol and triglyceride is preferred for measuring the CHD risk associated with lipid characteristics, but the appropriate statistical weighting remains to be determined.

► [In the 1977 YEAR BOOK (p. 297), the concept that serum high-density lipoproteins (HDL) are a negative risk factor for atherosclerotic heart disease was introduced, and this article provides substantial support for this theory. It would appear that HDL provide a mechanism for the transport of cholesterol out of cells and inhibit the uptake and degradation of low-density lipoproteins (LDL) in arterial smooth muscle cells.

Ischemic heart disease is a major cause of mortality among the Maori in New Zealand. Stanhope et al. (Lancet 1:968, 1977) showed that this race has lower serum HDL than whites, whereas LDL cholesterol levels do not show any race differences. I sus-

(1) Circulation 55:767–772, May, 1977.

pect that some mathematical relation between LDL and HDL (perhaps as simple as the LDL/HDL ratio or the difference between LDL and HDL) will prove to be a more useful expression of cardiovascular risk than the concentration of either alone. – Ed.] ◄

Regulation of Cholesterol Synthesis by Low-Density Lipoprotein in Isolated Human Lymphocytes: Comparison of Cells from Normal Subjects and Patients with Homozygous Familial Hypercholesterolemia and Abetalipoproteinemia. The ability of cultured human cells to utilize low-density lipoprotein (LDL) cholesterol depends on presence of a high-affinity cell surface receptor that binds LDL. Y. K. Ho, Jerry R. Faust, David W. Bilheimer, Michael S. Brown and Joseph L. Goldstein[2] (Univ. of Texas, Dallas) used a lymphocyte model to determine whether the LDL receptor plays a role in regulating cholesterol synthesis in nondividing cells freshly isolated from the body.

Studies were done in normal subjects, 4 patients with homozygous familial hypercholesterolemia (FH) and 2 patients with abetalipoproteinemia. Incorporation by intact lymphocytes of labeled acetate into cholesterol and of labeled oleate into lipids was determined.

Rate of cholesterol synthesis from ^{14}C-acetate was low in blood lymphocytes freshly isolated from 17 normal subjects and the 4 subjects with homozygous FH, but was twofold to fourfold above normal in cells from the 2 subjects with abetalipoproteinemia. Rate of cholesterol synthesis increased fivefold to 15-fold when lymphocytes from subjects in all three groups were incubated for 48 – 72 hours in the absence of lipoproteins. Addition of plasma LDL, but not HDL, rapidly suppressed

Fig 1. – Effect of LDL on cholesterol synthesis from ^{14}C-acetate in normal (*solid circles* and *solid triangles*) and FH homozygote (*open circles* and *open triangles*) lymphocytes previously incubated in the absence of lipoproteins. Lymphocytes were isolated in **A** from a healthy woman aged 23 years *(P. H.)* and a girl aged 13 years with homozygous FH *(K. W.)* and, in **B**, from a healthy boy aged 11 years *(D. C.)* and a girl aged 8 years with homozygous FH *(M. C.)*. After the cells had been incubated at 37 C for 55 hours in the absence of lipoprotein, each flask received the indicated final concentration of LDL. Incubation was continued for another 9 hours, and then incorporation of ^{14}C-acetate into ^{14}C-cholesterol was measured with a 4-hour labeling period. Each value represents the average of duplicate incubations. The 100% of control values for P. H., K. W., D. C. and M. C. were 370, 195, 392 and 1,171 pM, respectively, of ^{14}C-acetate converted to ^{14}C-cholesterol per hour per mg protein. (Courtesy of Ho, Y. K., et al.: J. Exp. Med. 145:1531 – 1549, June, 1977.)

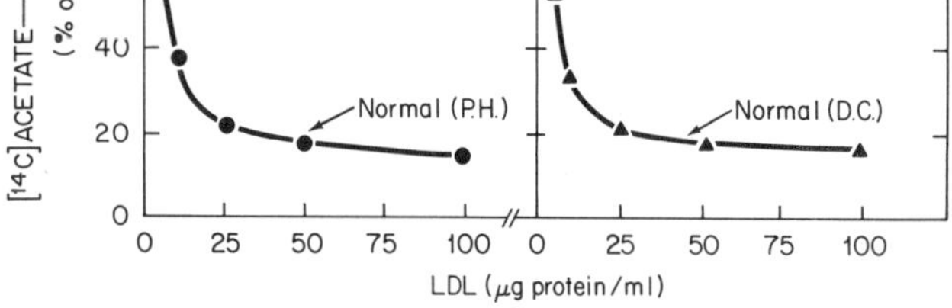

(2) J. Exp. Med. 145:1531 – 1549, June, 1977.

cholesterol synthesis in lymphocytes from normal subjects, but cells from the FH homozygotes were resistant to LDL-mediated suppression of cholesterol synthesis (Fig 1). Also, LDL suppressed induction of an enhanced rate of sterol synthesis when added to normal lymphocytes; this effect also occurred to a limited extent in cells from FH homozygotes. Only the FH lymphocytes could be made resistant to this action of LDL by inclusion of lipoprotein-deficient serum plus HDL in the incubation medium.

With previous data indicating a deficiency of LDL receptors in lymphocytes from FH homozygotes, the present findings support the hypothesis that the interaction of plasma LDL with its cell surface receptor serves to regulate cholesterol synthesis in human lymphocytes.

► [The interesting model utilized in this study results from the observation that rapidly divided cultured human cells, such as fibroblasts and lymphoblasts, can derive all of their required cholesterol from the LDL that is present in the culture medium. Cholesterol synthesis in human lymphocytes can be suppressed by the addition of LDL, but not HDL, to the incubation medium. However, the suppression of cholesterol synthesis requires LDL receptors which are severely deficient in the homozygous form of familial hyperlipoproteinemia. The exciting work carried out by Brown, Goldstein and their collaborators provides evidence that supports the hypothesis that cholesterol synthesis is regulated by the interaction of plasma LDL with its self-surface receptor and provides a molecular basis for the abnormalities existing in hyperlipoproteinemia, a principal risk factor in coronary artery disease.

These workers have demonstrated either a lack of LDL receptors (receptor negative) or a qualitative alteration in the LDL receptors (receptor defective) on the cell membrane of cultured fibroblasts of patients with familial hypercholesterolemia. The inability to bind LDL is associated with abnormalities of lipid and lipoprotein metabolism, including a lack of feedback inhibition of the rate-limiting enzyme of cholesterol biosynthesis, as well as decreased conversion of cholesterol to cholester ester. Chatterjee et al. (Proc. Natl. Acad. Sci. U.S.A. 73:4339, 1976) have demonstrated alterations of cell surface glycosphingolipids and of other major lipid classes in fibroblasts of patients with homozygous and heterozygous familial hypercholesterolemia, indicating that the defective regulation of lipid metabolism in this syndrome may be even more extensive than previously realized. – Ed.] ◄

Regression and Progression of Early Femoral Atherosclerosis in Treated Hyperlipoproteinemic Patients. Studies in hyperlipoproteinemic animals indicate that established atherosclerotic lesions can regress on dietary and clofibrate therapy, with cholestyramine therapy and after partial ileal bypass. Information on regression of atherosclerosis in treated hyperlipoproteinemic human beings is more limited. Robert Barndt, Jr., David H. Blankenhorn, Donald W. Crawford and Samuel H. Brooks[3] (Los Angeles) have studied patients with earlier atherosclerosis than previous workers, using a radiographic procedure more sensitive to small changes in lesions. Twenty-five outpatients aged 22–65 years, most often seen for inadequate lowering of blood lipids on drug therapy or difficulty in compliance with a diet, were studied. Nine had had an infarction or angina, but only 1 had claudication. Twelve had type IV and 13 had type II hyperlipoproteinemia. Hyperlipoproteinemic-type specific diet therapy was prescribed, with weight loss where indicated. Eight type IV patients received clofibrate, and 4 received tibric acid. Seven type II patients received clofibrate plus neomycin and 6, clofibrate alone.

---

(3) Ann. Intern. Med. 86:139–146, February, 1977.

The average interval between angiograms was 13 months. Density-matched, smooth vessel images were used as standards in detecting vessel edge roughness. A normal vessel segment was used as a reference for detecting changes in vessel lumen by a comparison procedure. Thirteen patients showed progression of disease, 3 showed no change and 9 showed regression. Patients showing regression had serum cholesterol changes that were significant at the 0.1% level, whereas those showing progression had no significant change in average serum cholesterol levels. Patients with regression also had changes in serum triglycerides and blood pressure that were significant at the 5% level, whereas those with progression did not. Glucose tolerance did not change significantly in either group. In patient-by-patient analysis of risk factors, the only variable significantly related to change in atherosclerosis per month was systolic blood pressure.

These results should not be interpreted too broadly, and they do not indicate whether treatment of hyperlipoproteinemia will improve more advanced arterial lesions in patients with symptomatic vascular disease. It seems encouraging, nonetheless, that early human atherosclerosis associated with hyperlipoproteinemia can improve with treatment.

► [Patients with more advanced atherosclerotic lesions treated by surgical partial ileal bypass show regression of coronary arterial lesions only occasionally. Perhaps the principal lesson of this extremely interesting study by Barndt et al. is that it is the *early* arterial lesions that regress after treatment of hyperlipoproteinemia. Perhaps this should not come as a surprise when one considers the massive changes in the arterial wall with advanced lesions. – Ed.] ◄

Cardiovascular Disease Mortality Trends and Oral Contraceptive Use in Young Women. Valerie Beral[4] (London) analyzed mortality trends in 1955 – 72 for twenty-one countries. Data on cardiovascular disease mortality and oral contraceptive use were collected from WHO reports. Since oral contraceptives became available, changes in mortality from nonrheumatic heart disease and hypertension, cerebrovascular disease and all nonrheumatic cardiovascular diseases in women aged 15 – 44 years have been strongly associated with changes in the prevalence of oral contraceptive use in each country. The relationship is highly specific for women of reproductive age. The relative risks of death from heart disease and hypertension, cerebrovascular disease and all cardiovascular diseases for oral contraceptive users were 5: 1, 2: 1 and 3: 1, respectively.

The findings suggest that the range of vascular diseases affected by oral contraceptive use and the size of the associated risks may be greater than previously recognized. The increased risks of cardiovascular disease may exist not only with pills containing high estrogen doses, but also with the new "low-dose" pills. There appears to be a true increase in the risk of death from myocardial infarction, hypertension, cerebrovascular diseases and possibly all cardiovascular diseases in women taking the pill. All the associations were evident for 1971 – 72, when oral contraceptives containing over 0.05 mg estrogen were no

(4) Lancet 2:1047 – 1052, Nov. 13, 1976.

longer being used in many countries. With 50 million women using oral contraceptives in 1973 and the number increasing annually, it seems particularly urgent to clarify the extent and size of the risks associated with oral contraceptive usage.

► [An excellent review of the association between oral contraceptives and myocardial infarction was provided by Ory (J.A.M.A. 237:2619, 1977). It appears that in women with other risk factors for coronary arteriosclerosis, such as cigarette smoking, oral contraceptive use increases the risk of myocardial infarction quite substantially. On the other hand, in women without other risk factors, oral contraceptive use increases the risk of myocardial infarction only slightly. Therefore, it is wise to question the use of oral contraceptives by women aged 40 years or older who have other risk factors for arteriosclerosis. The mechanism by which oral contraceptive usage may contribute to or precipitate myocardial infarction is unknown. These agents have been shown to raise the levels of arterial pressure, serum triglycerides, cholesterol, low-density lipoproteins and very-low-density lipoproteins; the arterial lesions in women taking oral contraceptives have shown intimal hyperplasia with luminal occlusion (Arthes: Chest 70:574, 1976).—Ed.] ◄

Alcohol Consumption and Blood Pressure: Kaiser-Permanente Multiphasic Health Examination Data. Several studies have raised the possibility that regular consumption of alcoholic beverages is associated with hypertension. Arthur L. Klatsky, Gary D. Friedman, Abraham B. Siegelaub and Marie J. Gérard[5] (Kaiser-Permanente Med. Center, Oakland, Calif.) present data showing an association between alcohol consumption and blood pressure in over 83,000 men and women of three races, 83.5% of them white. Health checkup questionnaire responses were used to classify subjects by drinking habits. Data on subjects having a multiphasic checkup in 1964–68 were analyzed. A total of 110,970 subjects aged 15–79 years were examined. A total of 83,947 white, black and yellow subjects were placed in definite drinking categories.

Among white men, systolic pressure was substantially and progressively higher in those taking three or more drinks daily. A similar difference was seen in yellow men, but the relationship was less marked in black men. A substantial relationship also was observed in women. Diastolic pressure showed a similar but less marked relationship to alcohol consumption. In whites and blacks, differences in mean blood pressure translated into substantial differences in the prevalence of a systolic pressure of 160 mm Hg or above or a diastolic pressure of 95 mm Hg or above. A relationship of three or more drinks a day to higher pressures was clear within different adiposity subgroups in both sexes. Adiposity was significantly and independently related to higher blood pressure in white men and women. The relationship of adiposity to blood pressure was of the same approximate magnitude in black and yellow men and women as in whites.

These findings suggest that there may be a "threshold level" of regular alcohol consumption (usual intake of three or more drinks daily in the present categorization above which blood pressure elevations are found, and below which pressures are not higher or perhaps are slightly lower than in nondrinkers. The data, along with earlier re-

---

(5) N. Engl. J. Med. 296:1194–1200, May 26, 1977.

ports, indicate a strong possibility that regular alcohol use in critical amounts results in higher blood pressure in a large proportion of persons.

► [Additional information concerning the association between alcohol intake and hypertension is provided in the review of Mathews (Clin. Sci. Mol. Med. 51:661S, 1976), who showed that: (1) death rates from hypertension were highest in groups with the highest death rate for liver cirrhosis in Wales and (2) there was a significant association between hypertension and a history of heavy drinking in Western Australia. Putting all of these data together suggests that up to 30% of the hypertension might be attributable to alcohol use and abuse. Beevers (Lancet 2:114, 1977) showed that in hypertensive patients there was a tendency for a higher incidence of biochemical abnormalities of liver disease than in normotensive controls. However, deaths from coronary artery disease may not rise as much as might be expected from the increased incidence of hypertension (Aust. N.Z.J. Med. 6:393, 1976); for further discussion of this paradox, see the following article. – Ed.] ◄

Coffee, Alcohol and Risk of Coronary Heart Disease among Japanese Men Living in Hawaii. Katsuhiko Yano, George G. Rhoads and Abraham Kagan[6] (Honolulu) recorded levels of coffee and alcohol consumption since 1965 in a large cohort of Japanese migrants and their descendants living in Hawaii and have related the findings to the incidence of coronary heart disease during a 6-year follow-up period. The Honolulu Heart Study is a prospective epidemiologic investigation of coronary disease and stroke in a cohort of men of Japanese ancestry, born in 1900–1919 and living on Oahu in 1965. Of 8,006 men examined in 1965–68, 301 were found to have definite evidence of coronary heart disease. Another 7,705 men were followed over 6 years. Definite coronary heart disease developed in 294 men during follow-up and 43 deaths were attributed to coronary heart disease, as were 136 nonfatal myocardial infarctions, 27 cases of acute coronary insufficiency and 88 cases of angina pectoris.

There was a positive association between coffee intake and the risk of coronary heart disease, but it became statistically insignificant when cigarette smoking was taken into account. A strong negative association was found between moderate alcohol consumption, up to 60 ml per day, mainly from beer and the risk of nonfatal myocardial infarction and death from coronary heart disease. The association re-

Age-Adjusted Six-Year Incidence Rate of Total Coronary Heart Disease according to Drinking Status

Status	Men at Risk	Cases	Incidence Rate*	Significance Test for Difference†
			per 1,000	
Never (A)	2,744	121	43.6	A vs B‡
Past (B)	821	47	55.7	B vs C§
Current (C)	4,026	119	30.0	C vs A§

*Age adjusted in 5-year groups by the direct method according to the age structure of the entire population at risk.
†Based on the χ-square values with 1 degree of freedom.
‡Not significant.
§P < 0.01.

(6) N. Engl. J. Med. 297:405–409, Aug. 25, 1977.

mained significant in multivariate analysis, taking smoking and other risk factors into account. The incidence of coronary heart disease was highest for ex-drinkers, lowest for current drinkers and intermediate for lifetime totalers (table). Alcohol consumption was significantly negatively associated with the risk of "hard" cases, deaths from coronary disease and myocardial infarction, and this association became stronger when smoking and other major risk factors were taken into account.

It seems possible that the correlation of alcohol consumption with levels of α-cholesterol (positive) and β-cholesterol (negative) may partly account for the negative association observed between alcohol and coronary heart disease.

► [Alcoholic intake has a significant effect on lipid metabolism, exhibiting a positive correlation with serum high-density lipoproteins and a negative correlation with low-density lipoproteins. This may explain the fact that alcohol appears to be a positive risk factor for the development of hypertension, but a negative risk factor for the development of coronary artery disease. As far as coffee consumption is concerned, Wilhelmsen and his colleagues (Acta Med. Scand. 201:547, 1977) reported that coffee consumption was significantly associated with cigarette smoking, but have not found a strong association between coffee consumption per se and the development of myocardial infarction. – Ed.] ◄

Left Ventricular Function after Cigarette Smoking by Chronic Smokers: Comparison of Normal Subjects and Patients with Coronary Artery Disease. Hemodynamic studies have suggested that smoking causes myocardial stimulation. Abnash C. Jain, Allen F. Bowyer, Robert J. Marshall and Hiroaki Asato[7] (West Virginia Univ.) used noninvasive systolic time interval analysis to evaluate left ventricular function in 45 male long-term smokers who underwent coronary angiography for evaluation of chest pain. All had smoked one to two packs of cigarettes daily for at least 5 years. Twenty-five had symptomatic coronary artery disease, with abnormal angiograms and exercise stress ECGs but normal left ventricular angiograms. Twenty patients were classified as being normal. Studies were done with the subjects supine 2 hours after a meal, after 4 or more hours without smoking. Subjects inhaled smoke from two cigarettes containing 20 mg nicotine, and measurements were repeated 5 minutes later.

Smoking raised the heart rate and blood pressure slightly in both groups of subjects. It did not alter ejection time. The preejection period increased in all but 2 of the patients with coronary artery disease. Changes in the ratio of preejection period to left ventricular ejection time are shown in Figure 2. The group difference in ratios was highly significant. All but 1 normal subject had a decrease in external isovolumetric contraction time after smoking, whereas all but 3 of those with coronary disease had an increase in the external isovolumetric contraction time.

Left ventricular performance is reduced after cigarette smoking in subjects with preexistent significant coronary artery disease. The increased cardiac work caused by smoking may not be accompanied by an equivalent rise in total coronary flow because of obstructive lesions,

(7) Am. J. Cardiol. 39:27–31, January, 1977.

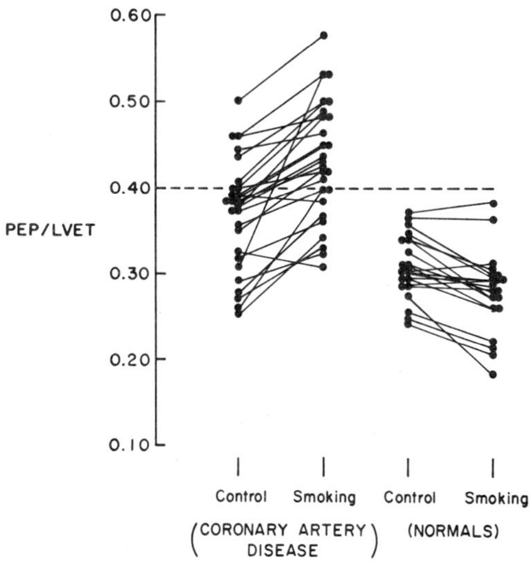

Fig 2.—Changes in preejection period *(PEP)*-left ventricular ejection time *(LVET)* ratio with smoking. (Courtesy of Jain, A. C., et al.: Am. J. Cardiol. 39:27–31, January, 1977.)

or an internal redistribution of myocardial flow may occur, leading to selective deprivation of flow to ischemic areas. Myocardial function may also be depressed by carbon monoxide.

► [It is widely recognized that cigarette smoking is an important risk factor for the development of arteriosclerotic coronary artery disease. Whereas smoking increases the degree of coronary arteriosclerosis found at autopsy, it also appears to precipitate acute events in patients with underlying coronary artery disease. It is interesting that persons who discontinue smoking have coronary heart disease rates only a little higher than persons who never smoked. The specific mechanism by which smoking triggers acute myocardial infarction is not known, but may include tissue hypoxia, acutely elevated carboxyhemoglobin concentration, increased platelet adhesiveness and sympathetic neural stimulation.

Cryer et al. (1977 YEAR BOOK, p. 270) demonstrated that smoking increases circulating levels of norepinephrine and epinephrine. The findings that smoking increases arterial pressure and pulse rate, as well as circulating levels of epinephrine and norepinephrine, combined with the observations presented by Jain et al., i.e., that patients with coronary heart disease show deterioration of left ventricular performance during smoking, may provide the basis for part of the increased risk.—Ed.] ◄

Community Education for Cardiovascular Health. The mass media, face-to-face instruction or combinations of the two may be used in community education campaigns for cardiovascular health. John W. Farquhar, Nathan Maccoby, Peter D. Wood, Janet K. Alexander, Henry Breitrose, Byron W. Brown, Jr., William L. Haskell, Alfred L. McAlister, Anthony J. Meyer, Joyce D. Nash and Michael P. Stern[8] (Stanford Univ.) used an untested combination of an extensive mass-media campaign plus a considerable amount of face-to-face instruction in a field study conducted in three northern California towns. In Gilroy and Watsonville, there were extensive mass-media campaigns over a 2-year period, and in Watsonville, face-to-face counseling was also pro-

(8) Lancet 1:1192–1195, June 4, 1977.

vided for a subset of high-risk subjects. The town of Tracy served as a control. Subjects were interviewed and examined before the campaigns began and 1 and 2 years afterward. Data were obtained from a random sample of men and women aged 35–59 years. The mass-media and counseling campaigns were designed to produce awareness of the probable causes of coronary disease and of the specific measures that may reduce risks.

The risk of cardiovascular disease increased over the 2-year period in Tracy but declined substantially in Gilroy and Watsonville. Initial improvement was greater in the community with face-to-face counseling, and health education was more successful in reducing cigarette smoking. The decrease in risk after 2 years, however, was similar in Gilroy and Watsonville. The results are shown in Figure 3.

The mass media can increase knowledge and alter health habits, but their power could be considerably enhanced if they were used to stimu-

Fig 3.—Percentage change from baseline (0) in risk of coronary heart disease after 1 and 2 years of health education among participants of three communities. Cardiovascular risk is measured by multiple logistic function of risk factors. To correct for bias resulting from exclusion of intensively instructed subjects, i.e., high-risk persons and their spouses, means for rest of subjects in high-risk and lower-risk groups were weighted to compensate for differential numbers of excluded subjects in the two risk strata. Resulting weighted means were called means of reconstituted sample, i.e., sample reconstituted after exclusion of intensively instructed subjects. Two thirds of Watsonville high-risk persons receiving face-to-face instruction were randomly assigned to intensive instruction treatment group, and one-third received health education through media only and were used as randomized control group. (Courtesy of Farquhar, J. W., et al.: Lancet 1:1192–1195, June 4, 1977.)

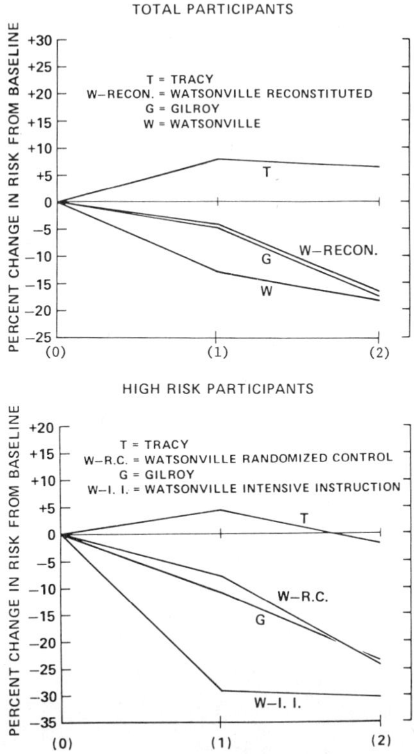

late and coordinate programs of interpersonal instruction in natural communities and to deliver forms of specialized training and counseling concerning weight loss and avoidance of smoking. Part of the prevention of premature cardiovascular disease in industrialized countries involves persuading persons to alter their life-styles, and this can be achieved at reasonable cost.

► [The interesting aspect of this study is that unlike the subjects of all previous investigations designed to reduce risk factors, in this study the participants were randomly selected from the total population, thereby providing a much more realistic basis for generalization about future public-health education efforts. It is reassuring that the changes in knowledge, behavior and physiologic end points that were observed in the 1st year of treatment were maintained through the 2d year. – Ed.] ◄

Earlobe Creases and Heart Disease. The diagonal earlobe crease is said to be correlated with coronary artery disease and thus a useful diagnostic tool, but some feel that the incidence of creases is a function of age rather than of a disease state. Carmen Doering, Chris Ruhsenberger and David S. Phillips[9] (Univ. of Oregon) evaluated these hypotheses in patients aged 30 – 80 years, admitted to a medical floor and the medical intensive-care unit of a 200-bed general hospital in a 10-week period. An earlobe crease was defined as a deep wrinkle in the lobular part of the auricle, extending for at least one third of the length of the earlobe. The findings in 50 patients with coronary heart disease (CHD) and those in 38 control patients were compared.

The two groups differed significantly in age and weight, but not in serum cholesterol, blood pressure or height. The CHD patients were older and heavier than the control patients. More CHD patients than controls had smoked. Earlobe creases were present in 88% of the CHD patients and in 36.8% of the controls, a highly significant difference. Diabetes was present in 16% of the CHD group and in 2.6% of the control group. Matching of eighteen pairs of patients and controls showed significant differences in weight and the presence of earlobe creases.

It appears that, although the incidence of earlobe creases increases with age, age alone does not account for the relationship between earlobe creases and CHD. The presence of these creases may be a useful diagnostic sign. It seems likely that, since both the incidence of creases and the incidence of CHD increase with age, both are functions of changes in the vascular system. The earlobe, being highly vascularized, may exhibit these changes by starting to crease and fold. If the changes occur early enough in the development of CHD, they might be used by the physician to screen patients for preventive measures before the disease advances. A prospective study to investigate the development of earlobe creases and CHD would be worthwhile.

► [I believe this article settles the issue of the usefulness of the earlobe crease as a simple, external marker that correlates with the presence of coronary heart disease. – Ed.] ◄

Acute Myocardial Infarction

Arteriographic Evidence of Coronary Arterial Spasm in Acute Myocardial Infarction. Coronary arterial spasm has been shown to

(9) J. Am. Geriatr. Soc. 25:183 – 185, April, 1977.

cause severe, reversible myocardial ischemia in patients with Prinzmetal's angina. In order to determine presence or absence of spasm within the first 12 hours of infarction, Philip B. Oliva and John C. Breckinridge[1] (Denver Genl. Hosp.) performed coronary arteriography before and after intracoronary nitroglycerin injection in volunteer patients who arrived at the emergency department of this hospital with historical and ECG evidence of acute infarction. Patients over age 70 and those with significant left ventricular dysfunction or significant arrhythmia or heart block were excluded from the study.

Seventeen patients who had 18 infarctions were studied. The dose of nitroglycerin injected into an acutely obstructed right coronary artery was 100 μg and that injected into an obstructed left coronary artery, 300 μg.

The 13 men and 4 women had an average age of 52 years. The interval from onset of symptoms to arteriography was less than 6 hours in 13 patients and 6 – 12½ hours in 5 patients. Three infarctions occurred in 2 patients with minimal or no coronary artery disease. Coronary arterial spasm was documented in 6 of the other 15 acute infarctions

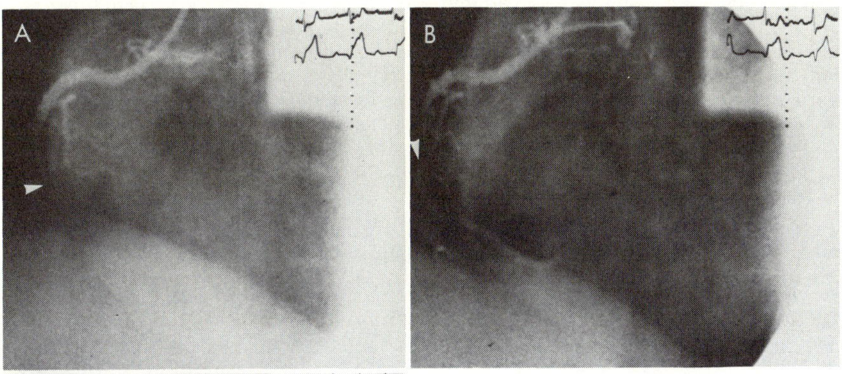

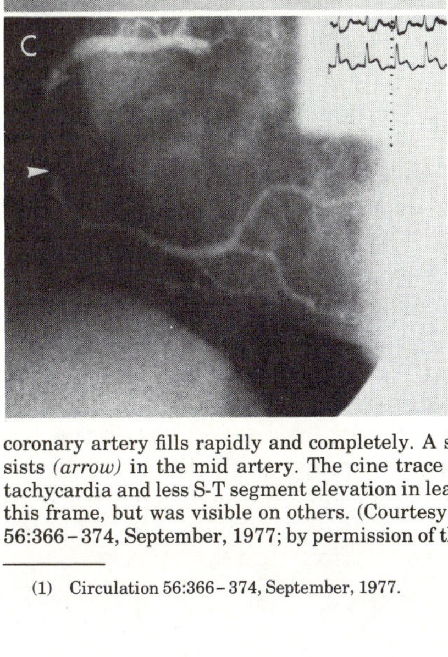

Fig 4. – Sequence of three right coronary arteriograms in the left anterior position in patient A. L., a woman aged 54. **A,** before nitroglycerin, complete occlusion of the mid right coronary artery is present *(arrow)*. The cine trace *(upper right corner)* shows complete heart block with junctional pacemaker and significant S-T segment elevation in lead II. **B,** 30 seconds after nitroglycerin, the right coronary artery is patent, although a severe obstruction persists at the point of previous occlusion *(arrow)*. Contrast medium slowly passes the obstruction, but the distal branches of the artery never fill. The cine trace again shows complete heart block with S-T segment elevation in lead II. **C,** 3 minutes after nitroglycerin, the right coronary artery fills rapidly and completely. A severe, presumably atherosclerotic, obstruction persists *(arrow)* in the mid artery. The cine trace shows a change from complete heart block to sinus tachycardia and less S-T segment elevation in lead II. The atrioventricular nodal artery is not seen on this frame, but was visible on others. (Courtesy of Oliva, P. B., and Breckinridge, J. C.: Circulation 56:366 – 374, September, 1977; by permission of the American Heart Association, Inc.)

(1) Circulation 56:366 – 374, September, 1977.

(40%). Four of the patients with spasm had an acute inferior infarction associated with total occlusion of the right coronary artery (Fig 4). Spasm always occurred at the site of atherosclerotic obstruction. No patient noted a change in intensity of chest pain after relief of spasm, but 1 patient (A. L.) had a marked reduction in S-T segment elevation and improvement in cardiac rhythm; simultaneous arteriographic and ECG changes are shown in Figure 4. No adverse cardiac effects resulted from the study, but 2 patients had femoral artery thrombosis at the puncture site.

This study establishes occurrence of spasm in acute myocardial infarction, but not the importance of spasm in the pathophysiology of acute infarction or whether relief of spasm has a beneficial or harmful effect on the ischemic myocardium. Further study is needed to determine if coronary patency can be maintained pharmacologically and, if so, whether such patency and restoration of some blood flow is beneficial.

► [As indicated in the articles by Selzer et al. and Mudge et al. in the chapter Chronic Coronary Artery Disease in this section, there is substantial evidence supporting the view that coronary arterial spasm plays an important role in the development of myocardial ischemia in patients with variant (Prinzmetal's) angina, as well as in other patients with chronic coronary artery disease. The present study extends this concept of coronary spasm to approximately one third of patients with acute myocardial infarction. This finding, if it can be confirmed, is potentially of great clinical importance, because the prevention or alleviation of spasm may well diminish the amount of myocardium that becomes infarcted after coronary occlusion. It is now known that the coronary vascular bed is extremely sensitive to vasoconstrictor stimuli and that the latter are mediated through the adrenergic nervous system. Fortunately, the latter can be blocked by catecholamine depletion or by α-adrenergic receptor blockade.—Ed.]

Comparison between Effects of Nitroprusside and Nitroglycerin on Ischemic Injury during Acute Myocardial Infarction. Cardiac failure is the major life-threatening complication of acute myocardial infarction in hospitalized patients. Massimo Chiariello, Herman K. Gold, Robert C. Leinbach, Michael A. Davis and Peter R. Maroko[2] (Harvard Med. School) studied the effects of nitroglycerin (TNG) and nitroprusside (NP) on the mechanical performance of the heart and the ECG ischemic injury in 10 patients with acute transmural anterior myocardial infarction. Nitroprusside was infused at a mean rate of 95 μg per minute for 10 minutes. Five patients then took 0.3 or 0.6 mg TNG sublingually. An experimental study was done in dogs in which the left anterior descending coronary artery or its apical branch was occluded. Both NP and TNG were given intravenously to reduce the mean arterial pressure by about 20 mm Hg.

Nitroprusside reduced the mean arterial pressure by 26 mm Hg in the patients and reduced the pulmonary capillary wedge pressure by 7 mm Hg, but the average S-T segment elevation increased. Hemodynamic effects were similar in the patients given both agents, but TNG reduced the S-T segment elevation by 1.4 mm, in contrast to the rise of 2.4 mm seen with NP. Cardiac output was reduced similarly by both drugs in the dog studies. The S-T segment elevation increased after NP administration and decreased after TNG infusion. Transmural blood

(2) Circulation 54:766–773, November, 1976.

flow declined after NP, but flow in the sites of ischemia rose after TNG. The endocardial-epicardial flow ratio rose significantly after TNG in the ischemic zone, whereas no significant change was seen after NP infusion.

Nitroglycerin reduced ECG myocardial injury in these studies and NP increased it. Both agents can produce important hemodynamic improvement in patients with acute infarction through reductions in preload and afterload, but their contrasting effects on the severity of ECG ischemic injury and their effects on collateral blood flow in dogs suggest that TNG may be preferable to NP when reductions in preload and afterload are desired in the early phase of acute myocardial infarction.

► [This study is important in view of the increasing use of vasodilators to improve ventricular function in patients with acute myocardial infarction. In addition, it should be noted that Capurro et al. (J. Clin. Invest. 60:295, 1977) compared the effects of nitroglycerin, nitroprusside and phentolamine on collateral function in dogs studied several weeks after an ameroid constrictor had been placed around the left anterior descending coronary artery. The authors also found that for a given reduction in systemic arterial pressure, nitroprusside is less effective in increasing retrograde flow than is nitroglycerin, whereas phentolamine actually exerts a deleterious effect on collateral function. — Ed.] ◄

Contrasting Influences of Alterations in Ventricular Preload and Afterload upon Systemic Hemodynamics, Function and Metabolism of Ischemic Myocardium. Studies that have used a model of total coronary occlusion have shown an increase in preload to increase ischemic injury and an increase in afterload to reduce it, but acute infarction in man is often associated with patent but stenotic coronary arteries. H. L. Wyatt, Protasio L. da Luz, David D. Waters, H. J. C. Swan and James S. Forrester[3] (Univ. of California, Los Angeles) determined the effects of primary increases in left ventricular preload and afterload on global and regional myocardial function and metabolism in the presence of a flow-limiting coronary stenosis. Studies were done in dogs in which left anterior descending artery stenoses of varying severity were produced with a screw clamp. Dextran was infused to increase the left ventricular end-diastolic pressure (LVEDP) from 5 to 11 and from 11 to 17 mm Hg, and angiotensin was given to augment the mean arterial pressure by about 30 mm Hg.

Reduction in coronary flow to 40–50% of control led to a 5–10% fall in cardiac output and mean arterial pressure and a 10–20% fall in stroke work. The magnitude of systolic shortening decreased in the ischemic zone and lactate extraction shifted to production. Volume loading led to increases in cardiac output and arterial pressure with no change in systemic vascular resistance. Smaller increases occurred with the secondary increase in LVEDP. Coronary flow rose significantly with initial volume loading, but regional lactate production also increased in most dogs. Angiotensin infusion led to a 100% increase in vascular resistance but little change in LVEDP. Cardiac output fell by 20%. Coronary flow increased but the magnitude of systolic shortening of the ischemic segment did not change significantly. Lactate production shifted to extraction.

(3) Circulation 55:318–324, February, 1977.

Left ventricular volume loading and pressure loading may have opposed effects on left ventricular performance and metabolism in the presence of a flow-limiting coronary stenosis. A primary increase in preload improves cardiac output at the expense of aggravated ischemia. A primary increase in afterload reduces cardiac output, but it may improve perfusion and lactate uptake of the ischemic myocardium. The extent to which these findings are applicable to man is unclear.

► [These experiments show nicely that in the presence of coronary occlusion efforts to diminish ischemia and improve myocardial performance may sometimes conflict. Thus, in these dogs without heart failure, a volume load increased myocardial performance, but only at the expense of intensifying ischemia, presumably because of further reduction of subendocardial blood flow or increased oxygen consumption of the ischemic myocardium, or both, as a consequence of increased mechanical performance. In contrast, the increase in afterload reduced ischemia, presumably by augmenting perfusion through collateral channels, but at the expense of reducing cardiac output. These observations cannot, of course, be transferred to the patient with acute myocardial infarction. Obviously, one would like both to augment ventricular performance and to reduce myocardial ischemia, but this may not be possible. I believe that a useful working principle is to exert major emphasis on the reduction of ischemia and thereby limit the amount of necrotic tissue during the first few hours after the occlusion, as long as the patient does not develop severe pump failure. Obviously, if the latter occurs, it must be treated promptly. Later on, i.e., perhaps 10–12 hours after the onset of the acute event, when the fate of the ischemic myocardium has been settled, it is less critical to worry about the ischemic process, and major attention can be directed to the function of the cardiac pump.

This important problem has also been addressed by Miller et al. (Am. J. Cardiol. 40: 504, 1977), who administered sublingual nitroglycerin to patients with multivessel coronary artery disease. This reduced arterial and left ventricular filling pressure, as well as coronary blood flow. On the other hand, phenylephrine raised coronary flow rates and reduced myocardial oxygen extraction, suggesting that the augmented coronary flow afforded by the enhanced myocardial perfusion gradient offset the increased oxygen requirements resulting from the phenylephrine-induced increase in ventricular afterload. In the setting of acute myocardial ischemia, the augmented coronary flow provided by phenylephrine might enhance the effects of nitroglycerin. These clinical observations support the earlier experimental findings of Borer et al. (N. Engl. J. Med. 293:20, 1975).

Poliner (Tex. Med. 73:53, 1977) has observed that isosorbide dinitrate, when given either by the oral or sublingual route, is of therapeutic value in patients with acute coronary insufficiency. The reduction of myocardial wall tension would be expected to benefit myocardial oxygen supply-demand relations. Similarly, Bussmann (Am. J. Cardiol. 39:91, 1977) studied the effects of oral isosorbide dinitrate in patients with acute myocardial infarction. Left ventricular filling pressure fell in all patients, while cardiac output declined in those with normal initial filling pressures and rose in those with elevated filling pressures. The favorable actions of this drug in acute myocardial infarction may result from the reduction in afterload, and the improved blood supply to the endocardium may be a consequence of the reduction of left ventricular filling pressure.—Ed.] ◄

Propranolol-Induced Reduction of Signs of Ischemic Injury during Acute Myocardial Infarction. Myocardial injury is reversible in the first hours after the onset of an ischemic event and conceivably its course can be modified. Herman K. Gold, Robert C. Leinbach and Peter R. Maroko[4] (Harvard Med. School) studied the effects of β-adrenergic blockade on ischemic injury in patients in the early hours after acute transmural anterior myocardial infarction. Twelve pa-

(4) Am. J. Cardiol. 38:689–695, Nov. 23, 1976.

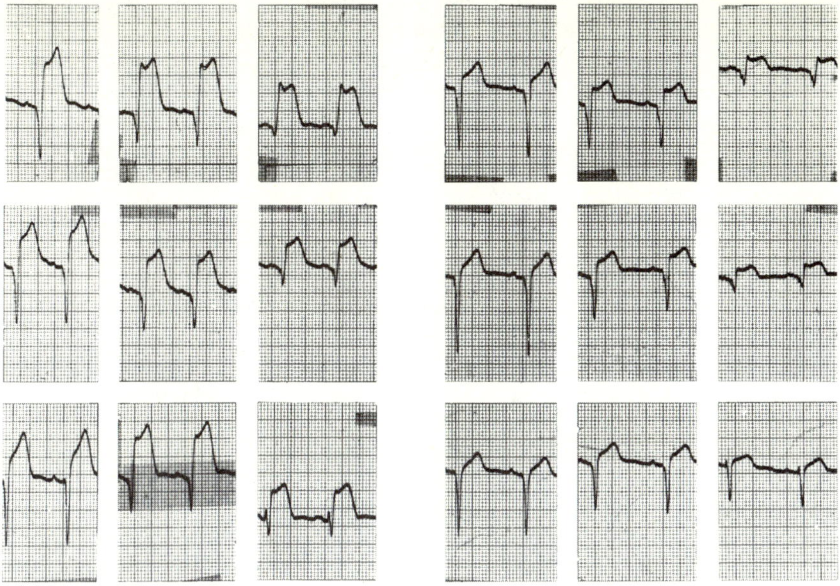

Fig 5.—The effect of propranolol on the reduction in S-T segment elevation in an average patient. The nine leads depicted are from the V_1, V_3 and V_5 positions and the corresponding sites one intercostal space above and below the standard positions. (Courtesy of Gold, H. K., et al.: Am. J. Cardiol. 38:689–695, Nov. 23, 1976.)

tients had propranolol infused at a rate of 1 mg/2 minutes; the target dose for β-blockade was 0.15/mg/kg. Precordial S-T segment mapping was carried out.

Mean arterial pressure fell from 112 to 95 mm Hg during propranolol infusion and the heart rate declined from 100 to 79 beats per minute. Pulmonary capillary wedge pressure fell in 6 patients and increased in the rest; no patient had pulmonary congestion. Cardiac output decreased on the average from 6.1 to 4.1 L/per minute; decrease was directly related to dose. A marked reduction in S-T segment elevation was apparent 30 minutes after propranolol administration (Fig 5). The group decrease in average S-T segment elevation over the left precordium recorded from multiple unipolar leads was 39%. The reduction persisted for 4 hours after propranolol administration, although the hemodynamic effects dissipated. The magnitude of S-T segment responses to propranolol varied within a wide range. Reductions were greatest in patients with angiographically demonstrable flow to the infarcted area, either through significant stenosis of the left anterior descending artery or by way of collateral vessels. Pain was reduced significantly or relieved in 9 of the 12 patients but persisted in the 3 patients with the poorest S-T segment responses. Ventricular ectopic beats decreased after β-blockade. No patient exhibited an atrioventricular condition defect. All patients survived and were discharged.

It is concluded that judicious intravenous administration of propranolol in the early phase of acute myocardial infarction reduces the signs of ischemic injury. This therapeutic approach, which is directed at interrupting ischemic injury, may play an important role in the management of these patients.

► [There is increasing interest in the notion of protecting the ischemic myocardium and thereby limiting myocardial infarct size. The precordial ECG provides a simple, though indirect, technique for assessing ischemic injury. The changes in S-T segment elevation demonstrated in this study with propranolol are extremely impressive; whereas they do not prove that the extent of myocardial necrosis was reduced, they certainly suggest that the intervention was beneficial. – Ed.] ◄

Influence of Time Interval between Coronary Artery Occlusion and Administration of Hyaluronidase on Salvage of Ischemic Myocardium in Dogs. Hyaluronidase limits myocardial necrosis when given 20–30 minutes after coronary artery occlusion and it appears to be of benefit to patients. L. David Hillis, Michael C. Fishbein, Eugene Braunwald and Peter R. Maroko[5] (Harvard Med. School) used hyaluronidase to examine the effects of the time interval from coronary occlusion to the application of interventions to salvage myocardium jeopardized by ischemia. Ten to 16 sites on the anterior left ventricular surface in mongrel dogs subjected to coronary occlusions for 24 hours were selected for recording unipolar electrograms. Some animals received 500 NF units of hyaluronidase per kg intravenously 20 minutes or 3, 6 or 9 hours after occlusion. Electrograms were recorded before and 15 minutes after occlusion.

There was good correlation among the three parameters of necrosis, depressed myocardial creatine phosphokinase (CPK) activity, histologic change and altered QRS configuration. The S-T segment elevation present 15 minutes after occlusion correlated well with the three reference parameters in control animals. When hyaluronidase was given 20 minutes or 3 or 6 hours after coronary occlusion, myocardial salvage was reflected in a significant reduction in myocardial CPK depression, less histologic evidence of infarction and less extensive changes in QRS configuration than in untreated dogs. It is notable that hyaluronidase does not simply delay necrosis but prevents its occurrence. There was a progressive reduction in tissue salvage as the interval between coronary occlusion and hyaluronidase administration increased. Treatment 9 hours after occlusion had no apparent effect on the development of myocardial necrosis.

Extrapolation of these findings to patients must be done cautiously but, since the histopathologic evolution of infarction in the dog is quite similar to that in man, the findings support the hope that patients reaching the hospital within a few hours after the onset of symptoms of infarction may benefit from interventions designed to limit ischemic injury. In pilot studies several agents, including hyaluronidase, propranolol and nitroglycerin, have proved effective in limiting ischemic injury in patients treated within several hours after the clinical event.

► [Myocardial necrosis after coronary artery occlusion can be limited by certain interventions designed to improve the balance between oxygen supply and demand. In

(5) Circ. Res. 41:26–31, July, 1977.

most early studies the intervention under investigation was applied either before or shortly after coronary artery occlusion, at a time when most cells are still reversibly injured. The potential clinical relevance of these observations are dependent on the time interval during which the intervention is effective. The results of the experimental studies presented in this article are encouraging because a beneficial effect of hyaluronidase was noted as long as 6 hours after coronary occlusion. Obviously, the interventions are most potent when applied prophylactically, i.e., prior to the coronary occlusion. Perhaps this can be done with drugs such as β-blocking agents or anti-inflammatory compounds, given to patients at high risk of developing coronary occlusion. In patients not protected in this manner, an intervention may still be useful in limiting myocardial damage as long as the patient is treated in the first few hours after the beginning of the event. – Ed.] ◄

Favorable Effects of Hyaluronidase on Electrocardiographic Evidence of Necrosis in Patients with Acute Myocardial Infarction. Clinical evaluation of many interventions that alter development of myocardial damage experimentally after coronary occlusion is difficult because of the need to use noninvasive techniques.

P. R. Maroko, L. D. Hillis, J. E. Muller, L. Travazzi, G. R. Heyndrickx, M. Ray, M. Chiariello, A. Distante, J. Askenazi, J. Salerno, J. Carpentier, N. I. Reshetnaya, P. Radvany, P. Libby, D. S. Raabe, E. I. Chazov, P. Bobba and E. Braunwald[6] (Harvard Med. School) determined the evolution of the QRS complex in hyaluronidase-treated and untreated patients with anterior or anterolateral transmural myocardial infarctions and chest pain of less than 8 hours' duration. Treated patients received 500 NF units per kg hyaluronidase intravenously, as a bolus every 6 hours for 48 hours. Forty-five patients were treated, and 46 were untreated.

Admission ECGs were similar in the two patient groups. Less evolution of QRS complexes occurred in the hyaluronidase-treated group

Fig 6. – Changes in scores for S-T segment elevation in hyaluronidase-treated and control groups. A, percentage of precordial sites with S-T segment elevations equal to or greater than 0.15 mV on the admission ECG with changes in QRS score of 1 or more in the tracing recorded on the 7th day. Numbers in columns represent number of patients in each group. Bars represent ±1 SEM. Control patients had 635 sites with S-T segment elevations, and hyaluronidase-treated patients had 591 sites. Note that control patients had significantly more sites with changed QRS morphology than did treated patients (* = $P < 0.05$). B, percentage of precordial sites with S-T segment elevations equal to or greater than 0.15 on admission ECG with changes in QRS score of 2 or more in the tracing recorded on the 7th day. Total number of vulnerable sites was 575 in control patients and 494 in treated patients. C, percentage fall in total R-wave voltage (ΣR) in sites with S-T segment elevations equal to or greater than 0.15 on initial ECG. Note that control patients had a significantly greater fall in ΣR-wave voltage than did treated patients. (* = $P < 0.01$; ** = $P < 0.01$). (Courtesy of Maroko, P. R., et al.: N. Engl. J. Med. 296:898–903, Apr. 21, 1977.)

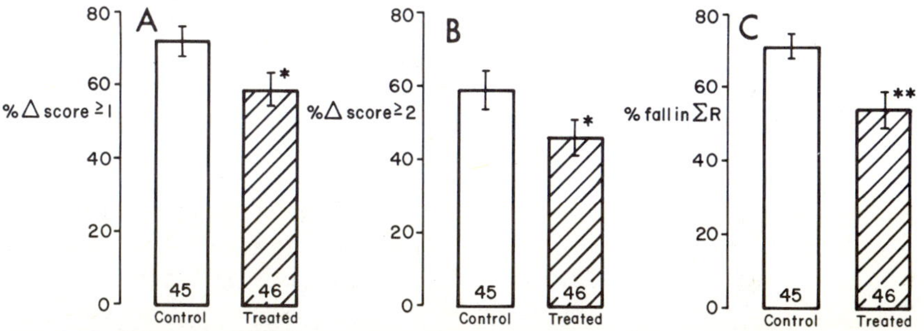

(6) N. Engl. J. Med. 296:898–903, Apr. 21, 1977.

(Fig 6), and also, significantly fewer sites with S-T segment elevation on admission showed increased scores after 1 week. Two patients had urticarial reactions to hyaluronidase that responded to treatment. None of the 10 treated patients skin-tested 6–24 months after discharge exhibited any reaction to hyaluronidase. Fewer treated patients were in congestive heart failure after treatment. The difference in mortality between the two groups was not significant.

These findings suggest that hyaluronidase, given within 8 hours after onset of the clinical event, reduces the extent of myocardial necrosis in patients with acute myocardial infarction. Hyaluronidase should now be tested in a much larger group of patients to determine its effects on morbidity and mortality and thus its role in treatment of patients with acute myocardial infarction.

► [It is relatively simple in patients with acute myocardial infarction to administer agents that have been shown to be helpful in preventing infarct size in dogs. It is much more difficult to determine the efficacy of these interventions. In the 1977 YEAR BOOK (p. 311), a technique based on an analysis of the QRS complex was proposed as a noninvasive means to evaluate the efficacy of interventions. This article by Maroko et al. is a follow-up report, demonstrating the application of this technique to the study of hyaluronidase, an agent that previously had been shown to be effective in experimental animals. This pilot study shows the effectiveness of hyaluronidase and suggests that a much larger trial should now be undertaken.

Techniques are available for estimating infarct size using serum creatine kinase (CK) curves. Bleifeld et al. (Circulation 55:303, 1977) demonstrated that infarct mass calculated from serial CK analysis, in conjunction with hemodynamic monitoring, is of considerable importance in the assessment of the hemodynamic function of the residual myocardium. Wackers et al. (ibid. 56:72, 1977) showed that thallium-201 scintiscans carried out in the acute phase of myocardial infarction correlated well with infarct size as determined post mortem. A third technique involves "hot spot" imaging with ^{99m}Tc-pyrophosphate, which can provide an index of infarct size as well. The latter technique is succinctly reviewed by Marcus and Kerber (ibid., p. 335). In addition, computerized tomography is likely to provide a potent method for measuring infarct size, but up to now its application has been limited to experimental preparations (Powell et al.: ibid. 55:99, 1977; and Wittenberg et al. Invest. Radiol. 12:215, 1977). – Ed.] ◄

Effectiveness of Coronary Care Units in Small Community Hospitals. Studies evaluating coronary care units have yielded conflicting findings. Jeoffrey K. Stross, Park W. Willis III, E. W. Reynolds, Jr., Ralph E. Lewis, Irwin J. Schatz, Luanne C. Bellfy and Jeanne Copp[7] (Univ. of Michigan) report a prospective study done in 1969–74 to evaluate a program establishing coronary care units in 29 community hospitals that had fewer than 150 beds and were located in an area without adequate coronary care facilities. Data were collected on 1,259 patients in community hospitals in 1972 and on 300 patients with a discharge diagnosis of acute infarction in an urban hospital coronary care unit.

The crude mortality rate from acute infarction in the small hospitals was 14.5%, slightly above the rate in three larger comparison hospitals (11.5%). Observed deaths exceeded those expected in small hospitals but were fewer than expected in comparison hospitals. Mortality was significantly greater in units admitting fewer than 60 patients with infarction annually than in those admitting more (20.9% vs. 10.7%).

---

(7) Ann. Intern. Med. 85:709–713, December, 1976.

No significant differences in the treatment of patients with ventricular arrhythmias were found among the different types of hospital. Most patients dying of ventricular arrhythmias had secondary arrhythmias. The overall mortality of patients with ventricular tachycardia or fibrillation was 45.6%.

Data from community hospitals in this study confirm that small coronary care units in areas of low population density allow effective acute coronary care if a minimum level of activity is exceeded, even though each unit may fail in one or more ways to meet minimum requirements contained in contemporary guidelines for the operation of coronary care units. Units provide less adequate coronary care when fewer than 60 patients with infarction are admitted yearly.

► [This interesting article demonstrates the relative effectiveness of coronary care in small community hospitals, compared to that existing in larger urban hospitals. However, it does not address the issue of the effectiveness of the coronary care unit concept, which has not been settled completely. Thus, Astvad et al. (Br. Med. J. 1:567, 1974) carried out a retrospective study of the rate of mortality due to acute myocardial infarction in two groups of comparable patients treated before and after coronary care units were established. No difference was observed. The complexity of this kind of analysis was discussed by Fabricius-Bjerre (Dan. Med. Bull. 23:163, 1976). O'Rourke et al. (Br. Med. J. 2:837, 1976) described a complex coronary care unit with facilities for fluoroscopy, hemodynamic monitoring, mechanical heart assistance and long-term ECG monitoring. The application of these techniques appeared to reduce the number of early deaths from cardiac arrest and cardiac failure, but had little effect on total mortality. An interesting article by Hunt et al. (ibid. 1:795, 1977) showed that there has been a significant reduction in mortality among consecutive patients with myocardial infarction treated in the coronary care unit of the Royal Melbourne Hospital between 1963 and 1975. Classifying patients in various risk groups showed that in each risk group mortality has decreased. This may reflect both the changing pattern and natural history of the disease, as well as the benefit of improved treatment. – Ed.] ◄

Chronic Coronary Artery Disease

Detection of Remote Myocardial Infarction in Patients with Positron Emission Transaxial Tomography and Intravenous ^{11}C-Palmitate. Ischemic myocardial injury has been detected in isolated perfused hearts and intact experimental animals with positron emitting ^{11}C-palmitate and reconstructive tomography, providing cross-sectional images of the heart free from superimposed activity in overlying structures. Burton E. Sobel, Edward S. Weiss, Michael J. Welch, Barry A. Siegel and Michel M. Ter-Pogossian[8] (Washington Univ., St. Louis) evaluated the applicability of this approach to detecting infarction in 10 normal subjects and 12 patients with myocardial infarction 3 – 12 months previously. Tomograms were obtained after the injection of 5 – 10 mCi ^{11}C-palmitate in 4% albumin.

Normal tomograms exhibited a characteristic distribution of activity dependent on the level at which the tomogram was obtained, from the apex to the base of the heart. Patients with anterior infarction showed decreased activity at the ECG site of infarction (Fig 7). Infarctions in the inferior and posterior regions of the heart were also detected. The distribution of activity in a series of cross sections of the heart in both normal subjects and patients with remote infarction was

(8) Circulation 55:853 – 857, June, 1977.

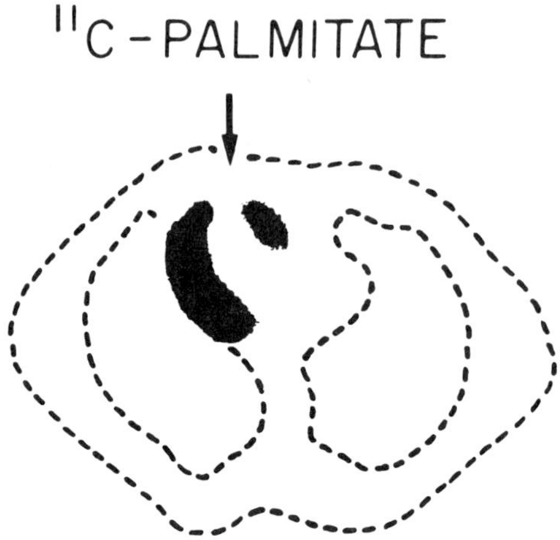

Fig 7.—A ^{11}C-palmitate tomogram from a patient with an anterior myocardial infarction. The characteristic horseshoe shape of the normal left ventricular emission tomogram at this level is interrupted anteriorly by a transmural defect. The dashed lines surrounding the emission tomogram were obtained from the transmission image obtained at the identical level. They delineate the pleural cavities and body wall. (Courtesy of Sobel, B. E., et al.: Circulation 55:853–857, June, 1977; by permission of the American Heart Association, Inc.)

analogous to that observed in normal dogs and animals with experimentally induced myocardial infarction.

Positron emission transaxial tomography provides a means of quantitatively detecting alterations in cardiac metabolism induced by ischemia of brief duration. The results obtained in animal preparations and in patients suggest that this technique will provide a useful means of evaluating myocardial ischemia and its sequelae in man.

► [Radiopharmaceuticals incorporated directly into the metabolic pathways of the myocardium provide a promising new means for evaluating myocardial metabolism. The basis of the method described in this article is that palmitic acid, a major physiologic substrate of myocardium, has a well-understood role in myocardial metabolism. Hoffman and his colleagues (J. Nucl. Med. 18:57, 1977) have shown that images obtained with ^{11}C-palmitic acid are comparable to those obtained with $^{13}NH_3$ and ^{11}CO-hemoglobin, which are excellent imaging agents. However, ^{11}C-palmitic acid is dependent not only on blood flow, but also on the uptake of the fatty acid by normally metabolizing myocardium. Presumably it is the decreased extraction of the fatty acid rather than the reduced flow which is responsible for diminished accumulation of ^{11}C-palmitate delineating regions corresponding to the ECG locus of infarction. Because of its short half-life, the use of ^{11}C-palmitate for positron emission transaxial tomography requires an extremely expensive cyclotron on the hospital premises. Hopefully, it will be possible in the future to carry out positron emission transaxial tomography with radionuclides such as gallium-68 or rubidium-82 that can be synthesized without a cyclotron.—Ed.] ◄

Thallium-201 Myocardial Perfusion Imaging at Rest and during Exercise: Comparative Sensitivity to Electrocardiography in Coronary Artery Disease. Evidence suggests that exercise-injected myocardial perfusion imaging (MPI) may be more sensitive than exercise electrocardiography in identifying patients with coronary artery disease. Ian K. Bailey, Lawrence S. C. Griffith, Jacques Rouleau, H.

William Strauss and Bertram Pitt[9] (Johns Hopkins Univ.), with the technical assistance of William Schafer and Henry Manspeaker, compared the sensitivity of MPI with ^{201}Tl, injected both at rest and during peak exercise, with that of simultaneously recorded 12-lead ECGs for detecting ischemia and infarction in 63 patients with proved coronary artery disease and 20 normal subjects. The patients included 52 men and 11 women with a mean age of 49 years. Forty-seven had a history of infarction and 40 had angina as a current symptom. The MPI was performed with an intravenous dose of 1.5 – 2 mCi ^{201}Tl. The rest and exercise studies were done at least a week apart and, like the ECGs, were interpreted by 2 independent observers without knowledge of the other findings.

No significant abnormalities were found in the normal group. Over half the patients with coronary disease developed new perfusion defects on exercise, and 38% developed ischemic S-T segment depression. When chest pain or S-T segment depression, or both, was considered to be an index of ischemia, however, the sensitivity of the two tests was similar. The greater sensitivity of MPI was due to patients with baseline ECG abnormalities and those who failed to achieve 85% of predicted maximum heart rate on exercise. Both positive ECGs and positive MPIs increased with the number of vessels involved. The MPI was the more sensitive study in patients with single-vessel disease. The combination of ECG and MPI studies and chest pain on exercise failed to identify 11% of patients with coronary artery disease.

Exercise ^{201}Tl MPI is more sensitive than S-T segment depression on the exercise ECG in detecting myocardial ischemia. Interpretation of exercise ECGs in patients with S-T segment elevation in a lead with a resting Q wave abnormality is difficult. There was no false positive MPI in this study, but greater experience is needed before the specificity of the technique is known.

► [Strauss and Pitt provide an excellent review of the use of thallium-201 as a myocardial imaging agent (Semin. Nucl. Med. 7:49, 1977). They point out that the limitation of technology at this time includes limited instrument resolution and a short effective half-life of thallium in the myocardium that virtually prohibits repeated imaging over a brief period. It must be remembered that the most common cause of a focal decrease in perfusion on the thallium scan is a healed myocardial infarction. It is also possible to use the thallium scan to predict which coronary vessels show obstructive lesions. Bulkley et al. (Circulation 55:753, 1977) have shown that thallium-201 imaging may be helpful in separating patients with ischemic from those with idiopathic congestive cardiomyopathy. In the former, defects of greater than 40% of the image circumference usually occurred, whereas in the latter the defects were much smaller. In general, there were good autopsy correlations between large thallium defects and transmural myocardial fibrosis. It is important to recognize, however, that thallium-201 scanning (or gated cardiac blood pool scanning) cannot distinguish between acute and chronic myocardial infarction. – Ed.] ◄

Angiographic Findings in Asymptomatic Aircrewmen with Electrocardiographic Abnormalities. Because of their previous medical examinations, Air Force crewmen manifest few of the typical and obvious cardiovascular diseases. Victor F. Froelicher, Jr., A. J.

---

(9) Circulation 55:79 – 87, January, 1977.

ANGIOGRAPHIC FINDINGS AND RISK FACTOR DATA IN 111 AIRCREWMEN WITH ABNORMAL TREADMILL TEST GROUPED ACCORDING TO ANNUAL RESTING ECG DATA

Annual Resting Electrocardiograms	Age* (yr)	no. (% of group) With Significant CAD†	no. (% of group) With No CAD	Serum Cholesterol (mg/100 ml)*	Serum Triglycerides (mg/100 ml)*	Blood Pressure (mm Hg)*	Positive Smoking History (% of group)	Positive Family History for CAD (% of group)
Normal (no. = 34)	44 ±8	8 (23.5%)	20 (58.8%)	241 ±48	145 ±73	130 ± 15 / 84 ± 9	32	32
Previous tracings with repolarization changes but current tracing normal (no. = 21)	43 ±6	5 (23.8%)	10 (47.6%)	226 ±46	162 ±86	130 ± 15 / 82 ± 10	71	50
Repolarization changes with persistent low amplitude T waves (no. = 24)	42 ±8	6 (25.0%)	15 (62.5%)	259 ±45	164 ±85	137 ± 18 / 87 ± 11	67	39
Persistent S-T segment depression or straightening (no. = 32)	44 ±6	15 (46.9%)	15 (46.9%)	250 ±47	160 ±98	136 ± 10 / 86 ± 10	50	34

*Values expressed as mean ±standard deviation.
†CAD, coronary artery disease.

Thompson, Roger Wolthuis, Robert Fuchs, Robert Balusek, Michael R. Longo, Jr., John H. Triebwasser and Malcolm C. Lancaster[1] (Brooks Air Force Base, Texas) determined the prevalence of angiographic coronary artery disease in asymptomatic apparently healthy aircrewmen with ECG abnormalities suggestive of heart disease. The 298 subjects were identified from annual ECGs and exercise tests used to screen for latent heart disease. Data also were obtained from 27 symptomatic subjects who had cardiac catheterization for probable mild angina pectoris.

The order of groups by increasing prevalence of coronary artery disease was: abnormal treadmill test (labile lead only), supraventricular tachycardia, right bundle-branch block, left bundle-branch block, abnormal treadmill test, ventricular irritability, probable infarct and angina. About 60% of the men were entirely free of angiographic coronary artery disease. The findings in 111 subjects with abnormal treadmill test findings are given in the table. Analysis of the 98 subjects with significant angiographic disease indicated a minimal increase in the percent of men with risk factors as the amount of disease increased. In men able to perform a maximal treadmill effort, there was very little difference in maximal oxygen consumption. The prevalence rate of significant coronary disease was 16.8% in 125 men under age 40 and 38.5% in 200 men aged 40 and over. A serum cholesterol level exceeding the 90th percentile for age was a more sensitive measure of risk in the younger subjects.

It appears that ECG abnormalities are poorer predictors of coronary artery disease in asymptomatic, apparently healthy men than in populations with a greater prevalence of coronary artery disease. Coronary angiography in aircrewmen has most often served to remove the diagnosis of coronary artery disease. False positive findings are a substantial problem in the ECG screening of apparently healthy men.

► [The principal lesson to learn from this article is that a positive exercise ECG does not usually signify coronary artery disease in totally asymptomatic young men. Indeed,

(1) Am. J. Cardiol. 39:32–38, January, 1977.

Kappes et al. (Curr. Probl. Cardiol. 7:3, December, 1977) have applied Bayes' theorem to assess the likelihood of coronary artery disease according to chest pain syndromes. In asymptomatic patients, 5% of whom have coronary artery disease, a positive exercise test raises the probability to only 27% (whereas a normal test in this group lowers it to 2%). – Ed.] ◄

Nature and Clinical Features of Myocardial Infarction with Normal Coronary Arteriogram. Andrew Rosenblatt and Arthur Selzer[2] (Pacific Med. Center, San Francisco) examined the clinical features of myocardial infarction without demonstrable coronary lesions. Seven such patients were encountered in 1970–75. The findings in 6 new cases in male patients and in 19 case histories collected from the literature (group I) were compared with those in 16 cases of infarction due to occlusive coronary disease in a comparable population (group II). Only male patients under age 40 were included in the study group.

Three patients were moderate smokers, none had hypertension and 1 had hyperlipoproteinemia. Five had typical attacks of pain at the onset of infarction; none had prodromal attacks. In 1 patient, the ECG showed typical changes of past infarction. Five of the 6 study patients had evidence of anterior wall infarction. In all patients, the course was benign. Coronary arteriography showed normal coronary arteries in 4 patients and minor lesions in 2. Three patients had abnormalities of left ventricular wall motion. No patient had effort angina or heart failure after the attack. One patient had another attack of infarction after 3 months and recovered uneventfully. All 16 control patients had risk factors. Ten had a history of effort angina, and 10 had prodromal attacks of pain. All but 3 patients had abnormal left ventricular wall motion. Eleven patients had angina or nonexertional chest pain after the infarction. One died of an arrhythmia some months later. The groups are compared in the table.

The unusually young age of some group I patients and the common absence of risk factors suggest a different population than that in group II. Myocardial infarction in group I may represent an "accident" of the coronary circulation, rather than chronic disease. The most at-

Comparison of Postmyocardial Infarction Patients with Normal Coronary Arteriograms (Group I) and Those with Arteriographic Evidence of Coronary Disease (Group II)*

	Group I (N = 25)	Group II (N = 16)	
Age	27.5	33.7	P <0.005
Range	14-37	26-39	
No Risk Factor (S,L,H)	15	0	P <0.0001
History of Effort Angina	0	10	P <0.0001
Unheralded Onset of MI	24	6	P <0.0001
Post MI Pain	5	11	P <0.001
Late Deaths (to 1 yr.)	1	1	NS
Multiple Documented MIs	2	3	NS

*Abbreviations: S = smoking; L = hyperlipoproteinemia; H = hypertension; MI = myocardial infarction.

(2) Circulation 55:578–580, April, 1977.

tractive hypothesis may be one assuming thromboembolism as a cause of infarction, with lysis of recanalization of the occluding thrombus. Infarction preceded by accelerating angina or followed by persistent angina, or both, is virtually certain to represent serious and premature coronary artery disease, probably with multivessel involvement.

► [Engel et al. (Br. Heart J. 39:477, 1977) described the occurrence of unequivocal myocardial infarction in 4 young women with normal or near-normal coronary arteries who had been taking oral contraceptives. These findings suggest that a primary thrombotic or thromboembolic event was responsible for the infarction. Fortunately, there is increasing evidence that patients with normal coronary vessels and coronary occlusion have a benign course. – Ed.] ◄

Clinical Syndrome of Variant Angina with Normal Coronary Arteriogram. Some patients with variant angina have been reported to have multivessel coronary artery disease or single-vessel lesions, whereas others have normal coronary angiograms. Arthur Selzer, Manly Langston, Charles Ruggeroli and Keith Cohn[3] (Pacific Med. Center, San Francisco) reviewed the findings in 29 patients with variant angina. Nine (group 1) had normal coronary angiograms or only minor lesions and the other 20 (group 2) had obstructive coronary artery disease. Seven group 1 patients had entirely normal angiograms, whereas 2 had plaques obstructing no more than 40% of the coronary artery lumen.

Six group 1 patients had a history of hypertension, and 2 had hyperlipoproteinemia. Anginal attacks generally occurred at rest. Recurrent attacks of rest pain had occurred for 5 weeks to 10 years. None had a history of infarction. The great majority of anginal attacks were nocturnal. None of four stress tests showed ischemic ECG changes. Five patients had arrhythmias during pain, and 4 had pain during angiography. No patient had notable abnormality of wall motion at ventriculography. All 4 patients followed have been well on medical therapy. Three group 2 patients had hypertension and 4 had hyperlipoproteinemia. Fifteen patients had typical effort angina. Ventriculograms showed abnormal wall motion in 6 patients, and 5 patients had had infarctions. The ECG was normal in only 6 patients. Both stress tests showed ischemia. Onset of variant angina was generally recent. Bypass surgery was performed on 13 group 2 patients. Four others had acute infarction after the study, and 3 of them died of pump failure. Tachyarrhythmias triggered by ischemia occurred in both groups.

Variant angina with normal coronary arteries generally has a benign course and is probably unrelated to atherosclerosis. Long-acting nitrates usually prevent attacks effectively in patients with this syndrome and are the first choice of therapy.

► [The principal thesis of this study is that variant (Prinzmetal's) angina in the absence of organic coronary artery disease is relatively benign. It is going to be important to confirm this in a series of patients studied prospectively because it has been my impression that patients in this category can be markedly disabled and go on to acquire acute myocardial infarction or serious tachyarrhythmias.

McLaughlin et al. (Am. J. Cardiol. 39:126, 1977) demonstrated the importance of coronary arterial spasm by carrying out arteriography before and after the intravenous administration of ergonovine maleate in demonstrating coronary constriction. Also,

(3) N. Engl. J. Med. 295:1343–1347, Dec. 9, 1976.

thallium-201 imaging during pain reproducibly revealed malperfusion in the region supplied by the artery with documented spasm. Indeed, Johnson and Detwiler (Circulation 55:947, 1977) demonstrated that three myocardial infarctions occurred in a 24-year-old man with angiographically normal coronary arteries in whom ergonovine caused spasm of the left anterior descending coronary artery. The results of surgical treatment of this lesion have been unimpressive. However, Grondin and Limet (Ann. Thorac. Surg. 23:111, 1977) proposed an interesting approach. In patients with organic stenosis and without spasm, operative treatment should consist of removal of the preaortic or pretracheal plexus in association with conventional coronary artery bypass grafting. However, in patients with intractable ventricular arrhythmias or with angina and normal coronary arteries, subject to spasm, bypass grafting, of course, should not be carried out, but cervical thoracic sympathectomy should be considered. In contrast to patients with S-T segment elevations, those patients with S-T segment depression during anginal pain at rest usually have advanced, obstructive, multivessel disease. – Ed.] ◄

Reflex Increase in Coronary Vascular Resistance in Patients with Ischemic Heart Disease. Variations in the tone of large coronary arteries have been documented in variant angina, but they have not been considered to be important in the usual forms of coronary artery disease. Gilbert H. Mudge, Jr., William Grossman, Roger M. Mills, Jr., Michael Lesch and Eugene Braunwald[4] (Harvard Med. School) measured changes in coronary vascular resistance during cold pressor testing in 24 patients with stable chest pain syndromes, 12 of whom had coronary disease. Vascular resistance was measured before and during the first 50 seconds of a cold pressor test, a stimulus known to produce systemic vasoconstriction. In 3 patients with coronary disease the test was repeated after intravenous administration of 5 mg phentolamine.

Baseline blood flows were similar in the two groups of patients, but coronary sinus flow after exposure to cold was lower in the patients

Fig 8. – Response of 3 patients with coronary artery disease to cold pressor test before *(solid line)* and after *(broken line)* phentolamine. After α-adrenergic blockade, expected hypertensive response to test was abolished, and coronary sinus flow did not change. (Courtesy of Mudge, G. H., Jr., et al.: N. Engl. J. Med. 295:1333–1337, Dec. 9, 1976.)

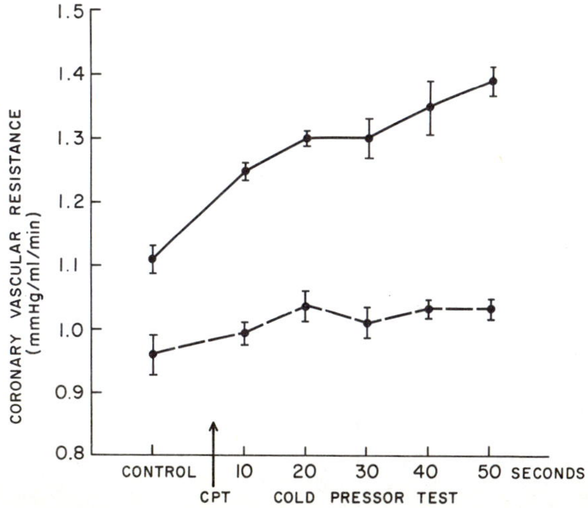

(4) N. Engl. J. Med. 295:1333–1337, Dec. 9, 1976.

with coronary disease. Coronary vascular resistance rose significantly by an average of 28% in these patients but was unchanged in those with normal coronary arteries. Most patients with coronary disease had little change in coronary sinus flow despite an increase in mean arterial pressure. Angina was precipitated by the test in 4 patients with coronary disease. Coronary vascular resistance increased by 49% in these patients, compared with 20% in those who did not have angina. Responses before and after phentolamine are compared in Figure 8.

Increased coronary vascular resistance may be an important determinant of coronary blood flow and is capable of eliciting transient ischemia in patients with coronary artery disease. The distinction between transient and permanent ischemia may merely reflect the intensity and duration of the constrictor stimulus. The existence of this mechanism suggests consideration of the use of α-adrenergic blockade in the treatment of transient ischemia and caution against the use of α-adrenergic agonists during the course of acute myocardial infarction.

► [The suggestion in this article, i.e., that coronary spasm is mediated by activation of α-adrenergic receptors, is supported by the study by Levene and Freeman (J.A.M.A. 236:1018, 1976) in which it was shown that striking stenosis of the right coronary artery could be abolished by treatment with intravenous phentolamine and that prolonged α-adrenergic receptor blockade with phenoxybenzamine improved exercise tolerance in a woman aged 41 with angina pectoris. When coronary vascular reactivity is considered, it must be recalled that there are β-adrenergic receptors that mediate vasodilatation in the coronary vascular bed and that treatment with β-blocking agents might produce paradoxical coronary vasoconstriction. Perhaps this accounts for the small number of patients with coronary disease who are propranolol failures. – Ed.] ◄

Hemodynamics and Antianginal Effects of High-Dose Oral Isosorbide Dinitrate after Chronic Use. Daniel T. Danahy and Wilbert S. Aronow[5] (Univ. of California, Irvine) conducted a double-blind crossover study of 19 patients with angina to evaluate side effects in the chronic use of oral isosorbide dinitrate (ISDN) in patients with angina and determine whether tolerance to the therapeutic effects of the drug will develop after chronic use. The patients were men aged 42–64 with typical effort angina and either a history of infarction or over 70% narrowing of at least one major coronary artery, or both. No patient had heart failure, hypertension or liver disease. Propranolol was gradually tapered before the study. Exercise testing was carried out at a 2-hour interval; 0.5 mg sublingual nitroglycerin or a placebo was given 2 minutes before exercise was begun. Subsequently tests were done in conjunction with oral ISDN or placebo administration. During follow-up, patients subsequently took a mean dose of 27.4 mg ISDN for a mean of 5.6 months before retesting.

Exercise time increased 56% initially and 51% on retesting after sublingual NTG, compared to placebo. Exercise times increased 58% and 58%, respectively, after ISDN. Mean exercise times initially and at retesting were not significantly different. Hemodynamic changes persisted for 5 hours after ISDN during both initial testing and retesting but the changes were significantly less during retesting. The S-T

(5) Circulation 56:205–212, August, 1977.

segment response to exercise and the duration of S-T depression after exercise were constant for most patients regardless of changes in the exercise time required to reach an anginal end point.

A partial tolerance to the hemodynamic effects of ISDN apparently develops after the chronic use of high oral doses, but the antianginal efficacy of both oral ISDN and sublingual nitroglycerin is unimpaired. Gradual reduction rather than abrupt discontinuance of chronic, high-dose nitrate therapy in anginal patients is strongly recommended. It is also recommended that continuous nitrate anti-anginal prophylaxis not be used in patients whose symptoms are readily controlled by less intensive nitrate therapy.

► [It is well known that orally and sublingually administered isosorbide dinitrate has significant hemodynamic and sustained anti-anginal effects. This study established the long-term efficacy of this agent. While it has been recognized that tolerance to the anti-anginal effects of sublingual nitroglycerin does not develop, it is reassuring that tolerance also does not develop after high doses of isosorbide dinitrate. — Ed.] ◄

Aspirin in Coronary Heart Disease is evaluated by the Coronary Drug Project Research Group.[6] Recent animal studies support the hypothesis that aspirin may have long-term therapeutic value in coronary heart disease. The Coronary Drug Project Aspirin Study was initiated in 1972 to test this hypothesis. The study population, at 53 clinical centers, consisted of men from groups originally given dextrothyroxine or estrogen therapy in the Coronary Drug Project. All had a past history of myocardial infarction. Follow-up ranged from 10 months to 28 months. A total of 1,529 patients were recruited and assigned on a double-blind basis to 324 mg aspirin 3 times daily or a placebo. A high level of adherence to the study protocol was found. There

Fig 9.—Life table cumulative rates for death (all causes). (Courtesy of Coronary Drug Project Research Group: J. Chron. Dis. 29:625–642, October, 1976.)

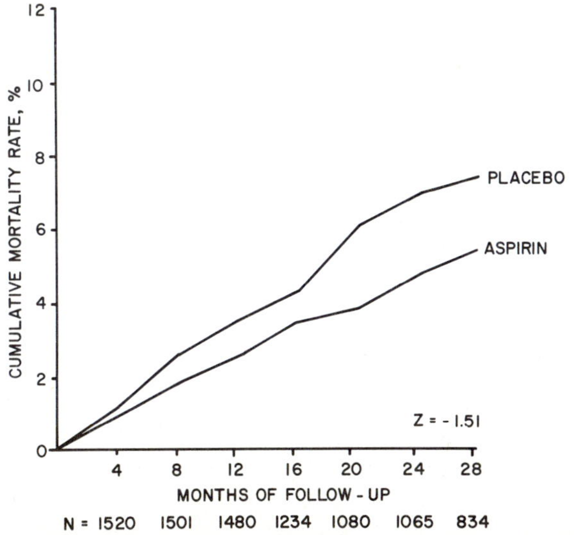

(6) J. Chron. Dis. 29:625–642, October, 1976.

were no major differences in the use of nonstudy medications in the two treatment groups. The study continued to early 1975.

Overall mortality was 5.8% in the aspirin-treated group and 8.3% in the placebo group, suggesting a beneficial effect of aspirin but one not marked enough to be conclusive. Cumulative life table rates for mortality are shown in Figure 9. The difference in the aspirin group relative to the placebo group for coronary deaths was 27% and that for sudden cardiovascular deaths, 19%.

More information is needed on the therapeutic value of aspirin in the management of coronary heart disease. Results available to date may lead to a further increase in the already massive use of aspirin, both via physician prescription and self-medication. The ready availability of aspirin and the general belief that its use poses little or no risk make this a potentially serious problem.

► [Jick and Miettinen first reported a negative association between regular aspirin intake and the risk of acute myocardial infarction based on a case-control study in 1974. This study has been updated (Br. Med. J. 1:1057, 1976) and now involves 658 patients with acute myocardial infarction, only 0.9% of whom were aspirin users, whereas 5% of a matched control group were regular aspirin users. As a consequence of these provocative observations, the National Heart, Lung and Blood Institute is now carrying out an aspirin-myocardial infarction study involving 4,500 patients who have had one or more documented myocardial infarctions. This study tests the hypothesis that regular administration of aspirin will reduce the risk of new heart attacks. The patients are randomized into placebo and drug groups, the latter receiving 1 gm aspirin (3 tablets) daily. The results of this study are anxiously awaited. – Ed.] ◄

Coronary Atherosclerosis in Valvular Heart Disease. Conflicting views have been expressed on the need for routine coronary angiography in patients undergoing cardiac catheterization for valvular heart disease. Jerome Lacy, Robert Goodin, Daniel McMartin, Ronald Masden and Nancy Flowers[7] (Univ. of Louisville) evaluated the usefulness of routine coronary angiography in a series of 201 adults who were primarily catheterized for the investigation of valvular heart disease over a 2½-year period. The series included 104 women and 97 men with respective mean ages of 49 and 53 years. Eighty-three patients (41%) were found to have coronary artery disease, and 22% had significant disease, with at least 50% obstruction of one or more vessels. The rates of significant disease were 27% for men and 18% for women.

The frequency of coronary disease rose with age. Significant obstructing lesions were present in 19% of patients with mitral stenosis, 18% of those with mitral regurgitation, 21% of those with aortic stenosis and 30% of those with aortic regurgitation. Five of 15 patients studied for prosthetic valve dysfunction had significant coronary disease. The distribution of coronary lesions by type of pain is shown in the table. Only 5 of the 45 patients with significant coronary disease had Q waves greater than 30 msec in the ECG. One patient developed ventricular fibrillation on angiography but was successfully defibrillated without sequelae. Risk factors for coronary disease were equally frequent in patients with and those without coronary disease and those with typical pain or without pain.

(7) Ann. Thorac. Surg. 23:429–435, May, 1977.

DISTRIBUTION AND SEVERITY OF CORONARY ARTERY LESIONS BY TYPE OF PAIN

Involvement and Degree	No Pain	Atypical Pain	Typical Pain	Total
No. of diseased vessels				
3	3	1	3	7
2	2	8	5	15
1	13	5	5	23
Total	18	14	13	45
Obstruction				
≥ 90%	4	4	8	16
70–90%	5	3	3	11
50–70%	9	7	2	18
Total	18	14	13	45

Radiologically significant coronary artery disease exists in an asymptomatic form in many patients with symptomatic, hemodynamically severe valvular heart disease. If angiographic data are important determinants of management, the present findings indicate that they can be obtained with minimal risk. They cannot be reliably deduced or extrapolated by noninvasive means. Coronary angiography should be a routine part of the presurgical data base.

► I agree with the authors' conclusion insofar as mitral valve disease is concerned. However, it has been my experience that patients with aortic valve disease (stenosis, regurgitation or mixed lesions) severe enough to warrant consideration of valve replacement who do not have angina pectoris usually do *not* have severe coronary artery disease. The converse, of course, is not true in that many patients with aortic valve disease and angina pectoris may well have normal coronary vessels. As a consequence, while I recommend coronary arteriography in the preoperative evaluation of most patients over age 40 with valvular heart disease, I do not believe that it is necessary in patients with aortic valve disease *without* angina. – Ed.] ◄

SURGICAL TREATMENT.

Treatment of Chronic Stable Angina: A Preliminary Report of Survival Data of the Randomized Veterans Administration Cooperative Study is presented by Marvin L. Murphy, Herbert N. Hultgren, Katherine Detre, James Thomsen, Timothy Takaro and participants of the VA Cooperative Study[8] (VA Hosp., Little Rock, Ark.). The study was developed in 1970 to determine the efficacy of saphenous vein bypass grafting in patients with chronic stable angina.

Males with chronic stable angina admitted to thirteen participating VA hospitals were considered for inclusion in the study. Excluded were those with acute infarction in the past 6 months, unstable angina or congestive heart failure. Angiographic criteria were a 50% or greater reduction in luminal diameter of at least one major coronary artery, a potentially graftable distal segment or segments and acceptable ventricular function.

(8) N. Engl. J. Med. 297:621–627, Sept. 22, 1977.

BASELINE VARIABLES OF 310 MEDICAL AND 286 SURGICAL PATIENTS

VARIABLE	MEDICAL %	SURGICAL %
New York Heart Association Classes II & III	94.2	95.4
History of previous myocardial infarction	59.3	64.0
Interpretation of infarction by electrocardiogram, definite or possible	36.1	40.5
Duration of angina >25 mo	50.0	51.8
History of hypertension	30.0	27.6
History of congestive heart failure	8.4	5.2
History of cerebral vascular episode	3.2	2.1
History of diabetes	12.9	12.2
Cardiothoracic ratio >0.49	10.4	12.2
Serum cholesterol >249 mg/100 ml	31.9	20.6*

*Difference significant to <0.05.

A total of 596 patients entered in the final phase of the study (1972–74) were available for analysis. The only significant difference in distribution of baseline variables in the medical and surgical groups was in the serum cholesterol (table). Adherence to assigned treatment remained over 90% at a minimal follow-up of 21 months. Operative mortality at 30 days averaged 5.6%. An average of 69% of grafts were patent about a year postoperatively. An average of 54% of patients had all grafts patent, and 88% had at least one graft patent; 12% had all grafts closed. Cumulative survival curves are shown in Figure 10. There was no significant difference in survival between any of the medical and surgical cohorts when cohorts with a similar extent of disease were compared.

Fig 10.—Cumulative survival rates for patients according to treatment assigned for the medical *(solid circles)* and the surgical *(open circles)* groups. Numbers of patients at risk in both groups at specific intervals after randomization are indicated below the survival curves (top numbers are medical group and bottom numbers, surgical group). (Courtesy of Murphy, M. L., et al.: N. Engl. J. Med. 297:621–627, Sept. 22, 1977.)

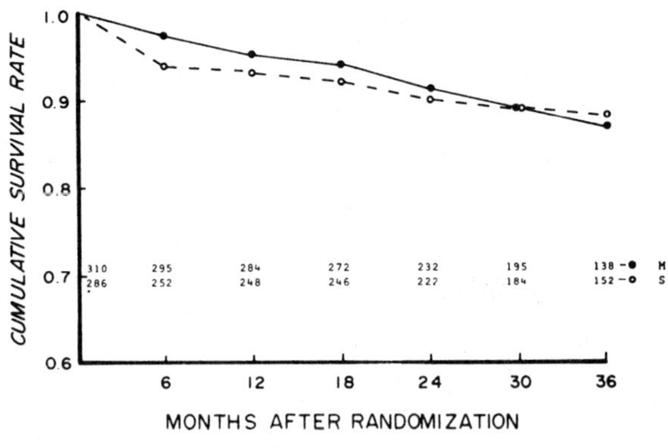

These results are preliminary, but indicate no significant difference in survival between patients managed medically for chronic stable angina and those undergoing saphenous vein bypass grafting. Ongoing detailed analyses of results are being performed, and in-depth analysis of clinical, ECG and angiographic subgroups and long-term follow-up observation are planned.

► [Previous studies have established that coronary bypass grafting is clearly effective in reducing angina pectoris in patients with one-, two-or three-vessel disease and in prolonging life in patients with obstructive disease involving the left main coronary artery. But a critical question remains: Does this operation prolong life in patients with chronic angina pectoris without left main coronary artery disease? In this, the first relatively large-scale prospective and randomized trial, the results at 3 years do not indicate any benefit of operation. This study has met with considerable criticism because of the relatively high mortality (5.6%) and the facts that only 69% of the grafts were patent a year postoperatively and revascularization was not complete in many patients. It is true that in many centers the mortality for coronary artery bypass grafting has now been reduced to the neighborhood of 1–3%, but, to be fair, these operations were carried out in 1972–74 when the mortality of 5.6% was comparable to what was observed in many institutions. Indeed, a review of surgical treatment of coronary artery disease in seven community hospitals in the New Orleans area (Richter et al.: South. Med. J. 70: 1052, 1977) reported an average mortality of 8.7%. Therefore, it is my impression that whereas the results of surgical treatment in some centers are superior to those in this VA cooperative trial, there are many institutions in which the surgery is inferior to what it was in those VA hospitals and perhaps this trial represents a reasonable picture of the effectiveness of surgery in the operation as a whole.

Attention is called to two other articles describing the same cooperative trial. Thus, Detre et al. (Am. J. Cardiol. 40:212, 1977) described the results of medical treatment. What is exciting is that the results of medical treatment in this group are superior to those in most previously published studies. In the VA trial the 2-year survival in patients with double-vessel disease was 90% and in previously widely quoted studies it ranged from 74% to 80%; in patients with three-vessel disease in the VA study it was 88%, whereas in earlier studies it ranged from 63% to 67%. Thus, either the natural history has improved as a consequence of modern treatment (β-blockers and long-acting nitrates, etc.) or patients in the earlier series assigned to medical therapy were unusually poor risks, or both. There is a suggestion in the VA data, although the results are not statistically significant, that patients with three-vessel disease and abnormal ventricular function have a better survival after surgical than after medical treatment (Read et al.: J. Thorac. Cardiovasc. Surg. 75:1, 1978). McNeer et al. (Circulation 49:606, 1974) have made a similar suggestion on the basis of retrospective evaluation of closely matched, although not intentionally randomized, patients.

It is likely that this debate will continue for some time. Fortunately, the VA patients are being followed and the long-term results of their survival will be of great interest. Also, the National Institutes of Health are conducting a coronary artery surgery study that undoubtedly will throw additional light on this critically important problem.

One thing is clear. It is not appropriate to draw conclusions concerning survival in this disease without concurrent randomized controls. A helpful summary of this entire problem is provided in a review article by Miller and Dodge (Arch. Intern. Med. 137: 1439, 1977).—Ed.] ◄

Survival Predictors in Coronary Artery Disease: Medical and Surgical Comparisons. Ronald E. Vlietstra, Jose L. Assad-Morell, Robert L. Frye, Lila R. Elveback, Daniel C. Connolly, Erik L. Ritman, James R. Pluth, Donald A. Barnhorst, Gordon K. Danielson and Robert B. Wallace[9] (Mayo Clinic) used linear discriminant function analysis to test the independent prognostic value of nine variables in patients with coronary artery disease. Comparison was made between

(9) Mayo Clin. Proc. 52:85–90, February, 1977.

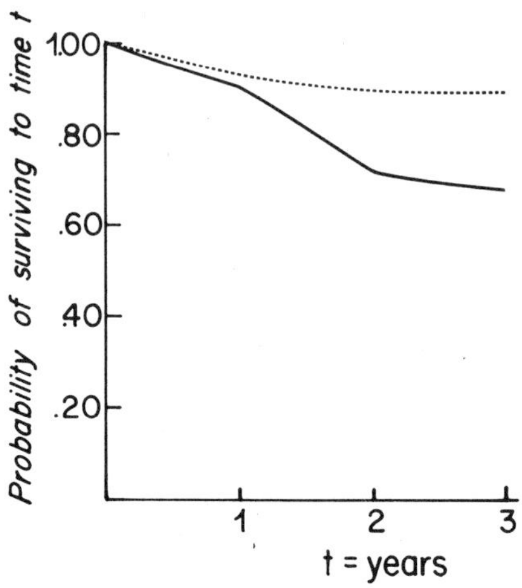

Fig 11.—Survival for 30 medical *(solid line)* and 56 surgical *(broken line)* patients with ejection fractions of 25–49%. (Courtesy of Vlietstra, R. E., et al.: Mayo Clin. Proc. 52:85–90, February, 1977.)

183 medically treated patients who would have been accepted for surgery on anatomical grounds and 520 patients undergoing aortocoronary saphenous vein bypass grafting in 1969–72. Survival status was established in 1974 for 98.9% of the medical group and 99.6% of the surgical group.

Medical patients more often had past symptoms of heart failure, larger hearts, higher left ventricular end-diastolic pressures and lower ejection fractions. The overall functional status of surgical patients was worse, and more had three-vessel disease. All but 1 of 44 deaths in the medical group were of cardiac origin, as were 33 of 40 deaths in the surgical group. The 30-day mortality in the latter group was 3%. In the medical group, the best discriminator between 2-year survival and death was the ejection fraction, and the best discrimination was provided by the combination of ejection fraction, left ventricular end-diastolic pressure and left main coronary stenosis. A discriminant function permitted correct classification of 91% of both survivors and deaths. Ejection fraction was also the best single factor in the surgical group, and maximal information was provided by the combination of ejection fraction and prior transmural infarction. Patients with ejection fractions below 25% did poorly. Survival at 3 years was better in surgical patients among those with ejection fractions of 25–49% (Fig 11).

The findings confirm the importance of left ventricular function for the outcome in patients with coronary artery disease. The data suggest a role for saphenous vein bypass grafting in prolonging the lives of patients with moderately impaired ventricular function.

► [As indicated in the comments following the preceding article, there is suggestive evidence that patients with moderate reduction of ventricular performance, i.e., ejection fractions between 25% and 49%, showed better survival after surgical treatment. On the other hand, in patients with normal ventricular function, i.e., with ejection fractions greater than or equal to 50%, or those with very poor ventricular function, that is, with ejection fractions less than 25%, surgical treatment did not appear to alter survival rate. Manley et al. (J. Thorac. Cardiovasc. Surg. 72:841, 1976) have suggested that surgery improves the prognosis in patients with poor left ventricular function. However, this conclusion came from an unrandomized study. Zubiate et al. (ibid. 73:84, 1977) also believe, on the basis of a comparison of nonrandomized, nonconcurrently treated patients with poor left ventricular function (ejection fractions less than 0.2), that surgery improves survival. – Ed.] ◄

Internal Mammary Artery Graft for Ischemic Heart Disease: Effect of Revascularization on Clinical Status and Survival. Floyd D. Loop, Manuel J. Irarrazaval, Johan J. Bredee, Wayne Siegel, Paul C. Taylor and William C. Sheldon[1] (Cleveland Clinic) have obtained a high rate of patency and a symptomatic response similar to that from vein grafting by internal mammary artery (IMA) grafting over a 5½-year period. A comparison was made between 400 consecutive patients given a single IMA graft, alone or combined with vein grafts, in 1971 and 1972 and 741 patients given venous autografts in 1967–70. Of the IMA graft patients, 80% had multivessel obstruction. Vein grafts were combined with IMA grafts in 279 patients. The IMA group included 360 men and 40 women with a mean age of 52 years. About half were in NYHA functional classes III and IV. The operative attempt was considered to be complete in 67% of patients. Three patients had IMA grafting as a reoperation.

Four patients (1%) died during or within a month after surgery, and 16 patients had intraoperative transmural infarction. Five of 10 late

Fig 12. – Comparison of survival of 741 patients receiving venous autografts in 1967–70 *(broken line)* and 400 receiving IMA grafts, alone or with venous autografts, in 1971 and 1972 *(solid line)*. Ninety-three percent of patients in earlier series were alive at 36 months, compared with 97% of those with IMA grafting ($P < 0.004$). (Courtesy of Loop, F. D., et al.: Am. J. Cardiol. 39:516–522, April, 1977.)

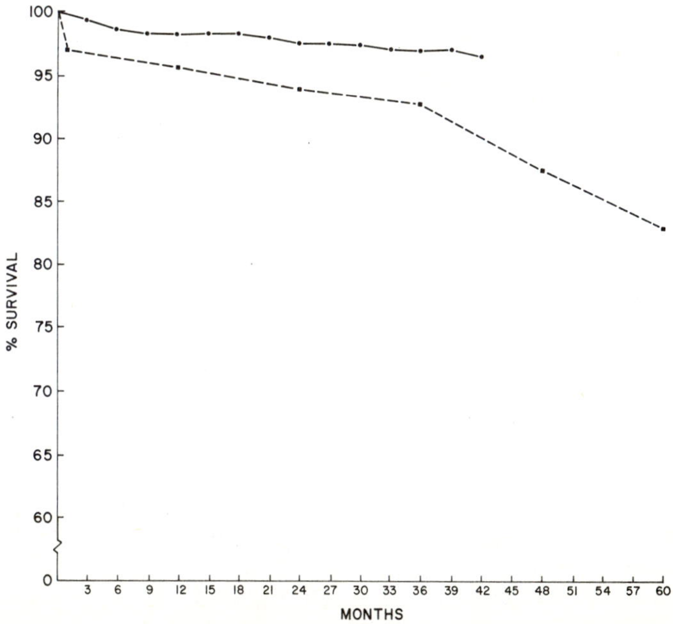

(1) Am. J. Cardiol. 39:516–522, April, 1977.

deaths were due to infarction and 2 were sudden deaths. Late infarction was documented in 4% of patients. At a mean follow-up of 38 months, 7% of patients were in functional classes III and IV. The 4½-year actuarial survival rate at a mean follow-up of 50 months was 95%. On angiographic evaluation of 254 patients a mean of 1 year after operation, 95% of IMA grafts and 82% of vein grafts were patent. Survival has been greater than in the comparison group given vein grafts only (Fig 12).

The factors responsible for improved survival in the IMA-vein graft group in this study include reduced operative mortality, fewer intraoperative infarctions, more complete revascularization and a higher patency rate of the IMA grafts. Internal mammary artery grafting has become a valuable addition to surgery for ischemic heart disease. When the technique of graft construction is mastered, the results are excellent and quite consistent.

► [Debate among cardiovascular surgeons continues as to the relative advantages and disadvantages of internal mammary anastomosis vs. saphenous vein grafting. Some surgeons believe that the internal mammary artery graft is superior insofar as postoperative patency is concerned. However, Angell and Sywak (Circulation 56 (Suppl. 2):22, 1977) analyzed 74 consecutive unselected patients with bypassable lesions of the left anterior descending coronary artery and randomized them to either saphenous vein bypass grafting or internal mammary artery anastomosis. The number of patent grafts was essentially equal in the two groups and the resulting flow in the internal mammary graft was less than in the saphenous vein bypass grafts. It should also be noted that many surgeons find the preparation of the internal mammary artery for grafting to be tedious and the anastomosis more difficult to perform than the saphenous vein bypass graft. All of this points to the superiority of the latter procedure. —Ed.] ◄

Improved Survival after Coronary Bypass Surgery in Patients with Poor Left Ventricular Function: Role of Intra-aortic Balloon Counterpulsation. The survival of patients with severe myocardial dysfunction due to occlusive coronary artery disease depends on the preservation of all viable myocardium and the arrest of further ischemic injury. Mario Feola, Leslie Wiener, Paul Walinsky, Hratch Kasparian, Peter Duca, Ronald Gottlieb, Albert Brest and John Templeton[2] (Thomas Jefferson Univ.) found that the operative mortality with aortocoronary bypass surgery in such patients can be significantly reduced with the aid of intra-aortic counterpulsation. The results in 23 patients with an ejection fraction of 0.3 or less who were operated on in 1973–74 without balloon assistance were compared with those in 25 patients treated in 1975–76 with balloon assistance. All patients were in NYHA classes III and IV and had at least 70% obstruction of three or more coronary vessels. About three fourths of the patients had had a previous myocardial infarct. The same surgical technique was used in both groups. Counterpulsation was instituted about 12 hours before operation and was discontinued gradually, usually over 2–5 days postoperatively.

The in-hospital mortality in the control group was 34.7%, 4 deaths being intraoperative and 3 due to postoperative pump failure. Two study patients died postoperatively, 1 of pump failure. The difference

(2) Am. J. Cardiol. 39:1021–1026, June, 1977.

in mortality was significant. The groups were similar in age, functional disability, condition of the left ventricle and degree of coronary artery disease. The duration of bypass and the total duration of anoxic cardiac arrest were also similar in the two groups. The effects of intra-aortic balloon counterpulsation in the preoperative period were characterized by "unloading" of the left ventricle and improved metabolic ability of the myocardium to tolerate the pacing stress. Blood flow in 12 vein grafts increased intraoperatively with counterpulsation from 82.9 to 102.5 ml/minute. The only balloon-related complication was leg ischemia due to thrombus formation at the site of the graft after removal of the balloon; a thrombectomy was done, and no residual damage occurred.

The operative mortality of aortocoronary bypass surgery in patients with poor left ventricular function can be significantly reduced by the perioperative use of intra-aortic balloon counterpulsation. This approach may give new hope to patients with otherwise intractable ischemic heart disease.

► [Obviously, since this was not a controlled randomized study (which is difficult, if not impossible, to carry out in such high-risk patients) the conclusions must be interpreted cautiously. It is possible that the surgeons improved with time and that the mortality might have declined even without the use of balloon assistance. Nonetheless, the results are strongly suggestive that the balloon was helpful in this important group of patients. Cooper et al. (Am. J. Surg. 133:463, 1977) also reported the effectiveness of preoperative intra-aortic balloon assist in revascularization of high-risk patients. – Ed.]

Use of Augmented Ejection Fraction to Select Patients with Left Ventricular Dysfunction for Coronary Revascularization. Some patients with coronary disease and severe left ventricular dysfunction have significant improvement in both angina and failure symptoms after myocardial revascularization, implying that the ventricular dysfunction may result from ischemia as well as ventricular fibrosis. Lawrence H. Cohn, John J. Collins, Jr., and Peter F. Cohn[3] (Harvard Med. School) determined whether a diagnostic determinant could be found to help separate patients with a high expectation of improvement from those with high operative risk and little hope of long-term improvement. Thirty-three patients (31 men) with left ventricular dysfunction and angina of varying intensity were studied. Their mean age was 52 years. All had multiple coronary artery obstruction and had had at least one infarction. All had symptoms of congestive failure. Coronary-venous anastomoses were performed, and left ventricular aneurysms were resected in 6 patients. Seven patients had intra-aortic balloon counterpulsation.

There were 24 patients in whom the systolic ejection fraction (SEF) was augmented more than 0.1 with postextrasystolic potentiation (group I) and 9 with less augmentation (group II). The mean resting ejection fraction (EF) was 0.31 in group I, the left ventricular end-diastolic pressure (LVEDP) was 20.3 mm Hg and the cardiac index was 2.38 L per minute per sq m. In group II, mean resting EF was 0.34, LVEDP was 16.3 mm Hg and cardiac index was 2.48 L per minute per sq m. Operative mortalities were 9% in group I and 33% in group II,

(3) J. Thorac. Cardiovasc. Surg. 72:835–840, December, 1976.

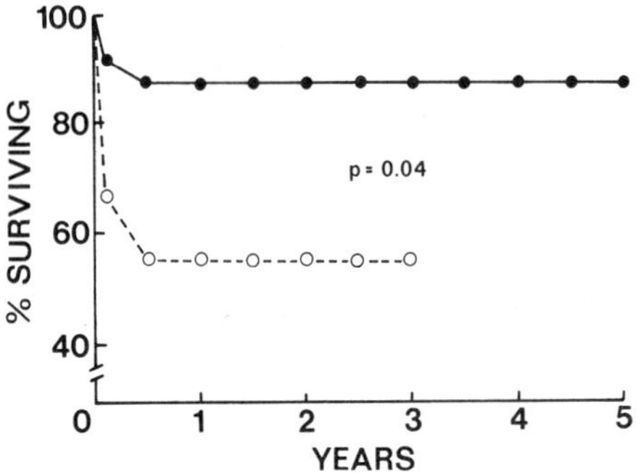

Fig 13. – Life-table curves for group I *(solid line)* and group II *(broken line)* patients after coronary revascularization for angina and congestive symptoms. (Courtesy of Cohn, L. H., et al.: J. Thorac. Cardiovasc. Surg. 72:835–840, December, 1976.)

and 1 late death in each group was due to infarction. Life-table curves are shown in Figure 13. Four group I patients had mild angina on follow-up at a mean of 24.9 months, and 1 is in class III. Only 1 of 5 group II survivors is entirely asymptomatic. Five of the 7 patients who required intra-aortic balloon counterpulsation died.

Significant augmentation of SEF by a premature ventricular contraction is a simple and useful indicator for selection of patients with left ventricular dysfunction to undergo coronary revascularization. More careful patient selection will obviate unnecessary operations and offer surgery safely to some patients who might not ordinarily be considered for operation.

► [Up to now, the most commonly used index for assessing operative risk and outcome has been the ejection fraction. However, the ejection fraction can be depressed not only by myocardial fibrosis due to previous myocardial infarction, but by ischemia as well. In the latter cases, this index can be improved by a variety of pharmacologic (isoproterenol, epinephrine and nitroglycerin) and physiologic (postextrasystolic potentiation) maneuvers. A depressed ejection fraction due to ischemia is associated with a more favorable outcome than a similar depression due to infarction. Therefore, study of the effects of postextrasystolic potentiation is useful in the selection of patients with serious depression of left ventricular function. – Ed.] ◄

M-Mode Echocardiography in Evaluating Left Ventricular Function and Surgical Risk in Patients with Coronary Artery Disease. Mortality during hospitalization after surgery for coronary artery disease is closely related to the preoperative state of ventricular function. Betty C. Corya, Susan Rasmussen, Suzanne B. Knoebel and Harvey Feigenbaum[4] (Indiana Univ.) evaluated the clinical usefulness of M-mode echocardiographic studies in assessing the extent of left ventricular dysfunction and identifying high-risk surgical patients. Study was made of 204 consecutive patients having 75% or greater narrowing of at least one coronary artery. The 172 men and 32 women had a mean age of 51. Half the patients had a history of myocardial infarction. Echographic left ventricular size and closure time of the mitral valve were measured. Eighty-six patients subsequently had operations with bypass and hypothermia.

(4) Chest 72:181–185, August, 1977.

Mitral valve closure alone was abnormal in 45 patients, 27 had an increased left ventricular dimension and 30 had both abnormalities. Extensive abnormalities of left ventricular contraction were found in 37 patients. The left ventricular end-diastolic pressure (LVEDP) and extent of contraction abnormality were significantly greater in patients with both echographic abnormalities. The LVEDP averaged 23 mm Hg in this group, and 80% of the 30 patients had extensive abnormalities of contraction on left ventriculography. The LVEDP averaged 11 mm Hg in the 174 patients without both echographic abnormalities, and only 7% of them had extensive contraction abnormalities. All 7 hospital deaths were related to left ventricular failure and ventricular arrhythmias. Mortality was significantly increased only in the group with both echographic abnormalities. Extensive left ventricular contraction abnormality and a LVEDP of 20 mm Hg or above were significantly related to mortality but a history of past infarction was not. Eight of 14 patients who had myocardial resection had both echographic abnormalities and 5 of them died.

An echocardiogram showing an increased end-diastolic left ventricular internal dimension and abnormal mitral valve closure indicates severe left ventricular dysfunction, and surgical mortality is significantly increased in patients with these findings. Echocardiography is useful both in assessing the extent of left ventricular dysfunction and in screening patients for further invasive studies when a significantly increased risk of mortality would not be clinically justified.

► [Standard (M-mode) echocardiography is useful in the preoperative assessment of patients with coronary artery disease. Abnormality of mitral valve closure, for the purpose of this study, was defined as an ECG P-R interval minus the echocardiographic A-C interval of 0.06 second or less. In addition to left ventricular size and mitral valve closure, echocardiography is useful for detecting regional abnormalities of left ventricular wall motion and/or thickening during systole in patients with impaired left ventricular function. Also, left ventricular wall thinning during systole may indicate acute ischemia or infarction, and thin, dense myocardial echoes indicate scar formation. On the other hand, echocardiography has not proved useful in determining graft patency in the postoperative period (Corya: Am. J. Med. 63:10, 1977). — Ed.] ◄

Accelerated "Atherosclerosis": Morphological Study of 97 Saphenous Vein Coronary Artery Bypass Grafts. Bernadine H. Bulkley and Grover M. Hutchins[5] (Johns Hopkins Univ.) examined 97 saphenous vein coronary artery bypass grafts from 55 patients on whom autopsy was performed to evaluate the sequence of development of intimal changes in transplanted veins. Average patient age was 55 years; 78% were men. Twenty patients died intraoperatively, and 9 died 1 – 54 months after surgery.

Forty grafts from intraoperative deaths showed minimal changes; 6 showed small fibrin microthrombi. None of these grafts was occluded by thrombus. Twenty-two early postoperative grafts showed focal laminar deposits of fibrin thrombus or circumferential fibrin deposits; none had occlusive thrombi. Of 21 grafts in place for 2 – 21 days, 2 were occluded by organizing thrombus. The others exhibited thin laminar fibrin deposits and a concentric fibrous plaque. Foci of laminar intimal

(5) Circulation 55:163 – 169, January, 1977.

fibrin were present in 74% of these grafts. Six of 14 grafts in place for 1–54 months had occlusive thrombi with organization and recanalization. Most of the other grafts in this group showed intimal fibrin thrombus, and all showed intimal fibrous plaque. Over half these grafts showed infiltration of the plaque by lipid-laden macrophages. Fibrous plaque tended to become more marked with longer periods of implantation and with narrowings of the distal vein-to-artery anastomosis. The plaque consisted of collagen fibrils and ground substance containing mesenchymal cells.

Significant alterations in saphenous vein grafts are confined to the intima and are evident in all grafts after 1 month. The lesions include occlusive thrombus, thin layers of circumferential intimal fibrin and platelet microthrombi, and concentric fibrous plaque. The plaque exhibits changes characteristic of atheromas. It is not a simple response to increased pressure or an "arterialization" of the vein. Early-appearing intimal thrombus is apparently converted into fibrous plaque. This early thrombus is a factor in the development of accelerated "atherosclerosis" in saphenous vein bypass grafts.

► [As stressed by these authors (J. Thorac. Cardiovasc. Surg. 73:660, 1977), a common cause of graft occlusion is thrombosis secondary to encroachment on the lumen resulting from sewing the inverted artery to the vein graft. Intimal atheromas also tend to develop at the anastomotic sites. Lawrie et al. (Am. J. Cardiol. 37:856, 1976) also concluded that most graft occlusions occur early and are usually due to thrombosis. Late graft occlusion is uncommon and when it does occur it is rarely due to intimal proliferation. The moderate to marked intimal proliferation that has been found to occur up to 75 months postoperatively suggests that this phenomenon is compatible with good graft patency. Batayias et al. (Circulation 56 (Suppl. 2):18, 1977) also concluded that: (1) during the 1st month after operation, graft occlusion is due to thrombosis; (2) intimal proliferation of the graft appears 4 weeks after bypass surgery; (3) a change in the morphological features of the intimal thickening from cellular to fibrotic and hyalin may occur after 1 year; and (4) typical atherosclerosis may develop in vein grafts after 3 years.—Ed.] ◄

Valvular Heart Disease

Long-Term Experience with Porcine Aortic Valve Xenografts. Edward B. Stinson, Randall B. Griepp, Philip E. Oyer and Norman E. Shumway[6] (Stanford Univ.) discontinued the use of "fresh" aortic allografts in 1971 because of the high rate of allograft dysfunction. Glutaraldehyde-preserved porcine aortic valve xenografts were used for isolated mitral valve replacement (MVR) in 243 patients in 1971–75. They were used as aortic valve replacement (AVR) in 167 patients and as double valve replacement in 51. Combined procedures were done in a third to half of the groups. Long-term anticoagulation was instituted in 34 patients having MVR, 7 having AVR and 4 having double valve replacement (AVR and MVR). The average follow-up was 1.6 years after MVR, 1 year after AVR and 0.9 year after double valve replacement.

The overall operative mortality rates were 7.8%, 6.0% and 11.8%, respectively, for MVR, AVR and double valve replacement. No death was attributed to xenograft dysfunction. Late postoperative survival was 85% in the MVR group 4.4 years postoperatively. Patients with associated coronary artery disease accounted for a substantial portion of both early and late deaths. Late survival after AVR was 90.6% at 3 years. Comparison of patients with coronary artery disease with those with significant coronary narrowing showed higher operative mortality for the former but equal numbers of late deaths. Three late deaths followed double valve replacement. Causes of xenograft dysfunction are given in the table. Two of 12 dysfunctional valves had features of primary involvement of xenograft tissue. The linearized rate of thromboembolism was 5.2% per patient-year after MVR, 2.0% after AVR and

Causes of Diagnosed Xenograft Dysfunction

Cause	*MVR (n =243)*	*AVR (n =167)*	*MVR +AVR (n =51)*
Insufficiency murmur			
Early	4	1	1
Late	1	0	0
Endocarditis	1	1	0
Valve stenosis	0	1	0
Primary tissue involvement	2	0	0
Totals	8	3	1

(6) J. Thorac. Cardiovasc. Surg. 73:54–63, January, 1977.

5.4% after double valve replacement. Most patients presently have greatly improved physical capacity, and a majority in all groups are in functional class I. Only 10 of 396 surviving patients are in functional class III or IV.

These findings support the use of glutaraldehyde-preserved porcine xenografts as bioprostheses carrying a low risk of thromboembolism without anticoagulation. The overall durability of the valves appears comparable to that of currently available mechanical prostheses. The continued clinical use of these valves is warranted.

► [There is a general tendency around the United States to replace prosthetic valves with porcine aortic valve xenografts (heterografts) because of the low incidence of thromboembolism and what appears to be excellent durability. Cevese et al. (Surg. 56 (Suppl. 2):111, 1977) described 564 patients who have undergone single or multiple heart valve replacement with the Hancock bioprosthesis and showed that the glutaraldehyde-preserved porcine valve is durable for up to 6½ years. In 2 patients, reoperation was required for mitral stenosis caused by tissue ingrowth; 2 patients acquired endocarditis and 8 acquired thromboembolism. Actuarial curves showed little, if any, decline in survival from 3 to 6½ years for patients who underwent replacement of the mitral valve. Spray and Roberts (Am. J. Cardiol. 40:319, 1977) have described structural changes in porcine xenografts; they noted that degeneration of the cusp tissue with resulting regurgitation was present in three valves, two in the mitral position with an implantation period of 56 and 75 months, respectively. Similarly, Fishbein et al. (Am. J. Cardiol. 40:331, 1977) also pointed out that valve dysfunction, i.e., infection, thrombosis or degeneration, while unusual in the late postoperative period may nevertheless occur. Some surgeons, such as Barratt-Boyes and his colleagues (Circulation 55:353, 1977) have no difficulty with antibiotic-sterilized homograft valves. In patients with a relatively small aortic root diameter (less than 24 mm), however, Barratt-Boyes has discontinued replacement of the mitral valve with stent-mounted antibiotic-treated aortic homografts because of the relatively high incidence of late postoperative complications.—Ed.] ◄

Valve Replacement with the Starr-Edwards and Hancock Prostheses: Comparative Analysis of Late Morbidity and Mortality. Philip E. Oyer, Edward B. Stinson, Randall B. Griepp and Norman E. Shumway[7] (Stanford Univ.) compared the long-term performance of patients given Starr-Edwards valve replacements and Hancock porcine xenograft prostheses. Starr-Edwards model 1260 aortic valves were used in 435 patients in 1968–74, and 251 patients received Hancock model 242 aortic xenograft prostheses in 1971–76. Starr-Edwards model 6120 mitral prostheses were used in 515 patients in 1964–74 and Hancock model 342 mitral xenografts were used in 338 patients in 1971–76. In corresponding periods, 121 patients received Starr-Edwards combined aortic and mitral prostheses, whereas 88 received combined xenograft valves. The groups were comparable in age, sex and preoperative hemodynamics. All patients given Starr-Edwards valves received warfarin indefinitely, whereas about half of those having xenograft mitral valve replacement received anticoagulant therapy for 3 months postoperatively. About one fourth of the xenograft aortic valve group also received short-term anticoagulant therapy.

Mortality and morbidity are given in the table. Total follow-up was 3944 patient-years for the Starr-Edwards patients and 947 patient-

(7) Ann. Surg. 186:301–309, September, 1977.

LINEARIZED MORTALITY AND MORBIDITY*

	Aortic Valves		Mitral Valves		Double Valves	
	Starr	Xenograft	Starr	Xenograft	Starr	Xenograft
Late Mortality	*6.3*	*3.4*	*7.9*	*4.5*	7.8	6.2
Thromboembolism						
Overall	*6.0*	2.6†	*10.9*	*4.1*†	6.6	3.1
Fatal	0.5	0.0	*1.0*	*0.0*	1.4	0.0
Hemorrhage						
Overall	*5.7*	*0.7*	*5.5*	*1.4*	*4.1*	*1.0*
Fatal	*0.7*	*0.0*	*0.9*	*0.2*	*0.2*	*0.0*
Valve failure	1.8	1.1	2.6	1.7	1.0	3.1
Endocarditis	1.2	1.4	0.4	0.2	0.9	1.0

*All values expressed as percent per patient-year. Significant differences are italicized ($P < 0.01$).

†Value skewed by uneven distribution of events in time.

years for the xenograft patients. Hospital mortality did not differ significantly in comparable groups. The rate of thromboembolism and that of hemorrhage were significantly lower in the xenograft groups, without offsetting increases in rates of valve failure or endocarditis.

The Hancock xenograft valves compare quite favorably to the Starr-Edwards prostheses with respect to durability and susceptibility to endocarditis and appear to be superior when thromboembolism, overall survival rates and morbidity and mortality from anticoagulant-associated hemorrhage are taken into consideration. The Hancock xenograft bioprosthesis appears to be the valve of choice.

► [Salomon (Circulation 56 (Suppl. 2):94, 1977) compared the long-term mortality and morbidity resulting from mitral valve replacement with a variety of prosthetic valves, allografts and xenografts. He found that 3 years after mitral valve replacement, 65% of patients with Starr-Edwards valves, 30% with homografts and 85% with heterografts were free of prosthesis-related deaths or complications. Starr's group now has follow-up data for up to 15 years on patients with caged-ball prostheses in the mitral position. Whereas most patients in whom the non-cloth-covered model used from 1960 to 1966 was placed have had emboli, approximately 50% are alive. The 10-year survival for prosthetic replacement of the aortic valve is 61%. Whereas the cloth-covered model is associated with a lower incidence of thromboembolism than the non-cloth-covered valves, they are also subject to a higher risk of reoperation because of cloth injury. Therefore, Starr has developed a "track" valve designed with exposed metal on the inner surface of each strut to prevent ball-cloth contact. This prosthesis maintains a low incidence of thromboembolism, and no reoperations for valve failure have been required (ibid., p. 133). The risk of anticoagulation in patients with prosthetic valves has been estimated; both serious and mild bleeds have been found to occur at an average rate of 1.4% per year. – Ed.] ◄

Pregnancy in Patients after Valve Replacement. The increasing use of artificial heart valves in the management of congenital and post-infective as well as rheumatic heart disease is resulting in a growing population of women of childbearing age who have had valve replacements. Celia Oakley and P. Doherty[8] (London) obtained questionnaire

(8) Br. Heart J. 38:1140–1148, November, 1976

data on 39 pregnancies in 34 patients who underwent valve replacement in the United Kingdom. Three other patients had valve replacement during pregnancy. Most patients had mitral, mitral plus aortic or tricuspid valve replacement, and half of these received anticoagulants. Patient age range was 18–38 years, and interval from cardiac surgery to conception ranged from 3 months to 5 years.

Thirty healthy infants were born. There were 3 spontaneous early abortions in women taking warfarin and 1 at 24 weeks in a patient who was not on anticoagulants. Two late intrauterine deaths occurred in women receiving phenindione. Two fetal deaths resulted from maternal death. Both women who survived valve replacement during pregnancy had malformed infants. The only fetal complications among 20 women not given anticoagulants were a spontaneous abortion at 24 weeks and 1 case of harelip and talipes. The other 19 patients had 23 successful pregnancies. Maternal complications were few, and no major complications were attributable to the use of anticoagulants. Two postpartum hemorrhages and 1 abdominal wall hematoma that followed cesarean section were attributable to anticoagulants. Two thromboembolic complications occurred. Congestive failure was observed in only 2 patients, and both recovered well on bed rest and diuretic therapy.

Most patients with artificial heart valves can safely undertake pregnancy, but patients on anticoagulants must know that there is an increased risk to the infant. Patients with tissue valves who do not require anticoagulation can expect a healthy infant, and biologic valves are therefore preferred for young women. An anticoagulant other than warfarin should be considered for young women who undergo valve replacement.

► [The overall results of pregnancy in these patients were really much better than I would have guessed. First of all, it is apparent that most patients can easily cope with the hemodynamic demands of pregnancy after valve replacement, since only 1 maternal death among 95 completed pregnancies has been reported up to the end of 1975 in patients with valve replacements. The relatively high fetal mortality in this series is not a necessary consequence of the maternal disease; rather, it is related to the use of oral anticoagulants. I suspect that this problem would vanish entirely with the more widespread use of tissue valves. Despite these relatively favorable results, it still seems worthwhile for women to undergo vigorous medical therapy in order to get through pregnancy before cardiac surgery is undertaken. Although open heart surgery can be carried out successfully during pregnancy, the risk to the baby is relatively high, so deferral of open heart surgery and the choice of closed rather than open mitral valvulotomy seems still to be wise at the present time in pregnant women with mitral stenosis who require immediate operation. – Ed.] ◄

Infective Endocarditis: Analysis of 54 Surgically Treated Patients. The mortality of surgically treated patients with infective endocarditis is about 30%. Arthur D. Boyd, Frank C. Spencer, O. Wayne Isom, Joseph N. Cunningham, George E. Reed, Anthony J. Acinapura and David A. Tice[9] (New York Univ.) reviewed experience with 54 patients operated on for infective endocarditis in 1970–75. They were among 177 patients admitted with the diagnosis in this period (Fig 14). The 37 men and 17 women had a mean age of 42 years. Fifteen patients

(9) J. Thorac. Cardiovasc. Surg. 73:23–30, January, 1977.

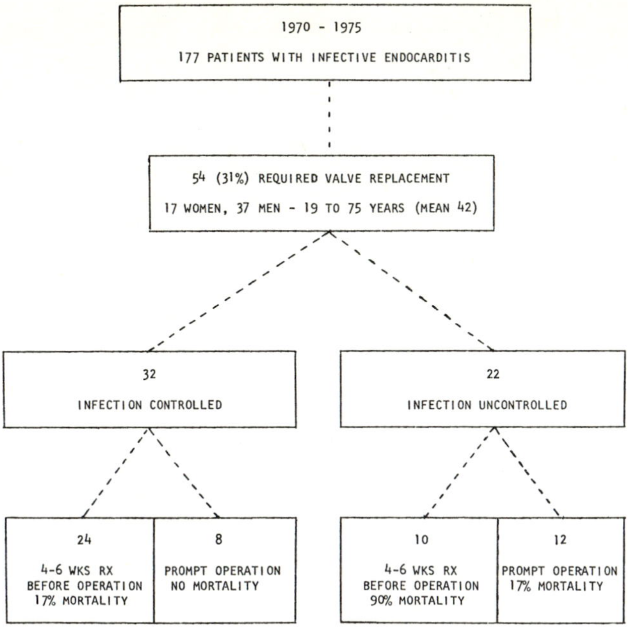

Fig 14.—Breakdown of patient population admitted for infective endocarditis in 1970–75. (Courtesy of Boyd, A. D., et al.: J. Thorac. Cardiovasc. Surg. 73:23–30, January, 1977.)

had a history of rheumatic fever, and 9 were drug addicts. The aortic valve was involved in 28 cases. Appropriate antibacterial and antifungous therapy was instituted, and surgery was performed 4–45 days later. The most common infecting organisms were staphylococci and streptococci. The primary indication for valve replacement was progressive heart failure in 26 patients, uncontrolled sepsis in 15 and systemic embolization in 13. Starr-Edwards prostheses were used in most patients. Antibiotic therapy was continued for 2 weeks after operation.

Endocarditis was controlled by antimicrobial therapy in 32 patients. Twenty-four were treated for 4–6 weeks before operation and 4 (17%) died. The other 8 patients were operated on within 10 days of the onset of heart failure or embolization, without a death. Ten patients were treated for 4–6 weeks despite continued evidence of infection and 9 of them died, 5 within 48 hours of surgery. Ten of the 12 patients with uncontrolled infection who were operated on within 10 days of the onset of embolization, worsening heart failure or progressive infection survived, although bacteria or fungi were present in the blood or valve tissue of each. Five of 6 patients in the series with fungous infections on the valve died.

If endocarditis can be controlled clinically, surgery can safely be delayed for 4–6 weeks, at which time valve replacement can be done if necessary. Otherwise prompt operation is indicated. Embolization or progressive heart failure at any time indicates a need for prompt valve replacement.

► [It is clear that the tide is turning to earlier operation. What was once considered to be a last-ditch stand is now used progressively earlier. The prompt surgical treatment of patients with advancing heart failure and persistent sepsis appears to reduce mortality. – Ed.] ◄

Long-Term Prognosis of Mitral Valve Prolapse. Peter Mills, John Rose, Jane Hollingsworth, Ingrid Amara and Ernest Craige[1] (Univ. of North Carolina) undertook a retrospective study of mitral valve prolapse based on phonocardiographic diagnostic criteria, with subsequent echocardiographic or pathologic confirmation. Follow-up was made of 53 patients (34 females) in whom mitral valve prolapse had been documented at least 10 years previously. Twenty-two presented with nonspecific chest pain, palpitation and lethargy and the

Fig 15. – Phonocardiographic and echocardiographic records from patient documenting no change in midsystolic click *(X)* over 19 years. Study in 1976 shows echocardiographic evidence of mitral valve prolapse *(arrow)*. Recording speed was 75 mm per second in both tracings; S_1, 1st heart sound; S_2, 2d heart sound. (Courtesy of Mills, P., et al.: N. Engl. J. Med. 297:13–18, July 7, 1977.)

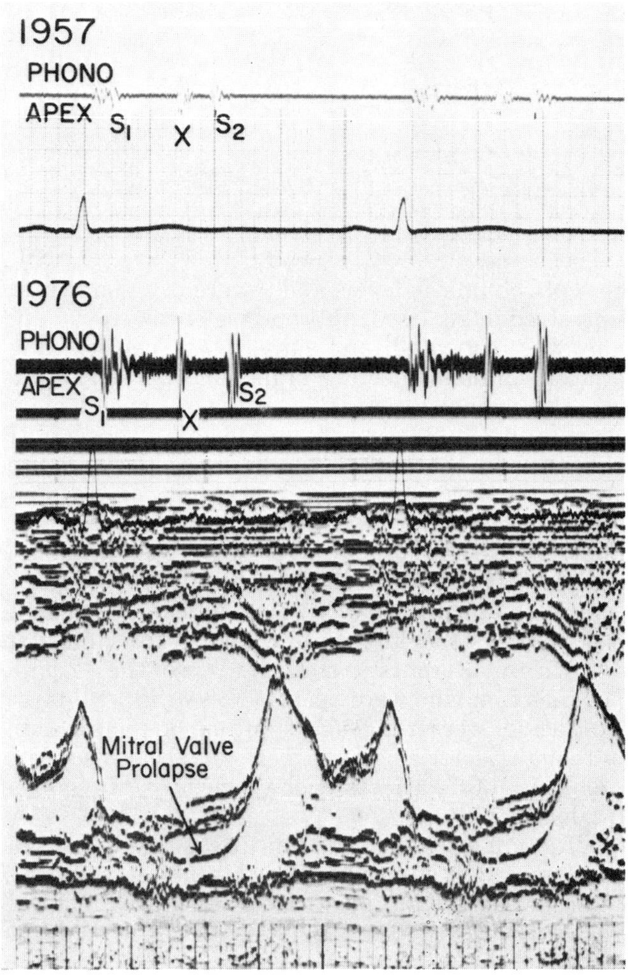

(1) N. Engl. J. Med. 297:13–18, July 7, 1977.

other 31 were asymptomatic. Systolic clicks were recorded in 22 patients, a late systolic murmur in 18 and both in 13. Nine patients died during follow-up, and the hearts were available for study in 3 instances.

Mean time from initial study to follow-up examination or death was 13.7 years. Only 2 deaths were related to the mitral valve abnormality; 1 was due to chord rupture complicating endocarditis. Complications included 3 cases of bacterial endocarditis, 5 of severe mitral regurgitation and 1 of ventricular fibrillation. Pathologic studies showed voluminous, thickened valve cusps exhibiting myxomatous degeneration. Symptoms had worsened at follow-up in 2 of 38 patients in NYHA classes 1 and 2. Echocardiographic features of mitral valve prolapse were found in 33 patients (Fig 15). In 3 patients with an isolated midsystolic click initially, echocardiography did not show prolapse. Compared with an isolated midsystolic click, a late systolic murmur was significantly associated with subsequent complications. Complications were more frequent in men and in older patients. An abnormal ECG was not a significant predictive factor for serious complications.

Bacterial endocarditis or progressive mitral regurgitation is more important in the spectrum of this disorder than is the dramatic but rare occurrence of sudden death. Patients with a late systolic murmur should receive antibiotic prophylaxis and be evaluated regularly. When antidysrhythmia agents are indicated, quinidine should be used with caution, especially in patients with atrial fibrillation and cardiomegaly or abnormalities of repolarization. Propranolol may be the drug of choice in these patients.

► [The relatively benign nature of mitral valve prolapse in this series of patients is noteworthy. It is important to recall that the prolapsing mitral valve leaflet syndrome may be responsible for the combination of angina and normal coronary arteriograms (Nakhjavan et al.: Chest 70:706, 1976). However, Crawford (Am. J. Med. 62:447, 1977) has pointed out that the myocardial damage from coronary artery disease can definitely cause mitral valve prolapse in patients without preexisting redundant mitral valve tissue. Clearly, in that group the prognosis of mitral valve prolapse is not as benign as it is in the idiopathic group. – Ed.] ◄

Strokes: Complication of Mitral Leaflet Prolapse? Although the syndrome of midsystolic click and murmur is thought to be generally benign, numerous reports have described a syndrome with many symptoms, including bacterial endocarditis and sudden death in rare instances. W. J. Kostuk, D. R. Boughner, H. J. M. Barnett (London, Ont.) and M. D. Silver[2] (Univ. of Toronto) report an association between cerebral ischemic events and mitral prolapse. A prospective trial of platelet-inhibiting drugs has been conducted in the past 4 years in patients with transient ischemic attacks and nonprogressive partial strokes. Fourteen patients had no significant atherosclerotic disease on cerebral angiography and the focal nature of their neurologic events suggested an embolic cause.

The study group included 7 men and 7 women with a mean age of 37. Only 1 woman was taking contraceptive pills when symptoms began and she had not taken the pill for 2 years when symptoms recurred. No

(2) Lancet 2:313–316, Aug. 13, 1977.

patient had hypertension, anemia or polycythemia. Ten patients had sudden hemiparesis or a major stroke. The carotid territory was thought to be involved in 9 patients. Attacks were multiple in 10 of the 14 patients; in 3 they involved the two hemispheres on separate occasions. Five patients had a history of palpitation and 5 had episodes of chest pain; 3 had midsystolic clicks and 5, apical midsystolic, late or pansystolic murmurs; 3 had both midsystolic click and a late systolic murmur. All 14 patients had cardiac symptoms or signs, or both. Echography showed definite mitral leaflet prolapse in 9 patients and probable prolapse in 2. Episodes of paroxysmal atrial fibrillation were monitored in 3 patients and bouts of ventricular tachycardia in 1. Five other patients had frequent premature beats. Left ventriculography showed posterior mitral leaflet prolapse in all patients; in 1 the anterior leaflet was also involved.

In another patient, a small antemortem left atrial thrombus was found at autopsy. The findings in this case support the thesis that a localized thrombus could be the source of the embolus in these patients. Cerebral ischemic events should be added to the many symptoms associated with mitral leaflet prolapse.

► [In addition to cerebrovascular accidents, ventricular arrhythmias are an important serious complication of patients with mitral valve prolapse (Campbell et al.: Br. Heart J. 38:1053, 1976). Continuous 24-hour ambulatory electrocardiography has revealed that serious ventricular arrhythmias occurred most frequently in patients with mitral valve prolapse with inferolateral S-T and T wave abnormalities in the resting ECG, suggesting that the ECG may be helpful in identifying those patients with this deformity of the mitral valve who are at risk from sudden death. Also intermittent complete atrioventricular block has been reported in this condition (Woodley et al.: Chest 72:369, 1977). —Ed.] ◄

Afterload Reduction

Oral Hydralazine Therapy for Chronic Refractory Heart Failure. Intravenous vasodilator therapy is impractical for the long-term management of heart failure. Nitrates may significantly reduce left ventricular filling pressure with little or no change in cardiac output. They may be less effective in patients in whom low output is the primary problem. Hydralazine significantly reduces arteriolar tone with little effect on capacitance vessels, and it can be given orally. Kanu Chatterjee, William W. Parmley, Barry Massie, Barry Greenberg, Jeffrey Werner, Steven Klausner and Anne Norman[3] (Univ. of California, San Francisco) studied the hemodynamic effects of oral hydralazine in 10 patients with severe chronic heart failure refractory to conventional medical therapy. The patients were aged 29 – 65 years. Heart failure was due to cardiomyopathy of unknown cause in 4 patients, ischemic cardiomyopathy in 2 and persistent failure after valve replacement in 4. Nine patients were in NYHA class IV and 1 was in class III. All patients were on adequate digitalis therapy and were taking furosemide. Hydralazine was given in a dose of 25 mg, followed by 50 mg 3 hours later and, if necessary, 75 mg. A dose of 50 or 75 mg was then given every 6 hours.

The maximum doses of hydralazine used were 50 mg in 2 patients and 75 mg in 8. Both systemic and pulmonary vascular resistances declined significantly and cardiac output and stroke volume rose markedly. The stroke work index increased despite some reduction in arterial pressure. There was no significant change in heart rate or pulmonary capillary wedge pressure. The maximum rise in cardiac output usually occurred at 24 hours. Two patients had some tachycardia. The mean arterial pressure fell only moderately in 5 patients. Changes in left ventricular filling pressure were inconsistent. All patients perceived lessening of fatigue. Urine output was satisfactory despite a reduced dosage of diuretics. Nine patients used hydralazine for 2 – 5 months and 7 were significantly improved clinically. One patient died suddenly after having improved markedly in effort tolerance. No patient developed postural hypotension or signs of the lupus erythematosus syndrome. Two gained weight slightly. Nausea disappeared on continued treatment.

Hydralazine can produce significant beneficial hemodynamic responses in patients with severe congestive heart failure. Oral hydralazine therapy may be a practical and effective means of managing patients with refractory heart failure.

► [Experiments on isolated cardiac tissue have established that myocardial fiber shortening is dependent on the preload, which determines the muscle's end-diastolic

---

(3) Circulation 54:879 – 883, December, 1976.

length, the contractile state of the myocardium and the afterload. At any level of the contractile state and preload, the extent of shortening varies inversely with the afterload. Although the geometric arrangement of myocardial fibers in the intact ventricle is far more complex than it is in strips of cardiac muscle, physiologic studies have demonstrated that the three factors that affect the extent of shortening of isolated cardiac muscle also influence the stroke volume of the intact heart; changes in afterload generally elicit reciprocal alterations in stroke volume. Vasodilators, i.e., afterload-reducing agents, have been demonstrated to improve the impaired dynamics of left ventricular failure. An important recent observation is that the salutary hemodynamic and clinical effects of vasodilator therapy may be sustained for periods of months and even years.

The available vasodilators vary in their hemodynamic effects, locus and duration of action and mode of administration. Some vasodilators, such as the α-adrenergic blocking agents and hydralazine, act predominantly on the arterial bed and, as such, tend to raise cardiac output, but have relatively little effect on left ventricular filling pressure and therefore tend not to relieve pulmonary congestion. When the primary defect is a reduction of cardiac output or mitral regurgitation, an arterial vasodilator such as hydralazine is the drug of choice; when pulmonary congestion is the principal defect, a venodilator that results in displacement of blood from the lungs to the peripheral venous bed would be preferable. When it is desired both to elevate cardiac output and to reduce pulmonary vascular pressure, an agent that acts on both the arterial and venous beds, such as prazosin, which is described in the following article, may be indicated. – Ed.] ◄

Sustained Reduction of Cardiac Impedance and Preload in Congestive Heart Failure with the Antihypertensive Vasodilator Prazosin. No single available oral vasodilator has been as effective as parenteral vasodilators in the long-term management of chronic heart failure. Richard R. Miller, Najam A. Awan, Kevin S. Maxwell and Dean T. Mason[4] investigated prazosin, which lacks the hazardous side effects of long-term hydralazine therapy, to determine if a single oral agent might obviate the need for combination therapy in chronic congestive heart failure. Six men and 4 women with a mean age of 51 who had severe ischemic cardiomyopathy and documented heart failure were studied. All were on digoxin and diuretics and 7 were also taking long-acting nitrate preparations. Studies were done with patients in the postabsorptive state. Forearm plethysmography was done in 9 patients. Prazosin was given orally in a dose of 2–5 mg to 9 patients, whereas 1 received a second 2-mg dose for a total of 7 mg.

Heart rate fell insignificantly after prazosin administration. The mean systemic arterial pressure fell from 95.3 to 86.1 mm Hg at 30 minutes and to 76.2 mm Hg at 2 hours and remained lowered, although gradually rising toward control. Left ventricular filling pressure was also reduced. The cardiac index increased, as did the stroke work index; myocardial oxygen demand was reduced. Total systemic vascular resistance was reduced by prazosin in all patients. Forearm blood flow was increased and remained so for 6 hours of study and forearm vascular resistance was reduced by prazosin. Venous tone in the forearm was also lowered by administration of the drug. The agent produced relatively more venous than arteriolar dilatation.

The sustained dual actions of prazosin on left ventricular impedance and preload suggest that this long-acting oral agent may be useful in ambulatory patients with severe congestive heart failure to make

(4) N. Engl. J. Med. 297:303–307, Aug. 11, 1977.

combinations of unloading drugs unnecessary. Extended evaluation in outpatients is needed to establish the chronic clinical efficacy of prazosin.

► [The same group of investigators (Awan et al.: Circulation 56:346, 1977) have studied the long-term efficacy of prazosin in patients with refractory heart failure due to chronic coronary disease. After 2 weeks of therapy, end-diastolic dimensions measured by echocardiography had fallen, whereas ventricular shortening increased, treadmill exercise duration increased and symptomatic improvement persisted. Thus, prazosin possesses a sustained, nitroprusside-like, balanced dilator action on the systemic arterial and venous systems and is effective in the ambulatory management of chronic severe heart failure.

Oral isosorbide dinitrate (Williams et al.: Am. J. Cardiol. 39:84, 1977) resulted in a reduction of pulmonary wedge pressure with little change in cardiac output. The principal hemodynamic action of the nitrates is marked and sustained reduction in left ventricular filling pressure. These drugs should be used primarily for the relief of congestive symptoms.

It is important to mention the value of vasodilators in the management of valvular regurgitation (Shah: Am. Heart J. 93:403, 1977). In patients with mitral regurgitation, nitroprusside results in lowering of the V waves and reductions of the regurgitant fraction. In patients with aortic regurgitation (Miller et al.: Am. J. Cardiol. 38:564, 1976) nitroprusside lowered left ventricular end-diastolic pressure and volume, as well as the regurgitant fraction, while effective cardiac index rose. Presumably oral prazosin should have a similar, though prolonged, effect. – Ed.] ◄

Comparative Hemodynamic Effects of Inotropic and Vasodilator Drugs in Severe Heart Failure. Recent studies revealed that infusion of a vasodilator drug can significantly improve left ventricular pump function in patients with heart failure. Esteban Mikulic, Jay N. Cohn and Joseph A. Franciosa[5] (Univ. of Minnesota) compared the functional response of the left ventricle to sodium nitroprusside, a potent vasodilator, and dobutamine, an inotropic agent relatively devoid of peripheral vascular effects, in 21 hospitalized patients with New York Heart Association class III or IV congestive heart failure. Ten patients had severe ischemic heart disease and 11, nonischemic myocardial disease. All had had symptomatic heart failure for at least 6 months and had not been totally relieved by digitalis and diuretic therapy. Twelve patients received nitroprusside to reduce the pulmonary arterial wedge pressure by 40% or the systolic arterial pressure to 95 mm Hg. After pressures and outputs returned to control levels, dobutamine was infused in increasing doses to a rate of 10 μg/kg/minute. Five patients received the two drugs singly and in combination. Plethysmographic studies were done in 4 other patients with heart failure.

The hemodynamic data for the patients receiving the drugs sequentially are given in the table. Symptomatic improvement was noted with both agents. Cardiac output rose significantly with both, and the hemodynamic responses to the two drugs were quite similar. Ejection time was significantly prolonged only by nitroprusside infusion. The heart rate-blood pressure product and tension-time index were higher with dobutamine infusion. When the two agents were given together to 5 patients, the effects were additive. Brachial artery infusion of nitroprusside produced a dose-dependent forearm vasodilation. Infusion of dobutamine exerted a mild vasodilator effect.

---

(5) Circulation 56:528–533, October, 1977.

HEMODYNAMIC EFFECTS OF NITROPRUSSIDE AND DOBUTAMINE IN 12 PATIENTS WITH CONGESTIVE HEART FAILURE*

		HR	Systolic AP	Diastolic AP	$\overline{AP}$	$\overline{PA}$	PCW	CO	CI	SVR	PVR
Control	Mean	97.3	126.1	81.8	95.1	39.9	29.1	2.9	1.6	2339	330
	SEM	±4.7	±4.8	±2.8	±3.2	±2.4	±1.9	±0.3	±0.1	±173	±62
Nitroprusside	Mean	95.3	116.0	73.0	86.2	27.1	16.6	5.0	2.8	1254	189
		±5.1	±3.9	±2.1	±2.6	±1.3	±1.6	±0.4	±0.3	± 99	±32
	P		<0.001	<0.001	<0.001	<0.001	<0.001	<0.001	<0.001	<0.001	<0.001
Recontrol	Mean	98.1	126.0	81.5	95.0	39.2	28.0	2.8	1.5	2388	341
		±4.6	±5.2	±2.7	±3.3	±2.5	±1.8	±0.2	±0.1	±179	±57
Dobutamine	Mean	102.5	141.2	82.2	99.3	34.1	20.2	5.8	3.1	1350	193
		±4.4	±6.1	±3.2	±3.9	±2.0	±2.0	±0.5	±0.3	±125	±32
	P		<0.05			<0.02	<0.01	<0.001	<0.001	<0.001	<0.001

*HR, heart rate (beats per minute); AP, arterial pressure, $\overline{AP}$, mean arterial pressure, $\overline{PA}$, mean pulmonary artery pressure, PCW, pulmonary wedge pressure (mm Hg); CO cardiac output (L/minute); CI, cardiac index(L/minute/sq m); SVR, systemic vascular resistance; PVR, pulmonary vascular resistance (dynes-second-cm^{-5}).

Potent inotropic and vasodilator drugs produce similar and additive augmentation of left ventricular performance in patients in heart failure. Reduction in vascular resistance with dobutamine is probably largely of reflex origin, but the vasodilation itself may be an important determinant of the rise in cardiac output that occurs. Oral treatment with both an inotropic and a vasodilator drug might be effective in patients who remain symptomatic despite digitalis and diuretic therapy.

► [When an inotropic agent, such as dobutamine, is given to patients with congestive heart failure, the cardiac output rises, and there is a secondary reduction in systemic vascular resistance. Thus, the hemodynamic effect resembles that resulting from the administration of a vasodilator, such as nitroprusside. With the latter, however, reduction of peripheral resistance is the primary event and elevation of cardiac output is secondary. When both drugs are given together, an additive effect occurs, as is seen in the following article. — Ed.] ◄

Combined Dopamine and Nitroprusside Therapy in Congestive Heart Failure: Greater Augmentation of Cardiac Performance by Addition of Inotropic Stimulation to Afterload Reduction. Patients with congestive heart failure gain enhanced cardiac performance from inotropic agents and afterload-reducing drugs, but it is not clear if the simultaneous use of both approaches would give more benefit. Richard R. Miller, Najam A. Awan, James A. Joye, Kevin S. Maxwell, Anthony N. DeMaria, Ezra A. Amsterdam and Dean T. Mason[6] (Univ. of California) studied the comparative individual and combined actions of dopamine and nitroprusside on cardiocirculatory function in 9 patients (mean age 53 years) with chronic congestive heart failure, in NYHA functional class III. The patients required digitalis glycoside and diuretic therapy. All had resting left ventricular end-diastolic pressures of 18 mm Hg or above, and 7 had reduced cardiac indices. Nitroprusside was infused at a mean rate of 68 μg per minute to reduce the systolic pressure to 110 – 120 mm Hg and/or the left ventricular end-diastolic pressure (LVEDP) to 10 – 15 mm Hg. Dopamine was then begun at a rate of 5 – 7 μg/kg/minute, and the two agents were infused concomitantly for 10 minutes, followed by continuation of the dopamine infusion alone for 20 minutes.

The mean arterial pressure was lowered by nitroprusside from 89.9

(6) Circulation 55:881 – 884, June, 1977.

to 77.7 mm Hg but was unchanged by dopamine. A reduction to 83.1 mm Hg occurred with the combined infusion. No treatment altered the mean heart rate significantly. The mean LVEDP fell from 25.4 to 14.1 mm Hg with nitroprusside but was unchanged by dopamine. The combined infusion reduced the pressure to 15.7 mm Hg. Cardiac index was augmented by both agents and more so by the combined infusion. Each drug reduced the systemic vascular resistance, but only nitroprusside lowered the pressure time per minute. Neither drug alone significantly altered the stroke-work index, but the combined infusion augmented it.

Combined dopamine and nitroprusside infusion affords maximal benefit to patients with congestive heart failure. Nitroprusside reduces the left ventricular preload, while dopamine augments cardiac output and maintains the systemic arterial pressure. This approach provides an effective means of treating severe chronic heart failure due to left ventricular dysfunction from a variety of causes. It is uniquely suited for use in patients with ischemic heart disease and reduced systemic blood pressure.

► [For an excellent review of the theoretical and practical basis of vasodilator therapy of cardiac failure, see the work of Cohn and Franciosa (N. Engl. J. Med. 297:27, 1977; and ibid., p. 254). —Ed.] ◄

Sudden Death and Arrhythmias

Sudden Death in Patients with Chronic Bifascicular Block. Sudden cardiac death (SCD) has become a severe problem despite a persistently low incidence of heart block. Sudden cardiac death in patients with bifascicular block could reflect either trifascicular block with failure of a subsidiary escape mechanism, resulting in asystole, or the occurrence of ventricular fibrillation. Pablo Denes, Ramesh C. Dhingra, Delon Wu, Christopher R. Wyndham, Fernando Amat-y-Leon and Kenneth M. Rosen[7] (Univ. of Illinois) reviewed the records of 277 adults seen in 1970–75 with chronic bifascicular block with intact atrioventricular conduction. Sudden cardiac death was defined as unexpected death due to natural causes and occurring within 24 hours of the onset of acute symptoms or within 24 hours of the patient being seen alive without symptoms.

Sixty patients had complete left bundle-branch block (LBBB), 196 had complete right bundle-branch block (RBBB) with left anterior fascicular block and 21 had complete RBBB with left posterior fascicular block. The mean follow-up was 555 days. Sixty-eight patients died, 30 of them suddenly. The latter patients were followed for a mean of 294 days after entry to the study. Cumulative SCD mortality was highest for the group with LBBB. Arteriosclerotic heart disease was more fre-

COMPARISON OF SELECTED ECG AND ELECTROPHYSIOLOGIC FINDINGS IN PATIENTS WITH BIFASCICULAR BLOCK WITH AND WITHOUT SUDDEN CARDIAC DEATH

	Sudden Cardiac Death (N=30)		Non-Sudden Cardiac Death (N=247)		
Variables*	No.	(%)	No.	(%)	P
LBBB	14	(47)	46	(19)	<.01
RBBB + LAH	15	(50)	181	(73)	<.05
RBBB + LPH	1	(3)	20	(8)	NS
Ventricular premature complexes	15	(50)	47	(19)	<.01
	Sudden Cardiac Death		**Non-Sudden Cardiac Death**		
	Mean + SEM	No. Patients	Mean + SEM	No. Patients	P
PR interval (sec)	0.202±0.007	30	0.193±0.002	238	NS
QRS duration (sec)	0.141±0.003	30	0.142±0.001	247	NS
AH (msec)	120±9.3	30	107±2.3	238	NS
HV (msec)	56±2.8	30	54±0.9	247	NS
Sinoatrial nodal recovery time (msec)	928±48	21	1,050±26	195	<.05

*LBBB, left bundle-branch block; RBBB + LAH, right bundle-branch block and left anterior hemiblock; RBBB + LPH, right bundle-branch block and left posterior hemiblock.

(7) Arch. Intern. Med. 137:1005–1010, August, 1977.

quent in the SCD group than in the other patients, whereas hypertensive heart disease was significantly less frequent. Electrocardiographic and electrophysiologic findings in the two groups are compared in the table. Six patients died suddenly in the hospital; 4 had been hospitalized for congestive heart failure. Ventricular fibrillation caused four SCDs where terminal ECG documentation was available. Bradyarrhythmias did not appear to potentiate ventricular fibrillation in these patients.

It is concluded that SCD is a major cause of mortality in patients with chronic bifascicular block. The association of SCD with coronary disease and ventricular dysrhythmia suggests ventricular fibrillation as a frequent mechanism. The findings indicate that cardiac pacing alone would not be helpful in preventing SCD in high-risk patients. The effectiveness of antiarrhythmic drugs and coronary revascularization in preventing SCD remains to be defined.

► [An important aspect of this study is that it was carried out in a prospective manner. The authors have not excluded that sudden trifascicular block with failure of a ventricular pacemaker was the cause of death in their patients, but it is unlikely. It is of great interest that in this study electrophysiologic investigation by His bundle electrocardiography with measurement of the H-V interval was not helpful in identifying patients at high risk for sudden cardiac death, presumably because the latter was not caused by a bradyarrhythmia. Perhaps patients with complete left bundle-branch block and evidence of ischemic heart disease should be placed in the same category as those who have suffered a myocardial infarction and who exhibit complex ventricular premature beats, as described in the following article. – Ed.] ◄

Ventricular Premature Beats and Mortality after Myocardial Infarction. Both clinical and epidemiologic observations have led to interest in ventricular arrhythmia as a forerunner of fatal ventricular fibrillation. William Ruberman, Eve Weinblatt, Judith D. Goldberg, Charles W. Frank and Sam Shapiro[8] (New York) assessed the role of ventricular premature beats (VPB) in mortality in coronary patients by monitoring 1,739 men, who had had myocardial infarction, for ectopic activity for 1 hour at baseline examination and following them for mortality during up to 4 years. The average follow-up was 24.4 months. The subjects were men aged 35–75 in a prepaid group-practice plan who had had a recent myocardial infarction or angina. Half the subjects had had their last infarction within 3 months before baseline examination and 20%, 9 months or more earlier.

The presence of complex premature beats (R on T, runs of two or more, multiform or bigeminal premature beats) in the monitoring hour was associated with a risk of sudden coronary death three times that of the men without complex VPBs. The corresponding risk of death from any cause was twice that of men without complex beats (table). The arrhythmias made an independent contribution to the increased risk of death that persisted over the length of follow-up.The 27% of the study group that manifested complex VPBs during monitoring produced half of all deaths and 59% of the sudden coronary deaths occurring during follow-up.

Among men recovered from myocardial infarction, it is possible from 1 hour of ECG monitoring at rest to select those with constellations of

(8) N. Engl. J. Med. 297:750–757, Oct. 6, 1977.

RELATIVE RISKS OF DEATH IN RELATION TO COMPLEX VENTRICULAR PREMATURE BEATS (VPBs) AND OTHER SPECIFIED CHARACTERISTICS: COMPARISONS OF MORTALITY OVER THREE YEARS AFTER BASELINE MONITORING OF MEN WITH PRIOR MYOCARDIAL INFARCTION (MI)*

OTHER VARIABLE	COMPLEX VS NO COMPLEX VPB'S, ADJUSTED FOR OTHER VARIABLE & AGE		OTHER VARIABLE PRESENT VS NOT PRESENT, ADJUSTED FOR COMPLEX VPB'S & AGE	
	ALL CAUSES	SUDDEN CORONARY DEATHS	ALL CAUSES	SUDDEN CORONARY DEATHS
CHF†	2.2++	3.3++	2.0++	2.0++
Diuretics‡	2.4++	3.7++	2.0++	2.0++
ST-segment depression§	2.4++	3.5++	2.0++	2.1++
Heart rate ⩾90	2.4++	3.6++	2.3++	1.8+
Digitalis‡	2.4++	3.7++	1.7++	1.2
T-wave abnormality§	2.4++	3.5++	1.7++	1.9+
Diabetes	2.4++	3.5++	1.6++	1.8+
CHF or shock with acute MI¶	2.0++	3.2++	1.7++	1.9+
Duration heart disease ⩾1 yr	2.5++	3.6++	1.5++	1.4
Elevated blood pressure**	2.5++	3.7++	1.5++	1.8++
Angina in mo before base line	2.5++	3.7++	1.4+	1.5 ×
⩾2 definite prior MI's††	2.4++	3.5++	1.5+	1.6
Definite vs possible MI††	2.4++	3.6++	1.3	1.0
Conduction defect or major left-axis deviation§	2.5++	3.7++	1.2	1.1
Q or QS abnormality§	2.5++	3.6++	1.2	1.2
<3 months vs 3–8 mo since last MI	2.4++	3.8++	1.1	1.2

*Differences in survival and relative risk of death are assessed with the Peto-Pike method. Relative mortality risks are shown for patients with complex VPBs in the monitoring hour as compared with those free of complex VPBs, adjusted for age and presence or absence of another specified variable and for patients with a specified variable present as compared with those without that variable, adjusted for age and presence of complex VPBs. Levels of statistical significance for the 1-degree-of-freedom chi-square values obtained are indicated by 2+ for $P < 0.01$, + for $0.01 < P \leq 0.05$ and × for $0.05 < P \leq 0.10$. A more detailed version of this table, presenting the values of the chi-squares associated with the relative risks, has been placed in the National Auxiliary Publications Service.

†A positive finding is here defined as congestive heart failure (CHF) experienced at any time before or at the baseline examination.

‡Diuretics and digitalis are considered positive among patients who are habitually taking these drugs as of the baseline date.

§Minnesota code criteria for the specified abnormalities have been applied to the 12-lead ECG taken at the baseline.

¶CHF or shock accompanying acute MI occurring within 9 months before preceding baseline. Only patients meeting criteria for definite MI are classified in this respect (see footnote †† below).

**Elevated blood pressure, definition: ≥3 readings before baseline are ≥160 systolic or ≥95 diastolic, or <3 such readings are present but there is a physician's diagnosis of hypertension, or casual blood pressure at baseline examination is ≥160 systolic or ≥95 diastolic.

††Criteria for diagnosis of MI were those developed for and earlier study of coronary heart disease incidence and prognosis among members of the Health Insurance Plan. The diagnosis of definite MI requires either highly specific or characteristic ECG abnormalities associated with a combination of appropriate clinical symptoms and acute-phase reactants. The diagnosis of possible MI is based on less specific ECG, clinical and symptomatic findings.

ventricular ectopic activity that signify a markedly increased risk of death, particularly sudden coronary death, independent of other important clinical characteristics. The findings offer a rationale for seeking prophylactic approaches to suppressing ventricular arrhythmias in patients with coronary heart disease and for controlled studies of whether significant reductions in mortality can be effected through such means.

► [An important finding in this article was that simple isolated ventricular premature contractions did not increase the risk of death during the follow-up period. Unfortunately, at present no antiarrhythmic agent is available that can be tolerated by most patients with complex ventricular premature beats after myocardial infarction. – Ed.]

Angiographic Findings and Prognostic Indicators in Patients Resuscitated from Sudden Cardiac Death. Sudden cardiac death accounts for a large proportion of deaths from coronary atherosclerosis.

ANGIOGRAPHIC AND HEMODYNAMIC OBSERVATIONS

	All patients N = 64 No. (percent)	VF × 1* N = 45 No. (percent)	RVF/SD† N = 14 No. (percent)
Coronary anatomy			
≥70% stenosis			
1 vessel	21 (33)	18 (40)	2 (14)
2 vessel	18 (28)	13 (29)	3 (21)
3 vessel	21 (33)	10 (22)	9 (64)
100% stenosis			
1 vessel	24 (38)	18 (40)	4 (29)
2 vessel	11 (17)	7 (16)	4 (29)
3 vessel	8 (12)	4 (9)	3 (21)
No. of collaterals	49 (75)	32 (71)	9 (64)
No. with anatomy suitable for total revascularization	34 (53)	25 (56)	3 (21)
Left ventricular function			
EDP >15 mm Hg	19 (30)	12 (27)	6 (43)
EDV >100 ml/m²‡	28 (55)	20 (53)	6 (67)
Ejection fraction <0.50§	30 (50)	20 (47)	9 (64)
Moderate mitral regurgitation	4 (6)	2 (4)	1 (7)
Extent of left ventricular contraction abnormality			
None (normal)	19 (30)	15 (33)	1 (7)
<25% abnormal	10 (16)	7 (16)	2 (14)
25-50% abnormal	15 (23)	14 (31)	1 (7)
>50% abnormal	20 (31)	9 (20)	10 (71)
Types of contraction abnormalities			
Normal	19 (30)	15 (33)	1 (7)
Hypokinesia only	16 (25)	12 (27)	3 (21)
Akinesia	18 (28)	14 (31)	3 (21)
Paradoxical wall motion	11 (17)	4 (9)	7 (50)

*VF × 1 = patients who survived during follow-up after VF.

†RVF/SD = patients who had recurrent VF or died suddenly after discharge from the hospital and during the follow-up period.

‡End-diastolic volume measurements possible in 51 patients.

§Ejection fraction determined 60 patients.

Abbreviations: EDP = end-diastolic pressure; EDV = end-diastolic volume.

Ventricular fibrillation (VF) might be prevented by prophylactic measures. W. Douglas Weaver, Gerald S. Lorch, Hernan A. Alvarez and Leonard A. Cobb[9] (Seattle) studied the coronary anatomy and left ventricular characteristics of 64 patients who were successfully resuscitated from out-of-hospital VF, 14 of whom had recurrent VF or sudden death during follow-up. Coronary arteriography preceded the episode of VF in 10 patients. The average follow-up of surviving patients was 20.4 months.

Nearly three fourths of the patients were known to have cardiovascular disease before the first episode of VF. Patients who survived out-of-hospital VF usually had extensive coronary artery disease. Collateral arteries were frequently observed at coronary angiography. The hemodynamic findings are given in the table. Patients who had recurrent VF or sudden death were similar in age to the others, but a history of heart failure was more frequent. Significantly more extensive coronary and myocardial abnormalities were present in these patients. Nearly two-thirds had triple-vessel disease, compared with 22% of the survivors. The mean ejection fraction was significantly lower in patients with recurrent VF or sudden death than in the survivors, and the former patients showed far greater impairment of contraction.

This study showed a strong association between certain angiographic and functional abnormalities and the development of VF and recurrent VF. Patients resuscitated from one episode of VF and who have high-risk coronary and left ventricular characteristics for a recurrence require rigorously controlled prophylaxis. Many such patients have coronary stenoses suitable for bypass grafting, and some might benefit from prophylactic bypass surgery or excision of akinetic or dyskinetic areas.

► [A subgroup of these survivors of sudden cardiac death underwent radionuclide angiography and myocardial imaging with thallium-201 (see Ritchie et al.: Am. J. Cardiol. 39:852, 1977). These noninvasive studies revealed a broad spectrum of ischemic and ventriculographic abnormalities. Hopefully, these noninvasive studies will be correlated with the arteriographic and angiographic findings in the observations made by Weaver et al. (Circulation 54:895, 1976) and can be used to identify a subset of patients at particularly high risk for the recurrence of sudden cardiac death. Unfortunately, what is beginning to come through from both of these studies is that from the point of view of myocardial perfusion, left ventricular function and coronary anatomy, these particular patients are not unique. Conceivably, the radioisotopic studies could be used simply to confirm the presence of impaired perfusion and thereby avoid invasive investigations unless it becomes clear that bypass grafting and excision of any detectable aneurysms reduce subsequent mortality in these patients. – Ed.] ◄

Cardiac Arrest Complicating Acute Myocardial Infarction: Predictability and Prognosis. If cardiac arrest can be shown to be related to mortality in hospital survivors of acute myocardial infarction, vigorous efforts to eliminate ventricular arrhythmias should become an integral part of the management of infarction. Martin J. Conley, J. Frederick McNeer, Kerry L. Lee, Galen S. Wagner and Robert A. Rosati[1] (Duke Univ.) reviewed experience with 905 consecutive patients admitted to a cardiac care unit for acute infarction in 1965–74. A monitored cardiac arrest occurred in 102 patients, with

(9) Circulation 54:895–900, December, 1976.
(1) Am. J. Cardiol. 39:7–12, January, 1977.

yearly arrest rates of 7–18%. Forty-five patients with arrest were in Killip class I for heart failure on admission, 42 were in class II and 15 were in class III. Few patients changed their functional class for heart failure before the episode of arrest.

The only significant individual predictors of arrest after hospitalization were admission class for heart failure, history of heart failure and history of infarction. Admission class for heart failure was the most important predictor. The rate of arrest was 17% for patients with signs of heart failure on admission (Killip class II or III) and 9% for those in Killip class I. Only 59% of the patients with cardiac arrest survived hospitalization compared to 88% of those without arrest, a markedly significant difference. Twenty-three patients were resuscitated from cardiac arrest but died before discharge. Postdischarge survival was significantly greater in the patients who had not had cardiac arrest than in those who had survived an episode of cardiac arrest. The worst heart failure class was the strongest predictor of long-term survival after hospitalization for acute infarction. Sudden or heart failure-related deaths did not differ significantly in the groups of survivors with and without cardiac arrest.

Cardiac arrest is a serious complication of acute infarction, even when occurring in a cardiac care unit. Many deaths among hospital survivors occurred in patients who had some degree of heart failure during hospitalization. Currently, vigorous antiarrhythmic prophylaxis and treatment are integral parts of the management of acute infarction at the authors' unit.

► [These findings confirm the report of Sloman (Chest 63:513, 1973) which suggests an excess mortality after hospital discharge of patients with acute myocardial infarction complicated by ventricular fibrillation. However, since the mode of death among hospital survivors did not differ between the groups who did and did not experience cardiac arrest, it would appear that prophylactic antiarrhythmic therapy is not indicated in these patients after discharge from the hospital unless, of course, they demonstrate complicated ventricular premature beats. I concur with the authors' notion that vigorous antiarrhythmic prophylaxis to prevent cardiac arrest in the course of acute myocardial infarction is desirable.—Ed.] ◄

Effect of a Digitalis Drug on Ventricular Premature Beats. The great frequency of ventricular arrhythmias in patients with coronary heart disease may predispose to sudden death. Current drugs used to suppress ventricular premature beats (VPBs) have little therapeutic utility and substantial toxicity. Bernard Lown, Thomas B. Graboys, Philip J. Podrid, Barry H. Cohen, Mark B. Stockman and Charles E. Gaughan[2] (Harvard Univ.) determined whether a digitalis drug, acetylstrophanthidin, effectively suppresses VPBs. Studies were done in 142 patients with more than 1 VPB per minute, 104 men and 38 women with mean ages of 61 and 62 years, respectively. About half had coronary heart disease, and 40 of these had had myocardial infarction. Thirteen patients had no heart disease. Digitalis drugs were being given to 98 patients. Acetylstrophanthidin was injected in 0.9% saline in a dose of 0.2 mg every 6–8 minutes to a total of 1 mg or until early digitalis intoxication was evident, when increments of 0.05 or 0.1 mg were used.

(2) N. Engl. J. Med. 296:301–306, Feb. 10, 1977.

In 65 patients (group 1), VPB frequency and grade were reduced during acetylstrophanthidin administration; in 37 (group 2), VPBs were unaltered; and in 40 (group 3), they increased during the test. Patients with cardiomyopathy and otherwise normal subjects predominated in group 1. Group 3 patients had less frequent VPBs than those in the other groups. The doses of acetylstrophanthidin required were 1.07 mg for group 1, 0.88 mg for group 2 and 0.61 mg for group 3. Serum digoxin levels were lowest in group 1 and highest in group 3. Reductions in heart rate and rises in blood pressure were similar in the three groups. Fewer than half of groups 1 and 2 but nearly all of group 3 had toxic manifestations with a dose of 1 mg or less.

Digitalis drugs may reduce the frequency of VPBs. The effect may be due to enhanced vagus nerve action. Acetylstrophanthidin has reduced or abolished VPBs in 17 of 29 patients with frequent, uncontrollable, life-threatening ventricular tachyarrhythmias. In 15 cases, digitalis glycosides in maintenance doses contributed to a reduction or complete control of paroxysmal ventricular arrhythmias. It appears that, in some patients, digitalis drugs may have a useful place in the management of difficult ventricular arrhythmias.

► [Lown and his colleagues have developed a technique for acute drug testing that is useful in determining the efficacy of antiarrhythmic drugs in patients with high-grade ventricular arrhythmias (Gaughan et al.: Am. J. Cardiol. 38:677, 1976). This method involves administering a single large dose of the antiarrhythmic agent, monitoring cardiac rhythm and determining blood drug levels at selected intervals. This approach appears to be particularly useful for patients who have been successfully resuscitated from ventricular fibrillation and who have ventricular arrhythmias. In such patients it is important to define an effective antiarrhythmic program, consisting perhaps of a combination of drugs.

It is quite clear that it is now possible to define patients at high risk of sudden death and, furthermore, to show how arrhythmias can be suppressed in such patients. Whether or not this will affect their survival is a critical question that has yet to be answered. Until an answer is forthcoming, however, it is clear that it is incumbent on us to try to suppress these arrhythmias. – Ed.] ◄

Ventricular Electric Instability in the Conscious Dog: Effects of Psychologic Stress and β-Adrenergic Blockade. The role of psychologic stress in predisposing to cardiac arrhythmias is well recognized clinically, but precise data documenting the relationship have been difficult to obtain. Raymond J. Matta, James E. Lawler and Bernard Lown[3] (Harvard Univ.) studied the effects of psychologic stress on ventricular electric stability in the conscious dog. The hypothesis was that a psychologically stressful environment would increase cardiac electric instability and susceptibility to ventricular fibrillation. Pacing and ECG catheters were installed in mongrel dogs and, after adaptation, 20-minute stress periods that required the animal to learn to avoid an electric shock were imposed. The repetitive extrasystole threshold was determined before and after the stress session and before and after the administration of Tolamolol, a β-adrenergic blocking agent, in a dose of 4 mg/kg intravenously.

Stress significantly reduced the repetitive extrasystole threshold in all 10 dogs tested. The threshold decreased by nearly 50% during 3

(3) Am. J. Cardiol. 38:594–598, Nov. 4, 1976.

days of exposure to the stressful environment. When Tolamolol was administered before a stress session, the threshold was unaltered from the control value. Significant decreases in the effective refractory period were also noted, but not when Tolamolol was administered. Measurement of the heart rate response to isoproterenol confirmed the establishment of effective β-blockade.

If ventricular fibrillation and sudden death in man are related to neural input by way of the sympathetic nervous system, β-blocking agents may prove to be of prophylactic value. The effect would result from prevention of a reduction in ventricular fibrillation threshold on increased sympathetic nervous traffic to the heart. No data are available that clearly formulate a relationship between cardiac vulnerablity and the presence of ventricular ectopy in man.

► [The behavioral stress in this study required the animal to learn to avoid a programmed electric shock. These observations are relevant to the clinical trial in which β-adrenergic receptor antagonists were administered to patients who had recovered from acute myocardial infarction and in which a statistically significant reduction in sudden death was observed. (Br. Med. J. 2:735, 1975). – Ed.] ◄

Cardiomyopathies

Evidence for Cardiomyopathy in Familial Diabetes Mellitus. A relatively high incidence of cardiac deaths in diabetic patients has been attributed to coronary atherosclerosis and its complications but not all cardiac deaths in diabetics are related to this process. Timothy J. Regan, Michael M. Lyons, S. Sultan Ahmed, Gilbert E. Levinson, Henry A. Oldewurtel, Mehmood R. Ahmad and Bunyad Haider[4] (Newark, N. J.) examined left ventricular function and coronary artery anatomy after the development of cardiac symptoms in 17 patients with familial-type adult-onset diabetes without hypertension or obesity and in 9 control subjects of similar age. The patients were generally well controlled without ketosis and were in good clinical condition at the time of study. None had evidence of myocardial infarction.

Twelve of the 17 patients had no significant coronary obstructive disease and 8 of these had no clinical evidence of heart failure. In these 8 patients the stroke volume index was reduced and the end-diastolic pressure elevated at rest compared with control subjects. Responses to angiotensin infusion were consistent with preclinical cardiomyopathy. The 4 patients with episodes of heart failure tended to have had diabetes longer than the others and to have ECG evidence of hypertrophy and minor repolarization changes. Stroke volume was reduced more than in the patients without heart failure and 3 of the 4 patients had diffuse hypokinesis. Stress tests with atrial pacing did not cause ischemic changes in these patients. Ventricular biopsy in 2 patients without ventricular decompensation showed interstitial collagen deposition and relatively normal muscle cells. Autopsy studies of 11 uncomplicated diabetics showed periodic acid-Schiff-positive material in the interstitium in those without significant coronary obstructive disease. Most of these patients died with heart failure. Enhanced triglyceride and cholesterol concentrations were found in samples of left ventricle and septum.

It is concluded that a diffuse extravascular abnormality may be a basis for cardiomyopathic features in diabetics.

► [There is increasing suspicion that many cardiac deaths in patients with diabetes are *not* related to atherosclerosis. For example, Ledet (Diabetologia 4:268, 1968) observed that at post mortem examination intramural vessels in patients with diabetes commonly exhibit accumulation of glycoproteins, but do not show excessive luminal narrowing. Also, it has been observed that the intimal surface area of coronary vessels involved by fibrous plaques is only modestly increased in patients with diabetes. It is interesting that even when patients with prior coronary or rheumatic heart disease were excluded, diabetic subjects have a four- to fivefold increased risk of congestive heart failure (Am. J. Cardiol. 34:29, 1974). This increased risk persists even after taking into account age, blood pressure, weight and cholesterol values, as well as clinical evi-

(4) J. Clin. Invest. 60:885–899, October, 1977.

dence of coronary heart disease. This epidemiologic finding suggests that diabetes is associated with a cardiomyopathy.

Doctor Regan's group has pioneered in studying the cardiomyopathy of diabetes mellitus; they have observed in a canine model with chronic diabetes that ventricular function and compliance are abnormal and that this is associated with an accumulation of periodic acid-Schiff-positive glycoproteins, as well as increments of triglyceride in the myocardium. In patients the functional abnormality is reflected in noncardiac adult diabetics with abnormal systolic time intervals, similar to those that occur in patients with a history of ethanol intake. Hamby and colleagues (J.A.M.A. 229:1749, 1954) have also addressed themselves to the problem of diabetic cardiomyopathy. They found a statistically significant increase in the frequency of diabetes in patients with idiopathic cardiomyopathy. There is some clinical evidence that the cardiomyopathy in diabetics is related to the microangiopathy. Seneviratne (Br. Med. J. 1:1444, 1977) found that patients with microangiopathy, as reflected in the presence of proteinuria or proliferative retinopathy, had impaired left ventricular function, measured by means of systolic time intervals and echocardiography, whereas those with uncomplicated diabetes had normal ventricular function. The association of microangiopathy and impaired left ventricular function may explain the high immediate mortality and high incidence of cardiogenic shock and congestive heart failure that occur after myocardial infarction in diabetics. — Ed.] ◄

Primary Restrictive Cardiomyopathy: Nontropical Endomyocardial Fibrosis and Hypereosinophilic Heart Disease. C. Y. C. Chew, G. M. Ziady, M. J. Raphael, M. Nellen and C. M. Oakley[5] (Hammersmith Hosp., London) describe a group of patients who share a diastolic abnormality of a type not seen in patients with other primary cardiomyopathies or in such rare specific disorders as amyloid heart disease. Eleven patients (7 men and 4 women, aged 20 – 58 years) were studied for a restrictive cardiomyopathy during 1972 – 75. Seven patients were white and had not lived in the tropics. Five patients presented with features of predominant right-sided heart failure with little or no cardiomegaly. Two had a constitutional illness, and 4 had chest pain. The most prominent sign was a loud and early 3d heart sound. The jugular venous pressure was elevated in 7 patients. Four patients had soft late systolic murmurs of mild mitral regurgitation. The ECG showed nonspecific, nonfocal abnormalities. Five patients had normal chest films, and the others had slight cardiomegaly or left atrial or biatrial dilatation.

Echography showed rapid diastolic closure of the anterior mitral leaflet in 7 patients. Left ventricular dimensions were within normal limits, and filling was rapid. Filling pressures in both ventricles were raised. The left ventricular end-diastolic pressure usually exceeded the right by over 12 mm Hg and ranged from 14 to 36 mm Hg. Four patients had left ventricular dysfunction only. The three biopsies showed a small, thick-walled left ventricle with increased myocardial fibrous tissue and some hypertrophy of myocardial fibers. Endomyocardial biopsies in 2 patients showed fibrous tissue with collagen and irregular elastic fibrils. The 1 autopsy examination showed features indistinguishable from tropical endomyocardial fibrosis.

Two patients in this series had eosinophilia and clinical features of Löffler's endocarditis. Four had disease apparently confined to the left ventricle. This spectrum of ventricular abnormalities appears to result

(5) Br. Heart J. 39:399 – 413, April, 1977.

from endomyocardial fibrosis of varying severity and probably differing cause. "Tropical" endomyocardial fibrosis may occur outside the tropics. Endocardial resection and valve replacement may be indicated in the most severely affected patients.

► [The principal hemodynamic defect in these patients is restriction of ventricular filling and stroke volume. The ability to empty the ventricle was not apparently affected, in that the ejection fraction was normal or even slightly elevated, whereas end-diastolic volume was normal or reduced. Angiocardiography in these patients shows that ventricular filling is essentially complete in the first 30–40% of diastole, with little or no further filling in late diastole; this is associated with a loud and early 3d heart sound. Restrictive cardiomyopathy resembles pericardial constriction in that the dip and plateau ("square root" sign) form of the diastolic portion of the ventricular pressure pulse is seen and the ventricular pressure in early diastole is normal. In contrast, in idiopathic hypertrophic subaortic stenosis and in amyloid heart disease the early diastolic pressure in the left ventricle usually is elevated. In contrast to constrictive pericarditis, in which the end-diastolic pressure is elevated in *both* ventricles, in restrictive cardiomyopathy the left ventricular end-diastolic pressure often exceeds that of the right, although in some instances they are equal.

There is bound to be some overlap in restrictive and obliterative cardiomyopathy. In the obliterative form there is impaired ventricular filling due to intracavitary space-occupying masses that restrict filling. This may be thrombus, fibrosis or an eosinophilic infiltrate. In restrictive cardiomyopathy there is impaired diastolic volume and stretch due to organic subendocardial or myocardial lesions.

The concept of restrictive cardiomyopathy is important because it indicates that a combination of a rapid x and y descent in the atrial pressure pulse and jugular venous pulse, elevated venous pressure, a pattern of early diastolic dip and plateau and sometimes pulsus paradoxus do not necessarily signify constrictive pericarditis, but may occur in myocardial disease. This term should not be used in patients with cardiomyopathy with left ventricular enlargement or in the presence of massive ventricular hypertrophy.

Most authorities, contrary to Chew et al., consider amyloid heart disease to be a restrictive cardiomyopathy. For further information on this subject see the following article, and for an excellent classification of the cardiomyopathies see Chapter 81A, written by J. Goodwin, in the 4th Edition of *The Heart* edited by J. Willis Hurst. – Ed.] ◄

Cardiac Amyloidosis, Constrictive Pericarditis and Restrictive Cardiomyopathy. Eduardo Meaney, Ralph Shabetai, Valmik Bhargava, Mary Shearer, Cathy Weidner, Lucia Maria Mangiardi, Richard Smalling and Kirk Peterson[6] (Univ. of Kentucky) reexamined data from a patient with cardiac amyloidosis who was misdiagnosed as having constrictive pericarditis, along with data from 2 other patients with cardiac amyloidosis and 2 with constrictive pericarditis. Pressures were measured with high-fidelity micromanometers simultaneously with left ventricular dimensions and the data were computer processed. In the study case (Case 1), cardiac amyloidosis was not suspected, even after cardiac catheterization, but was proved at autopsy.

Left and right ventricular filling pressures were elevated in all 5 patients despite diuretic therapy. In both patients with constrictive pericarditis and the study patient the diastolic pressure tracings from both ventricles showed the "square root" sign, with an early diastolic dip followed by a mid- and late diastolic plateau. In the cases of amyloid disease the heart rate was rapid and pressure rose steeply throughout diastole in both ventricles. Pressures were greater in the left ventricle throughout diastole in all patients with amyloidosis. Mitral re-

(6) Am. J. Cardiol. 38:547–556, Nov. 4, 1976.

VALUES OBTAINED AT CARDIAC CATHETERIZATION IN THREE PATIENTS WITH CARDIAC AMYLOIDOSIS AND TWO WITH CONSTRICTIVE PERICARDITIS*

	Amyloidosis			Pericarditis	
	Case 1	Case 2	Case 3	Case 4	Case 5
CI	1.5	2.4	1.9	2.14	. . .
Pressures (mm Hg)					
RA	(15)	(10)	(10)	(20)	(21)
RV	44/15	47/10	38/12	35/20	49/23
PA	44/21	47/20	38/12	35/20	49/23
	(30)	(38)	(31)	(27)	(30)
PCW	24	20	18	20	25
LV	80/23	118/20	93/25	88/22	90/23
A_0	80/23	118/65	93/58	88/58	. . .
	(74)	(100)	(73)	(64)	
dP/dt	1666	1455	853		1044
V_{pm}	0.86	0.82	0.9	1.19	0.83
V_{max}	1.5	1.05	0.9	2.69	1.63
EDVI	36	54.9	54.5	60.0	62
ESVI	11.0	23.4	33.8	15.1	29
SVI	25	31.5	20.7	48.3	34
EF	0.69	0.57	0.37	0.79	0.54
MCFSR	1.3	0.8	0.7	1.83	0.87
PLVFR	5.04	3.82	2.02	5.7	5.50
PLVER	5.40	3.72	2.54	6.96	2.70

*C1, cardiac index (L/minute/sq m); RA, right atrial; RV, right ventricular; PA, pulmonary arterial; PCW, pulmonary capillary wedge; LV, left ventricular; A_0, aortic; dP/dt, rate of rise of left ventricular pressure (mm Hg sec^{-1}); V_{pm}, peak velocity of contractile element; V_{max}, velocity of contractile element at zero load; EDVI, ESVI, SVI, end-diastolic, end-systolic and stroke volumes, respectively (ml/sq m); EF, ejection fraction; MCFSR, mean circumferential fiber shortening rate (circumferences per second); PLVFR and PLVER, peak left ventricular filling and ejection rates, respectively ($second^{-1}$) (normal, 3.38 ± 1.15 and 3.29 ± 0.86, respectively) (mean ±SE).

gurgitation was present in all 5 patients. The degree of impairment of left ventricular systolic function differed among the patients with amyloidosis (table). The peak rate of left ventricular filling was above normal in both patients with pericarditis and the patient (Case 1) with restrictive amyloid cardiomyopathy. Pulsus paradoxus was not found in any patient. A dicrotic pulse was recorded in all 3 patients with cardiac amyloidosis.

It is an oversimplification to state that the functional abnormality of cardiac amyloidosis is specific and is characterized by a small, poorly contracting left ventricle that is distinguished from the ventricle in constrictive pericarditis by its hypokinesia and the absence of rapid filling in early diastole. When patients with a large dilated left ventricle and increased end-diastolic pressure, such as subendocardial fibroelastosis or hypertrophic obstructive cardiomyopathy, are included in restrictive cardiomyopathy, the term loses its usefulness.

► [It is clear that cardiac amyloidosis is not characterized by a single hemodynamic pattern. There is a spectrum of findings; some patients have hemodynamics resembling restrictive cardiomyopathy (as described in the preceding article by Chew et al.), in which the diastolic pressure pulse exhibits the square root sign, as seen in constrictive pericarditis, and in which the end-diastolic pressures in the two ventricles are either equal or in which the left exceeds the right, but in which ventricular emptying is normal. In other patients with cardiac amyloidosis there is no diastolic dip in the ventricular pressure pulse, diastolic pressure is elevated throughout diastole and ventricular contractile activity is impaired. – Ed.] ◄

Hypertrophic Cardiomyopathy in Friedreich's Ataxia. An association of myocardial disease with progressive ataxia has been known for many years, but the hemodynamic findings in this rare syndrome are largely ignored. L. G. Van der Hauwaert and M. Dumoulin[7] (Univ. of Louvain) describe 2 siblings with Friedreich's ataxia who had clinical, hemodynamic and echocardiographic findings of hypertrophic cardiomyopathy. The patients were a boy first seen at age 14 years with a heart murmur and a brother who presented at age 12 with symptoms of mild ataxia and exertional fatigue. The clinical signs suggested hypertrophic obstructive cardiomyopathy, and at left ventricular catheterization a systolic pressure gradient across the left ventricular outflow tract was provoked by isoprenaline infusion. Angiocardiography and echocardiography showed gross thickening of the interventricular septum and, in 1 case, a systolic anterior motion of the anterior mitral valve leaflet.

These patients had a midsystolic murmur at the apex, which increased in intensity on amyl nitrite inhalation, and a prominent *a* wave on the apex cardiogram. The older subject had elevated right and left ventricular end-diastolic pressures. No resting outflow tract gradients were recorded. Echocardiography showed gross septal thickening in both patients, with septal-posterior left ventricular free wall ratios of 1.4 and 1.7. The end-diastolic transverse dimension of the left ventricle was reduced in each patient. Systolic anterior motion of the anterior mitral leaflet was seen in the older patient, who was more severely affected.

Outflow tract obstruction is not invariably associated with Friedreich's cardiomyopathy. It is unlikely that the condition is related to any specific metabolic or neurogenic disturbance. These patients may represent two stages of a slowly progressive form of hypertrophic cardiomyopathy, characterized by asymmetric septal hypertrophy and variable left ventricular outflow obstruction. Echocardiography is a good means of studying patients with Friedreich's ataxia.

► [The association between Friedreich's ataxia and cardiomyopathy is well established. Hewer (Br. Heart J. 31:5, 1969) found at postmortem examination that all 16 of his patients with Friedreich's ataxia showed muscle fiber hypertrophy and interstitial fibrosis. Indeed, most patients with Friedreich's ataxia die from cardiac complications, principally heart failure or arrhythmias, rather than from the neurologic disorder. The coronary arteries may be normal or diffusely involved with atheromatous lesions; the Purkinje system, atrioventricular node and conducting pathway may be infiltrated by fibrous tissue; atrial fibrillation and paroxysmal supraventricular tachycardia may occur. Both right and left ventricular hypertrophy may occur electrocardiographically. – Ed.] ◄

Sarcoidosis of the Heart: Clinicopathologic Study of 35 Necropsy Patients (Group I) and Review of 78 Previously Described Necropsy Patients (Group II) are reported by William C. Roberts, Hugh A. McAllister, Jr., and Victor J. Ferrans.[8] All patients had non-necrotic granulomas in lymph nodes and either sarcoid granulomas in

(7) Br. Heart J. 38:1291 – 1298, December, 1976.
(8) Am. J. Med. 63:86 – 108, July, 1977.

the heart (in 109 patients) or transmural myocardial scarring (in 4 patients) unassociated with coronary arterial narrowing. In 89 patients, cardiac dysfunction clearly was the result of sarcoid granulomatous infiltration of the heart. Death was sudden in 60 (67%) of these patients, secondary to progressive congestive heart failure in 20 (23%) and secondary to recurring pericardial effusion in 3 (3%). Sudden death was the initial manifestation of sarcoidosis in 10 (17%) of the patients who died suddenly. Other than premature ventricular beats, ventricular tachycardia was the most common arrhythmia and complete heart block the most common conduction disturbance. Ventricular aneurysm occurred in 8 patients, and papillary muscle dysfunction in 16.

Steroid therapy tends to cause fibrous replacement of myocardial sarcoid granulomas but a possible consequence of this treatment is the development of ventricular aneurysm. Most patients in this series with cardiac sarcoidosis causing dysfunction presented initially with manifestations related to the heart. Most patients with cardiac sarcoidosis have little or no clinical evidence of dysfunction of an organ system other than the heart. The course in patients with extensive cardiac sarcoidosis is usually not prolonged.

► [At autopsy about 20% of patients with sarcoidosis show cardiac involvement, which usually occurs late in the course of the disease. Sinus tachycardia, arrhythmias, conduction abnormalities, cardiac enlargement and congestive heart failure, as well as complete heart block, are common clinical findings. Unfortunately, the arrhythmias tend to be refractory to antiarrhythmic agents and are a frequent cause of death. Implantation of a permanent demand pacemaker is indicated in patients with sarcoidosis and atrioventricular conduction disturbances. – Ed.] ◄

Hypertension

Mild High-Renin Essential Hypertension: Neurogenic Human Hypertension? It is possible that elevated plasma renin activity in mild hypertension represents stimulatory neural influences on renin secretion. As such, the elevation could be a marker of a generalized increase in cardiovascular sympathetic nervous tone. Murray Elser, Stevo Julius, Andrew Zweifler, Otelio Randall, Ernest Harburg, Hermsworth Gardiner and Vincent DeQuattro[9] explored the possibility that mild high-renin essential hypertension is a neurogenic condition in which elevated renin activity reflects generalized sympathetic overactivity. Thirty-one men, aged 18 – 35 years, with essential hypertension were studied. There were 15 "normal-renin" and 16 "high-renin" patients. Twenty normal subjects were also studied. Sequential autonomic blockade was performed with atropine, propranolol and phentolamine. Five high-renin patients received oral propranolol on a chronic basis.

High-renin patients had a high heart rate and a shortened cardiac preejection period index. Mean cardiac output was not significantly elevated because of a limitation of stroke volume. Normal-renin patients had a normal heart rate and preejection period index, a significantly reduced cardiac index and pressure elevations maintained by an elevated peripheral vascular resistance. Plasma norepinephrine concentration was elevated in the high-renin patients. Hemodynamic changes were greater with propranolol in the high-renin patients. On α-blockade, peripheral resistance fell significantly only in the high-renin group. Mean blood pressure fell only in the high-renin patients with "total" autonomic blockade. The plasma norepinephrine concentration remained elevated when plasma renin activity was suppressed by propranolol in the high-renin group. Baroreceptor function testing showed underactivity of the heart rate baroreflex in the hypertensive patients, but this was unrelated to the renin status. Psychometric testing indicated "suppressed hostility" in the high-renin patients but not in the normal-renin group.

Mild essential hypertension in patients with high renin activity is neurogenic and possibly psychosomatic in origin. The extent, if any, to which the hypertension progresses to moderate or severe grades in these patients is uncertain.

► [In severe high-renin essential hypertension, renal function is commonly impaired and the elevated plasma renin activity presumably results from the arterial damage to the kidney. In the patients described in this study, who presumably had neurogenic hypertension, the hyperreninemia probably results from stimulatory neural influences. In these patients the elevation of blood pressure appears to be sustained by neural mechanisms rather than the renin-angiotensin system, and circulating angiotensin

(9) N. Engl. J. Med. 296:405 – 411, Feb. 24, 1977.

does not appear to be responsible for maintaining the pressure elevation. This notion is supported by the finding that low doses of propranolol, 40 mg daily, will depress plasma renin activity, but not return blood pressure to normal. What emerges from these studies is that abnormalities of the autonomic nervous control may be responsible in patients with mild borderline hypertension. Both α- and β-adrenergic blockades are likely to be useful in counteracting the autonomic hyperactivity.

Whereas the etiology of neurogenic hypertension is not clear, it is known that several kinds of emotional stress can produce a temporary rise in arterial pressure. Interestingly, however, prolonged exposure to a stressful auditory stimulus, severe and prolonged enough to cause a permanent loss of hearing, may be a contributing factor for the development of hypertension (Jonsson: Lancet 1:86, 1977). – Ed.] ◄

Accentuated Vascular and Endocrine Response to SQ 20881 in Hypertension. The relationship of activity of the renin-angiotensin system to the pathogenesis of hypertension remains controversial. Gordon H. Williams and Norman K. Hollenberg[1] (Harvard Med. School) assessed vascular and hormonal responses to inhibition of peptidyldipeptide hydrolase, which converts angiotensin I to angiotensin II (converting enzyme) and inactivates bradykinin (kininase II), in 9 normal and 6 hypertensive subjects given 10 mEq sodium to activate both systems and observed a striking influence on bradykinin catabolism in patients with essential hypertension. The patients had supine diastolic pressures over 90 mm Hg and evidence of hypertension for at least 6 months. Five patients had normal arteriograms and 1 had bilateral small-vessel disease and elevated plasma renin activity. Patients were off medications for at least 2 weeks before study.

Renal blood flow was significantly lower in the hypertensive subjects and less than predicted for the patients' age and salt intake. The nonapeptide peptidyldipeptide hydrolase inhibitor SQ 20881 in a dose of 10 μg/kg did not alter blood pressure, renal blood flow or plasma renin activity significantly in the normal subjects. Hypertensive patients had accentuated endocrine and vascular responses to dipeptidyl carboxypeptidase inhibition. The 10 μg/kg-dose significantly increased renal blood flow and reduced angiotensin II concentration and these differences were more apparent with 30 μg/kg. The mean blood pressure fell by 11 mm Hg at 3 minutes and remained significantly reduced at 20 minutes. The renal blood flow response was accentuated at both intervals. Bradykinin levels rose significantly in the hypertensive patients. The relationship between blood pressure change and angiotensin II and bradykinin levels was not consistent. Renin responses in the two groups did not differ significantly.

Since both the renin-angiotensin and kallikrein-bradykinin systems are influenced, vascular responses to SQ 20881 must be interpreted cautiously, but this agent has excellent antihypertensive characteristics, and many features make it attractive as a therapeutic agent. The concentration of a vasodilator is increased while the renin-angiotensin system is blocked, and the agent increases renal blood flow despite reducing the blood pressure.

► [The close interrelationship between the renin-angiotensin and kallikrein-bradykinin system is not widely appreciated. Thus, the enzyme that converts angiotensin I to angiotensin II also inactivates bradykinin. Inhibition of this enzyme would be expected

(1) N. Engl. J. Med. 297:184–188, July 28, 1977.

to lower arterial pressure by two separate mechanisms, i.e., augmenting the concentration of a circulating vasodilator and depressing the concentration of a circulating vasoconstrictor. It is also important to distinguish the angiotensin-converting enzyme inhibitors from the pharmacologic interruption of the renin-angiotensin system produced by saralasin, which blocks the angiotensin receptor and thus acts as an angiotensin antagonist. Interpretation of responses to this agent are complicated, because saralasin is a partial agonist.

Haber has provided an excellent summary of the role of renin in cardiovascular homeostasis (Circulation 54:849, 1976). He points out that angiotensin II does not have an obligatory role in blood pressure maintenance in the normal, sodium-replete individual, but is essential after sodium depletion. Also, angiotensin II is responsible for the initial pressor response in experimental renovascular hypertension and appears to be important in the initiation of chronic renovascular hypertension. In congestive heart failure, maintenance of arterial pressure and accumulation of edema appear to be dependent on angiotensin II. It may turn out that the angiotensin-converting enzyme inhibitors may be useful in the treatment of heart failure, since by lowering arterial pressure they would reduce afterload and thereby increase cardiac output and simultaneously interfere with the production of aldosterone, thereby exerting a diuretic effect.

The debate about the value of renin profiling continues. The proponent of this approach, Doctor Laragh, has provided us with an excellent summary of his views (Am. J. Med. 61:797, 1976). The opposite point of view is championed by Dr. Norman M. Kaplan (J.A.M.A. 238:611, 1977. – Ed.] ◄

Physiologic Evaluation of a New Antihypertensive Agent: Prazosin HCl. Prazosin is a new type of antihypertensive drug, which effectively reduces blood pressure in hypertensive patients and is relatively free from serious side effects. Its mechanism of action is not fully understood. M. C. Koshy, Diane Mickley, Jacques Bourgoignie and M. Donald Blaufox[2] (Albert Einstein College of Medicine) studied physiologic parameters of importance in the treatment of moderate essential hypertension with prazosin HCl. Twenty patients with sustained diastolic pressures of 90 – 130 mm Hg who had received no antihypertensive therapy for a month were studied as outpatients. A single oral dose of 0.5 – 1 mg prazosin was given, with subsequent dosages of from 2 mg twice daily to a maximum of 5 mg 4 times daily. Fourteen patients completed at least 8 weeks of prazosin therapy. Two were withdrawn because of initial reactions, 2 because of rapid acceleration of hypertension and 2 because of poor compliance.

The 5 women and 9 men who completed the trial had a mean age of 36 years. Ten had a reduction in systemic blood pressure. The mean pressure was 148/102 mm Hg before and 139/91 after treatment. The mean creatinine clearance rose from 108 to 127 ml per minute after treatment. Cardiac output increased from 6,564 to 7,029 ml per minute. Peripheral resistance declined. Five subjects had a fall in mean blood pressure of 10 mm Hg or more, and these patients had the greatest reduction in peripheral resistance and the most marked changes in cardiac output. Plasma renin activity did not change significantly after treatment. Urinary sodium excretion averaged 140 mEq/24 hours before and 182 after treatment. No patient reported a decrease in libido or failure of ejaculation.

The findings support the previously reported efficacy of prazosin in reducing elevated blood pressure, but the effect is more prominent soon after the start of therapy than after 8 weeks of treatment. The drug

(2) Circulation 55:533 – 537, March, 1977.

appears to act primarily as a peripheral dilator. Its effectiveness might be enhanced by simultaneous use of a diuretic.

► [Attention is being focused increasingly on two antihypertensive drugs that appear to be of substantial promise, prazosin, discussed in this article, and clonidine, discussed in the article that follows. The effectiveness of prazosin in reducing afterload in patients with congestive heart failure is discussed in the article by Miller et al. in the chapter Afterload Reduction in this section. Fortunately, unlike that of hydralazine, the hypotensive effect of prazosin is not usually accompanied by significant tachycardia. Whereas the precise mechanism of the hypotensive action of prazosin is not clear, data from isolated vascular preparations suggest that it acts as an α-adrenergic blocking agent. I suspect that it will find a role in the treatment of moderate and severe hypertension and might well replace hydralazine and minoxidil, which have significant adverse effects. – Ed.] ◄

Clonidine and the Vasodilating β-Blocker Antihypertensive Drug Interaction. The combination of vasodilators with β-blocking drugs controls elevated blood pressure in most severely hypertensive subjects with relatively few disabling side effects, but some patients cannot use propranolol because of asthma, cardiac enlargement and failure, bradycardia, drug eruption or sleep disturbances. Clonidine and propranolol have similar hemodynamic and endocrine effects that are mediated by different receptor mechanisms. William A. Pettinger, Helen C. Mitchell and Hans-Georg Güllner[3] (Univ. of Texas Southwestern Med. School) substituted clonidine for propranolol in 14 adult minoxidil-treated subjects with severe hypertension. The patients initially had diastolic pressures above 100 mm Hg on optimal doses of standard antihypertensive drugs. Minoxidil-propranolol therapy was given for 6–38 months. Clonidine, 0.4–0.6 mg, was substituted for propranolol in 3 patients, whereas in 11 patients the drug was added initially to the propanolol-minoxidil combination in doses of 0.2 mg daily to minimize sedation. A dose necessary to establish a diastolic pressure below 95 mm Hg was maintained.

Clonidine had a pressure-lowering effect at initial follow-up in the 11 patients in whom it was added to the propranolol-minoxidil combination. Serum renin activity increased but the pulse rate was not altered. The average weight fell by 2 kg. Five patients relapsed when propranolol was discontinued, and clonidine was discontinued in 2 of these patients because of mental obtundation or abdominal pain. Clonidine substituted satisfactorily for propranolol in long-term use in 8 patients. Cardiothoracic ratios decreased in 2 patients with the addition of clonidine. Plasma antidiuretic hormone levels were not suppressed by the drug and an elevation was seen in most patients. Most patients preferred propranolol because of the sedation, dry mouth and conjunctival irritation produced by clonidine.

Clonidine can be substituted for propranolol or, when added to a propranolol-vasodilator combination, supply an added blood pressure-lowering effect. An increase in side effects results and clonidine has a diuretic action in this setting.

► [Both clonidine and propranolol depress heart rate and cardiac output; clonidine accomplishes this by stimulating α-adrenergic receptors in the brain that inhibit the cardiovascular control center in the brain stem, whereas propranolol accomplishes

(3) Clin. Pharmacol. Ther. 22:164–171, August, 1977.

this by inhibiting β-adrenergic receptors in the heart. Clonidine also inhibits renin release by activating α-adrenergic receptors within the kidney. Myers (Br. Med. J. 2:802, 1977) demonstrated that clonidine augments the reduction of arterial pressure that results from electric stimulation of the carotid sinus nerves, presumably facilitating the central component of the baroreceptor reflex. The cardiovascular effects of clonidine are complex because there may be a transient hypertensive effect related to the α-adrenergic stimulating properties of the compound (Tangri et al.: J. Pharmacol. Exp. Ther. 202:69, 1977). However, in the brain it stimulates the vasomotor inhibitory pathway in the brain stem, thus reducing sympathetic vasomotor tone to the periphery.

The absence of a fall in blood pressure induced by clonidine in tetraplegic subjects (Reid et al.: Clin. Pharmacol. Ther. 21:375, 1977) suggests that its hypotensive action in man is dependent on intact descending bulbospinal pathways and is mediated by withdrawal of sympathetic tone, thus providing direct evidence that an antihypertensive drug may lower blood pressure by a direct action on the brain.

For the treatment of moderately severe hypertension, clonidine has the advantage over guanethidine of lowering recumbent blood pressure without creating orthostatic hypotension, and it is superior to methyldopa because it may be effective in the patient with severe hypertension incompletely responsive to maximal doses of methyldopa. One drawback to its action is that when it is discontinued, transient sympathetic hyperactivity, characterized by hypertension, tremor and tachycardia and by the excretion of substantial quantities of catecholamines, may occur (Hoobler: Mayo Clin. Proc. 52:395, 1977). This is particularly prominent in patients taking a daily dose of 1.2 mg or more. From a practical point of view it would appear that the drug can be given in two divided doses, with the larger dose at bedtime and the smaller before noon, thereby limiting unwanted drowsiness and combining the convenience of less frequent dosing with superior blood pressure control (Jain et al.: Clin. Pharmacol. Ther. 21:382, 1977).—Ed.]

Miscellaneous

Indications for Pericardiectomy in Uremic Pericardial Effusion. John P. Connors, Robert E. Kleiger, Richard C. Shaw, John D. Voiles, Richard E. Clark, Herschel Harter and Charles L. Roper[4] (Washington Univ.) reviewed experience with 16 patients with uremic effusions who underwent pericardiectomy since 1968. Of 295 patients admitted to a chronic hemodialysis program in the past 8 years, 8% developed clinical evidence of uremic pericarditis (table). Pericardiectomy was done in 16 of these patients, whereas the rest underwent daily dialysis with regional heparinization. The indications for surgery included cardiac tamponade in 12 patients, enlarging effusions or no change on dialysis in 3 and hypotension in 1. Age range was 20–55 years. Renal failure antedated pericarditis by an average of 10.4 years. Average duration of dialysis was 18.1 months. Pericardiocentesis was done in 10 patients. Daily dialysis was carried out for 4 or 5 days after surgery.

No fluid was obtained at pericardiocentesis in 3 patients and in the rest, relief from tamponade was transient. Two patients developed progressive cardiac tamponade after needle lacerations of the right ventricle. All patients had hemorrhagic pericardial fluid and fibrinous adhesions. No operative deaths occurred, but 3 patients had significant morbidity, including one recurrence of tamponade due to adhesion of the edges of a small pericardial window to the epicardial surface. No subacute or chronic pericarditis has developed an average of 34 months after operation.

Disappointing results and occasionally serious complications should limit the use of pericardiocentesis in patients with uremic pericarditis. Hemodynamic instability and echocardiographic evidence of a persistent or enlarging effusion on dialysis are indications for surgery.

► [It is clear that while the etiology of uremic pericarditis remains obscure, long-term intermittent hemodialysis decreases its frequency and effusions can often be managed with intensive hemodialysis. Whereas uremic pericarditis may be fatal, control of the severity of uremia has not abolished the incidence of this complication. Since uremic

Uremic Pericarditis: Experience

	No.	%
Chronic hemodialysis	295	
Uremic pericarditis	37	8
Conservative Rx	21	57
Pericardiectomy	16	43

(4) Surgery 80:689–694, December, 1976.

pericardial effusion is characteristically serosanguineous, fatal tamponade may occur when heparin is administered systemically. Pericardial construction appears to be more frequent in patients on chronic dialysis since it may be due, at least in part, to heparin-related bleeding. There is considerable debate about whether uremic cardiomyopathy is a specific entity (see Gueron et al.: Nephron 15:2, 1975; and Tosser: ibid., p. 4). – Ed.] ◄

Sympathetic Nervous System Defect in Primary Orthostatic Hypotension. Michael G. Ziegler, C. Raymond Lake and Irwin J. Kopin[5] (Natl. Inst. of Health) sought to elucidate the neurologic defect of idiopathic orthostatic hypotension and found that patients with severe, long-standing orthostatic hypotension of unknown cause fall into two distinct groups with different plasma norepinephrine levels. Ten patients with acquired orthostatic hypotension, 8 men and 2 women, with a mean age of 56 years, were studied. Ten controls, with a mean age of 53 years, were also studied.

All patients with hypotension had fatigability and other evidence of peripheral autonomic dysfunction. Six had such evidence of central nervous system (CNS) disorder as parkinsonism and signs of cerebellar dysfunction. Five each had a Babinski sign and tremor and 5 had cranial nerve defects. These patients had normal plasma norepinephrine levels while recumbent, whereas those without apparent CNS dysfunction had low levels. No patient had a rise in plasma norepinephrine concentration on standing or exertion. Failure to maintain a normal blood pressure on standing was similar in the two groups of patients. Patients had significantly lower reclining plasma values of dopamine β-hydroxylase than did controls.

Patients with orthostatic hypotension and signs of CNS involvement appear to have an intact peripheral sympathetic nervous system, but they are unable to activate the otherwise intact sympathetic nerves appropriately, and symptoms of autonomic insufficiency and an inadequate rise in plasma norepinephrine concentration with postural change or exertion are found. In patients with isolated autonomic insufficiency, the deficit appears to be at the sympathetic nerves, and plasma norepinephrine values are low even at rest. Indirectly acting sympathomimetic amines are ineffective, and there is supersensitivity to exogenous norepinephrine.

► [Orthostatic hypotension may be secondary to decreased blood volume, diminished cardiac output or the inability to increase peripheral resistance. The last may come about as a consequence of diabetes, thiamine deficiency or amyloidosis. In the absence of these disorders, there is a group of patients with so-called idiopathic orthostatic hypotension. This article has now dissected this group into those with and those without central nervous system abnormalities; the former patients have normal sympathetic activity and norepinephrine release at rest, but failure to augment it upon assuming the erect posture. – Ed.] ◄

Current Results of Human Heart Transplantation. Eugene Dong, Jr., and Norman E. Shumway[6] (Stanford Univ.) reviewed the results of heart transplantation in 109 patients given 114 transplants since 1968. The diagnosis was coronary artery disease in 72 patients and idiopathic cardiomyopathy in 33. Absolute contraindications include a high pulmonary vascular resistance, infection and a positive

(5) N. Engl. J. Med. 296:293–297, Feb. 10, 1977.
(6) World J. Surg. 1:157–164, March, 1977.

PRIMARY CAUSE OF DEATH IN 67 RECIPIENTS OF HEART TRANSPLANTS AT STANFORD UNIVERSITY

Cause of death	No. of patients
Pulmonary hypertension	3
Acute rejection	16
Infection	35
Graft arteriosclerosis	
Proliferative	3
Atherosclerotic	6
Lymphoma	2
Cerebrovascular accident	2
	67

cross-match between recipient serum and donor lymphocytes. Relative contraindications include advanced age, a long duration of severe heart disease and acute pulmonary disease. The influence of age on survival after transplantation is uncertain. Advanced renal or hepatic dysfunction makes a successful outcome unlikely. Immunosuppression has been used in all cases; the primary agents are prednisone and azathioprine or cyclophosphamide. Graft rejection is treated variably with high-dose methylprednisolone, actinomycin D, systemic heparinization and reinstitution of antithymocyte globulin therapy.

Patient survival calculated by the actuarial method is 52% at 1 year, 43% at 2 years, 33% at 3 years and 28% at 5 years. The 6-year rate is 17%. The 1- and 2-year survival rates for patients surviving 3 months are 80% and 66%, respectively. Five patients had second cardiac transplants. Primary causes of death are given in the table. No patient has died of pulmonary hypertension since the 1st year of the program. The incidence of graft arteriosclerosis has declined since the institution of antiarteriosclerosis measures in the 3d year of the program. Studies have shown that reactive pulmonary hypertension decreased, prehepatic and prerenal failure regressed after transplantation and the cardiac output increased. All but 5 of 51 patients surviving 6 months or longer are able to return to work or housekeeping functions.

Cardiac transplantation can be considered a worthwhile measure. The major problems are related to its cost and the logistics of wide application.

► [Doctor Shumway and his colleagues at Stanford University have described an important technique for control of graft arteriosclerosis in heart transplant recipients (Surgery 81:262, 1977). They believe that a prophylactic regimen of antithrombotic agents (warfarin and dipyridamole) and restriction of dietary lipids are useful. Presumably, inhibiting the intra-arterial thrombosis that occurs in response to endothelial injury helps to prevent the development of arteriosclerosis. This group (Copeland et al.: J. Thorac. Cardiovasc. Surg. 73:242, 1977) has also described cardiac retransplantation in 5 patients, with long-term survival and rehabilitation achieved in 2. The major indications for this heroic procedure appear to be intractable acute rejection and late postoperative graft atherosclerosis. – Ed.] ◄

PART FIVE

THE DIGESTIVE SYSTEM

NORTON J. GREENBERGER, M.D.

The Esophagus and Stomach

Controlled Trial of Metoclopramide in Symptomatic Gastroesophageal Reflux. Patients with chronic symptomatic gastroesophageal reflux have reduced mean lower esophageal sphincter (LES) pressures, and metoclopramide stimulates smooth muscle of the upper gastrointestinal tract. Accordingly, R. W. McCallum, A. F. Ippoliti, C. Cooney and R. A. L. Sturdevant[1] (Univ. of California, Los Angeles) evaluated metoclopramide in a dose of 10 mg 4 times daily versus placebo in the treatment of symptomatic reflux and determined the effects of 2 months' treatment on basal LES pressures. The trial included 32 men and 2 women with a mean age of 55.6, who had had chronic heartburn for a mean of 10 years. Eighteen patients completed a double-blind crossover study of two consecutive 8-week periods. Metoclopramide was taken 15 minutes before meals and 30 minutes before bedtime. Esophageal manometry was done before the study and within 48 hours after the completion of each 8-week study period.

The study and control groups had similar baseline symptom scores. Study patients on metoclopramide had significantly greater improve-

Fig 1 (left).—Improvement from prestudy baseline in symptom score for each patient during the first treatment period. The mean (±SEM) for metoclopramide treatment was 56.9 ± 10%, as compared to 32.7 ± 5.8% for placebo ($P < 0.05$).

Fig 2 (right).—Increase in lower esophageal sphincter pressure above basal levels after 10 mg metoclopramide given by mouth in individual patients plotted against improvement from prestudy baseline in symptom score during metoclopramide therapy. *Closed circles,* first treatment period; *open circles,* second treatment period.

(Courtesy of McCallum, R. W., et al.: N. Engl. J. Med. 296:354–357, Feb. 17, 1977.)

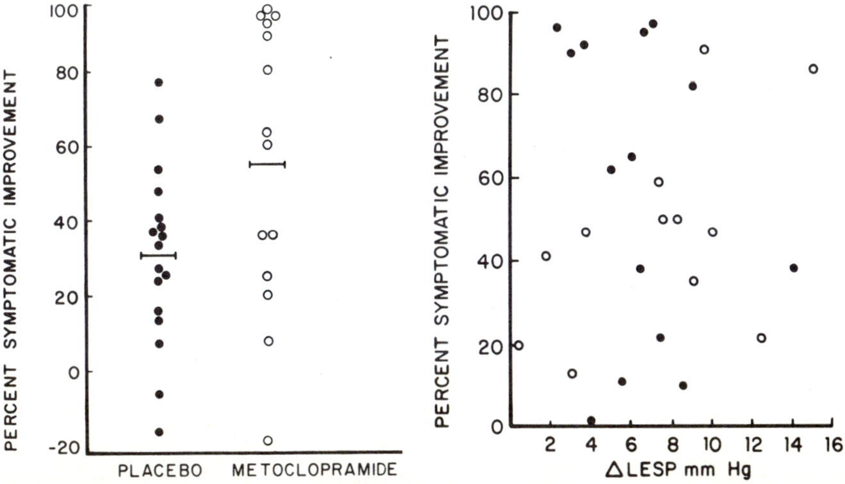

(1) N. Engl. J. Med. 296:354–357, Feb. 17, 1977.

ment in scores, 56.9% as compared with 32.7% for placebo patients (Fig 1). However, the mean antacid intake remained similar for the two groups. In the second study period, antacid intake was significantly less in the metoclopramide-treated group. Patients who improved with metoclopramide in the first test did not return to baseline symptom scores. No significant group differences in LES pressures were noted and pressures did not correlate significantly with changes in symptom scores. The peak pressure increase in response to metoclopramide did not correlate significantly with percent of symptomatic improvement during chronic metoclopramide therapy (Fig 2). One patient had marked anxiety during metoclopramide therapy; 3 patients required a reduction in dosage because of anxiety or lethargy. One patient developed gynecomastia. No significant changes occurred in laboratory tests and no patient developed a positive antinuclear antibody test during the study.

Metoclopramide-treated patients with gastroesophageal reflux had significantly more symptomatic improvement than control patients in this study. The treatment was not free of side effects. Metoclopramide may be indicated for patients who do not show substantial improvement in symptoms after a few weeks of intensive treatment with current agents.

► [In this study, the magnitude of the rise in lower esophageal sphincter pressure in an individual patient did not predict the subsequent symptomatic response of that patient to chronic metoclopramide therapy. Thus, metoclopramide may improve symptoms of gastroesophageal reflux by other mechanisms, such as: (1) increased rate of return to the stomach of refluxed material; (2) reduced duodenogastric reflux; and (3) increased rate of gastric emptying, especially in patients in whom emptying is delayed. The last possibility is supported by recent studies on the effect of metoclopramide in patients with diabetic gastroparesis (N. Engl. J. Med. 291:1257, 1974; and Ann. Intern. Med. 86:195, 1977). In a 19-year-old diabetic woman with severely impaired gastric emptying, metoclopramide strikingly increased the rate of gastric emptying, as evidenced by decreased gastric volume (344 ml on placebo vs. 13 ml after metoclopramide), and decreased recovery of ingested food solids (40.7% vs 1.2%, respectively) at 3 hours (ibid).

Cholestyramine has been used in the treatment of reflux esophagitis despite the absence of controlled trials of its use in this syndrome. I have not been impressed with its effectiveness in the treatment of reflux esophagitis. This prejudice has been heightened by a recent randomized, double-blind crossover study (Gastroenterology 73:441, 1977) which indicated that cholestyramine was ineffective in the symptomatic treatment of bile reflux gastritis.

Preliminary unpublished reports suggest that cimetidine, a histamine H_2-receptor blocker, may increase the rate of healing of reflux esophagitis. Controlled trials on this important question will be awaited with interest. – Ed.] ◄

Heartburn of Pregnancy. Reflux esophagitis with symptomatic heartburn is common in pregnant women and it has been suggested that hormonal events associated with pregnancy may be responsible. David H. Van Thiel, Judith S. Gavaler, Shobha N. Joshi, Rajinder K. Sara and John Stremple[2] (Univ. of Pittsburgh) evaluated this hypothesis directly by quantitating lower esophageal sphincter (LES) pressures serially during pregnancy and relating them to plasma steroid hormone concentrations in 4 pregnant women. The subjects, with a mean age of 19, were studied at 12, 24 and 36 weeks' gestation and 1–4

(2) Gastroenterology 72 (Pt. 1):666–668, April, 1977.

LOWER ESOPHAGEAL SPHINCTER (LES) PRESSURE, ACID SECRETORY RESPONSE AND HORMONAL LEVELS IN WOMEN DURING AND AFTER PREGNANCY*

Parameter	Duration of pregnancy			Postpartum
	12 wk	24 wk	36 wk	
LES (mm Hg)	10 ± 1.0†	9.0 ± 1.0 †	2.5 ± 1.3‡	22 ± 2.0
ΔLES§ (mm Hg)	0.5 ± 0.1†	0.5 ± 0.1†	0.2 ± 0.0†	2.0 ± 0.3
*p*H + reflux (no. with reflux)	2	2	4	0
Basal gastric *p*H (*p*H units)	2.8 ± 1.0	2.1 ± 0.4	2.2 ± 0.5	2.1 ± 0.5
Gastrin (pg/ml)	45 ± 14†	108 ± 18	87 ± 16	120 ± 18
Basal acid output (mEq/hr)	2.5 ± 0.8	1.0 ± 0.3	2.0 ± 0.3	1.6 ± 0.4
Peak acid output (mEq/hr)	25.0 ± 8.3	21.0 ± 10.0	28.0 ± 5.0	25.1 ± 4.0
Estrone (ng/ml)	2.6 ± 0.3‡	7.6 ± 1.6‡	9.0 ± 0.5‡	0.6 ± 0.5
Estradiol (pg/ml)	5.6 ± 0.6‡	19.0 ± 2.7‡	16.6 ± 2.3‡	2.3 ± 0.6
Progesterone (ng/ml)	108.1 ± 21.8	197.0 ± 28.4	217.9 ± 33.2	10.7 ± 5 3

*Values are means ±SEM.
†P < 0.05 compared to postpartum response.
‡P < 0.01 compared to postpartum response.
§In response to abdominal compression with a 2.3-kg weight.

weeks postpartum. Intraluminal pressures were recorded with the subjects supine.

Lower esophageal sphincter pressures were below the lower limits of normal for women at all intervals during gestation but postpartum pressures were normal. The difference was most significant at 36 weeks' gestation. At all times during pregnancy, the response of LES to abdominal compression was significantly less than in the postpartum period (table). Acid reflux was detected in all 4 subjects studied at 36 weeks' gestation; 2 patients had reflux at 12 and 24 weeks' gestation. None of the 4 postpartum subjects had reflux. Gestational gastric pH and plasma gastrin values were comparable to postpartum values in all subjects. Plasma estrone, estradiol and progesterone levels increased during gestation and, at each interval, were significantly greater than in the postpartum period. Basal and peak acid responses to pentagastrin during pregnancy were not different from those recorded in the postpartum period.

These findings are in accord with studies in women ingesting oral contraceptives, suggesting that an increase in plasma progesterone, alone or combined with estrogen, that occurs during pregnancies might be at least partly responsible for the reduction in LES pressure noted during pregnancy. This pressure reduction, acting with other factors, probably allows reflux to occur with the development of symptomatic heartburn. Progesterone has also been held responsible for reduced intestinal motility and reduced gallbladder contractility during pregnancy, and progesterone has been found to reduce gastrin-stimulated contraction of LES muscle in vitro.

► [Similar studies by Fischer (Clin. Res. 24:284A, 1976) support the hypothesis of Van Thiel et al. that elevated plasma progesterone either alone or in combination with estrogens is responsible for reduction of lower esophageal sphincter pressure (LESP) in pregnancy. Additional evidence supporting this concept is the earlier observation that oral contraceptives containing progesterone cause a reduction in LESP whereas ethinyl estradiol alone has no such effect (Gastroenterology 71:232, 1976). Other hormones potentially responsible for the reduction in LESP during pregnancy, such as specific prostaglandins, remain to be measured. — Ed.] ◄

Studies on Role of Cephalic-Vagal Stimulation in Acid Secretory Response to Eating in Normal Human Subjects. Charles T. Richardson, John H. Walsh, Kathleen A. Cooper, Mark Feldman and John S. Fordtran[3] determined the relative secretory potencies of cephalic-vagal stimulation, gastric distention with saline and distention with food in 9 normal subjects (6 men), with a mean age of 30 years. Secretory responses to 0.04 mg subcutaneous histamine acid phosphate per kg were determined. In vivo intragastric titration studies were performed during modified sham feeding (MSF) and test meal administration, and pentagastrin infusion studies were performed. In MSF, subjects chewed and expectorated appetizing food.

Acid secretion increased significantly and reproducibly during MSF. Serum gastrin concentration did not change significantly with MSF. Acid secretion was increased by gastric distention with saline but not by distention with food in the first 15 minutes; subsequently acid secretion was higher with food. Saline distention did not increase serum gastrin over basal concentrations. The findings are illustrated in Figure 3. Modified sham feeding did not augment maximally pentagastrin-stimulated acid secretion.

Within the limits imposed by maximal secretory capacity, the peak response to MSF is about the same regardless of the background rate of acid secretion or the background stimulus, whether saline, glucose or food. When the stomach is distended, as after a meal is ingested, the

Fig 3. — Acid secretion and serum gastrin concentration in 9 normal subjects in basal state and after 600 ml sodium chloride solution, glucose or homogenized food was infused into stomach. Each experiment was performed with and without MSF. Statistically significant differences ($P < 0.05$) by paired t test between each stimulus alone and with MSF is shown by asterisk. (Courtesy of Richardson, C. T., et al.: J. Clin. Invest. 60:435–441, August, 1977.)

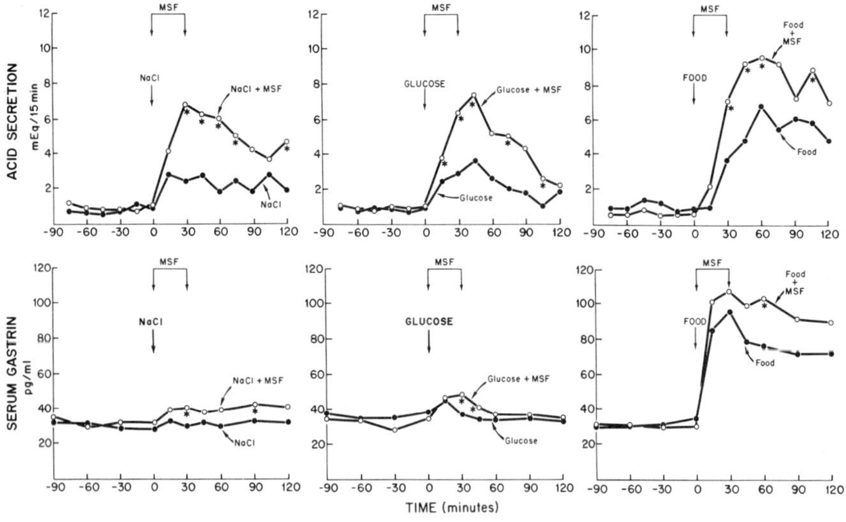

(3) J. Clin. Invest. 60:435–441, August, 1977.

secretory response to MSF is prolonged and continues for at least 90 minutes after sham feeding is discontinued. Cephalic-vagal stimulation accounts for about a third of the acid secreted when all mechanisms act simultaneously. Increased vagal activity secondary to cephalic influences is an important mediator of acid secretion while a meal is eaten and afterward.

► [A recent study on the effect of low-dose propantheline on food-stimulated gastric secretion is of considerable interest. Feldman et al. (N. Engl. J. Med. 297:1427, 1977) evaluated the widely held notion that anticholinergic drugs must be used in near-toxic doses to inhibit gastric acid secretion effectively. Nine patients with duodenal ulcer were studied after a low dose (15 mg) and after a near-toxic dose (averaging 48 mg) of the anticholinergic drug propantheline. Inhibition of food-stimulated acid secretion was identical with the two doses of propantheline: 29 ± 10 (mean ± 1 SE) and 29 ± 11% respectively. In addition, when 15 mg propantheline was combined with the histamine H_2-receptor antagonist cimetidine, acid secretion was suppressed to a greater degree than with either drug alone. These findings indicate that a *low dose* of propantheline is as effective as a *near-toxic dose* in suppressing food-stimulated acid secretion and augments the inhibitory effect of cimetidine. Since ingestion of this combination is convenient and well tolerated, it is worthy of trial in patients with duodenal ulcer and other acid peptic disorders that are resistant to treatment with H_2-receptor antagonists alone. – Ed.] ◄

Antacid and Placebo Produced Similar Pain Relief in Duodenal Ulcer Patients. Controlled double-blind studies supporting the efficacy of antacids in relieving duodenal ulcer pain have not been reported. Richard A. L. Sturdevant, Jon I. Isenberg, Donald Secrist and James Ansfield[4] (Univ. of California, Los Angeles) compared the effects of a liquid antacid and placebo in the acute relief of spontaneous duodenal ulcer pain. Twelve men with a mean age of 44 in whom a duodenal ulcer crater was demonstrated within 48 hours of study, who had had symptoms for a mean of 46.5 days, received a preparation containing 13% aluminum hydroxide and 12% magnesium trisilicate. Its buf-

TABLE 1.—STUDY A: NUMBER OF DOSES OF ANTACID OR PLACEBO PRODUCING VARIOUS LEVELS OF PAIN RELIEF IN 10 HOSPITALIZED SYMPTOMATIC DUODENAL ULCER PATIENTS

Pain relief	Day 1	Day 2	Day 3	Day 4	Day 5	Total
Complete						
Antacid	7	11	9	13	11	51
Placebo	4	7	13	15	11	50
Partial						
Antacid	34	21	34	23	2	114
Placebo	31	30	24	11	4	100
None						
Antacid	11	10	6	8	7	42
Placebo	13	11	10	12	7	53
Total						
Antacid	52	42	49	44	20	207
Placebo	48	48	47	38	22	203

(4) Gastroenterology 72:1–5, January, 1977.

TABLE 2.—STUDY B: COMPARISON OF DEGREE OF PAIN RELIEF PRODUCED BY SINGLE DOSES OF ANTACID (A) AND PLACEBO (P) IN 20 SYMPTOMATIC HOSPITALIZED DUODENAL ULCER PATIENTS*

Degree of pain relief	5 min		10 min		15 min		20 min		25 min		30 min	
	A	P	A	P	A	P	A	P	A	P	A	P
0	12	12	4	7	4	7	5	6	4	6	3	6
1+	4	4	9	8	5	3	4	4	4	3	4	2
2+	2	3	5	1	6	6	3	6	0	3	1	2
3+	2	0	1	2	4	2	5	2	8	6	5	6
4+	0	1	1	2	1	2	3	2	4	2	7	4
Total	20	20	20	20	20	20	20	20	20	20	20	20

*Patients' estimates of degree of relief: 0, none; 1+, 1–24%; 2+, 25–75%; 3+, 76–99%; 4+, 100%. The numbers of patients with various degrees of pain relief at 5-minute intervals after ingestion of the test drug are shown.

fering capacity is similar to that of Gelusil-M and Amphogel. Patients were hospitalized during the study and received a regular diet excluding milk. Twenty other males with a mean age of 48 received a single dose of antacid or placebo; 7 of these patients were hospitalized. A commercial antacid was used.

In the 5-day, multiple-dose inpatient study, no differences were noted between the antacid and placebo in ability to relieve pain. The results are presented in Table 1. In the single-dose study, the time course and degree of pain relief did not differ significantly between antacid and placebo treatments (Table 2). In data from the two studies combined, neither minimal nor strict criteria resulted in a significant difference in pain relief between the antacid and placebo treatments.

These findings do not necessarily prove that antacids have no effect on duodenal ulcer pain, but they indicate that factors other than gastric acid neutralization are important in the relief of ulcer pain. Because millions of dollars are spent each year for antacids in the treatment of duodenal ulcer and because antacids have some inherent untoward effects, the present findings suggest a need for further clinical trials to define the efficacy, if any, of antacids in the treatment of duodenal ulcer.

Gastric and Duodenal Ulcer Healing under Placebo Treatment. It has been impractical in therapeutic trials to assess ulcer size continuously. Ulrich Scheurer, Lothar Witzel, Fred Halter, Hans-Martin Keller, Rolf Huber and Renato Galeazzi[5] (Bern, Switzerland) used fiberoptic endoscopy to observe peptic gastroduodenal ulcer healing under placebo treatment in 41 patients, 38 of whom completed the study. Twenty-four had gastric and 14, duodenal ulcers. All were aged 16–70 and had had their most recent attack less than 4 weeks before the study. Patients took inert placebo tablets 3 times daily before meals and a few took a liquid antacid as well. They were advised to

(5) Gastroenterology 72 (Pt. 1):838–841, May, 1977.

take a bland diet and to moderate their smoking habits. Ulcer size was measured by endoscopy on day 1 and day 21 and in the absence of healing, also on day 42.

At 3 weeks, 53.3% of duodenal and 26.6% of gastric ulcers had healed completely. At 6 weeks the respective figures were 73.3% and 83.3%. The mean time to 50% size reduction of gastric ulcers was 1.7 weeks and of duodenal ulcers, 1.9 weeks. The average percentage reduction in size of incompletely healed lesions within 3 weeks was 71% for gastric and 82% for duodenal ulcers and within 6 weeks, 83% and 89%, respectively. The ulcers that healed initially were similar in size regardless of their location, but overall the initial size of gastric ulcers was significantly greater than that of duodenal ulcers. The smaller ulcers required less time to heal completely in both ulcer groups.

Repeated measurements of ulcer size before complete healing contribute to optimal characterization of the healing process. The time to 50% reduction in ulcer size is a reasonable parameter for judging healing. Since small ulcers heal quite rapidly, ulcer size should be assessed at intervals of less than 2 weeks. If ulcers are not matched for size, the use of number of ulcers healed in a fixed time can give rise to inaccurate conclusions as to the efficacy of a given form of treatment.

► [To recapitulate, the important findings in this study were: (1) at 3 weeks 53.3% of duodenal and 26.6% of gastric ulcers had healed completely as judged by endoscopy, (2) at 6 weeks the respective figures for healing were 73.3% and 83.3% and (3) the mean time to 50% reduction in size was 1.7 weeks for gastric ulcers and 1.9 weeks for duodenal ulcers. These results are impressive in view of the fact that the patients received inert placebo tablets and apparently only a few patients took additional liquid antacids for dyspeptic symptoms. That the persistence of symptoms in such patients may bear little relationship to the presence or absence of residual ulceration is discussed in the following article. – Ed.] ◄

Healing of Duodenal Ulcer with an Antacid Regimen. The effect of antacid therapy on healing of duodenal ulcer has been evaluated by only one controlled double-blind study, which showed no benefit, according to Walter L. Peterson, Richard A. L. Sturdevant, Harold D. Frankl, Charles T. Richardson, Jon I. Isenberg, Janet D. Elashoff, James Q. Sones, Robert A. Gross, Richard W. McCallum and John S. Fordtran.[6] They therefore carried out a 28-day double-blind trial to determine whether a large-dose antacid regimen is effective in promoting healing of duodenal ulcer.

Subjects were sought among outpatients at three medical centers: University of Texas Southwestern Medical School, Dallas, Wadsworth Veterans Administration Hospital, Los Angeles, and Kaiser Hospital, Los Angeles. Eighty-eight patients with proved duodenal ulcer were accepted and randomly assigned to treatment with antacid or placebo. All were examined endoscopically before and after 4 weeks of treatment with 30 ml liquid antacid or placebo taken 1 and 3 hours after meals and at bedtime. A magnesium-aluminum hydroxide liquid identical to Mylanta II was used. Uncoded antacid tablets were supplied to be taken only for relief of ulcer pain.

Thirty-eight patients in the placebo group and 36 in the treatment

(6) N. Engl. J. Med. 297:341–345, Aug. 18, 1977.

CHANGE IN ULCER SIZE WITH EACH TREATMENT REGIMEN*

GROUP	74 PATIENTS COMPLETING FULL 28 DAYS		ALL 80 PATIENTS HAVING 2 ENDOSCOPIES	
	ULCER HEALED	ULCER NOT HEALED	ULCER HEALED	ULCER NOT HEALED
Placebo	17 (45%)	21 (55%)	17 (40%)	25 (60%)
Antacid	28 (78%)	8 (22%)	29 (76%)	9 (24%)
P value†	<0.005		<0.005	

*Data expressed as number of patients with percent of total group in parentheses.

†Difference between placebo group and antacid group.

group completed the study. Complete healing was observed in significantly more antacid patients (table). Four placebo and 5 antacid patients had at least a 50% reduction in ulcer size without complete healing. One antacid and 4 placebo patients were withdrawn because of intolerable ulcer pain, and 1 antacid patient was withdrawn because of nausea and vomiting.

There was little relation between freedom from ulcer symptoms in the final week of treatment and ulcer healing (Fig 4). Differences in use of antacid tablets by placebo and antacid patients were not significant. Stool frequency was greater in the antacid group. Smoking was associated with less ulcer healing in the placebo group. No changes in serum gastrin or pepsinogen levels were observed.

These data provide supportive evidence for the importance of gastric acid in the pathogenesis of duodenal ulcer and justification for use of antacids in its treatment. Healing of ulcers was enhanced with large doses of antacids to about the same degree as has been reported with histamine H_2-receptor antagonists, colloidal bismuth and carbenoxolone. Combinations of these agents may prove the best approach to treatment of duodenal ulcer. Choice of medical therapy at present

Fig 4.—Final symptom score versus ulcer healing. (Courtesy of Peterson, W. L., et al.: N. Engl. J. Med. 297:341–345, Aug. 18, 1977.)

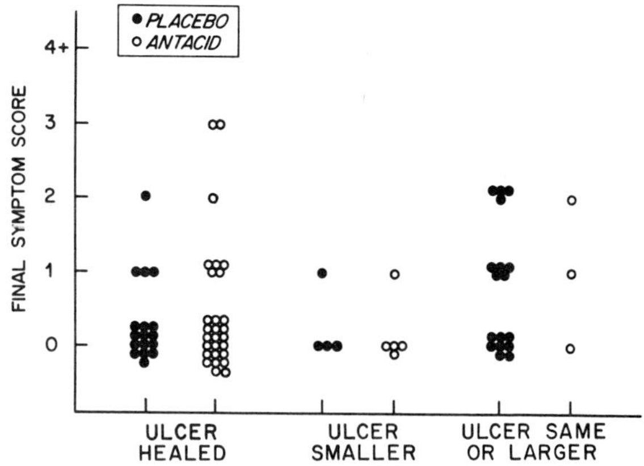

should be based on such considerations as availability, cost, potential toxicity and patient acceptance.

► [An important finding in this study was the dissociation between ulcer symptoms and ulcer healing. Presence or absence of symptoms during the 4th treatment week was a poor predictor of presence or absence of an ulcer crater. Of the patients who were *symptom free,* the ulcer had not *healed* in 16 of 44 (33%); of those who were *not symptom free,* the ulcer had *healed* in 12 of 25 (48%). These findings raise a question as to the validity of previous trials of antacids in peptic ulcer disease in which symptoms or x-ray findings were used as therapeutic end points. – Ed.] ◄

Comparison of an H_2-Receptor Antagonist and a Neutralizing Antacid on Postprandial Acid Delivery into the Duodenum in Patients with Duodenal Ulcer. Timothy B. Deering and Juan-R. Malagelada[7] (Mayo Clinic) measured postprandial rates of acid delivery into the duodenum for direct evaluation of the efficacy of two different acid-reducing treatments for duodenal ulcer disease – cimetidine, which inhibits secretion of gastric acid, and Maalox (magnesium and aluminum hydroxides), which neutralizes acid already secreted. Both were given with an identical solid meal.

Eighteen studies were done in 6 patients with duodenal ulcer, 5 men and 1 woman aged 23–63 years. None had evidence of gastric outlet obstruction. Each patient took 400 mg cimetidine at the start of the meal on the 1st day, 30 ml Maalox (liquid) at 1 and 3 hours after the meal on a 2d day and no treatment on a 3d day. The duodenum was perfused continuously with saline containing ^{14}C-polyethylene glycol.

The intragastric pH was significantly higher with both treatments than with the control meal alone beyond the 1st hour. Only sporadic significant differences occurred between the Maalox and cimetidine treatments. Cimetidine continually reduced the total postprandial acid content of the stomach, whereas Maalox had a comparable effect only in the hour after each dose. However, the total titratable acid emptied in the first 4 hours after the meal did not differ significantly. Both treatments significantly reduced the hydrogen ion delivered to the duodenum for most periods after the 1st hour. Cimetidine decreased the 4-hour delivery of titratable acid and hydrogen ion into the duodenum by 63% and 86%, respectively. Liquid Maalox reduced 4-hour delivery of acid by 47% and 74%, respectively, versus control values.

An oral dose of 400 mg cimetidine is necessary to match the reduction in postprandial duodenal acid load produced by Maalox taken 1 and 3 hours after meals. Liquid antacid still provides a rational alternative therapy for duodenal ulcer disease during daytime. Antacid, however, stays only briefly in the empty stomach and would not match the prolonged nocturnal inhibition of gastric acid secretion produced by cimetidine. Treatment combining liquid neutralizing antacid and histamine H_2-receptor antagonists may find clinical application in management of duodenal ulcer disease.

► [Numerous reports have demonstrated that cimetidine is an effective agent in the treatment of gastric and duodenal ulceration and, indeed, accelerates the rate of ulcer healing. Side effects are minimal and include headache, dizziness, rash, transient increases in serum alkaline phosphatase and serum glutamic-pyruvic transaminase lev-

(7) Gastroenterology 73:11–14, July, 1977.

els, and leukopenia. Perforation of peptic ulcer also has been reported after abrupt cessation of cimetidine therapy (Br. Med. J. 2:865, 1977).

Whereas cimetidine is clearly an effective agent, two important questions need to be raised. First, what is the long-term effect of cimetidine on serum gastrin levels and gastric acid secretion? For example, is there a rebound acid hypersecretion after cimetidine is discontinued? Second, does long-term cimetidine therapy reduce the rate of duodenal ulcer relapse? There are some preliminary reports bearing on these questions. Spence et al. (Gut 18:A949, 1977) determined the effect of 2 and 12 months of treatment with cimetidine on fasting and peptone meal-stimulated serum gastrin concentrations and integrated gastrin response in 22 duodenal ulcer patients. One year's treatment with cimetidine produced an approximately threefold increase in the integrated gastrin response to a meal. However, this did not result in a rebound of acid secretion on discontinuation of treatment nor in an increased severity of symptoms in the 2 patients who subsequently have relapsed.

Blackwood et al. (ibid., p. A420) determined whether relapse of duodenal ulcer disease can be prevented by long-term maintenance therapy. Before entering the maintenance trial, patients were treated with 400 mg cimetidine or placebo 4 times daily. Thirty-one patients with endoscopically confirmed healed ulcers then entered a double-blind maintenance trial of either 800 mg cimetidine or placebo taken at bedtime. At 6 weeks, 1 of 13 cimetidine-treated and 9 of 14 placebo-treated patients had endoscopic relapse; at 3 months, 2 of 9 cimetidine-treated and 8 of 9 placebo-treated patients had relapsed. Finally, at 6 months, 2 of 7 cimetidine-treated and all 7 placebo-treated patients had relapsed. In another trial not yet published, 1 of 20 cimetidine-treated and 15 of 20 placebo-treated patients relapsed. These preliminary results suggest that cimetidine may prove to be an effective long-term prophylactic agent against duodenal ulcer relapse. — Ed.] ◄

Effect of Graded Amounts of Acid Instilled into the Duodenum on Pancreatic Bicarbonate Secretion and Plasma Secretin in Duodenal Ulcer Patients and Normal Subjects. Impaired secretin release or bicarbonate secretion, or both, in response to duodenal acidification could contribute to a lower duodenal pH in patients with duodenal ulcer. Jon I. Isenberg, Robert Cano and Stephen R. Bloom[8] studied the effects of graded doses of HCl, instilled into the duodenum, on plasma secretin and pancreatic bicarbonate secretion in 9 patients with duodenal ulcer and 9 normal subjects, having respective mean ages of 50 and 45. None of the patients had ulcer complications or symptoms at the time of the study. The duodenum was acidified with use of a Dreiling tube after overnight fasting, graded doses of HCl being instilled in doses of 0.94 – 7.50 mEq/5 minutes, equivalent to 11.25 – 90 mEq per hour. Plasma secretin was measured by radioimmunoassay.

Bicarbonate output was significantly greater in the ulcer patients under basal conditions and after 0.94 mEq HCl. Outputs were similar in both groups after the three largest doses of acid (Fig 5). Peak secretin values at rest and after acid were somewhat greater in the ulcer patients than in normal subjects but the differences were not significant. Like bicarbonate output, secretin values were linearly related to the log dose of acid instilled. Secretin-acid dose-response curves were similar in the ulcer patients and normal control subjects.

Graded amounts of acid instilled into the duodenum produce graded increases in pancreatic bicarbonate output in both duodenal ulcer patients and normal subjects and comparable increases in plasma secretin in the two groups. Increased gastric acid secretion coupled with

(8) Gastroenterology 72:6 – 8, January, 1977.

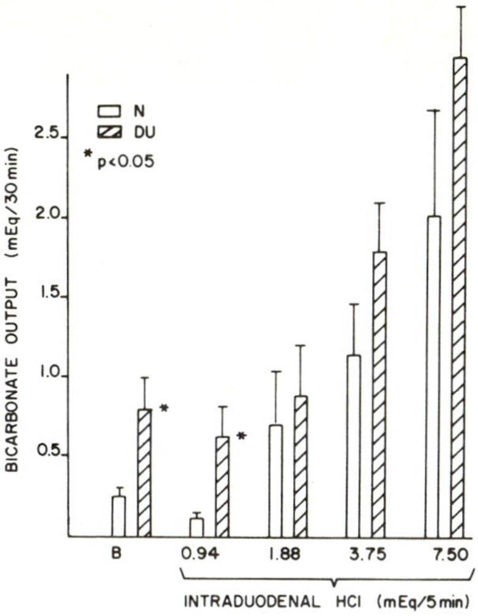

Fig 5.—Mean 30-minute bicarbonate output before *(B)* and in response to instillation of 4 graded doses of hydrochloric acid into the duodenum. *Open bars,* mean of 9 normal subjects; *hatched bars,* mean of 9 duodenal ulcer *(DU)* subjects. Vertical lines indicate mean ±1 SE. (Courtesy of Isenberg, J. I., et al.: Gastroenterology 72:6-8, January, 1977.)

rapid gastric emptying results in an increased duodenal acid load in ulcer patients and is probably the major cause of the reduced duodenal bulb pH. The present study revealed no defect in either secretin release or pancreatic bicarbonate secretion in response to duodenal acidification in duodenal ulcer patients.

► [In an interesting parallel study, Murthy et al. (Gastroenterology 73:758, 1977) studied the effect of smoking one unfiltered cigarette every 15 minutes for 1 hour on basal gastric acid and pancreatic secretion as well as plasma gastrin and secretin levels in patients with duodenal ulcer disease and control subjects. Smoking induced a transient rise of basal acid output that was more pronounced in the duodenal ulcer group. In addition, smoking markedly inhibited fluid and bicarbonate secretion during the smoking period, but there was no difference in the degree of inhibition of pancreatic secretion between the two groups. Importantly, immunoreactive gastrin and secretin in peripheral venous blood did not change significantly during smoking. Rather, the degree of inhibition of basal pancreatic secretion correlated well with plasma concentrations of nicotine. These findings strengthen a possible causal association between cigarette smoking and duodenal ulcer disease. The transient increase of basal acid secretion associated with a marked and prolonged inhibition of pancreatic bicarbonate secretion may create a highly acidic pH in the duodenal bulb for long periods of time. As Murthy et al. emphasize, smoking incessantly is common among heavy smokers and because inhaled nicotine accumulates in the blood, it is likely that even more prolonged inhibition of pancreatic secretion occurs than what was demonstrated with just 1 hour of smoking.—Ed.] ◄

Use of Calcium and Secretin in Diagnosis of Gastrinoma (Zollinger-Ellison Syndrome). Clifford W. Deveney, Karen S. Deveney, Bernard M. Jaffe, Rayford S. Jones and Lawrence W. Way[9] (San Francisco) evaluated the role of calcium and secretin tests in diagnosis of gastrinoma in 65 patients with peptic ulcer disease. In 38 of these, gastrinoma was suspected because of marked acid hypersecretion, high indeterminant gastrin levels, recurrent ulcer disease after surgery, or a combination of these findings. All patients had active peptic ulcer disease when studied.

(9) Ann. Intern. Med. 87:680-686, December, 1977.

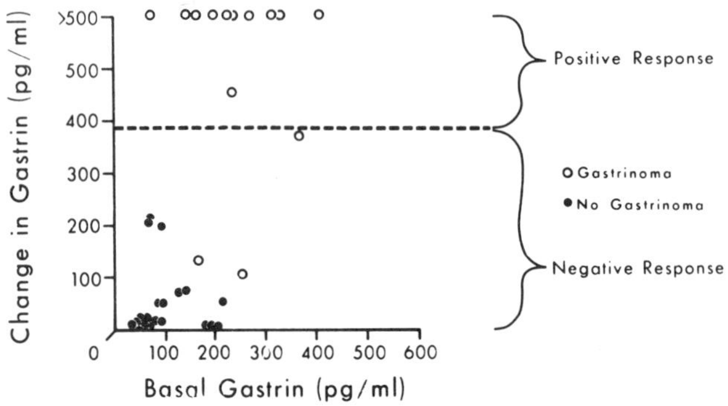

Fig 6.—Distribution of 34 patients with suspected gastrinoma according to basal gastrin *(abscissa)* and change in gastrin with calcium *(ordinate)*. Note that basal gastrin does not permit separation of patients with and without the disorder, but that change in gastrin with calcium permits such separation. A level of 395 pg or more was chosen to define patients with gastrinoma. Note that false negative responses occur but not false positive responses. (Courtesy of Deveney, C. W., et al.: Ann. Intern. Med. 87:680–686, December, 1977.)

The patients were divided into three groups for study: (1) 11 with known gastrinoma; (2) 16 unlikely to have gastrinoma; and (3) 38 with suspected gastrinoma. Calcium gluconate was given by intravenous infusion of 4 mg Ca^{2+} kg/hour for 3 hours. Secretin was given as an intravenous bolus of 2 units per kg. Serum gastrin was measured by radioimmunoassay.

Only 1 patient had an elevated serum calcium and hyperparathyroidism at the time of study. The average rise in serum calcium was 2.95 mg/dl; neither the basal nor postinfusion calcium levels differed in the three patient groups.

Serum gastrin rose markedly during calcium infusion in the patients with known gastrinoma. All 8 patients studied had at least a

Fig 7.—Distribution of 27 patients with suspected gastrinoma according to basal gastrin and change in gastrin with secretin. A change of 110 pg or more characterizes patients with gastrinoma. With this criterion, false positive responses should not occur, and incidence of false negative responses should be 5% or less. (Courtesy of Deveney, C. W., et al.: Ann. Intern. Med. 87:680–686, December, 1977.)

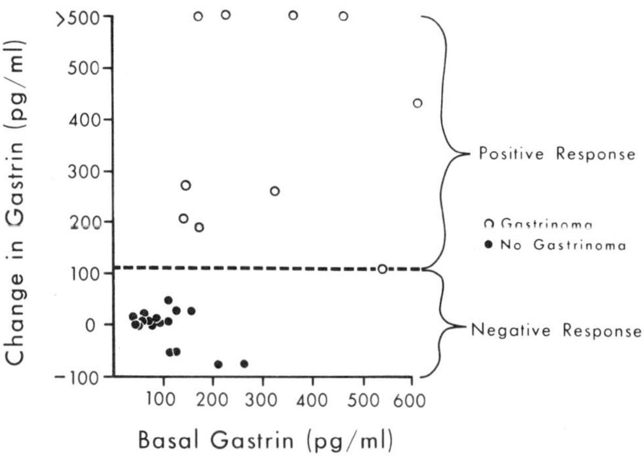

twofold increase over basal levels and an absolute response exceeding 1,000 pg/ml. After secretin, the serum gastrin rose to high levels in all 8 patients. The minimal absolute rise was 1,400 pg/ml.

The serum gastrin rose slightly in 9 patients in whom gastrinoma was considered unlikely. No marked changes were seen after secretin injection.

Among the patients with suspected gastrinoma, all 12 whose gastrin levels rose more than 300 pg/ml after calcium stimulation are now thought to have gastrinoma. Five of the 10 patients operated on for ulcer disease had histologically confirmed gastrinomas; the other 5 continue to have elevated gastrin levels after total gastrectomy. Diagnosis of gastrinoma in suspected patients by use of calcium is illustrated in Figure 6 and by use of secretin in Figure 7.

Stimulation by calcium and secretin proved to be highly useful in diagnosis of gastrinoma. The diagnostic limits will vary with the radioimmunoassay used. With use of criteria of serum gastrin increases of over 395 pg/ml after calcium and of 110 pg/ml after secretin, there were no false positive tests with either substance. False negative responses have been seen with both agents. Bolus injection of secretion is the preferred single provocative screening test for gastrinoma because it is less time consuming and more reliable than calcium.

► [Secretin-stimulated serum gastrin levels were measured in 23 patients with hyperparathyroidism from 6 families with multiple endocrine adenomatosis (MEA-1) syndrome (Ann. Intern. Med. 86:719, 1977). In 9 cases this led to increases in serum gastrin levels ranging from 298 to 13,300 pg/ml, whereas the maximum rise in gastrin in the other 14 patients was 32 pg/ml. In all 9 patients with marked gastrin responses to secretin, the Zollinger-Ellison syndrome (ZES) was diagnosed by gastric acid hypersecretion and large increases in gastrin after calcium administration. In 34 normal subjects, 23 nonaffected members of families with MEA-1 syndrome and 42 patients with various diseases, the maximum gastrin response to secretin was 21 pg/ml.

Lamers et al. (Gut 18:128, 1977) evaluated the usefulness of calcium and secretin provocation tests in the diagnosis of the ZES in 15 patients with histologically proved or suspected ZES. These tests were also performed in normal subjects and in patients with duodenal ulcer, antrectomy, total gastrectomy and achlorhydria. All tests were considered to be positive if a more than 50% increase in serum gastrin was found. The secretin test and calcium infusion test were both positive in 13 of 15 ZES patients. Lamers et al. feel that secretin stimulation is the provocation test of first choice in the diagnosis of ZES for the following reasons: (1) there were few (2 of 15) false negative test results in ZES patients; (2) there were no false positive tests in 69 patients without gastrinoma; (3) it was easy and quick to perform; and (4) there were no adverse reactions. The 2 ZES patients with negative secretin stimulation tests had negative calcium provocation tests as well, despite histologically proved gastrinoma.

The secretin and calcium infusion tests are useful adjuncts in the diagnosis of ZES, especially when basal serum gastrin levels are only slightly elevated. The two tests complement each other as neither is invariably positive. – Ed.] ◄

H_2-Histamine Receptor Blocking Agents in the Zollinger-Ellison Syndrome: Experience in Seven Cases and Implications for Long-Term Therapy. D. M. McCarthy, E. J. Olinger, R. J. May, B. W. Long and J. D. Gardner[1] (Natl. Inst. of Health) evaluated the H_2-histamine receptor blocking agents metiamide and cimetidine in 7 patients with Zollinger-Ellison syndrome, evidenced by a fasting immunoreactive serum gastrin of over 300 pg/ml, a basal acid output of over 15

(1) Ann. Intern. Med. 87:668–675, December, 1977.

mEq/hour, a ratio of basal to maximal acid output of over 0.5 and radiographic or endoscopic evidence of peptic ulcer disease.

Metiamide in 0.9% saline was infused intravenously in doses of 2 and 4 mg/kg/hour on successive days in a double-blind sequence. Cimetidine (300 mg) and metiamide (200, 300 and 400 mg) were given orally during gastric aspiration studies.

Infusion of metiamide, 4 mg/kg/hour for 90 minutes, reduced acid secretion strikingly (at least 70%) in all 5 patients studied. Both metiamide and cimetidine orally also reduced gastric acid output substantially in all patients. The marked reduction in volume of gastric juice secreted after the drugs resulted in marked reduction in chloride and potassium output without great changes in the concentrations of the ions. A relatively minor fall in total sodium output was noted when the drug was maximally active.

Three patients were treated only with metiamide, 2 with only cimetidine and 2 with both agents. Later, 6 patients were treated orally for 3–15 months, and 1 patient was treated intravenously for 1 month. The treatment abolished symptoms in all 7 patients and diarrhea in 5 of them and allowed ulcer healing in 6. No patient had adverse effects from the medication. No patient failed to respond, although 1 died of progressive tumor and 2 required total gastrectomy.

Patients with Zollinger-Ellison syndrome can be managed medically and, in view of current mortality trends, gain little from the added risks attending total gastrectomy. The problem of gradual loss of efficacy of the drugs remains. Three of 9 patients from the literature who took oral metiamide on a long-term basis appeared to develop tolerance to the drug.

► [It is not generally appreciated that gastric emptying is accelerated in patients with Zollinger-Ellison syndrome (ZES). Dubois et al. (J. Clin. Invest. 59:255, 1977) demonstrated that the fraction of gastric contents emptied per minute (fractional rate of emptying) was increased in ZES patients but unchanged or actually decreased in normal subjects receiving pentagastrin. It is of interest that the increased fractional rate of gastric emptying in patients with ZES persisted despite abolition of gastric acid hypersecretion by the H_2-receptor blocking agent metiamide. Thus, the increased fractional gastric emptying seen in ZES patients is not attributable to hypergastrinemia or to gastric hypersecretion per se. Instead, it appears to be caused by an undefined nervous or humoral factor. – Ed.] ◄

Does Early Endoscopy Benefit the Patient with Active Upper Gastrointestinal Bleeding? Gregory L. Eastwood[2] (Harvard Med. School) points out that prompt fiberoptic endoscopy has been enthusiastically adopted by most physicians who care for actively bleeding patients, on the assumption that an early, accurate diagnosis would lead to reduced morbidity and mortality. Four prospective controlled studies comparing early endoscopy with less aggressive approaches to upper gastrointestinal bleeding have appeared in the past 2 years. In the first two studies, the aggressive approach, which included emergency endoscopy followed by barium contrast radiography, did not reduce mortality or lead to differences in the frequency of surgery or duration of hospital stay as compared with selective endoscopy and barium studies. In the third trial, endoscopy patients had a shorter

(2) Gastroenterology 72 (Pt. 1):737–739, April, 1977.

time to diagnosis, but the need for emergency surgery and duration of hospitalization were no different between the two groups. The fourth study failed to show whether early endoscopy benefits the active gastrointestinal bleeder, because both groups had both endoscopy and barium contrast studies within 24 hours of each other.

The assumption that a prompt endoscopic diagnosis leads to reduced morbidity and mortality has not been verified. The necessity of making a definite diagnosis before treating active upper gastrointestinal bleeding has not been proved. It is assumed that the putative benefit of endoscopy outweighs the risks of the procedure, but adverse reactions do occur. Endoscopy of the bleeding patient is expensive and benefit to the patient that would justify the expense has not been proved. These aspects of endoscopy must be clarified if the procedure is to be relied on in the management of active upper gastrointestinal bleeding. Appropriate studies will not be easy to design. It is clear that endoscopy is diagnostically superior to other methods, but the issue is whether this superior accuracy confers any therapeutic advantage that will ultimately reduce morbidity and improve survival.

► [Doctor Eastwood's thesis in this article is that we should question the value of emergency endoscopy in active upper gastrointestinal bleeding (UGIB) since in the few controlled studies there is little evidence that emergency endoscopy benefits the patient. Two additional recent articles also have assessed the impact of endoscopy on the management and outcome of UGIB (Lancet 1:1167, 1977; and Gut 18:A987, 1977). In the former article, 318 patients admitted to the hospital with UGIB were entered into a prospective randomized comparison of investigation by either endoscopy or radiology. Although the diagnostic yield was higher in the endoscopy group than the radiology group, there was no difference between the two groups in management or survival. In the latter article, 108 patients with UGIB underwent endoscopy and were compared with an earlier group of 98 patients studied in 1970–73. The average duration of stay in hospital fell slightly from a mean of 14.8 to 13.0 days. Blood transfusion requirements were not significantly affected (2.5 vs. 2.7 units) but in 87% a bleeding site was identified as opposed to only 55% in the group studied earlier. The diagnosis was also made more quickly (2.0 vs. 4.1 days) and surgery was performed earlier and more frequently (32 vs. 9%). Despite this, the overall mortality was not improved.

In assessing all these studies, one key factor is missing, namely, a subgroup analysis. The impact of endoscopy might well be different in patients with duodenal ulcer, gastric ulcer, erosive gastritis, Mallory-Weiss syndrome and esophageal varices. Inclusion of patients with other than massive bleeding can have an artifactual leveling effect on the data. For example, if a series of patients with UGIB includes a large number with alcohol-associated erosive gastritis and Mallory-Weiss syndrome, the overall mortality and morbidity rates will be low, and it is doubtful that endoscopy would show any impact on the outcome. Conversely, in patients with liver failure and bleeding esophageal varices, the mortality rate is inordinately high even when the diagnosis is known with certainty, and it is difficult enough to evaluate the effect of different treatments. In this setting, it is also unlikely that early endoscopy will change the outcome. Another key variable is age; UGIB in patients older than 55 years is associated with a fourfold to fivefold increase in mortality.

In view of these limitations in previously published articles, a properly designed prospective study of UGIB with appropriate subgroup analysis and the requisite number of patients would be instructive. Obviously, endoscopy does have an important place in the management of patients with UGIB and should be considered especially in those patients in whom therapy and outcome will change as a function of the lesion(s) identified.—Ed.] ◄

Diagnostic Accuracy of Fiberendoscopy in Detection of Upper Intestinal Malignancy: Follow-up Analysis. The combination of endoscopy with directed biopsy can potentially determine whether or not a malignancy is present with great accuracy, and modern fiberendoscopy is safe and well tolerated. W. Dekker and G. N. Tytgat[3] (Univ. of Amsterdam) reviewed results of 1,096 upper fiberendoscopic studies made on 1,005 consecutive patients in 1971–73. Patients were referred with a radiologic abnormality in the upper gastrointestinal tract or with persistent digestive symptoms. A forward-viewing endoscope was utilized, with supplementary use of a lateral-viewing instrument where indicated. Multiply directed biopsy specimens were obtained when abnormality was observed. Ten or more specimens were obtained in cases of gastric ulcer.

In 9 patients with obvious malignancy the lesion could not be reached for anatomical-technical reasons. In 83.2% of the other patients either a benign lesion or no disease was diagnosed. Malignancy was diagnosed in 16.8% of patients. On follow-up of 990 patients, all endoscopy-biopsy diagnoses of malignancy proved to be correct. Two malignancies occurred in the "benign" group, both initially presenting as gastric ulcers. The overall rate of correct diagnosis was 99.8%. The rate of correct diagnosis of malignant lesions was 98.8%. Seven of the 135 gastric adenocarcinomas appeared to be early gastric cancers; 5 presented as benign-looking ulcers. Not infrequently, only 1 or 2 among about 10 biopsies appeared to be definitely abnormal in cases of malignancy. Endoscopic diagnosis was correct in 94.6% of all patients. An incorrect endoscopic diagnosis was made in 2.1% of all patients. Most errors were in patients with gastric ulcer. An overall incorrect endoscopic interpretation was made in 7.3% of ulcer cases, and in 8.2% no firm endoscopic conclusion could be reached.

Endoscopy supplemented by multiply directed biopsies is a reliable method for diagnosis of upper digestive tract malignancy. Multiple biopsies are necessary to obtain high accuracy. The endoscopic aspect of a lesion offers no certainty about its nature. Endoscopy should be considered merely as a convenient way of adequately sampling tissue.

► [Weinstein (Gastroenterology 73:1160, 1977) has written a provocative article on the role of gastroscopy in gastric ulcer. What follows has been abstracted from this article. Weinstein questions whether gastroscopy should be done at the outset in all patients who have a benign-appearing gastric ulcer on barium x-ray. The main argument for this is that some benign-appearing gastric ulcers on x-ray are really malignant—3.3% in the cooperative Veterans Administration study (ibid. 61:598, 1971). The main argument against it is that the vast majority of gastroscopies done in patients with benign-appearing gastric ulcers will simply confirm the x-ray findings. Furthermore, provided the patient is available for follow-up examination, the risk of overlooking a cancer is remote (0.6%) even if one relies solely on the criterion of "x-ray healing." I agree with Weinstein that it is a waste of patient and physician time to do early gastroscopy in *all* patients who have clinical findings and an x-ray compatible with a benign gastric ulcer.

A second important question is whether endoscopy should be used to insure that the benign ulcer defect has closed over. It is widely acknowledged that some benign gastric ulcers may take several months to heal. It is also recognized that an x-ray may show "complete healing" whereas gastroscopy may show a residual small ulceration. In the name of insuring "complete healing," patients are now having repeated endoscopies (and biopsies) while receiving treatment for benign gastric ulcer. For the time being, it should be considered perfectly acceptable to rely primarily on barium x-ray for the healing test, provided good quality x-ray is available, and assuming that the clinical course of the patient is uncomplicated.

---

(3) Gastroenterology 73 (Pt. 1):710–714, October, 1977.

A number of studies have attempted to define the optimal number of biopsies required in order to insure that gastric malignancy is correctly diagnosed. Opinion may vary, but in most centers the average number taken is probably five. Insufficient emphasis has been placed on the quality of the biopsy. After the first few biopsies, succeeding biopsies may contain significant amounts of clotted blood.

The value of gastroscopy in clinical diagnosis has recently been reviewed by Cameron and Ott (Mayo Clin. Proc. 52:806, 1977), who surveyed the results of more than 6,000 gastroscopic examinations during a 5-year period. Overall, gastroscopy resulted in an altered diagnosis in 18% of 1,368 examinations. When the radiologist suspected a gastric ulcer, something different was found on gastroscopy in 27% of such patients. Twenty percent had no ulcer and 5% had gastric malignancy. Gastroscopy also has its limitations: in 3% of this group, the visual gastroscopic diagnosis of benign gastric ulcer or cancer was proved wrong at surgery. This underscores the importance of taking multiple biopsies, as emphasized by Dekker and Tytgat.

The lowest incidence of significant gastroscopic findings, 7%, occurred in the group who had abdominal pain not typical for ulcer and no other indication for the procedure. By contrast, 21% of patients who had ulcer-like pain and negative x-ray films had significant findings on gastroscopy. Recurrent ulcers and one carcinoma were found in 9% of patients who had negative x-ray films after Billroth I or II gastrectomy and who had pain as the only indication for gastroscopy. Gastric ulcers found only at gastroscopy were usually small, about 5–10 mm wide, and they had shallow craters. –Ed.] ◄

Mucosal Changes in the Gastric Stump 20–25 Years after Partial Gastrectomy. In most countries with a low or moderate rate of gastric cancer, the rate of gastric carcinoma is higher in patients having partial gastrectomy for peptic ulcer than in matched controls. Stump carcinomas are difficult to diagnose at an early stage.

E. Schrumpf, A. Serck-Hanssen, J. Stadaas, S. Aune, J. Myren and M. Osnes[4] (Ullevål Hosp., Oslo) evaluated the benefit of routine endoscopy combined with multiple biopsies in 320 patients born after 1900 who underwent a Billroth type II partial gastrectomy at an average age of 39 years in 1950–54. The ratio of duodenal to gastric ulcers was 4:1. Complete gastroscopy was carried out in 108 patients. Multiple biopsies, usually 20, were taken from the distal part of the gastric stump within 2 cm of the anastomosis, at equal intervals about the stoma. Five patients were operated on after a histologic diagnosis of malignancy was made, by removal of the entire remnant in 4 and by resection in 1.

In 2 patients, the history suggested malignant disease. Endoscopy showed mucosal folding and reduced thickness in most cases and a small polypoid lesion near the anastomosis in 1 case. Infiltrating carcinoma was found histologically in 4 patients and severe dysplasia in 3 others. Only 1 patient had a near-normal mucosa (table). In patients with carcinoma or severe dysplasia, malignant or premalignant changes were found in 28 (12%) of 226 biopsy specimens. Malignant disease was misjudged by gross examination of the resected stomachs. Generally, changes were most marked in the posterior wall near the efferent loop and along the magenstrasse.

Patients who have had partial gastrectomy for benign lesions are at high risk of gastric-stump carcinoma. The findings indicate either that the rate of stump carcinomas has been underestimated or that their slow growth allows some patients to die with undiagnosed carcinoma.

(4) Lancet 2:467–469, Sept. 3, 1977.

Histologic Diagnosis	
Histology	No.
Normal	1
Gastritis (degree of atrophy not recorded)	12
Intestinal metaplasia	24
Slight dysplasia	52
Moderate dysplasia	12
Severe dysplasia (carcinoma-in-situ)	3
Infiltrating carcinoma:	
a. Advanced (i.e., with infiltration deeper than the submucosa)	1
b. Early (i.e., with infiltration limited to mucosa/submucosa)	3

It is important to obtain multiple specimens and to examine all specimens carefully. If surgery is to be done, the entire gastric remnant should be removed. Severe dysplasia is managed by total gastrectomy in patients with a life expectancy of 10–15 years since the specimens may not represent the most severe disease.

► [Stump carcinoma occurring later than 5 years after operation for benign ulcer disease is emerging as a distinct clinical entity. The findings of Schrumpf et al. have been confirmed by Domellof et al. (Gastroenterology 73:462, 1977), who reviewed data on 459 patients who underwent resection for benign ulcer disease from 1952 to 1956. Among 140 patients dead at follow-up, 3 patients with stump carcinoma were found. An endoscopic follow-up was performed in 214 of the other 319 patients; 6 carcinomas, among which 2 were early carcinomas, were diagnosed in this follow-up group. Thus, the total incidence of stump carcinoma in this study was 9/459 or 2.0%. All carcinomas were found in men. The macroscopic and microscopic changes were most severe in the stoma, which seems to be a preferential site for carcinoma. There was little evidence obtained to indicate that histologic findings such as chronic atrophic gastritis, intestinal metaplasia or cystic dilatation of the gastric glands can be regarded as earlier indicators of malignant transformation.

To achieve early detection of stump carcinoma, it seems reasonable to recommend repeat gastroscopy in combination with multiple biopsies at 10–15 years after surgery. As Domellof et al. emphasize, special attention should be given to patients with mucosal polyps.—Ed.] ◄

The Small Intestine

Gastric Emptying of Liquid Meals and Pancreatic and Biliary Secretion after Subtotal Gastrectomy or Truncal Vagotomy and Pyloroplasty in Man. Few studies have been devoted to the intraluminal digestive events occurring in symptomatic postgastrectomy patients. I. MacGregor, J. Parent and J. H. Meyer[5] (Univ. of California, San Francisco) determined pancreatic and biliary secretion and gastric emptying rates of a liquid test meal (LTM) in 6 normal men with a mean age of 49, 11 men having subtotal gastrectomy (STG) without vagotomy and 5 patients having vagotomy and pyloroplasty (V-P) at least a year previously for peptic ulcer disease. Five STG patients had had a Billroth I gastroduodenostomy (STG-BI) and 6 a Billroth II gastrojejunostomy (STG-BII). All surgical patients were thought to have had very good to excellent results; none had significant symptoms. A test meal of nonfat milk powder, glucose and corn oil was used. An infusion of secretin and cholecystokinin was given during part of the test.

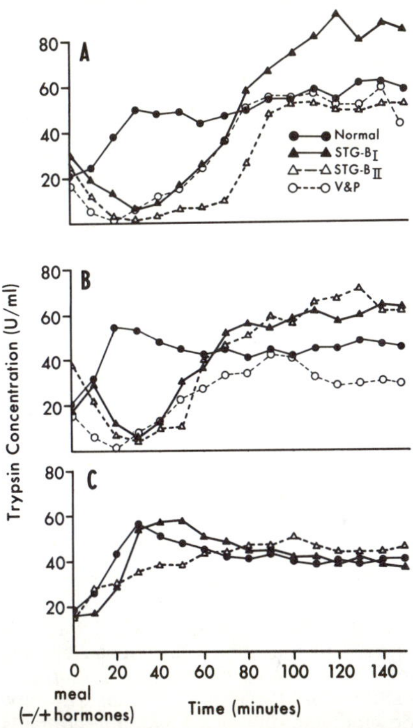

Fig 8.—Mean trypsin concentration at proximal jejunal sampling site: **A,** after liquid test meal *(LTM)* alone; **B,** after LTM plus hormone; **C,** after hormone alone. Meals were taken and intravenous hormone infusion started at zero time. Trypsin concentration was significantly lower than normal ($P < 0.05$): STG-BI, **A,** 30 minutes, **B,** 20 and 30 minutes; STG-BII, **A,** 20, 30, 60 and 70 minutes, **B,** 20, 30, 40 and 50 minutes; V-P, **A,** 20 and 30 minutes, **B,** 20 minutes. (Courtesy of MacGregor, I., et al.: Gastroenterology 72:195–205, February, 1977.)

(5) Gastroenterology 72:195–205, February, 1977.

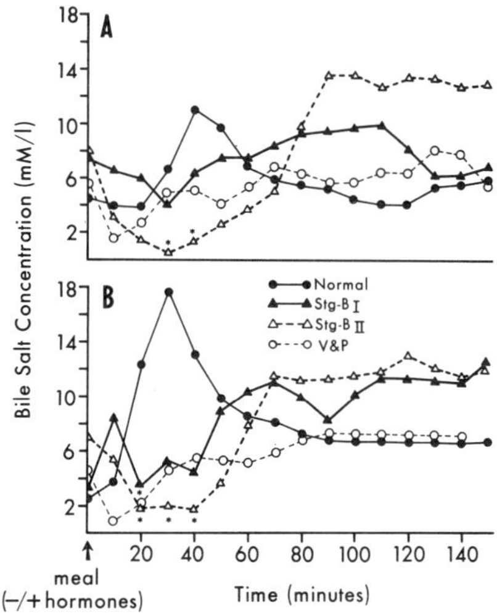

Fig 9.—Mean bile salt concentrations at proximal jejunal sampling site: **A,** after liquid test meal (LTM) alone and **B,** LTM plus hormones. Meals were taken and intravenous hormone infusion began at zero time. Bile salt concentration was significantly below normal ($P < 0.05$): **A,** STG-BII, 30 and 40 minutes; **B,** STG-BI, 20 minutes, STG-BII, 20, 30 and 40 minutes, V-P, 10, 20, 30 and 40 minutes. (Courtesy of MacGregor, I., et al.: Gastroenterology 72:195–205, February, 1977.)

Rapid gastric emptying diluted the intraluminal contents in all operated patients, with resultant subnormal concentrations of trypsin (Fig 8) and bile salts (Fig 9) initially. This pattern was not corrected by giving an intravenous infusion of the hormones secretin and cholecystokinin at the time the LTM was started (Figs 8 and 9). Trypsin output after the LTM was depressed to 40% of normal in V-P patients, but was normal in the STG-BI patients. Delay in reaching normal trypsin and bile salt concentrations was most marked in the STG-BII group due to sequestration of secretions in the afferent loop.

Low luminal levels of digestive secretions after a LTM are attributable to rapid gastric emptying in all surgical groups and to a depressed pancreatic enzyme response as well in V-P patients. In STG-BII patients, afferent-loop sequestration exaggerates the delay in attaining normal intraluminal concentrations and results in greater abnormalities than are seen in STG-BI patients.

In summary, the major problem after STG is not pancreatic and biliary secretory insufficiency, but rather abnormally rapid gastric emptying. This rapid emptying of LTM results in passage of the bulk of the test meal into the gut before the pancreas and biliary tract are able to secrete large amounts of bile and enzymes. By contrast, in normal subjects gastric contents are slowly delivered into the gut over a period of hours and the ratio of secretory rates to rates of passage of food normally remains high throughout the alimentary period.

► [It has generally been accepted that a form of "functional" pancreatic insufficiency is a major factor responsible for steatorrhea in patients with a subtotal gastrectomy and Billroth II type of anastomosis. Since the duodenum is bypassed there is decreased entry of stomach contents in the proximal duodenum and afferent loop. It was reasoned that this resulted in decreased stimulation of the duodenal mucosa by acid chyme and decreased release of secretin and cholecystokinin, in turn resulting in a *reduced output* of pancreatic enzymes. The studies of MacGregor et al. clearly show that this is not the case. Rather, rapid gastric emptying dilutes intraluminal contents with consequent abnormally low concentrations of trypsin and bile salts. In addition, in patients with vagotomy and pyloroplasty, however, there is a depressed pancreatic enzyme response. This latter abnormality was not demonstrated in patients with subtotal gastrectomy and either a Billroth I or Billroth II type of anastomosis. – Ed.] ◄

Use of Breath Hydrogen (H_2) to Quantitate Small Bowel Transit Time Following Partial Gastrectomy. Postprandial diarrhea is a common problem after partial gastric resection. It has been attributed to rapid transit through the small intestine, but this has not been documented. John H. Bond and Michael D. Levitt[6] (Univ. of Minnesota) used breath H_2 excretion as an indicator of small bowel transit time in evaluating 20 patients 9–38 months after partial gastrectomy with Billroth II anastomosis for peptic ulcer and 40 normal subjects. Eighteen patients had duodenal and 2 had gastric ulcer disease. All patients but 1 had had a vagotomy. Ten patients had persistent diarrhea for at least 6 months after surgery and 10 had normal, formed bowel movements. Patients ingested 10 gm lactulose in 100 ml water (280 mOsm/L) for the breath H_2 test. Glucose absorption was measured directly and by measuring H_2 excretion by the lungs after ingestion of a glucose test meal.

The mean transit time for patients with diarrhea was significantly shorter than for the other patients or for the normal subjects. All patients with diarrhea had a transit time below 50 minutes, whereas all but 1 of the other patients had longer transit times. Seven of the 40 normal subjects had transit times below 50 minutes. Transit time was not influenced by gastric emptying. Transit time is correlated with glucose absorption as shown in Figure 10.

It appears that rapid transit in gastrectomized patients is secondary to rapid gastric emptying, rather than to a primary intestinal abnormality. Presumably the shortened time of exposure of the luminal contents to small bowel mucosa results in malabsorption and hence diarrhea. Since transit time depends on the size of the small bowel bolus, it

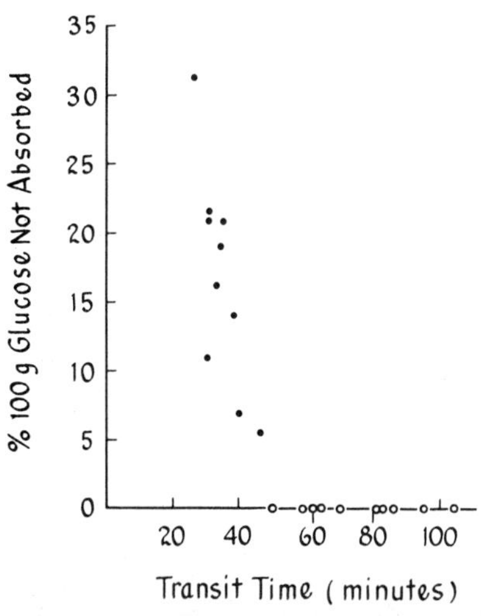

Fig 10. – Correlation of small bowel transit time with glucose absorption in postgastrectomy patients with *(solid circles)* and without *(open circles)* diarrhea. (Courtesy of Bond, J. H., and Levitt, M. D.: J. Lab. Clin. Med. 90:30–36, July, 1977.)

(6) J. Lab. Clin. Med. 90:30–36, July, 1977.

TABLE 1.—CLINICAL DIFFERENTIATION OF FOODBORNE DISEASE OUTBREAKS

Predominant type of symtomatology	Median incubation period (Hr)				Median duration (days)		Fever frequent	Other differentiating features
	<2	2–7	8–14	>14	<1	>1		
Upper gastrointestinal								
Staphylococcus aureus		×			×			Often causes explosive vomiting, prostration
*Bacillus cereus**		×			×			May simulate staphylococcal food poisoning
Heavy metals	×				×			Often causes metallic taste
Lower gastrointestinal								
Clostridium perfringens			×		×			Often causes severe abdominal cramps
*B. cereus**			×		×			May simulate *C. perfringens* food poisoning
Vibrio cholerae				×		×		May cause profuse, watery diarrhea, and dehydration
Enterotoxigenic *Escherichia coli*				×		×		May resemble mild and sometimes severe cholera
Shigella spp.				×		×	×	May cause blood or mucus in stool, tenesmus
Invasive *E. coli*				×		×	×	Resembles shigellosis;
Vibrio parahaemolyticus†				×		×	×	May resemble shigellosis
Both upper and lower gastrointestinal								
Salmonella spp.‡				×		×	±	Lower gastrointestinal symptoms are usually more prominent
V. parahaemolyticus†				×		×	±	May resemble Salmonella enterocolitis
Extragastrointestinal								
Scombrotoxin	×				×			Burning of mouth and throat, flushing, headache, urticaria, generalized pruritis
Shellfish toxin	×				×			Paresthesias—oral, perioral, extremities—floating sensation
Puffer fish toxin	×					×		Paresthesias—oral, perioral, extremities—floating sensation, loss of proprioception, numbness
Ciguatoxin		×			×			Paresthesias—oral, perioral, extremities—sensation of looseness and pain in teeth, paradoxical temperature sensation
Mushroom toxins§								
Rapid onset	×				×			Altered mental status, visual disturbances; sometimes associated with alcohol (disulfiram-like compounds)
Delayed onset			×			×		Often causes triphasic disease: gastrointestinal period, asymptomatic period, hepatic and/or renal failure period
Clostridium botulinum				×		×		Symmetrical descending motor paralysis
Group A Streptotoccus				×		×	×	Pharyngitis; upper respiratory infection
Trichinella spiralis				×		×	×	Gastrointestinal illness followed by orbital edema, eosinophilia, myalgias
Nongastrointestinal								
Brucella				×		×	×	Malaise, lymphadenopathy, anorexia, weight loss, arthralgias
Toxoplasma gondii				×		×		Malaise, lymphadenopathy
Hepatitis				×		×	×	Malaise, hepatomegally, jaundice, dark urine
Anisakidae				×				Results frequently in regurgitation of nematode
Monosodium glutamate	×				×			Burning sensations—chest, neck, abdomen, extremities—sensations of lightness and pressure over face, heavy feeling in chest

*One clinical syndrome resembles staphylococcal food poisoning and is characterized by abrupt onset of nausea, vomiting and abdominal cramps, and another resembles *Clostridium perfringens* food poisoning and is characterized by abdominal cramps and diarrhea.

†One clinical syndrome resembles *Salmonella* enterocolitis and is characterized by nausea, vomiting, abdominal cramps and prominent watery diarrhea, and another syndrome resembles shigellosis and is characterized by fever, abdominal pain and bloody, mucoid stools.

‡Information in this table refers to acute enterocolitis syndrome of *Salmonella.*

§Rapid-onset group includes mushrooms containing ibotenic acid and muscimol, muscarine, psilocybin and psilocin, miscellaneous gastrointestinal irritants or disulfiram-like compounds. Delayed-onset group includes mushrooms containing phallotoxin and amatoxin or gyromitrin.

might be postulated that treatment should consist of limiting the volume of liquid ingested with meals and using small feedings, which will have limited osmotic activity in the bowel. This treatment has been empirically used successfully for many years in managing patients with postgastrectomy diarrhea.

In conclusion, diarrhea in some postgastrectomy patients is, in part, the result of malabsorption of carbohydrate due to excessively rapid small bowel transit which is secondary to rapid gastric emptying.

► [Bond and Levitt previously reported the use of breath hydrogen measurements to quantitate small bowel transit time as well as carbohydrate absorption (J. Lab. Clin. Med. 85:546, 1975; and J. Clin. Invest. 51:1219, 1972). They have now applied this technique to study intestinal transit time, glucose absorption and development of diarrhea in patients with partial gastrectomy and Billroth II anastomosis. All postgastrectomy patients with diarrhea failed to absorb a portion of a 100-gm dose of glucose, but all patients without diarrhea and 10 healthy control subjects absorbed the entire dose. The major finding in this study is that the malabsorption of carbohydrate is due to excessively rapid small bowel transit which is secondary to rapid gastric emptying. These observations tie in extremely well with the findings in the preceding article indicating that rapid gastric emptying is responsible for dilution of pancreatic enzymes and bile salts, an important factor in the development of steatorrhea. – Ed.] ◄

Specific Diagnosis of Foodborne Disease. Marcus A. Horwitz[7] (Center for Disease Control, Atlanta, Ga.) observes that single cases of foodborne disease are generally more difficult to identify than are outbreaks. Three hundred or more outbreaks are reported to the Center for Disease Control annually and are believed to represent only a minute fraction of the total number that occur. An etiology is confirmed in about 45% of instances. It is important to determine the specific etiology of an outbreak to offer specific treatment where indicated, to institute appropriate precautions for contacts of patients and to control the outbreak and prevent recurrence. The clinician can play a critical role in the control of foodborne disease by recognizing and reporting outbreaks to health authorities.

The median incubation period (MIP) provides the first and often the most important clue to the etiology of an outbreak. Differences in MIP in different types of outbreak are shown in Table 1. The cause of an outbreak with an extremely short MIP is almost certainly chemical, whereas that of an outbreak with an MIP of 2–7 hours is probably

TABLE 2. – Criteria for Laboratory Confirmation of Bacterial Foodborne Disease

Bacteria	Isolation of organisms from epidemiologically incriminated food	Isolation of $\geq 10^5$ organisms/g from epidemiologically incriminated food	Isolation of organism from stool (or other source) of ill persons	Isolation of organism of same serotype from epidemiologically incriminated food and stool of ill persons	Isolation of organism of same serotype from stool of most ill persons and not controls	Positive serological test
Bacillus cereus		×	×			
Brucella spp.			× (blood)			×
*Clostridium botulinum**	×		×			
Clostridium perfringens		×		×	×	
Escherichia coli†		×		×	×	
Salmonella spp.	×		× ‡			
Shigella spp.	×		×			
Staphylccoccus aureus §		×				
Group A Streptococcus	×		× (throat)			
Vibrio cholerae	×		×			×
Vibrio parahaemolyticus	×		×¶			

*More important tests are detection of botulinal toxin in food, feces and serum.

†If possible, organisms should be tested for enterotoxigenicity and invasiveness by special laboratory techniques.

‡In *Salmonella* enteric fever syndrome, most frequently caused by *S. typhi*, *S. paratyphi A*, *S. paratyphi B* and *S. choleraesuis*, organism may also be cultured from blood, bone marrow and urine.

§Other tests: (1) demonstration that organism of same phage type is in stool or vomitus of ill persons and food, skin or both or nose of food handler; (2) demonstration of enterotoxin in epidemiologically incriminated food.

¶Organism should be Kanagawa positive.

(7) Gastroenterology 73:375–381, August, 1977.

staphylococcal food poisoning. Other clinical clues include the clinical syndrome, median duration of illness, vehicle of transmission, geographic location and time of year that the outbreak occurs. Certain foods are more likely to transmit some foodborne diseases than others, and some diseases are more likely to be transmitted by certain foods. Some foodborne diseases, such as botulism, have geographic predilections. Certain diseases have seasonal predilections. Criteria for laboratory confirmation of bacterial foodborne disease are given in Table 2. If not immediately available locally, most tests can be done at state health department laboratories.

► [This fine article should be read in its entirety as it contains a large amount of clinically useful information. For a comprehensive review of viral gastroenteritis, see the article by Schreiber et al. (Gastroenterology 73:174, 1977). — Ed.] ◄

***Yersinia* Enteritis and Enterocolitis: Gastroenterologic Aspects.** *Yersinia enterocolitica* is a gram-negative rod which causes zoonoses in several animal species and has been recognized with increasing frequency as a human pathogen in many countries in recent years. Gastroenteritis, terminal ileitis or mesenteric lymphadenitis occurs in most symptomatic *Yersinia* infections in man. G. Vantrappen, E. Ponette, K. Geboes and Ph. Bertrand[8] (Univ. of Leuven) reviewed the records of 37 patients seen in 4 years with *Y. enterocolitica* infections. The diagnosis was based on isolating the bacterium from stools in 36 cases and on changing antibody titers in 1. The 25 men and 12 women had a mean age of 35. Eight had to be hospitalized.

The symptoms are summarized in Table 1. Symptoms of colicky pain and diarrhea were usually present for 1 – 2 weeks before the diagnosis was established. Some 40% of patients had symptoms suggestive of appendicitis syndrome. All patients received tetracycline or chloramphenicol. Symptoms usually resolved within 2 – 4 weeks, but 1 patient relapsed and is symptomatic 20 months after initial treatment. All infections but one were due to organisms of serotype 0 : 3. The radiologic signs are given in Table 2. Ulceration mimicked a meniscus sign in one instance (Fig 11). The earliest mucosal abnormalities were thickened mucosal folds or nodular filling defects, or both. Biopsy specimens showed chronic nonspecific inflammation, mostly with mononuclear cells and lymphocytes. Plasma cells were rare and no giant cells or sarcoid-like granulomas were found. The ulcers healed both grossly and microscopically in 4 – 5 weeks under treatment.

Yersinosis is not a rare human disease in many countries. A differentiation from Crohn's disease is usually not difficult. Abscess, fistula formation, stenosis, skip lesions and signs of marked thickening of the intestinal wall are not observed in yersinosis. In doubtful cases, presence of *Y. enterocolitica* antibodies in the serum is important. Systematic endoscopy will probably reveal a much greater incidence of gastric and colonic involvement in *Y. enterocolitica* infections than is presently apparent.

► [Reports such as this one are a useful reminder that infection with *Yersinia entero-*

(8) Gastroenterology 72:220 – 227, February, 1977.

TABLE 1.—CLINICAL SYMPTOMS IN 37 PATIENTS WITH *Y. enterocolitica* INFECTIONS

Symptoms	Incidence %
Abdominal pain	84
Diarrhea	78
Fever	43
Anorexia	22
Weight loss	16
Nausea	13
Vomiting	8
Headache	8
Fatigue	8
Arthritis	2.6
Pharyngitis	2.6
Erythema nodosum	2.6

TABLE 2.—RADIOLOGIC SIGNS OF TERMINAL ILEITIS CAUSED BY *Y. enterocolitica* (24 CASES)

Radiological signs	Incidence %
Abnormalities of mucosal pattern	
Coarse folds	67
Nodules	45
Granules	45
Distorted pattern	33
Transverse pattern	20
Ulcerations	
Oval	12
Longitudinal	29
Aphthoid	4
Meniscus sign	4
Other abnormalities	
Dilation of terminal ileum	50
Hypercontractility of terminal ileum	25
Extrinsic compression	17
Thickening of wall	12

colitica may be responsible for terminal ileitis and mesenteric lymphadenitis. It is puzzling, however, why there are no such reports originating in the United States. We are looking for *Yersinia* infection, albeit not with the vigor of Vantrappen et al., yet keep coming up empty-handed. Perhaps what is needed is a systematic study of patients with acute ileitis and mesenteric lymphadenitis with appropriate cultures and serologic studies being done on all patients. In this manner, we might gain a better appreciation of the magnitude of this problem in the United States. Occult *Yersinia* infection could account for an appreciable number of the patients with mesenteric lymphadenitis and acute terminal ileitis. Older reports suggest that approximately one fourth of teenagers found to have acute ileitis on surgical exploration for presumed appendicitis have no further difficulty with inflammatory bowel disease. It is tempting to speculate

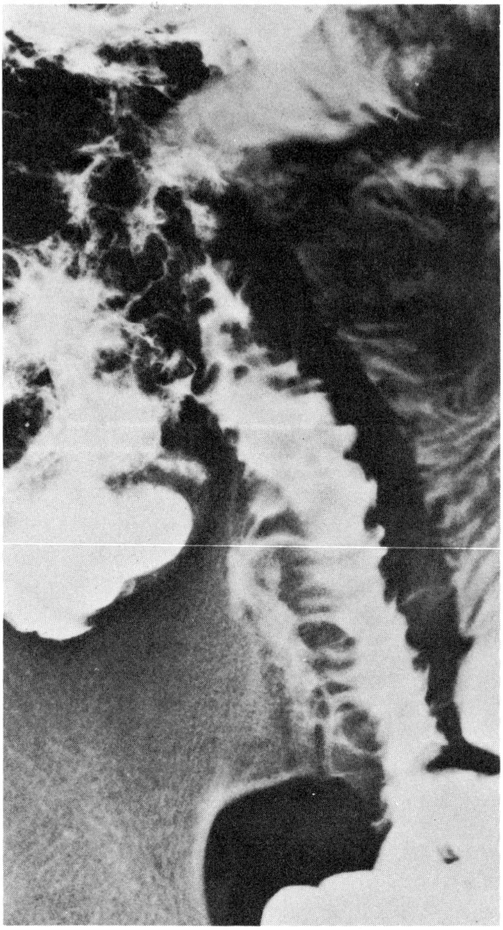

Fig 11.—Large ulceration of terminal ileum mimicking meniscus sign in patient with *Y. enterocolitica* infection. (Courtesy of Vantrappen, G., et al.: Gastroenterology 72:220–227, February, 1977.)

that some of these patients had an infection with *Yersinia enterocolitica* and thus a transient disease.—Ed.] ◄

Idiopathic Bile Acid Catharsis. Ileal mechanism is critical for intestinal bile acid reabsorption, although a minor fraction of the molecules normally escapes into the colon. If ileal absorption fails, high concentrations of bile acids may flood the colon to induce net secretion of fluid and watery diarrhea. Until recently, bile acid catharsis or choleretic enteropathy has been described only as a sequel to ileal surgery or inflammatory disease but a similar syndrome may result from a functional ileal disorder. E. Hess Thaysen and L. Pedersen[9] (Aalborg, Denmark) add 10 cases to the 5 initially reported of possible idiopathic bile acid malabsorption. Three patients with chronic persistent monosymptomatic diarrhea and confirmed bile acid malabsorption were

(9) Gut 17:965–970, December, 1976.

TABLE 1.—^{14}C-CHOLYLGLYCINE TESTS AND SCHILLING TESTS IN PATIENTS STUDIED

Patient	*Cholestyramine ingestion (months follow up)*	*Breath maximal concentration of $^{14}CO_2$ (% $^{14}CO_2$/mmol CO_2)*	*Faeces 24hr ^{14}C excretion (% dose)*	*Schilling test (%)*
LM		0·21	19	15
	31*	0·82	12	
EH		0·30	18	22
	12	0·14	18	
IC		0·86	8	16
	6	0·76	13	
Reference values		<0·1	<8	⩾10

*The reexaminations were performed during cholestyramine withdrawal.

studied in detail. Bile acid sequestration relieved the diarrhea in these cases and diarrhea recurred after the treatment was discontinued.

Woman (LM), 57, had had nearly continuous, usually watery diarrhea for some 35 years, as well as frequent headaches diagnosed as migraine. The symptoms were refractory to anticholinergics, constipating drugs, sedatives and various dietary regimens. All medication was withdrawn on admission and the diarrhea continued. Bile acid studies showed excess detergent loss (Table 1). Cholestyramine ingestion led to cessation of diarrhea and the patient's bowel habits were normal for 2 years on treatment with 4 gm cholestyramine 3 times daily. Diarrhea reappeared whenever the dose was reduced. After the patient went 1 week without medication, a ^{14}C-cholylglycine test indicated bile acid malabsorption as before.

These patients appeared to have selective bile acid malabsorption in the absence of conventional ileopathy. The bile acid half-life was reduced and the synthetic rate enhanced (Table 2). Chronic inflammatory disease of the ileum is quite unlikely because of the maintenance of near perfect health for many years, normal small intestinal x-rays and normal vitamin B_{12} absorption. Bile acid sequestration is helpful in these cases. Twelve more cases have been diagnosed in the past 3 years, in a unit serving a population of about 200,000. Cholestyramine should be given only to those patients in whom bile acid malabsorption is confirmed.

► [These studies indicate that a selective defect in bile acid reabsorption can be responsible for irritable bowel symptoms. This diagnosis should be considered in patients with a long history of watery diarrhea refractory to conventional therapy without other systemic symptoms or signs such as anorexia, fever, weight loss and anemia. The presence of watery diarrhea and increased stool weight (≥300 gm/24 hours) should raise the question of a secretory diarrhea. Bile acid malabsorption can be confirmed by an abnormal breath test with the use of a ^{14}C-labeled bile salt and measurement of $^{14}CO_2$ and ^{14}C excretion in the feces.

Because cholestyramine binds bile salts, it is not surprising that it is effective in

TABLE 2.—KINETICS OF CHENODEOXYCHOLIC ACID (CDC) IN THREE PATIENTS STUDIED

Patient	*CDC half life (days)*	*CDC synthesis rate (mmol/24 h)*
LM	0·8	1·7
EH	1·1	1·6
IC	0·8	6·8
Controls (n = 10)		
Mean ± SD	3·0 ± 0·8	0·4 ± 0·2

ameliorating the diarrhea associated with bile salt malabsorption. The studies of Thaysen and Pedersen confirm earlier observations of Schapiro et al. (Gastroenterology 58: 973, 1970) that cholestyramine is effective in certain patients with refractory irritable bowel syndrome, quite possibly patients with selective bile salt malabsorption. Recent studies (ibid. 73:550, 1977) suggest that aluminum hydroxide binds dihydroxy bile salts, and antacids containing aluminum hydroxide warrant exploration in therapeutic solutions in which bile acid binding is sought.

Finally, two recent controlled trials (Gut 18:531, 1977; and Br. Med. J. 1:674, 1977) demonstrated that cholestyramine produced a significant improvement in frequency, urgency, consistency of stool and episodes of diarrhea in patients with postvagotomy diarrhea. Fecal bile acid excretion was significantly higher in the postvagotomy group when compared with normal controls. These findings confirm the effectiveness of cholestyramine and support the concept of a bile-acid-mediated etiology in postvagotomy diarrhea. – Ed.] ◄

Comparative Susceptibility of Latin American and United States Students to Enteric Pathogens. Herbert L. DuPont, Jorge Olarte, Dolores G. Evans, Larry K. Pickering, Emma Galindo and Doyle J. Evans[1] undertook a study at a Mexican university for students from various countries to verify the importance of toxigenic *Escherichia coli* and other etiologic agents in travelers' diarrhea. Diarrhea was defined as bowel movements at twice the usual daily rate, associated with symptoms of enteric infection. Ninety-five students with diarrhea provided stool samples within 24 hours of the onset of illness and 94 asymptomatic students were also examined. The groups were matched for country of origin and length of time in Mexico. The ill group included 37 newly arrived summer students from the United States, 40 full-time United States students who had been present for over 1 year, 12 Mexican students and 6 Venezuelans.

The findings are given in the table. Significantly more students with diarrhea had pathogens isolated from their stools. The highest rate of recovery was 60% in the new United States students. Two or more pathogens were isolated in the first 24 hours of illness from 12% of the students with diarrhea. Toxigenic *E. coli* and *Shigella* strains were recovered from all student groups. Toxin-positive *E. coli* were more frequent in both symptomatic and asymptomatic United States students than in Latin Americans. No *Shigella* strains or toxin-positive *E. coli* were isolated from asymptomatic Latin students. Heat-stable toxin-

RECOVERY OF ENTERIC PATHOGENS FROM STUDENTS WITH AND WITHOUT DIARRHEA

STUDENT STATUS	NO. OF PATIENTS		≥1 PATHOGENS ISOLATED		MULTIPLE PATHOGENS	
	ILL	NON-ILL	ILL	NON-ILL	ILL	NON-ILL
US:						
Summer	37	30	22 (60)*	6 (20)	4 (11)	0
Full-time	40	37	23 (58)	10 (27)	5 (13)	1 (3)
Mexican	12	16	5 (42)	0	1 (8)	0
Venezuelan	6	11	4 (67)	1 (9)	1 (17)	0
Totals	95	94	54 (57)	17 (18)	11 (12)	1 (1)

*Figures in parentheses are percentages.

(1) N. Engl. J. Med. 295:1520–1521, Dec. 30, 1976.

only strains of *E. coli* were recovered from 6 United States students with diarrhea and from 2 United States controls. The intensity of diarrhea correlated with the recovery of an enteric pathogen.

It is likely that local intestinal immune mechanisms are important in immunity to enteric infection. Immunity in toxigenic *E. coli* infection appears to occur after repeated or chronic exposure. The immunity may be organism directed. Toxigenic *E. coli* and shigellae are of widespread occurrence in Latin America. *Giardia lamblia* has been commonly found in symptomatic and asymptomatic Latin students, suggesting that repeated exposure to *Giardia* may not lead to protective immunity.

► [Infection with toxigenic *E. coli* is an important problem for newly arrived United States students traveling to Mexico. However, it is less commonly associated with diarrhea among United States students who have remained in Mexico for a year or longer. Toxigenic *E. coli* is not an important cause of diarrhea among Latin American students. Similarly, while toxigenic *E. coli* strains are commonly found in stools of asymptomatic United States students, they are rarely isolated from Latin American students without disease. Thus, this study provides evidence that immunity in toxigenic *E. coli* infections occurs after repeated or chronic exposure.

In a companion article (Gastroenterology 73:715, 1977), Dupont and his associates evaluated the effect of bismuth subsalicylate or placebo in the treatment of 169 students attending a Mexican university who developed diarrhea. It was found that a 3½-hour course of therapy with either a 4.2-gm (30 ml every ½ hour for 8 doses) or an 8.2-gm (60 ml every ½ hour for 8 doses) regimen effectively decreases the number of unformed stools passed as well as the subjective complaints of diarrhea, nausea and abdominal cramping. This favorable effect was delayed in onset and appeared to occur generally after the 3½-hour treatment period. The number of unformed stools was decreased throughout the 48-hour surveillance period even though the drug was administered for only 3½ hours. – Ed.] ◄

Gastrointestinal Myoelectric Activity in Idiopathic Intestinal Pseudo-obstruction. Intestinal pseudo-obstruction is a clinical syndrome characterized by signs of intestinal obstruction without demonstrable organic occlusion of the bowel lumen. An esophageal motor abnormality is usually present, besides varying degrees of bowel distention. Pathogenesis is unknown. Mark A. Sullivan, William J. Snape, Jr., Stephen A. Matarazzo, Robert J. Petrokubi, Graham Jeffries and Sidney Cohen[2] examined the motor function of the intestinal tract basally and after neurohumoral stimulation in 4 patients aged 28–64 years with signs of long-standing obstruction. Obstructive lesions were excluded in all patients. All had had multiple laparotomies. Esophageal and duodenal motility studies were carried out, and sigmoidoscopy and anal manometry were also performed to evaluate myoelectric and motor function.

All patients had abnormal esophageal function (table). An increase in duodenal slow waves with associated spike potentials was observed in patients, compared with normal subjects (Fig 12). Motility increased less after secretin administration in the patients. Colonic dilatation was observed to respond to neostigmine injection. Colonic slow waves were similar in patients and normal subjects and responses to neostigmine were comparable. One patient exhibited elevated internal anal sphincter pressure, which failed to resolve after rectal distention.

---

(2) N. Engl. J. Med. 297:233–238, Aug. 4, 1977.

	Esophageal Motility				
Case No.	LES* Pressure (Mm Hg)	LES* Relaxation (% Relaxation)	Peristalsis		Simultaneous Contractions
			Primary	Secondary†	
1	11	25	No	No	Yes
2	39	40	No	No	Yes
3	17	65	No	No	Yes
4	11	80	No	No	Yes
Normal	15–30	96	Yes	Yes	No

*Lower esophageal sphincter.
†Induced by balloon distention with 15–30 ml air in upper esophagus.

The findings suggest that chronic idiopathic intestinal pseudo-obstruction is a generalized disorder of gastrointestinal motor function. A disorder of the control mechanisms initiating gastrointestinal motor function may be present, rather than a primary disorder of enteric smooth muscle. Many aspects of myogenic activity appear to be normal in this condition, but potential neurally mediated responses such as esophageal peristalsis and small bowel contraction after distention are abnormal. The contrast between intact myogenic and abnormal neuro-

Fig 12. – Duodenal spike and motor activity in basal state, after water distention (75 ml) or after secretin administration in normal subjects *(open bars)* and in patients with chronic idiopathic pseudo-obstruction *(hatched bars)*. Each bar and line represents mean ±SE. (Courtesy of Sullivan, M. A., et al.: N. Engl. J. Med. 297:233–238, Aug. 4, 1977.)

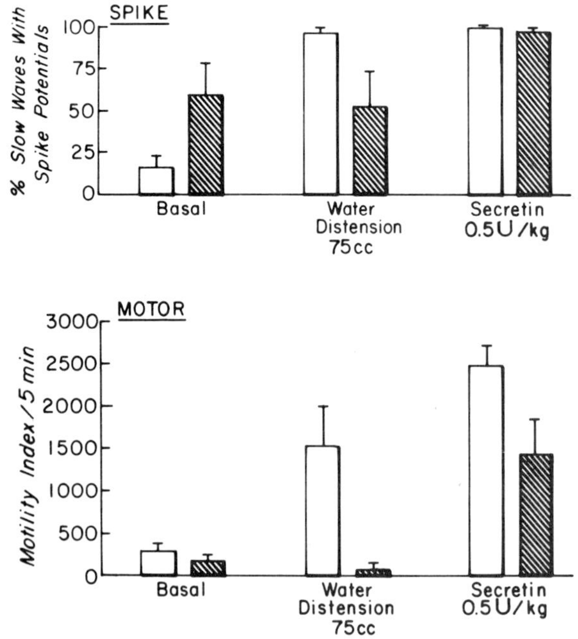

genic properties of the gut strongly supports the hypothesis of a primary disorder in neural function.

► [Intestinal pseudo-obstruction mimics intestinal obstruction. At exploratory laparotomy the bowel is greatly distended but no point of obstruction is found. Pseudo-obstruction has been associated with scleroderma (Am. J. Med. 45:301, 1968), myxedema (Arch. Intern. Med. 115:145, 1965) and amyloidosis (Gut 11:764, 1970). If the condition is chronic and no underlying disease is found, the term "idiopathic intestinal pseudo-obstruction" (IIP) is applied. The condition is frequently misdiagnosed. Recurrent attacks of abdominal pain, distention and vomiting may result in repeated laparotomies for suspected obstruction.

Schuffler et al. (Am. J. Roentgenol. 127:729, 1976) studied 6 patients with IIP who underwent extensive radiographic evaluation of the gastrointestinal tract. Propulsive activity was consistently absent. All had smooth muscle dysfunction of the esophagus, small bowel and colon, and 2 had abnormal gastric emptying. Two forms of the syndrome were observed, characterized by either hyperactive or hypoactive smooth muscle. In the hyperactive form, chaotic, spontaneous contractions of the esophagus and small intestine occurred and extensive diverticular disease of the colon was present. In the hypoactive form the esophagus was atonic, and there was marked widening and hypomotility of the small intestine and colon. These findings suggest that the IIP syndrome has a heterogenous basis.

Further support for this concept comes from additional studies also done by Schuffler et al. (Gastroenterology 73:327, 1977). In contrast to earlier reports (Am. J. Med. 49: 203, 1970) in which no significant gut histopathologic alterations were noted, Schuffler et al. demonstrated, by light and electron microscopic studies of excised small intestine, a marked thinning and degeneration of smooth muscle with replacement by fibrous tissue. The myenteric plexus was normal. This particular case suggests that a degenerative disease of smooth muscle may be *one cause* of IIP. It is of interest that of 12 relatives of the patient with this index case of IIP studied by esophageal manometry, 4 had esophageal motor dysfunction and mild dysphagia (Gastroenterology 73:339, 1977). In addition, 2 of these 4 patients had either a flaccid bladder or bilateral ureteral reflux. These provocative findings suggest that IIP in this family is secondary to a generalized disease of smooth muscle which is transmitted as a dominant trait.

To summarize, IIP should be considered in any patient with persistent obstructive symptoms. If x-rays of the esophagus, stomach, small bowel and colon show that motor abnormalities are diffuse and no underlying disease is present, a diagnosis of IIP is likely.—Ed.] ◄

The Colon

Cancer in Colitis: Assessment of Individual Risk by Clinical and Histologic Criteria. J. E. Lennard-Jones, B. C. Morson, Jean K. Ritchie, D. C. Shove and C. B. Williams[3] (St. Mark's Hosp., London) correlated the cancer risk in 229 patients seen during 1966–76 with extensive ulcerative colitis with length of history and histologic findings in rectal and colonic biopsies. All patients had disease extending proximally from the rectum to include the hepatic flexure on a double-contrast barium enema study.

Incidence of cancer was calculated according to duration of colitis. A total of 1,570 biopsies were reviewed and classified according to changes as severe dysplasia (32), moderate or mild dysplasia (73) or no dysplasia. Abnormalities of tubular architecture are illustrated in Figure 13.

Five patients are known to have developed carcinoma. No patient developed cancer within 10 years of onset of colitis, but the risk increased with time, being about 1 in 200 patient-years in the 2d decade and 1 in 60 patient-years in the 3d decade (table). No carcinoma has developed in patients without biopsy evidence of dysplasia. Of 20 patients with moderate dysplasia, 1 developed a carcinoma. Among 13

Fig 13.—Diagrammatic illustration of abnormalities of tubular architecture. *A*, normal; *B*, villous change; *C*, tubular budding. Mild (+) and severe (+++) changes are shown. (Courtesy of Lennard-Jones, J. E., et al.: Gastroenterology 73:1280–1289, December, 1977.)

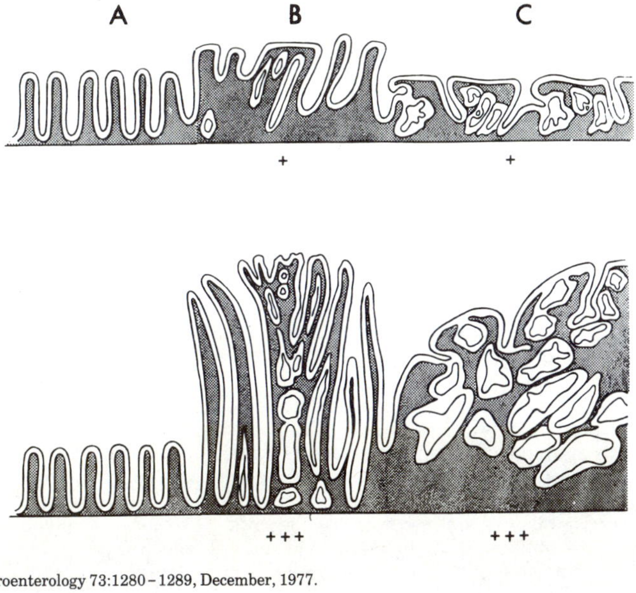

(3) Gastroenterology 73:1280–1289, December, 1977.

RISK OF CANCER CORRELATED WITH LENGTH OF HISTORY IN ENTIRE SERIES COMPARED WITH EXPECTED INCIDENCE IN A MATCHED GROUP OF THE GENERAL POPULATION

Periods since onset of colitis	No. of patients	Patient-years of follow-up	No. of patients with cancer	Risk of cancer per patient-year	Expected no. of patients with cancer	Excess risk
yr						
<10	159	578	0		0.1029	
10–20	105	392	2	0.0051	0.0874	×23
≥20	43	181	3	0.0166	0.0949	×32

patients with severe dysplasia, carcinoma was found in 4 of 7 operative specimens after severe dysplasia was found in sequential biopsies. No clear evolution of dysplastic change with time was observed in this series.

There is evidence that colitis starting in childhood is more likely to be complicated by carcinoma than is colitis developing in adult life. Sigmoidoscopy appears to be an adequate procedure in the first 10 years after onset of colitis. Thereafter, regular sigmoidoscopy should be supplemented by colonoscopy with multiple biopsies every 2 years, or more often if dysplasia is suspected. Histologic findings should be considered an indication for colectomy only if dysplasia is severe, consistent in more than one biopsy obtained at different sites or sequentially and preferably present in the absence of marked inflammation. Once consistent and severe dysplasia is recognized, carcinoma is often present, and the likelihood of surgical cure of early tumors is high. Endoscopists may be able to develop techniques for recognizing areas of dysplastic or early neoplastic change so that directed biopsies or cytologic preparations can be obtained.

► [Dobbins (Gastroenterology 73:1431, 1977) has critically analyzed the current status of the precancer lesion in idiopathic ulcerative colitis (IUC). His summary is based on a review of eleven reports; nine are retrospective analyses of biopsies and colectomy specimens and two are prospective analyses of multiple biopsies obtained during colonoscopy. Of 453 total colectomies in patients with IUC, colonic carcinoma was found in 108 specimens whereas 345 specimens were free from carcinoma. Precancer was present in 95 (88%) of the colectomies in which cancer was present and absent in 13 (12%). Thus, most patients with IUC and cancer of the colon have the precancer lesion. In 345 patients uncomplicated by colonic carcinoma, 46 (13%) had the precancer lesion.

The data on incidence of precancer in rectal biopsy specimens from patients with ulcerative colitis are similar. Overall, approximately 5.7% of patients with IUC had precancer. However, the incidence is much lower (2.4%) if disease duration is less than 10 years and much higher (15%) if it is greater than 10 years. The finding of precancer in a rectal biopsy specimen is not a reliable guide to the presence of colonic carcinoma. Conversely, negative rectal biopsies are not of value in excluding the presence of carcinoma since precancer is irregular in distribution and often spares the rectum.

The finding of precancer alone should not be taken as an indication for colectomy. Other features such as (1) onset of disease before age 15; (2) duration of disease greater than 10 years; (3) involvement of the entire colon, i.e., "universal colitis"; and (4) continuous active disease are important risk factors. However, in equivocal situations, the finding of precancer may tip the balance in favor of colectomy.

Finally, no discussion of colon cancer would be complete without citing recent data that indicate a change in site distribution of colorectal cancer. The proportion of colorectal cancer occurring above the rectosigmoid junction has been increasing over time. The 40,771 cases of colorectal carcinoma reported to the Connecticut Tumor Registry from 1940 through 1973 were analyzed to determine the incidence in the ascending, transverse, descending and sigmoid colon and the rectum (Am. J. Dig. Dis. 22:791, 1977). The number of cases, the proportion and the incidence rates of cancer in the ascending colon and sigmoid have increased over the 34 years. Only about half of colorectal cancer can now be identified with the rigid sigmoidoscope. Other tests must be used for early diagnosis of the increased numbers of cancers in the upper parts of the colon. – Ed.] ◄

Importance of the Colon in Enteric Hyperoxaluria. Patients with Crohn's disease have an increased prevalence of calcium oxalate urolithiasis, and many have increased absorption of dietary oxalate with resultant hyperoxaluria. It has been proposed that steatorrhea itself is the important factor in the increased oxalate absorption or, alternately, that unabsorbed fatty acids and bile salts increase the permeability of the colon to oxalate. John W. Dobbins and Henry J. Binder[4] (Yale Univ.) determined fecal fat and urinary oxalate excretion in 26 patients with gastrointestinal disease, 5 other patients and 10 normal subjects. The patient group included 10 without steatorrhea (group 1), 11 with steatorrhea and an intact colon (group 2) and 5 with steatorrhea and an ileostomy (group 3). All group 3 patients had Crohn's disease with ileal and colonic resections. Eight of the 10 group 1 patients had Crohn's disease with ileal involvement. Several pa-

URINARY OXALATE AND FECAL FAT EXCRETION IN PATIENTS WITH STEATORRHEA AND INTACT COLONS (GROUP 2) AND PATIENTS WITH STEATORRHEA AND ILEOSTOMIES (GROUP 3)

CASE NO.	DIAGNOSIS	FECAL FAT	URINARY OXALATE
		g/24 hr	*mg/24 hr*
Group 2:			
1	Chronic pancreatitis	14.5	127
2	Chronic pancreatitis	44.3	142
3	Chronic pancreatitis	22.3	65
4	Chronic pancreatitis	7.4	71
5	Crohn's disease	45.5	138
6	Crohn's disease	37.7	39
7	Crohn's disease	14.3	38
8	Crohn's disease	27.2	113
9	Jejunoileal bypass	15.0	74
10	Extrahepatic biliary obstruction	27.8	85
11	Pancreatic exocrine insufficiency	16.0	30
	Mean ±SEM	24.7±3.9	83.7±12.3
Group 3:			
12	Crohn's disease	11.8	45
13	Crohn's disease	23.1	40
14	Crohn's disease	14.3	33
15	Crohn's disease	41.9	42
16	Crohn's disease	35.0	18
	Mean ±SEM	25.2±5.8	35.6±4.8
Normal values:		<6	<45

(4) N. Engl. J. Med. 296:298–301, Feb. 10, 1977.

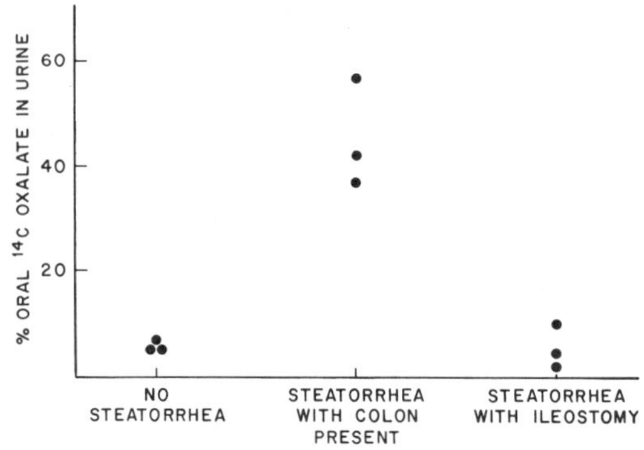

Fig 14. – ^{14}C-oxalate absorption studies (expressed as urinary excretion of percent of oral dose in 24 hours) in patients with and without steatorrhea and ileostomies. The 3 patients with steatorrhea and intact colons have an increased ^{14}C-oxalate excretion (48%) as contrasted with that in 3 patients with steatorrhea and an ileostomy. The ^{14}C-oxalate excretion parallels urinary oxalate excretion in these patients. (Courtesy of Dobbins, J. W., and Binder, H. J.: N. Engl. J. Med. 296:298–301, Feb. 10, 1977.)

tients were given a 300-mg oxalate, 800-mg calcium diet during the study. Urinary excretion of orally administered ^{14}C-oxalate was measured in some patients in each group.

Only one group 1 patient had hyperoxaluria. The findings in the other groups are given in the table, and the excretion of oral oxalate is shown in Figure 14. The 3 patients with increased oxalate excretion who were placed on a 3-gm fat diet had a decrease in oxalate excretion. No correlation between fecal fat and urinary oxalate excretion was noted in group 2 patients, but a direct correlation was found when the data for all group 1 and group 2 patients were analyzed.

Hyperoxaluria occurs in patients with steatorrhea of various causes. Steatorrhea, although important, is not the only determinant in the pathogenesis of hyperoxaluria. The colon appears to be necessary for enteric hyperoxaluria to develop in patients with steatorrhea. A possible explanation for hyperoxaluria is malabsorption of bile salts with a resultant increase in the permeability of the colon to oxalate. This could account for hyperoxaluria in patients both with and without steatorrhea.

► [Recent studies by Fairclough et al. (Gut 18:240, 1977) have clarified the mechanism for enteric hyperoxaluria. These investigators used a perfusion technique to study the effect of chenodeoxycholate on the absorption of oxalate from the surgically excluded colon in 2 patients with chronic liver disease. Colonic absorption of oxalate increased at least fivefold when sodium chenodeoxycholate was incorporated in the perfusion solutions. Thus, these studies show unequivocally that oxalate absorption from the excluded colon is increased by the presence in the lumen of an unconjugated bile salt. Normal feces contain only small amounts of bile salt bound to solid material but after ileal resection or bypass, the colon may be presented with high concentrations of bile salts.

The observations of Dobbins and Binder and Fairclough et al. also help explain the beneficial effects of cholestyramine in enteric hyperoxaluria. The bile acid-binding property of cholestyramine rather than the assumed direct binding of oxalate by cholestyramine may be responsible for the therapeutic effect of cholestyramine in enteric hyperoxaluria. Such bile salt binding might well result in decreased colonic absorption of oxalate.

In addition to ileal resection, hyperoxaluria has been well documented after jejunoileal bypass. Gregory et al. (J. Urol. 117:631, 1977) reported on 543 jejunoileal bypass patients screened for the presence of urinary calculi 1–6 years postoperatively. Of these patients, 9% had one or two calculi during the follow-up and 3% had multiple calculi. Ninety-four percent of the recovered calculi consisted entirely of calcium oxalate.—Ed.] ◄

Human Rectal Mucosa: Proctoscopic and Morphological Changes Caused by Laxatives. Opinions vary as to the effects, if any, of the use of enemas or suppositories on evaluation of the rectal mucosa. J. L. Meisel, D. Bergman, D. Graney, D. R. Saunders and C. E. Rubin[5] investigated the effects of Fleet's Phospho-Soda enema and of rectal bisacodyl on the proctoscopic appearances and histologic structure of the rectal mucosa in 10 subjects, aged 23–29 years, who were studied at weekly intervals. Isotonic saline by enema and oral mannitol-induced watery diarrhea served as alternative methods of treatment. The dose of rectal bisacodyl was 10 mg, used as a suppository or a solution of 100 or 200 ml. Ethanol was required to solubilize bisacodyl in saline and was incorporated in a control enema. Rectal biopsy specimens were taken from an area 5–10 cm proximal to the anus.

Mannitol and saline treatments did not alter the proctoscopic appearances (Table 1). Fleet's enema and rectal bisacodyl led to mucosal hyperemia and obliteration of the vascular pattern and, in some cases, mucosal friability. The rectum became normal within a week after each test. The light microscopic findings are given in Table 2 and shown in Figure 15. Fleet's enema disrupted the surface epithelium in 17 of 21 biopsy specimens, which were otherwise normal. Bisacodyl altered the superficial epithelium and also reduced goblet cell mucus. The scanning electron microscopic findings were consistent with the light microscopic results. With transmission electron microscopy, bisacodyl treatment caused a striking decrease in numbers of cytoplasmic organelles and in the density of the cytoplasm and nucleus. Mitochondria were abnormal in appearance, and profiles of endoplasmic reticulum were dilated.

These findings support the performance of sigmoidoscopy without preparation and also the use of saline enemas, if needed, to cleanse the rectum. It is possible that Fleet's enemas or bisacodyl suppositories

TABLE 1.—PROCTOSCOPIC FINDINGS AFTER LAXATIVES

Treatment	N[a]	Normal	Abnormal	
			Vascular pattern	Mucosal friability
No treatment	10	10	0	0
Mannitol orally	9	9	0	0
Saline 0.9% enema	10	10	0	0
Fleet's enema	10	0	10	1
Bisacodyl rectally	11	0	11	4

[a]N, number of observations.

(5) Gastroenterology 72:1274–1279, June, 1977.

TABLE 2.—LIGHT MICROSCOPIC FINDINGS AFTER LAXATIVES

Treatment	No. of biopsies	Normal	Abnormal: Epithelium, Surface	Abnormal: Epithelium, Crypt	Abnormal: Lamina propria inflammation
No treatment	35	35	0	0	0
Mannitol orally	17	17	0	0	0
Saline 0.9% enema	21	18	3	0	0
Fleet's enema	21	4	17	0	0
Bisacodyl rectally	25	2	21	16	3

might intensify the abnormalities found in patients with underlying mucosal disease.

► [In addition to causing proctoscopic and morphological changes, contact laxatives such as bisacodyl also alter fluid and electrolyte fluxes in the small bowel as well as the colon. Such effects may be more important than irritant effects in promoting laxation.—Ed.] ◄

► ↓ The following article provides some provocative information on the effect of bisacodyl on water and electrolyte fluxes in the bowel.—Ed. ◄

Fig 15.—Light microscopy of rectal mucosa. **A,** normal control at low power. **B,** normal control at high power. The surface epithelium is intact. **C** and **D,** effects of Fleet's Phospho-Soda enema. The surface epithelium is disrupted. Hematoxylin-eosin; **A** and **C,** reduced from ×100. **B** and **D,** reduced from ×400. (Courtesy of Meisel, J. L., et al.: Gastroenterology 72:1274–1279, June, 1977.)

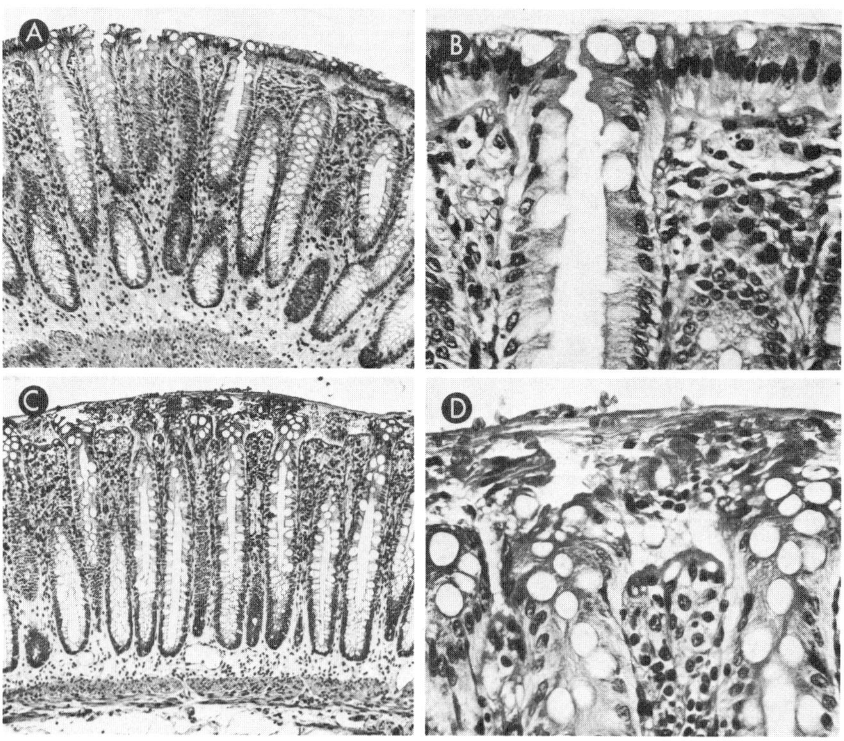

Effect of Bisacodyl on Structure and Function of Rodent and Human Intestine. Bisacodyl has been found to inhibit water and electrolyte absorption in rat bowel sacs but is not thought to alter water absorption in the human small bowel. D. R. Saunders, J. Sillery, D. Rachmilewitz, C. E. Rubin and G. N. Tytgat[6] assessed the relative potency of bisacodyl in three regions of rat intestine and attempted to determine by light and electron microscopy whether the agent alters the absorptive cells of rat intestine. The effect of bisacodyl on water absorption by human small bowel also was examined. Bisacodyl was infused with ^{14}C-polyethylene glycol into isolated intestinal segments of male Sprague-Dawley rats, with the use of the single-pass technique, and segments of rat jejunum and ileum that had been infused with 2 mg/100 ml bisacodyl were examined microscopically. Segments of human upper jejunum were studied by the triple-lumen tube technique and by the occluding balloon technique. The effect of 5 mg bisacodyl every 6 hours on ileostomy output was assessed in 5 patients. Two patients were studied for another 3 days immediately after the discontinuance of bisacodyl.

Bisacodyl inhibited water absorption in all regions of rat intestine, and alterations appeared in the surface cells of rat colon, including ballooning of cells and a decrease in density of the cytoplasmic and nuclear contents. In some areas of infused colon, the microvilli of surface cells were shortened, less numerous or absent, and the cells contained fewer organelles. Mitochondrial cristae were widened, and nuclear density was reduced. Bisacodyl induced net water secretion by human upper jejunum. The effects of bisacodyl on ileostomy output are shown in the table. Ileostomy output returned to baseline levels after bisacodyl was stopped.

The laxative action of bisacodyl is probably related to its ability to inhibit net water transport (Fig 16). The agent does not have to be absorbed, metabolized and excreted in bile before exerting a cathartic effect. Bisacodyl alters the surface epithelium of human rectum, and this may explain its laxative effect in the colon. Stimulation of cyclic

EFFECTS OF BISACODYL ON DAILY ILEOSTOMY OUTPUT*

Patient no.	Clinical diagnosis†	Control			Bisacodyl			Control		
		Wt	Na^+	K^+	Wt	Na^+	K^+	Wt	Na^+	K^+
		g	*mEq*		*g*	*mEq*		*g*	*mEq*	
1	CC	2075	196	31.0	2216	205	32.5			
2	CC	1420	199	12.2	1717	232	14.9	1422	180	14.5
3	CC	740	96	5.7	881	107	6.8			
4	UC	744	91	7.1	874	110	8.8			
5	UC	528	61	4.1	584	69	4.5	519	60	4.0

*Patients who had no clinical evidence of active mucosal disease were given bisacodyl (5 mg every 6 hours) or placebo while they continued their customary free-choice diets. Each value is the mean of three collections, each of 24 hours.

†CC, Crohn's colitis; UC, ulcerative colitis.

(6) Gastroenterology 72 (Pt. 1):849–856, May, 1977.

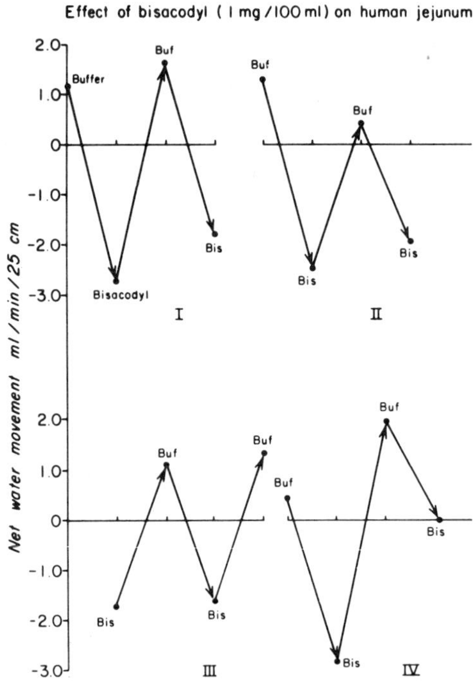

Fig 16.—The effect of bisacodyl, 1 mg/100 ml, on net water transport in human jejunum. The arrows indicate the sequence of the infusions. One of the 3 subjects was studied by the triple-lumen tube technique (**I**) and by the occluding balloon technique (**III**). (Courtesy of Saunders, D. R., et al.: Gastroenterology 72 (Pt. 1):849–856, May, 1977.)

adenosine monophosphate is not excluded; it may be operative along with an alteration of the absorptive surface.

Nature and Etiology of Vascular Ectasias of the Colon: Degenerative Lesions of Aging. Vascular lesions of the cecum and ascending colon are being increasingly recognized as a cause of lower intestinal hemorrhage in the elderly. They occur mostly in patients over age 60, are not associated with angiomatous lesions of the skin or other viscera, produce intestinal hemorrhage or anemia and can usually be diagnosed only by angiography. They are small and are rarely identified at surgery or by the pathologist using standard techniques. Scott J. Boley, Robert Sammartano, Anne Adams, Anthony DiBiase, Sylvain Kleinhaus and Seymour Sprayregen[7] (Albert Einstein College of Medicine) examined colons from patients with clinical and angiographic diagnoses of cecal vascular lesions by injection with a silicone rubber compound and clearing and histologically as well. Nineteen specimens from right colons were obtained from patients who had apparently bled from a colonic vascular lesion.

Mucosal vascular ectasias were found in all 12 specimens after injection. The mucosal lesions appeared to be secondary to dilated, tortuous submucosal veins, which were often present without mucosal ectasia.

(7) Gastroenterology 72 (Pt. 1):650–660, April, 1977.

The earliest and most marked distortion of the mucosal vessels involved the venules and veins that joined the capillary rings with large, dilated, tortuous veins in the submucosa. The lesions appeared to be ectasias of normal vascular structures, not malformations. In a second study, submucosal components of vascular ectasias were found in 53% of colons from 15 elderly patients with carcinoma of the colon but no history of gastrointestinal bleeding. A mucosal ectasia was also present in 27% of these specimens.

The ectasias appear to be due to chronic, partial, intermittent, low-grade obstruction of the submucosal veins, especially where they pierce the muscle layers of the colon. Obstruction occurs repeatedly over many years during muscular contraction and distention of the cecum and right colon; this ultimately results in dilation and tortuosity of the submucosal veins and later of the venules and capillaries of the mucosal units draining into it. Finally, as the capillary rings dilate, the competence of the precapillary sphincters is lost and a small arteriovenous communication is produced (Fig 17). This is responsible for the "early filling veins" noted on angiography. Prolonged increased flow through this communication can produce changes in the arteries supplying the area as well as in the extramural veins draining it. Life-

Fig 17.—Diagrammatic illustration of proposed concept of the development of cecal vascular ectasias. **A**, normal state of vein perforating muscular layers. **B**, with muscular contraction or increased intraluminal pressure the vein is partially obstructed. **C**, after repeated episodes over many years the submucosal vein becomes dilated and tortuous. **D**, later the veins and venules draining into the abnormal submucosal vein become similarly involved. **E**, ultimately the capillary ring becomes dilated, the precapillary sphincter becomes incompetent and a small arteriovenous communication is present through the ectasia. (Courtesy of Boley, S. J., et al.: Gastroenterology 72 (Pt. 1):650–660, April, 1977.)

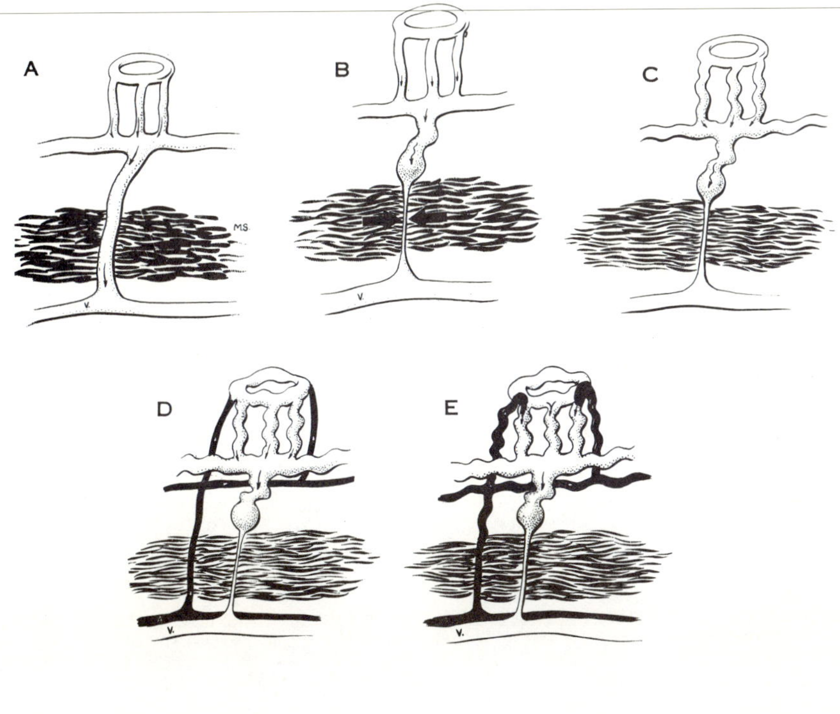

threatening recurrent bleeding can be avoided by prompt angiography and the performance of right hemicolectomy when an ectasia is identified.

► [These provocative studies suggest that vascular ectasia of the colon, also termed "hemangiomas" or "angiodysplasia" (1) develop as a degenerative process of aging, (2) are present with or without bleeding in a considerable portion of the population over 60 years of age, (3) are multiple more often than single lesions and (4) may represent a common cause of major lower intestinal bleeding in the elderly.

The barium enema examination will obviously be of no value when the vascular lesion is in the submucosa and does not produce a gross mucosal deformity, and this is the usual situation. The radiologic abnormality is best seen through early roentgenographic opacification during the venous phase of the angiographic study; demonstration of small lesions is possible but more difficult. Colonoscopy may demonstrate the lesions after arteriography has failed. Vascular ectasias often appear as bright red, flat lesions. Such lesions have been successfully treated by electrocoagulation (Gastroenterology 71:1079, 1976). Occasionally, vascular ectasias can be noted at laparotomy from the serosal surface (ibid. 73:195, 1977).—Ed.] ◄

The Liver

Does Gilbert's Disease Exist? A chance finding of elevated serum bilirubin often causes alarm, and Gilbert's disease, or constitutional hyperbilirubinemia, is often diagnosed. The nature of this disease is in dispute, and many workers believe that patients with the condition are abnormal. Alan Bailey, David Robinson and A. M. Dawson[8] (St. Bartholomew's Hosp., London) attempted to learn whether such subjects are a separate group from the normal population. Serums from 18,454 men and 5,471 women routinely screened were analyzed. Twelve men had a serum bilirubin of over 25 μM/L (1.5 mg/dl); 7 of these agreed to further investigation and underwent clinical examination and estimation of serum bilirubin before and after a 36-hour fast.

Both men and women had a frequency distribution of serum bilirubin with a skew to the right. The median value for men, 9.6 μM/L, was significantly higher than that for women (7.7 μM/L). The serum bilirubin exceeded 25 μM/L in 2% of men and 0.6% of women. The data for men showed that only one population was being studied. The mean serum glutamic-oxaloacetic transaminase was slightly higher in subjects with high bilirubin levels, but no difference in alkaline phosphatase levels was apparent. The mean age of subjects with elevated bilirubin was significantly lower (44 years) than that of the other subjects (46.7 years).

Total bilirubin remained outside the normal range of 0 – 20 μM/L in 6 of the 7 subjects who were restudied, and all levels increased after a 36-hour fast. The bilirubin was mainly unconjugated. Excessive hemolysis was excluded. One subject had an elevated γ-glutamyl transpeptidase and a palpable liver and probably drank to excess. All subjects were free of symptoms.

Cases now diagnosed as Gilbert's disease may constitute the upper end of the normal range for serum bilirubin levels rather than a disease state. The frequency of symptoms in patients with Gilbert's disease probably reflects the way they are diagnosed. The term "constitutional hyperbilirubinemia" is preferable to "Gilbert's disease." The patient can be assured that no symptoms will result and that unnecessary investigations will not be ordered during future unassociated illnesses. Treatment with phenobarbitone seems unwarranted.

► [This article has evoked considerable comment. Metreau et al. (Lancet 1:1319, 1977) object to the implication that all patients with unconjugated hyperbilirubinemia in the absence of overt bilirubin overproduction belong to a homogeneous group. These investigators cite their data and those of others that suggest that there are at least two types of "constitutional unconjugated hyperbilirubinemia" – one associated with a reduced bilirubin-uridine diphosphate glucuronosyltransferase activity and one related to a defect in hepatic uptake of bilirubin.

(8) Lancet 1:931 – 933, Apr. 30, 1977.

Powell et al. (ibid, p. 1256) state, "the concept of this condition being a variant of normal is not new but whether it represents an extreme expression of normality still remains conjectural. Whether these groups are abnormal or normal is semantic to some but practical to others. The importance of Gilbert's syndrome surely lies in the diseases with which it may be confused and not where the upper limit of normality exists. Indeed, few authors use the term 'disease' but retain 'Gilbert's syndrome' in preference to more cumbersome terms such as 'constitutional hyperbilirubinemia' which do not advance our understanding of the problem or help us further in explaining the nature of the problem to the patient." – Ed.] ◄

Liver during and after Fulminant Hepatitis. The histologic changes in the liver during and after recovery from fulminant hepatitis with coma have been examined in only a limited number of patients. John T. Horney and John T. Galambos[9] (Emory Univ.) studied 15 consecutive surviving patients who were in grade 3 or grade 4 coma from fulminant acute viral hepatitis. The 8 female and 7 male patients were aged 16 – 45 years. Six were drug addicts and 3 were sex partners of addicts. Eight patients were hepatitis B surface antigen (HB_sAg) positive during the fulminant illness. Chronic HB_s-antigenemia persisted in only 1 patient. Nine patients were in stage 4 coma. All patients were jaundiced or had a prothrombin time over 22 seconds during coma. Liver biopsies were made 5 – 14 days after the onset of coma

PATIENT CHARACTERISTICS AND BIOPSY RESULTS

Patient no.	Sex	Age	Stage of coma	Initial	Follow-up[a]	Interval	HB_sAg[b]	Drug abuse
		yr				*mo*		
1	F	17	3	Confluent zonal necrosis[c]	Normal (B)	12	Negative	None
2	F	18	4	Confluent zonal necrosis[c]	Normal (B)	20	Negative	Mate[d]
3	F	21	3	Confluent zonal necrosis[c]	Normal (B)	24	Positive	None
4	F	17	4	Confluent zonal necrosis[c]	Normal (B)	33	Positive	Mate[d]
5	F	25	4	Confluent mutilobular necrosis	Normal (B)	6	Positive	Mate[d]
6	F	29	4	Confluent multilobular necrosis	CAH, and cirrhosis (B)	10	Positive	Yes
7	M	38	3	Confluent mutilobular necrosis	CAH, mild portal granulomas (B)	60	Positive	Yes
8	M	45	3	Confluent zonal necrosis[c]	CAH, mild portal fibrosis (B)	10	Negative	No
9	M	16	4	Portal inflammation	Portal inflammation (A)	4	Negative	No
10	M	21	4	Confluent multilobular necrosis	Normal architecture; microabscesses (A)	4	Positive	Yes
11	M	28	3		Normal (B)	60	Negative	Yes
12	F	30	4	Confluent zonal necrosis[c]	None[e]	24	Negative	No
13	M	21	3	Confluent zonal necrosis[c]	Lost to follow-up		Positive	Yes
14	M	24	4	Confluent zonal necrosis[c]	Recent acute illness		Negative	No
15	F	22	4	Confluent zonal necrosis[c]	Recent acute illness		Positive	Yes

[a]B, biopsy; A, autopsy; CAH, chronic active hepatitis.
[b]During acute illness, hepatitis B surface antigen.
[c]Bridging portal tract with hepatic (central) venule or hepatic venules with each other; it is zonal because necrosis is in zone 3 of hepatic acinus.
[d]Sex partner used intravenous drugs, but patient did not.
[e]Clinical recovery is incomplete; patient refused follow-up biopsy.

(9) Gastroenterology 73 (Pt. 1):639 – 645, October, 1977.

in 14 patients, and follow-up biopsies were done 6 – 60 months after the fulminant illness. Two autopsies were done at 4 months.

The biopsy findings are given in the table. Hepatitis resolved in 7 of 9 patients who had follow-up biopsies. Six of 7 asymptomatic patients had normal biopsies on follow-up, but 1 had piecemeal necrosis, inflammation and fibrosis 10 months after acute illness. Two drug addicts who continued drug abuse had abnormal liver tests on follow-up. Chronic HB_s-antigenemia persisted in 1. Neither liver examined at autopsy showed evidence of chronic hepatitis or septum formation. In all, chronic hepatitis developed in 3 patients and cirrhosis in 1 of these.

If fulminant hepatitis is the result of vigorous cell-mediated immune attack on hepatocytes, the process cannot always eradicate chronic hepatitis B surface antigenemia, nor can it always prevent the development of chronic (active) hepatitis or cirrhosis. Confluent necrosis was not associated with vigorous cellular inflammation in fulminant hepatitis, but marked inflammation was present in confluent necrosis due to nonfulminant hepatitis, suggesting that it is a component of the inflammatory reaction that induces collagen synthesis, which in turn may lead to fibrosis.

► [Fulminant hepatic failure (FHF) is the most serious complication of viral hepatitis, the mortality of patients with stage IV coma being approximately 80 – 90%. Most survivors recover completely (Gastroenterology 67:870, 1974), apparently because of the capacity of the liver to regenerate. Numerous supportive measures have been used in an attempt to sustain life until spontaneous regeneration could occur. Treatment with corticosteroids, levodopa, exchange transfusion, plasmapheresis, total body washout and hemoperfusion through a pig liver or through suitable columns containing active charcoal, although of some short-term benefit, has not resulted in a convincing improvement in overall survival rate. A recent study (Ann. Intern. Med. 86:272, 1977) evaluated an intravenous hepatitis B immune globulin in the therapy of fulminant type B hepatitis; the study showed no benefit of treatment with exogenous antibody.

As Sherlock (N. Engl. J. Med. 295:1535, 1976) has emphasized, the "nitty-gritty" of the problem in FHF is to encourage the remaining viable liver cells to regenerate. Since earlier studies (Proc. Natl. Acad. Sci. U.S.A. 72:1157, 1975) in laboratory animals showed that hepatic regeneration can be enhanced by the synergistic action of the pancreatic hormones insulin and glucagon, Farivar and his associates (N. Engl. J. Med. 295:1547, 1976) examined the effectiveness of these two hormones in an animal model of FHF, namely, fulminant murine hepatitis. Considerable benefit, as indicated by survival, extent of hepatic necrosis and serum transaminase levels, was shown in the insulin-glucagon-treated group. These exciting preliminary findings suggest a promising approach to the problem of encouraging liver cell regeneration in patients with FHF. Obviously, it should be extended to controlled clinical trials in patients with FHF. – Ed.]

Immune Responses to Hepatitis B Surface Antigen and Liver-Specific Lipoprotein in Acute Type B Hepatitis. It has been postulated that T lymphocytes reacting with hepatitis B surface antigen (HB_sAg) on the surface of infected hepatocytes may destroy the cells and also initiate an autoimmune reaction responsible for continued liver damage in chronic active hepatitis. W. M. Lee, W. D. Reed, C. G. Osman, J. Vahrman, A. J. Zuckerman, A. L. W. F. Eddleston and Roger Williams[1] (London) tested this hypothesis in a serial prospective study of immune responses to HB_sAg in 21 patients with acute hepatitis type B, followed from presentation until antigen clearance was

(1) Gut 18:250 – 257, April, 1977.

complete. Leukocyte migration was examined with HB_sAg as antigen in 4 normal subjects over a 3-month period.

The patients had moderately severe hepatitis. Serum HB_sAg by complement fixation declined exponentially during the illness in all patients and was not detectable in any patient by immunoelectrophoresis after 6 weeks. Radioimmunoassay was also negative by 13 weeks. Anti-HB_s was sometimes detected when antigenemia was present, but only when antigen levels were low. Antibody was eventually detected in 12 of 13 patients followed for 20 weeks or longer. Migration inhibition was detectable at admission in 62% of patients, and in all patients as the serum HB_sAg level fell during recovery. Higher peak aspartate aminotransferase levels were associated with higher antigen titers, and there was some association between enzyme levels and the minimal migration index. Eight of 16 patients having the leukocyte migration test done with liver-specific lipoprotein as antigen had abnormal migration indices at admission; this sensitization was transient. Minimal migration indices with HB_sAg were lower in patients with sensitization to the lipoprotein.

These findings suggest that HB_sAg, or possibly antigen-antibody complexes, may interfere with the demonstration of cellular immunity in vitro. The severity of the illness appears related to both the number of infected hepatocytes and the intensity of the immune response to HB_sAg. The findings of migration inhibition with liver-specific lipoprotein as antigen and its disappearance within weeks are consistent with the suggestion that viral infection might temporarily stimulate a response to this membrane component.

Contagiousness of Acute Hepatitis B: Secondary Attack Rates in Household Contacts. Person-to-person contact has been postulated to be an important mode of spread of hepatitis B in the general population and episodes of household spread of acute hepatitis have been observed. Raymond S. Koff, Martha M. Slavin, Lorna J. D. Connelly and Deborah R. Rosen[2] (Boston) attempted to define the hazard resulting from household exposure to patients with acute hepatitis B in the absence of persistent hepatitis B surface antigen (HB_sAg). Of 90 patients admitted in 1972–75 with acute viral hepatitis, 42 men with acute hepatitis B comprised the index case group. Thirty-seven patients had HB_sAg transiently and 5 acquired antibody to HB_sAg within 6 months of the acute illness. Household contacts were tested for antigen, antibody and serum transaminases and followed for a period of 12 months.

The average age of study patients was 27.3 and of controls, 28.1. Parenteral use of illicit drugs and parenteral heroin use were more common in the study group. Of 98 household contacts of hepatitis patients, 14 had anti-HB_s and were considered immune; none of them had circulating HB_sAg detected. Three other contacts were HB_sAg positive and 2 were found to be persistent carriers of HB_sAg with elevated transaminase levels; 1 had acute hepatitis within 2 weeks and was considered as having a coprimary infection. Of 13 susceptible spouses

(2) Gastroenterology 72:297–300, February, 1977.

or sexual partners, 2 acquired acute HB_sAg-positive hepatitis during follow-up and 1 acquired anti-HB_s at 6 months. No evidence of hepatitis B infection was found in 68 parents, siblings and other contacts after follow-up for over 6 months.

These findings confirm the contagiousness of hepatitis B for household contacts of acute cases and suggest that the risk is confined to spouses and sexual partners. These persons appear to be prime candidates for prophylaxis with hepatitis B immune globulin. Further studies are needed to assess the risk of transmission of hepatitis B by patients who have become persistent carriers of HB_sAg. The potential value of hepatitis B immune globulin for household contacts of patients with acute hepatitis B who become persistent carriers remains to be determined.

► [Several recent studies have been concerned with the epidemiology of viral hepatitis. One study of particular interest (Ann. Intern. Med. 87:1, 1977) dealt with the etiology of sporadic HB_sAg-negative hepatitis. During the 9 months of the study there were 417 patients with a discharge diagnosis of viral hepatitis. Of these, 210 (50.4%) were HB_sAg positive and 207 (49.6%) were HB_sAg negative. Of the latter, 45 completed the study Two cases were due to hepatitis B, as demonstrated by the appearance of antibody to hepatitis B core antigen, and in 3 other patients the serologic pattern was inconclusive. Of 40 non-B hepatitis cases, 20 were type A hepatitis and 20 were non-A, non-B hepatitis. Clinically, type A and non-A, non-B hepatitis were indistinguishable. The type A cases were more frequent in young adults, with affected men predominating over affected women. On the other hand, non-A, non-B disease predominated in women aged 35 years or older. Epidemiologic backgrounds were generally similar, including illicit self-injection of drugs. However, transfusion-associated cases were limited to the non-A, non-B group. These studies indicate that hepatitis A virus and non-A, non-B viruses are both important in acute non-B disease. – Ed.] ◄

Multiple Hepatitis Viruses in Multiple Attacks of Acute Viral Hepatitis. Patients seen during two episodes of acute viral hepatitis usually have one bout identifiable as type B hepatitis, and occasional

SEROLOGIC EVALUATION OF THREE PATIENTS WITH THREE OR FOUR EPISODES OF VIRAL HEPATITIS

Patient	Status when Observed	Date (Mo/Yr)	Antibody to Hepatitis A*	HB_s Ag	Anti-HB_s†	Anti-HB_c‡	Antibody to Cytomegalovirus‡	Evaluation
A	1st bout	11/71	(−)	(−)	(−)	(−)	16	"Non-A, non-B"
	Follow-up	12/72	(−)	(−)	(−)	(−)	16	
	2d bout	3/72	(−)	+	(−)	±	16	Type B
	Follow-up	5/72	(−)	+	(−)	1+	32	
	3d bout	12/72	(−)	(−)	128	2+	128	"Non-A, non-B"
	Follow-up	1/73	(−)	(−)	256	2+	64	
B	1st bout	6/71	(−)	(−)	(−)	(−)	8	Type B
	Follow-up	7/71	(−)	(−)	(−)	+	8	
	2d bout	8/71	(−)	(−)	32	2+	4	"Non-A, non-B"
	Follow-up	10/71	(−)	(−)	32	2+	AC§	
	3d bout	4/72	(−)	(−)	64	2+	8	Type A
	4th bout	4/73	2-3+	(−)	16	2+	(−)	"Non-A, non-B"
	Follow-up	5/73	3+	(−)	32	2+	16	
C	1st bout	5/68	NT¶	NT	NT	NT	NT	Not studied
	2d bout	5/70	NT	+	NT	NT	NT	Type B
	Follow-up	10/70	(−)	(−)	16	2+	(−)	
	3d bout	11/71	(−)	(−)	32	2+	(−)	"Non-A, non-B"
	Follow-up	2/72	(−)	(−)	(−)	2+	(−)	
	4th bout	6/72	(−)	(−)	(−)	2+	(−)	"Non-A, non-B"
	Follow-up	7/72	(−)	(−)	(−)	1+	(−)	

*Quantity of antibody on a scale of 0 to 4+ as judged by immune electron microscopy.
†Reciprocal titer.
‡Quantity of antibody on a scale of 0 to 2+ as judged by radioimmunoassay blocking.
§Anticomplimentary.
¶Not tested.

patients with three or four separate episodes have been encountered. James W. Mosley, Allan G. Redeker, S. M. Feinstone and R. H. Purcell[3] evaluated the causes of 30 episodes of acute viral hepatitis in 13 patients having two or more attacks. The technique of immune electron microscopy was used in which hepatitis A antigen is agglutinated by an antibody appearing in convalescence. Serums were also tested for hepatitis B surface antigen (HB_sAg) by radioimmunoassay.

Two patients (7%) had one episode each caused by hepatitis A virus and 12 (40%) had one caused by hepatitis B virus, but no patient had more than one attack with the serologic features of type A or type B disease. Sixteen bouts (53%) were not attributable to either of the two recognized hepatitis viruses. None of these non-A, non-B episodes could be attributed to infectious mononucleosis or cytomegalovirus infection. The findings in 3 patients having three or four bouts of hepatitis are given in the table.

From this evidence, it appears that the clinical syndrome of viral hepatitis is produced not only by the two viruses (hepatitis A virus and hepatitis B virus) recognized since the 1940's, but also in all probability by a third non-A, non-B virus and a fourth agent, immunologically distinct from the third.

► [It is important to reemphasize that over half (53%) of the attacks of acute viral hepatitis in this group of patients with multiple bouts of disease could not be attributed to hepatitis A, hepatitis B, infectious mononucleosis or cytomegalovirus infection. Rather, these bouts were due to one or more hepatitis viruses collectively termed "non-A, non-B hepatitis virus(es)." That 3 patients had at least three or four separate episodes of viral hepatitis suggests that more than one agent is responsible for non-A, non-B hepatitis.—Ed.] ◄

Hepatitis and Pregnancy. Disparate results have been reported from studies of the effects of pregnancy on the course of viral hepatitis and of the effects of the disease on the outcome of gestation. Most data were obtained before serologic tests for type B hepatitis were generally available. J. Patrick Hieber, David Dalton, James Shorey and Burton Combes[4] (Univ. of Texas Southwestern Med. School) reviewed the outcomes of pregnancies complicated by acute viral hepatitis from 1970, when screening for hepatitis B surface antigen was begun at their institution, through 1974. Fifty pregnancies, or about 1 per 700, were complicated by acute hepatitis. Serum hepatitis B surface antigen (HB_sAg) was determined by counterimmunoelectrophoresis, reverse passive hemagglutination and radioimmunoassay, and antibody to HB_sAg was determined by radioimmunoassay.

The findings are summarized in the table, in which means are accompanied by standard deviations. Twenty cases (40%) were HB_sAg positive. The peak serum bilirubin and serum glutamic-oxaloacetic transaminase (SGOT) values tended to be higher in patients with type B hepatitis. One type B case was associated with a spontaneous abortion and 1 non-type B case with stillbirth. The groups were comparable in gestational age, birth weight and intrauterine growth and nutrition. All 18 children assessed in 1975 were physically normal and had no history of hepatic illness. Five of the 12 born to women who had had

(3) N. Engl. J. Med. 296:75–78, Jan. 13, 1977.
(4) J. Pediatr. 91:545–549, October, 1977.

ACUTE VIRAL HEPATITIS IN 50 PREGNANT WOMEN

	No.	Mean maternal age (yr)	Mean peak serum bilirubin (mg/dl)	Mean peak serum SGOT (IU/ml)	Trimester of onset: First (0-12 wk)	Second (13-24 wk)	Third (25-term)	Maternal outcome: Complete resolution	Residual liver disease
Total group	50 (100%)	20.2*	7.1†	1,465‡	10 (20%)	14 (28%)	26 (52%)	49 (98%)	1 (2%)
Type B	20 (40%)	19.2 (±2.3)	8.6 (±3.8)	2,350 (±1,433)	4 (20%)	5 (25%)	11 (55%)	20 (100%)	0 (0%)
Non-type B	30 (60%)	21 (±3.1)	6.1 (±4.2)	875 (±931)	6 (20%)	9 (30%)	15 (50%)	29 (97%)	1 (3%)

*P < 0.1.
†P < 0.05.
‡P < 0.001.

type B hepatitis had elevations of SGOT or serologic markers of type B hepatitis or both. One of two cord blood determinations of HB_sAg in infants born to affected mothers revealed the antigen. This infant had a normal SGOT value when examined subsequently and showed no HB_sAg or anti-HB_s.

The findings support previous observations of a good maternal outcome after gestational hepatitis. Pregnancies complicated by acute hepatitis are unattended by increased rates of congenital malformations, fetal wastage or intrauterine growth retardation. The prognosis of infants who become chronic carriers of HB_sAg is uncertain, but the chronic HB_s-antigenemic state has been associated with hepatic tumors, chronic active hepatitis, cirrhosis and systemic vasculitis. Prospective studies are needed to determine the significance of mild SGOT elevations.

Liver Involvement in the Syndrome of Mixed Cryoglobulinemia. Yoram Levo, Peter D. Gorevic, Hanna J. Kassab, Hillel Tobias and Edward C. Franklin[5] (New York Univ.) found evidence of hepatitis B virus exposure in two-thirds of 36 patients with mixed cryoglobulinemia and no well-defined connective tissue disorder, lymphoproliferative malignancy or chronic infection. The patients presented with purpura, arthralgia, weakness and, at times, kidney involvement. Only 2 had overt liver disease at the time of diagnosis.

Two thirds of the patients were women. The average age was 53.4 years. Nearly half had evidence of kidney involvement. The average follow-up from onset of cryoglobulin-related symptoms was 7.4 years for patients without renal involvement and 4.6 years for those with renal disease. All cryoprecipitates contained IgM and polyclonal IgG; the IgM was monoclonal with kappa light chains in 29% of cases and polyclonal in the rest.

The clinical and laboratory findings are given in the table. Group I consisted of 4 patients with clinical liver disease, group II of 28 patients with occult subclinical liver disease and group III of 4 patients with no evidence of hepatic involvement. Groups I and II did not differ in rate of hepatitis B surface antigen (HB_sAg) or its antibody (HB_sAb). None of the group I patients had renal involvement, whereas the kidneys were affected in half of the other patients.

(5) Ann. Intern. Med. 87:287–292, September, 1977.

Clinical and Laboratory Determinants of Liver Disease in 36 Patients with Essential Mixed Cryoglobulinemia*

Group†	Patient	Age	Hepatomegaly	Splenomegaly	Liver Disease	Liver Biochemical Tests‡			HBsAg	HBsAb	Cryoglobulin§		Biopsy
						Alkaline Phosphatase	Bilirubin	SGOT			IgA	IgMκ	
		yrs											
I	1‖	57	+	+	+	+	+	+	−	+	+		Cirrhosis
	2‖	46	+	+	+	+	N	+	+	−	+		CAH × 2
	3	55	+	+	+	N	+	++	−	−			CAH + cirrhosis
	4	63	+	+	+**	+	+	++	−	−		+	CAH + cirrhosis × 2
II	5	50	+	+	−	+	N	N	−	−		+	N
	6	63	+	+	−	++	N	+	+	+			CAH + cirrhosis
	7	69	+	−	−	+	N	N	+	+			
	8	29	+	+	−	++	+++	+++	−	−			
	9	49	+	+	−								
	10	51	−	−	−	+	N	N	−	−		+	
	11	43	−	−					−	+			
	12	59	+††	+	−	+	N	+	−	−			
	13	44	+††	−	−	+	N	++	−	−		+	Portal fibrosis
	14	47	−	−	−	+	N	++	−	−		+	
	15	57	+	+	−				−	+			
	16	64	+	+††	−	+	N	+	+	+			
	17	69	+	+	−	+	N	++	+	+			
	18	68	+††	+††	−	++	+	+			+		Cirrhosis
	19	75	+	−	−	++	++	N					
	20	67	+	−	−	+		++	−	+		+	Portal fibrosis
	21	63	+	+††	−	N	N	N	−	+		+	
	22	48	+	+	−				+	+			N → Portal fibrosis × 2
	23	45	+	+	−								
	24	61	+	−	−				−	−			
	25	55	+	+	−	N	N	N	+	+		+	
	26	44	−	−	−	+	N	+	−	+			CPH
	27	54	+	+	−			+					
	28	50			−				−	+		+	
	29	39	+	−	−	++	N	+	−	−	+		Minimal nonspecific
	30	39	+	−	−	+	+	N					
	31	30	+	−	−				+	−		+	
	32	55	+	−	−	N	N	N	−	+			
III	33	54	−	−	−	N	N	N					
	34	55	−	−	−	N	N	N	−	+			
	35	55	−	+	−	N	N	N	−	−			
	36	60	−	−	−	N	N	N	−	−			
Total above normal/total number			27/35	19/35	4/36	19/27	7/26	16/28	8/29	15/29	4/36	10/36	13/15
Percent positive			77	54	11	70	27	57	28	52	11	28	87

*N = normal; CAH = chronic active hepatitis; CPH = cirrhosis, persistent hepatitis; SGOT = serum glutamic-oxalacetic transaminase.

†Group I, overt liver disease; group II, occult liver disease; group III, no evidence of liver disease.

‡+ = above normal, ++ > 3 times normal, +++ > 6 times normal; − = no evidence of liver disease.

§All cryoprecipitates were IgG-IgM; + = those with IgA or monoclonal IgM.

‖Patient presenting with liver disease.

**Fatal liver disease.

††Detected by scan only.

Mixed cryoglobulinemia is a distinct clinical syndrome. Nearly all patients have liver involvement, although only a few have overt liver disease. All but 2 of 15 liver biopsies in the present series showed abnormalities, ranging from minimal lesions to chronic persistent and active hepatitis with piecemeal necrosis and cirrhosis. Mixed cryoglobulinemia should be considered a distinct connective tissue disorder associated with hepatitis B virus infection. Other viral agents are likely implicated in other cases of mixed cryoglobulinemia. Studies of immune complexes may prove of value in identifying possible etiologic agents in this and other disorders.

► [Essential mixed cryoglobulinemia (EMC) is a syndrome characterized by the clinical triad of purpura, arthralgia and weakness, frequently accompanied by renal involvement. Histologic examination reveals widespread vasculitis with immune-complex deposition. Levo et al. (N. Engl. J. Med. 296:1501, 1977) reviewed the clinical and laboratory features of a large series of patients with essential mixed cryoglobulinemia and were struck by the high frequency of clinical or laboratory evidence of liver involvement. Accordingly, these investigators looked for evidence of hepatitis B virus infection in 25 serum specimens and 19 cryoprecipitates obtained from 30 patients. Thirteen of 25—or more than 50%—of the serum specimens contained either HB_sAg or anti-HB_s. By contrast, only 5 of 28 serum specimens from patients with systemic lupus erythematosus contained either HB_sAg or anti-HB_s

The frequency of positive results in EMC was increased when cryoprecipitates were examined, and 14 of 19 (74%) of the cryoprecipitates were positive for either HB_sAg or anti-HB_s. Electron microscopy of four cryoprecipitates showed structures resembling the 20-nm and 27-nm spheres, tubules and the Dane particles characteristic of hepatitis B virus infection. Because such infection appears to be involved in the pathogenesis of the syndrome, Levo et al. feel the term "essential mixed cryoglobulinemia" should be replaced by "mixed cryoglobulinemia secondary to hepatitis B virus" or perhaps to other viral infections.—Ed.] ◄

Significance of Suspected "Chronic Aggressive Hepatitis" in Acute Hepatitis. It is important to recognize the transition from acute to chronic hepatitis, but the range of reported intervals is large. Lis Fauerholdt, Stig Asnaes, Leo Ranek, Torben Schiødt and Niels Tygstrup[6] (Univ. of Copenhagen) investigated the prognostic significance of the histologic criteria defined by De Groote et al., irrespective of time criteria, in 17 patients seen consecutively in 1965–71 with a clinical picture of acute viral hepatitis after previous health and first liver biopsy changes compatible with chronic aggressive hepatitis with "superimposed hepatitis."

All initial biopsies showed marked portal infiltration with lymphocytes and plasma cells, extending into the parenchyma as active septa, as well as piecemeal necrosis, focal parenchymal necroses, Kupffer cell proliferation and, in most instances, acidophilic bodies. Bridging necrosis and multilobular necroses were not seen in any biopsies, including those of 2 patients whose follow-up biopsies showed cirrhosis. One follow-up biopsy showed chronic persistent hepatitis. Initial biopsy and clinical and laboratory data did not distinguish the patients who developed cirrhosis or persistent hepatitis, and no histologic differences were apparent. One patient went into hepatic coma during the acute phase. All 3 patients who developed chronic liver disease were treated with steroids or azathioprine.

Cases in which active chronic hepatitis develops can be distinguished from fully reversible cases only by follow-up studies, including liver biopsies. The development of chronic liver disease in patients with histologic signs of chronicity is the exception rather than the rule. The highly optimistic results of some uncontrolled therapeutic trials in active chronic hepatitis may be explained by many reversible cases having escaped recognition. The transition from acute to chronic hepatitis cannot be recognized with any certainty by present methods. If the diagnosis of chronic active hepatitis is based on histologic findings

---

(6) Gastroenterology 73:543–548, September, 1977.

alone in patients with prolonged acute hepatitis, the incidence of this condition will be grossly overestimated.

► [Time has been used as one of several criteria for discrimination between protracted acute and chronic active hepatitis. Several intervals have been suggested, including 10 weeks (Gastroenterology 55:724, 1968), 3 months (N. Engl. J. Med. 284: 1154, 1971), 6 months (Gastroenterology 70:1161, 1976) and even 1 year. Most authorities now believe that at least 6 months should elapse before concluding that a patient has chronic active liver disease.

That liver biopsies from patients with acute hepatitis may show features of chronic active hepatitis is further illustrated in the follow-up by Miller and Klatskin of a series of patients with halothane hepatitis who exhibited benign resolution of a severe lesion (ibid. 73:1234, 1977). Whereas the initial liver biopsy in patients showed acute hepatitis with bridging necrosis and subsequent biopsies showed changes consistent with chronic active hepatitis, later biopsies at 10–14 months demonstrated only patchy mild fibrosis or minor portal fibrosis. – Ed.] ◄

Randomized, Double-Blind Controlled Trial of the Efficacy of Immune Serum Globulin for Prevention of Posttransfusion Hepatitis: Veterans Administration Cooperative Study. Posttransfusion hepatitis (PTH) is a major public health problem in the United States. L. B. Seeff, H. J. Zimmerman, E. C. Wright, J. D. Finkelstein, P. Garcia-Pont, H. B. Greenlee, A. A. Dietz, C. M. Leevy, C. H. Tamburro, E. R. Schiff, E. M. Schimmel, R. Zemel, D. S. Zimmon and R. W. McCollum[7] report the results of a double-blind trial reevaluating the efficacy of immune serum globulin (ISG) that was initiated by the Veterans Administration (VA) at 11 hospitals during a 49-month period. Nonaddicts who received whole blood or packed cells and were thought likely to survive for 5 months were included in the trial. Two 10-ml injections of either ISG or placebo were given, the first one as soon as possible but no more than 96 hours after the initial transfusion and the second 28 days after the first.

Of 2,204 patients entering the study, 1,094 received ISG. Posttransfusion hepatitis developed in 107 of those who had ISG and 134 of those who had placebo, a difference that was not significant. The significant reduction in incidence of icteric hepatitis applied only to those who acquired icteric type non-B hepatitis only. The incidence of icteric hepatitis was 2.5% in placebo subjects and 1.3% in ISG recipients. The rates of type B hepatitis and type non-B hepatitis were comparable in the two groups, as were rates of anicteric hepatitis. Totally inapparent hepatitis (biochemical and serologic) occurred 15 times as frequently as did overt, icteric hepatitis. Adverse reactions were rare and ISG did not alter the incubation period or duration of the disease significantly.

Despite the long-held belief that type B hepatitis is responsible for most instances of PTH, type B hepatitis constituted less than 20% of cases of hepatitis in each year of the study. The lack of identification of type A hepatitis in other studies, the effect of ISG manufactured in 1944 against type non-B hepatitis, age-attack rates, incubation periods and duration of disease – all support the probability that an undefined agent has been responsible for PTH for many years. Thus, the screening of donor blood for hepatitis B surface antigen, (HB_sAg), as might be

(7) Gastroenterology 72:111–121, January, 1977.

expected, has had a limited impact in reducing the incidence of PTH. The use of commercial blood was the most important risk factor in the development of PTH; elimination of commercial blood would have reduced the incidence of hepatitis by 75% from 10.9% to 2.6%.

In summary, the incidence of PTH can be most effectively reduced by eliminating commercial donor blood and by continuing to screen volunteer donors for HB_SAg by sensitive procedures. The agent or agents responsible for type non-A, non-B hepatitis must be defined in order to eradicate post-transfusion hepatitis completely.

► [This is an important study and the major findings can be summarized as follows:

1. Posttransfusion hepatitis developed in 107 of the 1,094 (9.8%) recipients of immune serum globulin (ISG) and 134 of the 1,110 (12.1%) recipients of placebo.

2. Inapparent or anicteric hepatitis occurred 15 times as frequently as did overt, icteric hepatitis.

3. There was no significant difference in the hepatitis incidence between ISG and placebo recipients among those whose disease was defined as type B hepatitis, type non-B hepatitis, hepatitis with incubation periods less than 40 days, hepatitis with incubation periods greater than 40 days and anicteric hepatitis.

4. There was a significantly lower incidence of icteric hepatitis among recipients of ISG (1.3%) vs. those who had received placebo (2.5%). *However, this reduction in the incidence of icteric hepatitis applied only to those who developed icteric non-B hepatitis.*

5. Immune serum globulin led to a reduction in the incidence of icteric hepatitis in recipients of commercial blood, but only among those who received 3 or more units of commercial blood.

6. Recipients of HB_sAg-positive blood had a greater incidence of hepatitis than recipients of HB_sAg-negative blood (27% vs. 10%).

Blumberg has recently reviewed non-A, non-B hepatitis (Ann. Intern. Med 87:111, 1977). Non-A, non-B hepatitis is more similar to hepatitis B than to hepatitis A. It is often preceded by transfusion or other forms of parenteral infection. There appears to be a carrier state. It is less likely to be accompanied by fever, headaches and myalgias as compared to hepatitis A. Another feature common to both hepatitis B and non-A, non-B hepatitis is the development of chronic active hepatitis, whereas hepatitis A does not appear to cause chronic hepatitis. There may be a difference in the prophylactic effect of γ-globulin on hepatitis B and hepatitis non-A, non-B, but further trials are needed to clarify this point. – Ed.] ◄

► ↓The following article describes the development of chronic active liver disease after non-A, non-B hepatitis. – Ed. ◄

Development of Chronic Liver Disease after Acute Non-A, Non-B Posttransfusion Hepatitis: Role of γ-Globulin Prophylaxis in Its Prevention. Hepatitis A virus has been proposed as a likely cause of cases of hepatitis B surface antigen (HB_sAg)-negative acute and chronic liver disease. Robert G. Knodell, Marcel E. Conrad and Kamal G. Ishak[8] reviewed 44 cases of non-A, non-B hepatitis encountered in a recent posttransfusion study in which the efficacy of γ-globulin prophylaxis in preventing this type of hepatitis was suggested. Twenty-eight patients had no symptoms of hepatitis or liver enzyme abnormalities 6 months after the acute illness, whereas 16 had enzyme elevations for 6 months or longer. Six of the latter patients had normal liver enzyme levels on two occasions a month apart when follow-up was begun, whereas 10 had continued enzyme abnormalities consistent with chronic hepatitis 12–36 months after initial elevations were recorded.

---

(8) Gastroenterology 72 (Pt. 1):902–909, May, 1977.

EFFECT OF PREOPERATIVE IMMUNE SERUM GLOBULIN (ISG) ON PROGRESSION OF ACUTE NON-A, NON-B HEPATITIS TO CHRONIC LIVER DISEASE

Treatment*	Progression	Resolution	Significance as compared to placebo (*P*)
Placebo (n = 92)	9	13	
Combined commercial and high titer anti-HB_s ISG treatment groups (n = 184)	1	21	0.009

*Number in parentheses represents total number of patients at risk of developing non-A, non-B posttransfusion hepatitis.

The 10 patients with evidence of chronic liver disease did not differ from the others with respect to age, sex or prevalence of preoperative antibodies. They had received more blood transfusions than the patients whose hepatitis resolved. Symptoms were more frequent in the study group, but there was no difference in the severity of hepatitis. The effects of preoperative immune serum globulin (ISG) on progression of chronic liver disease are shown in the table. Of 22 hepatitis patients who received the placebo, 9 developed evidence of chronic hepatitis. Only 1 of 11 hepatitis patients who received conventional ISG and none of 11 hepatitis patients who received high-titer ISG developed evidence of chronic hepatitis. Regarding hepatic histologic changes, 8 patients had chronic active hepatitis. One had a mixed macronodular and micronodular cirrhosis that was relatively inactive, and the other patient had chronic persistent hepatitis. No viral particles were seen on electron micrographs.

Hepatitis B virus clearly plays an important role in the development of chronic liver disease. Acute non-A, non-B posttransfusion hepatitis often progresses to chronic active hepatitis. Preoperative γ-globulin prophylaxis significantly reduces this progression. Identification and characterization of the viral agent or agents will aid the prevention of this complication of blood transfusion.

► [A key finding in this study was the high incidence of chronic liver disease after non-A, non-B hepatitis. Hoofnagle and associates (Ann. Intern. Med. 87:14, 1977) have also reported that patients who had acute non-A, non-B hepatitis developed chronic hepatitis. Indeed, the incidence may well be higher than that which obtains after hepatitis B infection. In this regard, approximately 10% of patients with acute hepatitis B infection develop chronic hepatitis (Am. J. Med. Sci. 270:9, 1975). Although the data of Knodell et al. and Hoofnagle et al. are obviously preliminary, combining their studies gives an incidence of chronicity of approximately 25%.

By contrast, hepatitis A does not appear to cause chronic liver disease. This conclusion is supported by several lines of evidence, the most recent being a study by Rakela et al. (Gastroenterology 73:1241, 1977), who looked for hepatitis A virus (HAV) infection as an etiologic agent among patients with chronic active hepatitis (CAH). They studied 13 cases of HB_sAg-positive and 22 HB_sAg-negative cases of CAH. The HB_sAg-negative cases were presumed to be viral in etiology. Serial serums collected over a period of 2–6 years were tested for antibody to HAV. The authors also examined stools for fecal shedding of HAV by immune electron microscopy. Anti-hepatitis A was found in 4 of 13 (31%) of HB_sAg-positive cases and in 7 of 22 (32%) of the HB_sAg-negative cases. No fecal shedding of HAV was found in any of the HB_sAg-negative CAH patients studied. The findings that the frequency of anti-HA was the same in patients with HB_sAg-positive as in HB_sAg-negative chronic active hepatitis and the failure to find hepatitis A virus in fecal specimens weigh against an important role of chronic hepatitis A infection in HB_sAg-negative chronic active hepatitis. – Ed.] ◄

Contrasting Features and Responses to Treatment of Severe Chronic Active Liver Disease with and without Hepatitis B_s Antigen. The specific features of chronic active liver disease (CALD) associated with hepatitis B surface antigen (HB_sAg) in CALD are poorly defined. S. W. Schalm, W. H. J. Summerskill, G. L. Gitnick and Lila R. Elveback[9] compared patients having HB_sAg-positive CALD with those chosen by identical clinical, functional and morphologic criteria in whom HB_sAg and anti-HB_s were absent. Postpuberal patients whose liver biopsy specimens had features of CALD, who had been ill for at least 10 weeks or had cirrhosis were included in the study. A total of 136 patients were randomized to treatment with 20 mg prednisone daily, 10 mg prednisone and 50 mg azathioprine daily or alternate-day prednisone therapy in a mean dose of 20 mg. Eighteen patients had serum HB_sAg on at least one occasion and 6 had anti-HB_s; 112 were repeatedly negative for both HB_sAg and anti-HB_s.

Men predominated among HB_sAg-positive patients and women in those who were negative. The HB_sAg-positive patients were older. Abnormalities in serum bilirubin and γ-globulin were less in the patients with HB_sAg. The histologic findings were similar in the two groups. Responses to prednisone therapy are given in the table. Treatment failure and death were significantly more frequent in HB_sAg-positive patients. On conventional maintenance doses, biochemical deterioration was less frequent in HB_sAg-negative patients (Fig 18). Treatment with higher doses of prednisone resulted in biochemical improvement in both groups. Survival was better in HB_sAg-positive patients given prednisone than in control patients who received azathioprine or placebo. In 8 of 10 HB_sAg-positive patients followed for over 1 year, HB_sAg has persisted.

In summary, HB_sAg-positive patients with severe CALD enter remission significantly less frequently and fail therapy significantly more frequently than do HB_sAg-negative patients when treated with prednisone. These data, however, suggest that therapy is indicated and that higher doses of medication given over longer periods may be nec-

Response to Prednisone Therapy in HB_sAg-Positive and HB_sAg-Negative CALD

	HB_sAg neg (82)	*HB_sAg pos (13)*	*HB_sAg neg† (13)*
Clinical and biochemical resolution	66 (80)*‡	6 (46)	11 (85)
Histological remission	56 (68)*	2 (15)	10 (77)*
Treatment failure	13 (16)*	6 (46)	1 (8)*
Death, total	9 (11)*	4 (31)	1 (8)

*$P < 0.05$.
†Matched for morphology and treatment (type and duration), sex, age and immunoserology and number of patients.
‡Percentages in parentheses.

(9) Gut 17:781–786, October, 1976.

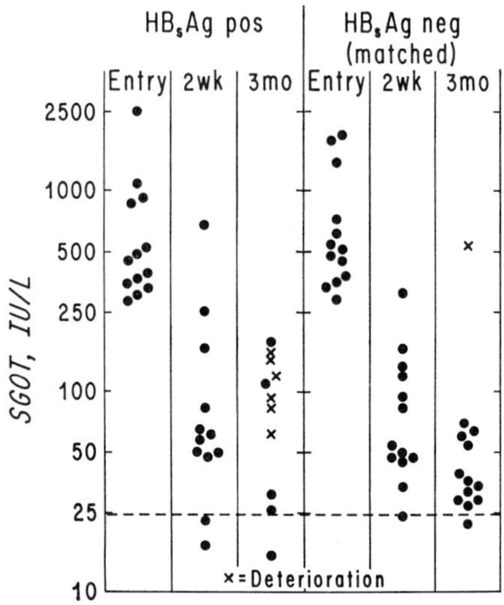

Fig 18.—Effect of prednisone (with or without azathioprine) on SGOT concentration in HB_sAg-positive and HB_sAg-negative CALD treated with prednisone. (Courtesy of Schalm, S. W., et al.: Gut 17:781–786, October, 1976.)

essary, but the benefits and risks of such therapy await evaluation in a controlled trial.

► [It is currently believed that the response to corticosteroid therapy is better in HB_sAg-negative patients with chronic active liver disease (CALD). As Sherlock (Lancet 2:354, 1976) has emphasized, the immunologic disturbance is much more marked in the HB_sAg-negative group and hence the effect of corticosteroids might be expected to be greater.

Czaja and Wolf (Gastroenterology 73:1217, 1977) have attempted to identify those features of HB_sAg-related disease that influence early prognosis. Twenty patients with HB_0Ag satisfied preestablished criteria for severe disease and were treated with prednisone. Seventeen patients, including 10 positive for e antigen, satisfied a therapeutic end point or were treated for at least 6 months (mean, 27 months). Eight patients deteriorated while receiving conventional doses of prednisone, including 5 who died of liver failure. Three patients failing initial therapy responded to higher doses of corticosteroid and are alive (mean 40 months); 1 had achieved remission. Eight patients responded to conventional therapy, including 2 who cleared their antigen. Four entered sustained remission, surviving without manifestation of disease for up to 4½ years. Four others achieved clinical and biochemical resolution but remain on treatment (mean, 43 months) because of continual histologic activity. Patients who died were (1) older, (2) usually had encephalopathy prior to therapy and (3) succumbed rapidly (mean, 5 months). Initial histology, biochemical findings and e antigen status did not distinguish these patients. Nine of the 12 patients without pretreatment signs of liver failure responded to conventional or high-dose therapy, although cessation of medication has only been possible in 5 so far. It is concluded that early prognosis of HB_sAg-positive patients with severe CALD who are treated with prednisone is influenced mainly by the clinical severity of the disease prior to treatment. Death usually occurs in the older patient with coma. Czaja and Wolf feel that biochemical and symptomatic improvement can be anticipated in most patients receiving conventional or high-dose therapy. The presence of HB_sAg does not preclude a satisfactory clinical response to steroid therapy—Ed.] ◄

Prednisone for Chronic Active Liver Disease: Pharmacokinetics, Including Conversion to Prednisolone. Most patients with chronic active liver disease (CALD) will experience remission on pred-

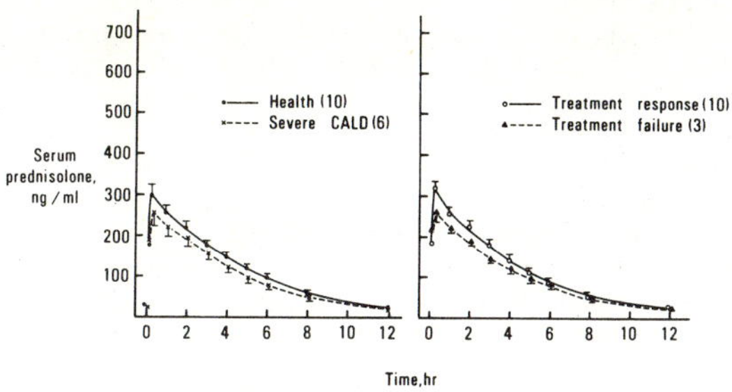

Fig 19.—Appearance of prednisolone after prednisone, 10 mg by vein, in normal volunteers, patients with untreated chronic active liver disease (CALD), those with treatment response and those with treatment failure. Each point represents mean ±SE. (Courtesy of Schalm, S. W., et al.: Gastroenterology 72 (Pt. 1):910–913, May, 1977.)

nisone therapy, but about 20% fail to improve or will deteriorate, despite treatment. S. W. Schalm, W. H. J. Summerskill and V. L. W. Go[1] (Mayo Found., Rochester, Minn.) determined the effect of impaired liver function on the conversion of prednisone to prednisolone and investigated the relationship of this to responses to treatment in 19 patients with severe CALD and 10 healthy subjects. Six patients were untreated, whereas 13 had received prednisone for 1 month to 8 years. Ten patients had responded with biochemical resolution or histological remission, whereas 3 were deteriorating, despite treatment. No patient had taken drugs (other than prednisone) known to induce microsomal enzymes. A dose of 10 mg prednisone in 50% ethanol was given intravenously in a 5-minute period with a rapid infusion of physiologic saline.

No striking group differences in serum prednisone levels were found after injection, and pharmacokinetic measurements were not significantly different among the various groups. Severe impairment of liver function did not affect prednisone pharmacokinetics, but previous treatment was associated with a smaller apparent volume of distribution. Times of appearance and subsequent disappearance of prednisolone did not differ significantly in the various groups (Fig 19). Severely impaired liver function was associated with about 15% lower serum prednisolone levels, and prednisolone half-life was more often 3.2 hours or less in treated patients than in untreated patients. Patients with untreated severe CALD or failing treatment had higher percentages of free prednisolone in serum than did healthy subjects or treatment responders.

Failure to respond to prednisone therapy can hardly be attributed to the small differences in conversion of prednisone to prednisolone associated with severe impairment of liver function in patients with CALD. No major defect of prednisone metabolism occurs in CALD and failure of this condition to respond to therapy with prednisone is caused by other factors. No practical advantage of either prednisone or prednisolone is apparent in the treatment of these patients.

► [In four controlled trials carried out to evaluate the effect of corticosteroids on sur-

(1) Gastroenterology 72 (Pt. 1):910–913, May, 1977.

vival in alcoholic hepatitis, two studies (Ann. Intern. Med. 74:311, 1971; and N. Engl. J. Med. 284:1350, 1971) showed an apparent increased survival rate in steroid-treated patients, and two (ibid. 79:625, 1973; and Am. J. Dig. Dis. 22:477, 1977) showed no difference in survival rates. It is pertinent to note that *prednisolone* was used in the former two studies and *prednisone* in the latter two studies. These findings have raised the question as to whether there is impaired conversion of prednisone to prednisolone in the presence of severe parenchymal liver disease; such a defect could account, at least in part, for the divergent results cited above. However, the findings of Schalm et al. indicate that no major defect of prednisone metabolism occurs in chronic active liver disease. Extrapolating these data to alcoholic hepatitis, it appears unlikely that a defect in prednisone metabolism can account for the failure of such patients to respond to corticosteroid therapy.

On the other hand, decreased metabolic clearance of prednisolone may be a factor in the development of corticosteroid side effects. Kozower et al. (J. Clin. Endocrinol. Metab. 38:407, 1974) measured the metabolic clearance rate (MCR) and serum half-life (T½) of prednisolone in 13 patients being treated with prednisone and in 7 normal subjects. Tritiated prednisolone was studied since it is the metabolically active form to which administered prednisone is rapidly converted. Steroid side effects, hirsutism and facial and truncal obesity correlated with a slow rate of prednisone catabolism. Prednisolone T½ was longer and MCR lower in patients who acquired side effects than in those who did not. Therapeutic response did not correlate with the rate of catabolism of prednisolone. These data suggest that patients who acquire side effects on synthetic corticosteroid treatment may be those who fail to adapt to such treatment by increasing their rate of catabolism of the administered corticosteroid. – Ed.] ◄

Alcoholic Hyalin Antigen (AHAg) and Antibody (AHAb) in Alcoholic Hepatitis. Preliminary studies indicated that alcoholic hyalin (AH) evoked humoral immunity. Natarajan Kanagasundaram, Shinichi Kakumu, Thomas Chen and Carroll M. Leevy[2] (New Jersey Med. School) attempted to characterize AH isolated from human postmortem liver and to determine the diagnostic value of AHAg and AHAb in serum and occurrence of tissue immune complexes in alcoholic hepatitis.

METHOD. – Alcoholic hyalin antigen and antibody were studied in serum from 7 healthy subjects, 42 patients with alcoholic liver disease (26 with alcoholic hepatitis) and 28 patients with evidence of nonalcoholic hepatic disorders. Purified AH was prepared; serum from patients with advanced alcoholic hepatitis gave a positive reaction to it. Complement fixation tests were used to detect AHAg (rabbit antiserum added to heat-inactivated human serum) and AHAb (purified AH added to test serum). The Mayumi technique was used for immune adherence hemagglutination studies. Tissue elution studies were also carried out.

Complement fixation tests for AHAg were positive in titers of 8–64 in 12 patients with early and 3 with advanced alcoholic hepatitis. Two of 3 patients with early phase alcoholic hepatitis who had negative tests had marked anticomplementary activity. Complement fixation for AHAg was negative in 8 of 11 patients with advanced alcoholic hepatitis who exhibited AHAb and in all patients with other hepatic disorders. Immune adherence hemagglutination tests were positive in 15 patients with early and 4 with advanced alcoholic hepatitis. The AHAg by this technique was negative in 7 patients with advanced alcoholic hepatitis with antibody and in all patients with other hepatic disorders.

Complement fixation tests for AHAb were positive in all patients

(2) Gastroenterology 73:1368–1373, December, 1977.

SERIAL STUDIES OF ALCOHOLIC HYALIN ANTIGEN (AHAG) AND ANTIBODY (AHAB) BY IMMUNE ADHERENCE HEMAGGLUTINATION IN PATIENTS WITH EARLY-PHASE ALCOHOLIC HEPATITIS

Patient	Course	Date	AHAg	AHAb
E. I.	Hospital treatment	8/5/75	2048	Neg.
		8/13/75	256	Neg.
	Recurrent alcoholism	9/2/75	1024	Neg.
		9/9/75	512	1024
	Hospital treatment	11/26/75	128	Neg.
		12/3/75	Neg.	Neg.
		12/16/75	Neg.	1024
Sp. R.	Hospital treatment	7/11/74	64	Neg.
		8/21/74	Neg.	Neg.
		9/8/74	Neg.	1024
	Recurrent alcoholism	—*		
	Hospital treatment	2/11/75	512	2048
		2/19/75	Neg.	Neg.
Ch. J.	Hospital treatment	4/18/75	512	1024
		5/2/75	Neg.	2048
		9/19/75	Neg.	Neg.

*Patient failed to return for follow-up.

with advanced alcoholic hepatitis and negative in those with other hepatic disorders. Immune adherence tests for AHAb were positive in advanced cases and in 3 early phase cases and negative in patients with other hepatic disorders. Tissue elution studies were positive for AHAb only in patients with advanced alcoholic hepatitis or active cirrhosis.

Serial studies showed AHAg to be present in early alcoholic hepatitis and to persist with continued intake of alcoholic beverages. Recurrent alcoholic hepatitis led to reappearance of AHAg and/or AHAb (table). One patient in whom alcoholic hepatitis converted to active cirrhosis despite cessation of alcoholism had AHAb in liver, although the initial serologic abnormalities disappeared.

Immunoglobulins eluted from the livers of patients with alcoholic hepatitis or active alcoholic cirrhosis exhibit reactivity to AHAg. Therefore, AHAg and AHAb may produce some of the manifestations of alcoholic hepatitis by forming immune complexes, which when deposited in the liver may induce chemotaxis and cell necrosis. Antibody-dependent tissue toxicity may foster progressive liver cell destruction.

► [Two recent studies dealing with immunologic alterations in alcoholic hepatitis and chronic hepatitis in the alcoholic are of interest.

In the first, Kakumu and Leevy (Gastroenterology 72:594, 1977) undertook studies to evaluate the cytotoxicity of peripheral lymphocytes obtained from patients with alcoholic hepatitis. Lymphocyte cytotoxicity to Chang live cells was investigated by a microcytotoxicity test and that to antologous liver cells obtained by percutaneous liver biopsy was studied with the use of a ^{51}Cr release assay. Lymphocytes from patients with alcoholic hepatitis were found to be highly cytotoxic to Chang liver cells and antologous liver cells when compared with those from healthy subjects. Cell-free supernatant fluid of lymphocytes from patients with alcoholic hepatitis incubated with purified alcoholic hyalin was significantly cytotoxic to Chang liver cells. It is concluded that ethanol toxicity and hyperactivity of lymphocytes independently contribute to development of cirrhosis in patients with alcoholic hepatitis who continue to imbibe alcohol.

In the second study, Goldberg and his associates (ibid., p. 598) describe 10 alcoholic patients with biopsy-proved chronic active or chronic persistent hepatitis. Goldberg et al. suggest several possible mechanisms that could explain the association between chronic alcoholism and chronic hepatitis. First, alcohol may be a direct initiator of liver injury in a manner similar to that observed with other drugs. Second, alcohol may increase the susceptibility of the person to viral hepatitis and in this manner influence the initiation of chronic liver disease. Third, alcohol might indirectly initiate active liver disease through the formation of a complex protein, alcoholic hyalin, which then serves as a "neoantigen" or "autoantigen." – Ed.] ◄

Deficiency of Carnitine in Cachectic Cirrhotic Patients. Carnitine is a trimethylated γ-amino acid present in all mammalian tissues, which is essential in fatty acid oxidation. The manifestations of human carnitine deficiency include muscle weakness and atrophy and hepatic and cerebral dysfunction. Protein deficiency is prevalent in the hospital population, and the rapid development of carnitine deficiency observed in rats fed a diet deficient in essential amino acids suggested that unrecognized carnitine deficiency could be endemic in patients with nosocomial malnutrition. Daniel Rudman, Charles W. Sewell and Joseph D. Ansley[3] (Emory Univ.) evaluated this idea by measuring the serum carnitine level in 247 inpatients with various diseases and 16 normal subjects and by investigating causes of subnormal levels in 6 cirrhotic patients. Tissue levels of carnitine were determined in the 7 of 14 hypocarnitinemic cirrhotic patients who died. A diet containing less than 10 μM carnitine daily was given, followed by an oral supplemen

The average total serum carnitine in normal subjects was 79 μM and the normal range was defined as 55 – 103 μM. The average serum free carnitine was 49 μM (25 – 73 μM). Values were normal in nonhepatic diseases, but in cirrhotics both the total and the free carnitine concentrations were significantly depressed. Fourteen of 36 cirrhotics had a serum level below the normal range. Advanced protein-calorie starvation was documented in these patients, as was severe hepatocellular disease. The hypocarnitinemic cirrhotics were markedly anorectic. Carnitine supplementation increased L-carnitine excretion in the cirrhotics. Autopsy studies showed total and free carnitine levels 16 – 40% of normal in the muscle, heart, liver, kidney and brain of cirrhotics.

Hypocarnitinemic cirrhotics have subnormal tissue contents of carnitine. Myopathy, fatty liver and cerebral disorder are frequently observed in patients with advanced cirrhosis, and carnitine deficiency might play a role in the pathogenesis of these manifestations of acquired liver disease. If so, correction of carnitine deficiency by oral supplements may be beneficial.

Abnormal Fibrin Polymerization in Liver Disease. The disturbance of blood coagulation in liver disease is not fully understood; the common occurrence of a prolonged thrombin time is puzzling. G.

(3) J. Clin. Invest. 60:716 – 723, September, 1977.

CLINICAL GROUPS SHOWING NUMBER OF PATIENTS AND CONTROLS STUDIED AND INCIDENCE OF ABNORMAL FIBRIN POLYMERIZATION

Group	*Diagnosis*	*No. studied*	*Incidence of abnormal FMP**
1	Controls	34	0
2	Cirrhosis	32	16 (50%)
3	Chronic active liver disease	15	7 (47%)
4	Obstructive jaundice	26	0
5	Primary liver tumour	3	2 (66.6%)
6	Acute hepatic failure	8	8 (100%)
7	Miscellaneous liver disorders	37	0
Total		155	

*FMP: fibrin monomer polymerization.

Green, Jean M. Thomson, I. W. Dymock and L. Poller[4] (Univ. of South Manchester) investigated the possibility that a qualitative rather than a quantitative abnormality of fibrinogen might cause prolonged thrombin times by examining the polymerization of fibrin in 121 consecutive patients with clinical or laboratory evidence of hepatic dysfunction. Studies were also done in 34 healthy subjects, in all of whom the maximum rise in optical density in the fibrin polymerization test occurred by 10 minutes.

Thrombin-fibrinogen time was significantly prolonged in 28 of 32 cirrhotic patients and reptilase times were also prolonged. Quantitative fibrinogen was normal, but 16 patients exhibited abnormal fibrin polymerization (table). Fibrin polymerization was also abnormal in 7 of 15 patients with chronic active liver disease but not in patients with obstructive jaundice. Two of 3 patients with primary liver tumors and all 8 with acute liver failure had abnormal fibrin polymerization. No impairment of fibrin polymerization was found in 37 patients with miscellaneous liver disorders. In patients with abnormal fibrin polymerization, the clot opacity test underestimated the quantitative fibrinogen, as measured by the method of Ratnoff and Menzie. Dilutions of abnormal plasmas for the polymerization test, based on the clot opacity test results, were less than optimal for quantitative estimation of abnormal fibrin polymerization.

Laboratory findings favor the presence of an acquired abnormality of the fibrinogen molecule as the cause of impaired fibrin monomer polymerization in liver disease. The clinical importance of the biochemical defect is apparent from its frequency in patients with liver disease. The abnormality can easily be demonstrated in patients with parenchymatous liver disease. Its relation to other measures of hepatocellular function is under review.

► [These results have been confirmed by Palascak and Martinez (J. Clin. Invest. 60:89, 1977), who also tested the possibility that a functionally abnormal fibrinogen exists in some patients with liver disease. These investigators studied the plasma and purified fibrinogens of 5 patients whose plasma thrombin times were prolonged at least 40% over normal controls. In no patient was there evidence of disseminated intravascular

(4) Br. J. Haematol. 34:427–439, November, 1976.

coagulation or fibrinolysis. No abnormalities were detected by immunoelectrophoresis of plasmas or purified fibrinogens. Increasing amounts of thrombin progressively shortened the clotting times of patient fibrinogens, but not to normal levels. Importantly, addition of equal amounts of patient fibrinogen to normal fibrinogen resulted in a prolongation of the thrombin time of the normal protein. Fibrin monomers prepared from patient plasmas and purified fibrinogens demonstrated impaired aggregation at low and high ionic strength.

These studies demonstrate that some patients with liver disease and prolonged plasma thrombin times have a dysfibrinogenemia functionally characterized by an abnormality of fibrin monomer polymerization.—Ed.] ◄

Survival in Patients with Postnecrotic Cirrhosis and Laennec's Cirrhosis Undergoing Therapeutic Portacaval Shunt. There is little information regarding survival in patients with postnecrotic cirrhosis who have therapeutic portacaval shunting. Gary C. Kanel, Marshall M. Kaplan, John K. Zawacki and Allan D. Callow[5] (Boston) reviewed experience with 82 patients who had therapeutic portacaval shunt surgery in 1950–70 and were followed for 5 years after shunting or until death. Survival rates were calculated by life-table methods. All patients had at least one major upper gastrointestinal hemorrhage and had varices documented. All patients had Laennec's cirrhosis, postnecrotic cirrhosis or primary biliary cirrhosis. Eleven of 29 patients with postnecrotic cirrhosis had signs of chronic aggressive hepatitis in liver biopsy specimens. Eight patients had primary biliary cirrhosis. Most patients had end-to-side shunts. Based on Child's criteria for the severity of liver disease, 30 patients were in class A, 31 in class B and 21 in class C.

About three fourths of alcoholic cirrhotic patients were men whereas

Fig 20.—Survival after therapeutic portacaval shunt in patients with Laennec's, postnecrotic and primary biliary cirrhosis. *Vertical bars,* mean survival ±SEM. (Courtesy of Kanel, G. C., et al.: Gastroenterology 73 (Pt. 1):679–683, October, 1977.)

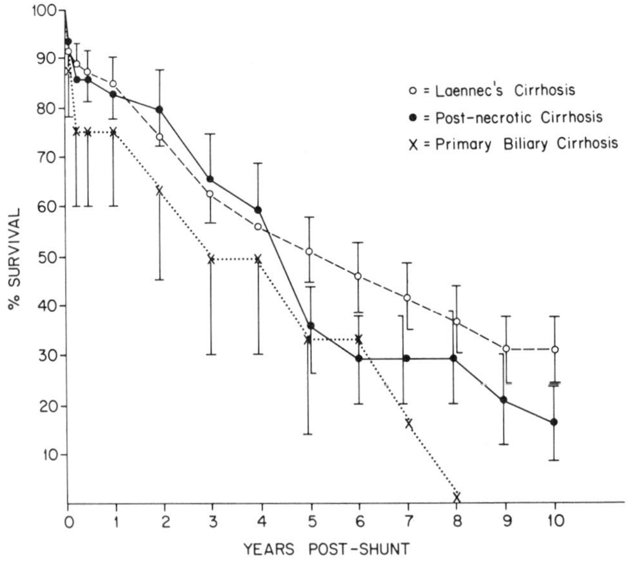

(5) Gastroenterology 73 (Pt. 1):679–683, October, 1977.

most of the others were women. Survival rates were similar in the three groups of patients (Fig 20). Survival was not influenced by the histologic activity of liver disease in alcoholic cirrhotic patients, but in postnecrotic cirrhosis, active inflammation and piecemeal necrosis were associated with a higher operative mortality and a resultant lower survival rate. The Child's classification provided better criteria for predicting survival than did liver function tests alone or liver histology. Child's class C patients did significantly worse than class A or B patients. The Child's classification was most predictive in patients with postnecrotic cirrhosis. The nature of the shunt was not an important factor in survival. The major cause of death in all groups was hepatic failure.

These findings indicate that once a patient has bled from esophageal varices, the cause of liver disease is not a factor in determining survival after a therapeutic portacaval shunt. The major determinant of survival in these patients is the state of hepatic functional reserve, as defined by Child's criteria.

► [The comparable survival rates in patients with biliary cirrhosis, postnecrotic cirrhosis and alcoholic cirrhosis after portacaval shunt is somewhat surprising. It has generally been accepted that patients with alcoholic liver disease have a poorer prognosis after portacaval shunt compared to patients with postnecrotic cirrhosis. In part, this is presumed to be due to the effects of continued ingestion of alcohol. Conversely, improved survival in early or moderately advanced cirrhosis is suggested after alcohol withdrawal (Am. J. Med. 44:406, 1968). However, some recent studies could find no evidence that continued alcoholism contributed significantly to morbidity, prevalence of ascites, bleeding varices and encephalopathy once a patient with alcoholic liver disease had been randomized into a portacaval shunt trial (Gastroenterology 74:64, 1978; and Lancet 2:65, 1973). Reynolds (Gastroenterology 74:153, 1978) is skeptical of these findings and cites his own as yet unpublished data suggesting that most patients with alcoholic liver disease who maintain their improvement are persons who have stopped drinking.—Ed.] ◄

Presentation and Course of Asymptomatic Primary Biliary Cirrhosis. R. G. Long, P. J. Scheuer and Sheila Sherlock[6] (London) report data on 20 patients with asymptomatic primary biliary cirrhosis (PBC) who have been followed for 2–11 years. The goal of the study was to assess the presentation and course of the disease and define markers distinguishing patients who had symptoms early from those who had a long asymptomatic course. Liver biopsy was repeated at least once in 18 patients. All patients but 2 were women. The mean age at diagnosis was 47. Five patients presented with hepatomegaly and 2 with hepatosplenomegaly. In 12 patients the diagnosis was suggested by an elevated serum alkaline phosphatase and in 1 patient by a positive mitochondrial antibody.

Ten patients (Fig 21) remained asymptomatic for 2–10 years, the mean period being 4½ years; 4 remain asymptomatic after 6–10 years. Eight patients are still alive. Ten patients had symptoms a mean of 2.2 years after presentation. In all of them the first symptom was pruritus. The mean age at presentation was 51, compared with 44 years for the patients who remained asymptomatic. Three patients in this group died of liver failure after variceal hemorrhage a mean of 6.7

(6) Gastroenterology 72:1204–1207, June, 1977.

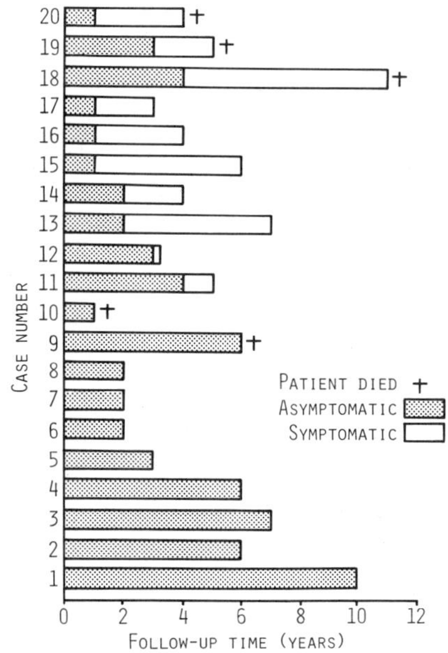

Fig 21.—The course of the 20 patients is depicted diagrammatically. (Courtesy of Long, R. G., et al.: Gastroenterology 72:1204–1207, June, 1977.)

years from diagnosis. Liver enzymes and bilirubin levels were higher in the patients who had symptoms but there was much overlap between the two groups for all biochemical tests. Eighteen patients had elevated serum IgM levels and 18 had positive mitochondrial antibody tests. All initial liver biopsy specimens were diagnostic or suggestive of PBC or compatible with the diagnosis. There was little difference in the histologic features of the two groups at presentation. Stage 3 or 4 was found at onset or in later biopsy specimens in 6 patients who remained asymptomatic and in 8 of those who had symptoms.

It appears that asymptomatic PBC is a stage through which many PBC patients pass but at which only a minority are discovered. In some patients the histologic stage remained static for many years even when symptoms developed. The course of asymptomatic PBC is variable. No means of arresting or decelerating the course of PBC is known. Asymptomatic patients should be assessed clinically and by liver function testing at 6-month intervals. Controlled trials of such drugs as D-penicillamine are reasonable.

► [Kayser-Fleischer rings are pigmented corneal rings at the limbus of the cornea in Descemet's membrane that have been deemed pathognomonic of Wilson's disease. However, pigmented corneal rings have been described in 3 patients with primary biliary cirrhosis (Ann. Intern. Med. 86:285, 1977). The rings were seen only by slit-lamp examination.

A randomized controlled trial of D-penicillamine therapy in primary biliary cirrhosis has been reported (Lancet 1:831, 1977). Nineteen patients received D-penicillamine (900 mg/day) and 13 received placebo. The two groups were similar in age, duration of illness, liver function tests and liver histology. Before entry into the trial, liver copper concentration was raised in 25 of the 27 patients in whom it was measured. After 3 months, patients taking D-penicillamine showed a significant reduction in serum asparate transaminase concentrations compared with the placebo group. In the 4 patients on D-penicillamine for a year, a second liver biopsy showed that mean liver copper concentration fell from 310 ± 128 (± 1 SEM) to 84 ± 36 mg/gm dry liver, compared with a reduction from 511 ± 169 to 454 ± 128 in 7 patients in the placebo group. Liver histology demonstrated a comparative improvement in cholestasis in patients on penicillamine, but the degree of inflammation, necrosis and the histologic stage of disease remained similar in both groups. In 5 of the 19 patients in the D-penicillamine group the drug was discontinued because of side effects. D-penicillamine seems to be a promising treatment for patients with primary biliary cirrhosis. It may produce its effect by reducing liver copper concentration. – Ed.] ◄

Antimicrobial Activity of Human Ascitic Fluid. Spontaneous bacterial peritonitis (SBP) occurs in about 8% of cirrhotic patients with ascites. A wide variety of organisms has been isolated, supporting the postulate that ascitic fluid is an ideal bacterial culture medium. John J. Fromkes, Fred B. Thomas, Hagop S. Mekhjian and Martin Evans[7] (Ohio State Univ.) studied the existence of humoral antimicrobial activity of human ascitic fluid for organisms commonly seen in SBP, as well as for rarely incriminated, predominantly enteric species. Five men and 2 women with a mean age of 49 years who had stable, biopsy-proved Laennec's cirrhosis were studied. None had received antibiotics for a month before. Ascitic fluid was obtained under aseptic conditions by abdominal paracentesis for bactericidal assays.

Bactericidal activity for *Escherichia coli* and *Klebsiella pneumoniae* was seen in 4 of the 7 fluids studied (table). All fluids were bacteriostatic for *Bacteroides fragilis,* but no antimicrobial activity for either *Streptococcus pneumoniae* or *S. faecalis* was seen in any fluid. Both heat inactivation and zymosal incubation abolished bactericidal activity in all fluids tested. Complement components and lysozyme were present in all specimens. Immunoglobulin concentrations varied widely. All serum immunoglobulin concentrations were normal or above normal. Two of 3 patients in the nonbactericidal group had subnormal serum levels of both C′3 and C′4, whereas all patients with ascitic fluid bactericidal activity had normal complement concentrations in serum.

Ascitic fluid possesses humoral antimicrobial activity for gram-negative organisms. The bactericidal activity seems to be complement

EFFECT OF ASCITIC FLUID ON MICROBIAL GROWTH IN 7 CIRRHOTIC PATIENTS*

Patient no.	Gram-negative			Gram-positive	
	Escherichia coli	*Klebsiella pneumoniae*	*Bacteroides fragilis*	*Streptococcus pneumoniae*	*Streptococcus faecalis*
1	++	++	+	0	0
2	++	++	+	0	0
3	++	++	+	0	0
4	++	++	+	0	0
5	+	0	+	0	0
6	0	0	+	0	0
7	0	0	+	0	0

*0, no inhibition; +, bacteriostatic; ++, bactericidal.

(7) Gastroenterology 73 (Pt. 1):668–672, October, 1977.

mediated, and alternate pathway activation may be particularly important. Susceptibility to gram-negative SBP may be related to low C'3 concentrations in ascitic fluid, resulting in a lack of bactericidal activity. Absence of humoral antimicrobial activity against gram-positive organisms may in part explain their relative prevalence in SBP. Gram-positive infections and septicemia may be especially dangerous for cirrhotic patients with ascites.

► [These interesting findings provide an explanation as to why some cirrhotics with ascites are prone to develop spontaneous bacterial peritonitis (SBP).

In reported series of patients with SBP, facultative gram-negative bacilli and streptococci account for most of the isolates whereas obligate anaerobes are rare. Targan et al. (Am. J. Med. 62:397, 1977), in their literature review of SBP, found that only 6 of 126 cases had involved anaerobes. This contrasts with peritonitis associated with bowel perforation in which anaerobes are almost universal. The paucity of anaerobes in SBP is puzzling. Conn (Medicine (Baltimore) 50:161, 1971) has explained the infrequency of anaerobes in SBP as due to their failure to penetrate the bowel lumen, failure to survive transit in the bloodstream or inability to replicate in large volumes of ascites fluid. Scheckman et al. (Lancet 2:1223, 1977) suggested that the environmental conditions, rather than available nutrients, are inadequate for initiation of growth. To test this hypothesis, they measured the P_{O_2} of ascites fluid collected by paracentesis from 10 cirrhotic patients without evidence of SBP and with negative ascitic fluid cultures. The mean P_{O_2} (43 mm Hg) approximated that of mixed venous blood, suggesting that there is free exchange of gases between the systemic circulation and body fluids. In earlier experiments (Appl. Environ. Microbiol. 31:168, 1976), these investigators found that 10–12% dissolved oxygen induced a complete metabolic shutdown in *Bacteroides fragilis,* an organism that is common in the intestine and in intra-abdominal sepsis. Scheckman et al. concluded that anaerobic bacteria are rare in SBP because the oxygen level in the ascitic fluid stops anaerobic growth. A similar oxygen concentration is found in urine, which may explain why anaerobes are rarely found in urinary tract infections (N. Engl. J. Med. 269:115, 1963).—Ed.] ◄

Complications of Diuresis in the Alcoholic Patient with Ascites: Controlled Trial. It is widely believed that diuresis in the patient with ascites causes marked electrolyte disturbances, hepatic encephalopathy, azotemia and hepatorenal syndrome. Peter B. Gregory, Peter H. Broekelschen, Malcolm D. Hill, Andrew B. Lipton, C. Michael Knauer, Marlene Egger and Rupert Miller[8] (Stanford Univ.) determined whether complications arise from careful diuretic treatment in the usual clinical setting. Patients with decompensated alcoholic liver disease and ascites of recent onset were randomized to salt and water restriction alone (control group) or salt and water restriction plus diuretics (diuresis group). All patients received a 20-mEq sodium, 1,500-ml water-restricted diet, and some received diuretics in increasing dosage until a daily reduction in weight of 1–2 lb was achieved. Spironolactone was used, in an initial dosage of 25 mg 4 times daily, and furosemide was added if necessary in an initial dosage of 40 mg daily. Twenty-two of the 43 patients received diuretics. The groups were comparable with respect to a wide array of clinical and laboratory data.

Seven control and 5 diuretic-treated patients died during the 8-week study. Weight loss was marked and ascites disappeared more often in the diuretic-treated group. Encephalopathy developed in 6 patients and hepatorenal syndrome in 4 during the study. The rates were com-

(8) Gastroenterology 73:534–538, September, 1977.

parable in the two treatment groups. A significant rise in blood urea nitrogen occurred in survivors given diuretics; it was reversed when the dosage was reduced or the drug was discontinued. Serum sodium and potassium values were similar in the two groups by the end of the study. Significant hypokalemia did not develop in any patient. Hospital stays were of comparable length for the two groups. Diuretics were stopped for modest hyponatremia in 1 patient and for hyperkalemia in another.

Diuresis can be achieved in critically ill alcoholic patients with ascites without serious complications attributable to the diuretic treatment. Further study is needed to determine whether complications of diuretics are more common in the occasional patient with chronic refractory ascites and inactive liver disease.

► [A small fraction of patients with cirrhosis and ascites will begin a spontaneous diuresis within a few days after initiation of sodium restriction. In a recent study by Fuller et al. (J.A.M.A. 237:972, 1977) only 2 of 48 (4%) subjects demonstrated such a diuresis. More prolonged (3–6 months) strict dietary sodium restriction (10 mEq/day) may well avoid some of the complications of diuretic therapy, but it may be successful in only up to 40% of the patients (Davidson: ibid., 159:1257, 1955). These findings underscore the need to reevaluate the effectiveness of diuretic therapy and hence the importance of this article by Gregory et al.

Fuller et al. (ibid. 237:972, 1977) carried out a two-part crossover study to evaluate the safety and efficacy of spironolactone and furosemide in cirrhotics with ascites. In the first part of the study it was demonstrated that a 6-day diuretic regimen with dietary sodium restriction of 10 mEq/day is safe and more effective than sodium restriction alone. In the second part, the duration of diuretic therapy was safely extended from 6 to 9 days, with mobilization of significantly more fluid. Only 2 of 18 (11%) subjects completing the studies had a complication attributable to the diuretic treatment (encephalopathy in 1 patient and azotemia in 1 patient). The low complication rate is due in part to the exclusion of a large number of patients with encephalopathy, gastrointestinal hemorrhage, renal failure, sepsis, hyponatremia ($Na^+ < 130$ mEq/L), hypokalemia ($K^+ < 3.4$ mEq/L) and inability to cooperate. In general, however, the results are similar to those of Gregory et al.

In the past 3 years there has been considerable interest in the LeVeen peritoneal-jugular shunt in the management of ascites, especially ascites refractory to conventional medical therapy. Wapnick et al. (ibid., p. 131) studied 30 patients with cirrhosis of the liver complicated by refractory ascites, hepatorenal syndrome or both given a LeVeen peritoneal-venous shunt. After surgery, these patients demonstrated a decreased abdominal girth (108 vs. 93 cm), decreased body weight (80 vs. 70 kg) and increased urinary flow (607 vs. 4,254 ml). All patients had previously failed to show substantial benefit with 7–124 days of medical therapy. The mean blood urea nitrogen value decreased from 39 to 23 mg/dl. Blendis et al. (Gastroenterology 73:1222, 1977) report similar findings but in addition noted that furosemide was necessary to initiate the diuresis. Blendis et al. also reported (1) increased cardiac output reflecting increased intravascular volume, (2) increased GFR and (3) decreased plasma renin and aldosterone levels after a LeVeen shunt. A few points bear special emphasis. First, patients receiving a LeVeen shunt mobilize large amounts of ascitic fluid, have a marked increase in intravascular volume and, indeed, may develop pulmonary edema. Second, it is often necessary to give intravenous furosemide to initiate a diuresis as well as prevent pulmonary congestion. Third, a LeVeen shunt alone may result in a marked decrease in plasma aldosterone levels without occurrence of a diuresis until a diuretic is given. –Ed.] ◄

Comparison of Lactulose and Neomycin in Treatment of Chronic Portal-Systemic Encephalopathy: Double-Blind Controlled Trial. The management of chronic, recurrent portal-systemic encephalopathy (PSE) is difficult and unsatisfactory. It consists primarily of restriction of dietary protein and antibiotic suppression of

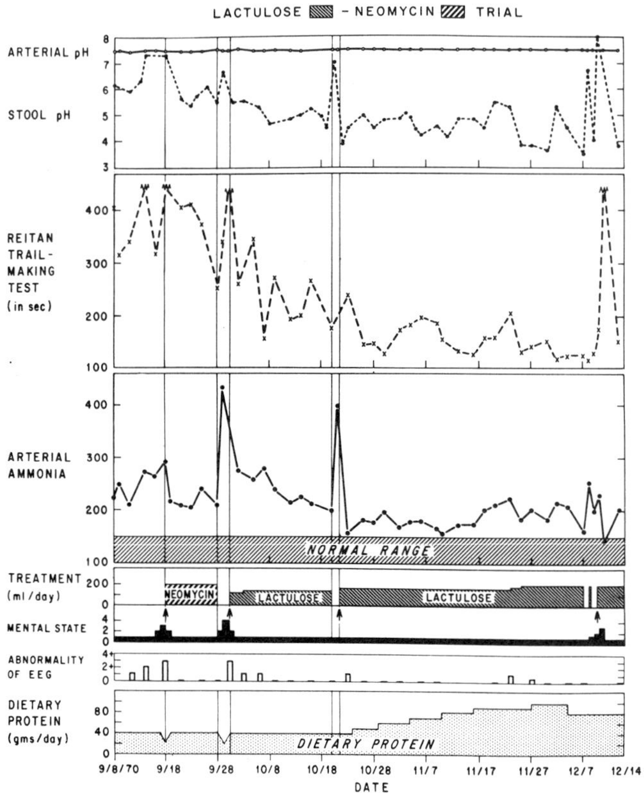

Fig 22.—Diagram of clinical and laboratory features of PSE of 1 patient during double-blind crossover study. During control period I *(9/8–9/18)* while on no therapy, the patient showed progressive deterioration in mental state, trailmaking test time, EEG and arterial ammonia concentration. During treatment period A *(9/18–9/28),* neomycin-sorbitol caused improvement in each of these parameters. Stool pH fell modestly. Control period II was abbreviated because of the rapid appearance of severe PSE after neomycin-sorbitol was stopped. The patient had deep coma, very slow ECG, marked hyperammonemia and inability to do the trailmaking test. During treatment period B *(9/30–10/20),* lactulose induced progressive return to normal of mental state, EEG, trailmaking test times and a large decrease in arterial ammonia levels. This was accompanied by a sharp and sustained fall in stool pH to approximately 5.0. Control period III lasted only 2 days during which stool pH returned to normal and all evidences of PSE began to recur. The double-blind study was terminated at this time. At this point investigation of the patient's dietary protein tolerance while on lactulose was begun. Throughout the 43 days of the double-blind study dietary protein had been kept constant at 40 gm per day. Lactulose was reinstituted *(10/22)* and the dietary protein increased by 10 gm per day at weekly intervals. The patient tolerated 80 gm of protein well, but at 90 gm daily the blood ammonia tended to increase and mild EEG abnormalities were noted. The patient was discharged on lactulose and normal dietary protein intake of 75 gm daily. (Courtesy of Conn, H. O., et al.: Gastroenterology 72:573–583, April, 1977.)

intestinal bacteria, usually by "nonabsorbable" antibiotics such as neomycin. Lactulose has been reported by a number of workers to be effective in treating nitrogenous PSE, but only a few studies have been objectively controlled and none has compared lactulose with neomycin in a controlled manner. H. O. Conn, C. M. Leevy, Z. R. Vlahcevic, J. B. Rodgers, W. C. Maddrey, L. Seeff and L. L. Levy[9] report a randomized

(9) Gastroenterology 72:573–583, April, 1977.

double-blind comparison of neomycin and lactulose in 33 cirrhotic patients with PSE at seven hospitals. Sorbitol syrup was used as a control solution along with neomycin. Twenty-nine patients participated in a crossover study after a 10-day control period. The dosage of neomycin was 1.5 gm 4 times daily. Liquid medications were started at 30 ml 3 times daily and adjusted to doses that induced two or three bowel movements daily. Dietary protein was kept at 40 gm daily.

Lactulose was effective in 15 of 18 patients (83%) and neomycin-sorbitol in 13 of 15 patients (87%) in the initial course of treatment. In the crossover comparison, lactulose was effective in 26 of 29 courses of therapy (90%) and neomycin-sorbitol in 24 of 29 (83%). In the crossover comparison, both treatments produced significant improvements in mental state, asterixis and EEG abnormality. Arterial ammonia levels were reduced more by lactulose therapy. Lactulose reduced the stool pH more dramatically than did neomycin-sorbitol. Both agents increased cathartic activity. Both were free from toxicity. Occasionally diarrhea occurred in the first few days of treatment. Several patients with severe encephalopathy tolerated large doses of lactulose or sorbitol poorly.

Lactulose is effective in the management of PSE. The course of 1 patient is shown in Figure 22. Neomycin is also effective in the treatment of chronic PSE. The medications act differently but, unfortunately, their mechanisms of actions appear to be mutually exclusive.

► [This controlled trial provides convincing evidence that neomycin-sorbitol and lactulose are both quite effective in the treatment of chronic portal systemic encephalopathy (PSE). Reported side effects with lactulose have generally been minor in nature and have included diarrhea, nausea and emesis. However, the cathartic response may be excessive and cause dehydration. In this regard, a case report (Ann. Intern. Med. 86: 745, 1977) documented severe hypernatremia (serum sodium = 175 mEq/L) after lactulose therapy and the patient required 6 L of fluid replacement therapy. This case illustrates that hypernatremia and dehydration may occur in situations where lactulose dosage is not excessive by published standards. – Ed.] ◄

► ↓ The following article illustrates an additional therapeutic approach to the patient with chronic PSE, namely, the use of a diet rich in vegetable rather than animal protein. – Ed. ◄

Effect of Vegetable and Animal Protein Diets in Chronic Hepatic Encephalopathy. There is considerable evidence that methionine and its intestinal breakdown products are important in the pathogenesis of hepatic encephalopathy. Norton J. Greenberger, James Carley, Steven Schenker, Irene Bettinger, Connie Stamnes and Pete Beyer[1] studied the effects of a vegetable protein diet (low in methionine) compared to an animal protein diet (high in methionine) on the clinical and laboratory parameters in patients with chronic hepatic encephalopathy.

Three patients with postnecrotic cirrhosis, status postportal systemic shunt and chronic recurrent hepatic encephalopathy were studied at the University of Kansas Medical Center and the Ohio State University Hospital. Diets containing vegetable or meat protein were given for 5 days after 2 days of equilibration. The diets were comparable in calo-

---

(1) Am. J. Dig. Dis. 22:845–855, October, 1977.

DIET THERAPY OF CHRONIC HEPATIC ENCEPHALOPATHY IN CASE 1

Date	Diet	Neomycin	Calories	Protein (g)	Methionine (mg)	CHO (g)	Encephalopathy indices: Asterixis (0–4+)	Fetor hepaticus (0–4+)	Arterial NH_3 ($\mu g/100\ ml$)	Reitan test (sec)	EEG 0–20 points	Confusion, disorientation	Stage (0–4)	Hepatic encephalopathy (points)
5/74	Vegetable*	(−)	2474	24	295	496	0 (0)†	1+ (3)	184 176 (6)	15 18 (0)	4 8 (4)	0	0 (0)	13
	Animal	(−)	2509	26	615	509	1+ (5)	1+ (3)	180 237 (12)	14 14 (0)	3 3 (2)	0	0 0 (0)	22
6/74	Animal	(−)	2935	63	1562	496	1+ (5)	1+ (3)	179 (6)	10–11 (0)	7 (4)	0	0 (0)	18
	Vegetable	(−)	3240	58	698	568	0 (0)	1+ (3)	133 (3)	12–12 (0)	7 (4)	0	0	10
9/74	Vegetable	(−)	2328	43	566	433	0 (0)	1+ (3)	194 (9)	14 (0)	8 (4)	0	0 0	16
	Animal	(−)	2429	45	1118	450	1+ (5)	1–2+ (3)	257 308 (15)	14 21 (5)	8 (4)	+	1+ (2)	34

*Randomized diet period.
†Numbers in parentheses refer to calculations used in tabulating the hepatic encephalopathy index.

ries, fat, carbohydrate and total protein content. The methionine content and amino acid composition of each diet were calculated daily.

In the 3 patients, liver function tests did not change much with the different diets. The vegetable protein diet resulted in lower hepatic encephalopathy index scores and reduced arterial ammonia levels in the first patient, a man aged 33 years (table). The second patient, a man aged 34 years, remained stable on the vegetable protein diet, deteriorated markedly on the meat protein diet and returned to baseline condition when the vegetable protein diet was repeated. In the third patient, a woman aged 62 years, both the vegetable protein diet and lactulose were effective in modifying the course of encephalopathy, and the beneficial effects of the two were additive.

A vegetable protein diet resulted in clinical improvement, improved performance on intellectual tasks and, in 1 case, improved protein tolerance in this study of patients with postnecrotic cirrhosis and chronic hepatic encephalopathy. The beneficial effects are not clearly understood, but probably the vegetable protein diet contains lower amounts of amino acids and other putative materials that may be important in the pathogenesis of hepatic encephalopathy. The data are encouraging enough to recommend that further controlled trials of a vegetable protein diet be carried out, both with and without lactulose, in patients with chronic recurrent hepatic encephalopathy.

► [Two recent studies suggest that subclinical portal systemic encephalopathy (PSE) is fairly common in cirrhotics, especially after portacaval shunt (Digestion 14:548, 1976; and Gastroenterology 72:1119, 1977). In the first study, two thirds of cirrhotic patients with portal hypertension without clinical evidence of PSE had impairment of cerebral function on psychometric testing. In the second study, 30 cirrhotic patients 35 ± 14 months (mean ± 1 standard deviation) after portosystemic shunt surgery were evaluated while on the 40-gm protein diet and compared to 14 normal subjects without liver disease. The metabolic and neuropsychologic evaluation included ammonia tolerance tests, antipyrine clearance, detailed neurologic and mental status examination, EEG and several quantitative psychometric tests. Approximately one third of the patients without obvious clinical evidence of PSE had impairment of cerebral function. These studies indicate that occult PSE is more common than generally is appreciated. – Ed.] ◄

The Biliary Tract

Biliary Lipid Secretion in Cholesterol Gallstone Disease: Effect of Cholecystectomy and Obesity. Eldon A. Shaffer (McGill Univ.) and Donald M. Small[2] (Boston Univ.) investigated the factors regulating bile composition and the effects of cholecystectomy by measuring bile salt pool size and biliary lipid secretion rates simultaneously in control subjects, patients with pigment stones, nonobese patients with cholesterol gallstones and very obese subjects without radiologic evidence of gallstones. The control groups consisted of 14 subjects without hepatobiliary disease and 12 patients with pigment stone disease, 6 of whom were studied before and 6 after cholecystectomy. There were 10 nonobese patients with cholesterol gallstones and

Fig 23.—Mean biliary lipid secretion (±SEM) before and after cholecystectomy. Bile salt and phospholipid secretion rates significantly ($P < 0.01$) increased after cholecystectomy in the nonobese patients with cholesterol gallstones. Bile salt secretion also increased in the extremely obese patients ($P < 0.01$), but the increase was not significant in patients with pigment stones. Cholesterol secretion was not affected by cholecystectomy. (Courtesy of Shaffer, E. A., and Small, D. M.: J. Clin. Invest. 59:828–840, May, 1977.)

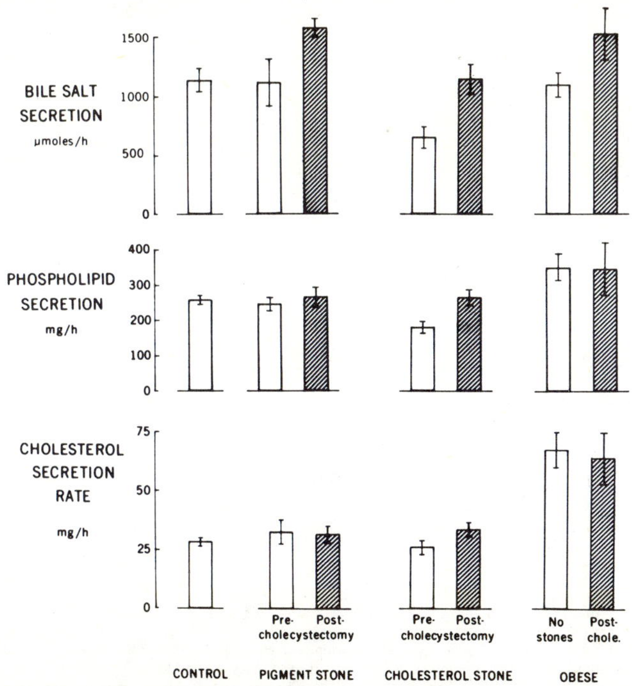

(2) J. Clin. Invest. 59:828–840, May, 1977.

13 other patients who had had cholecystectomy. Seven obese patients did not have gallstones, whereas 4 had had cholecystectomy for cholesterol stone disease. An Indian woman with cholesterol stones was evaluated before and after surgery. Bile salt pool size was estimated with the use of 2,4-^{3}H-cholic acid and 24-^{14}C-chenodeoxycholic acid.

Obese subjects without stones had the highest molar percentage cholesterol in gallbladder bile, whereas pigment stone patients had the lowest relative concentration. Both obese and nonobese patients with cholesterol stones produced an abnormal hepatic bile with excess cholesterol relative to the solubilizing agents, bile salts and phospholipids. Two different secretory mechanisms were found to be responsible for the abnormal bile in patients with cholesterol stones. Nonobese patients with cholesterol gallstones had a significantly reduced bile salt and phospholipid secretion compared with the controls. Cholesterol secretion was strikingly elevated in grossly obese subjects without gallstones. The effects of cholecystectomy on biliary lipid secretion rates are shown in Figure 23, and the size of the circulating bile salt pool is given in the table. The cycling frequency more than doubled after cholecystectomy in both gallstone groups and also in the obese patients. The relationship between hepatic bile salt secretion and that of cholesterol and phospholipid is shown in Figure 24. All groups showed improvement in biliary lipid composition after cholecystectomy but this was significant only in nonobese patients with cholesterol stones.

Bile salt and phospholipid secretion rates are both reduced in non-

EFFECT OF CHOLECYSTECTOMY ON MEAN BILE SALT SECRETION, POOL SIZE AND CYCLING FREQUENCY

Patient	No.	Bile salt secretion		Bile salt pool size		Cycling frequency
		μmol/h	*μmol/kg-h*	*mmol*	*μmol/kg*	*fraction cycled/h*
Subjects without hepatobiliary disease	11	1,246	17.7	6.48*	92.1	0.19
Pigment stone patients	4	1,219	19.3	7.03	111.8	0.17
Pigment stone patients after cholecystectomy	5	1,628	24.0	4.58‡	67.5	0.36§
Nonobese cholesterol stone patients	5	660	6.6	4.52	54.7	0.12
Nonobese cholesterol stone patients after cholecystectomy	12	1,149	16.9	3.64*	52.8	0.32§
Obese subjects without gallstones	7	987	7.5	7.07	53.1	0.14
Obese cholesterol stone patients after cholecystectomy	4	1,528	14.2	4.88‡	45.1	0.32§

*Group t test comparison that nonobese cholesterol stone patients had a significantly ($P < 0.05$) smaller bile salt pool than subjects without hepatobiliary disease.

‡Group t test comparison of bile salt pool size in pigment stone and obese patients with cholesterol gallstones showed a significant ($P < 0.05$) reduction in each group after cholecystectomy.

§Group t test comparison of cycling frequency in all three groups demonstrated a significant ($P < 0.05$) increase after surgery.

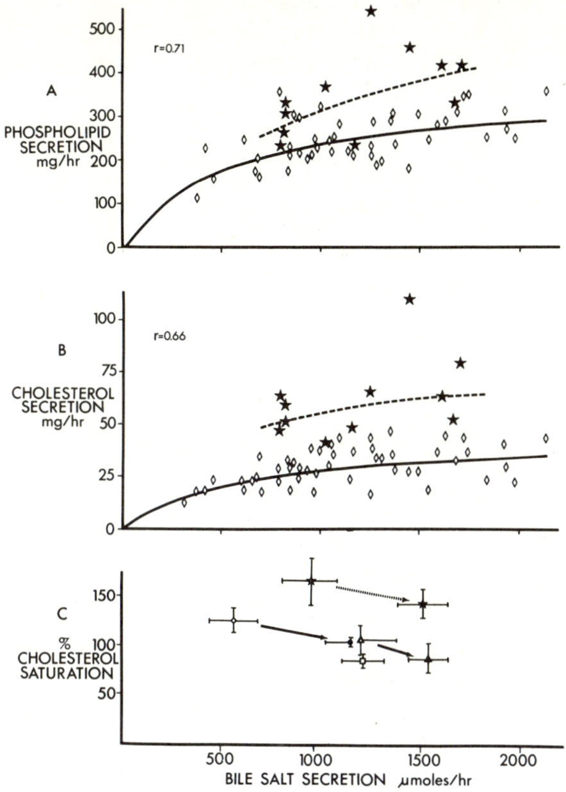

Fig 24.—Interrelations between bile salt and biliary lipid secretion; the effect of cholecystectomy. Comparison of hepatic secretion of bile salts to that of phospholipid and cholesterol is shown respectively in *A* and *B*. Data points represent individual secretory rates for all studies. The 11 extremely obese patients are depicted by stars with a dashed line. All others are represented by diamonds; the *r* values shown have been calculated for the corresponding solid regression lines. The nonlinear regression used was in the form $\gamma = x/(a + bx)$. In these nonobese subjects, a curvilinear relation was found between bile salt secretion and both phospholipid and cholesterol secretion. The rates of secretion were quantitatively different in the patients with morbid obesity, with higher phospholipid and especially cholesterol secretion. In *C*, the percent cholesterol saturation in bile is plotted against the bile salt secretion rate for each patient group. Mean values ±SEM are shown as open symbols for patients with functioning gallbladders and as closed symbols for patients after cholecystectomy. The respective groups are joined by arrows. Stars represent obese patients; circles, nonobese cholesterol gallstone patients; triangles, pigment stone patients; and squares, nonstone control subjects. The percent saturation was calculated by using the maximum cholesterol solubility in systems with 3.5% solid, which is the total concentration for the three components in hepatic bile. An inverse relation existed between bile salt secretion rate and cholesterol saturation. The obese patients, however, formed more saturated bile at any given rate of bile salt secretion. Cholecystectomy in all groups resulted in higher bile salt secretion rates and hence less saturated bile. (Courtesy of Shaffer, E. A., and Small, D. M.: J. Clin. Invest. 59:828–840, May, 1977.)

obese patients with cholesterol gallstones, whereas grossly obese subjects have increased cholesterol secretion. Cholecystectomy increases bile salt and phospholipid secretion in nonobese patients with cholesterol stones, but cholesterol secretion is unaffected by surgery. The improvement in bile composition after cholecystectomy is due to more rapid cycling of the pool around enterohepatic circulation. The defect causing lithogenic bile formation is ameliorated but not eliminated by cholecystectomy.

► [This article provides important new insights into the pathogenesis of cholesterol gallstone disease and the effect of cholecystectomy. It should be read in its entirety. In initiating these studies, the authors posed three questions. (1) What were the mechanisms for cholesterol gallstone disease in normal nonobese whites? (2) How did obese patients differ? (3) What were the effects of the standard surgical treatment, i.e., cholecystectomy? The last question is important because previous studies had suggested that removal of the gallbladder caused bile to revert to a more normal composition. There are conflicting data, however, as to whether the more normal composition of bile postcholecystectomy is due to an expanded bile salt pool or to more rapid recycling of bile salts, hence the authors' interest in this question.

I think it would be useful to briefly summarize the major findings in this article. (1) Whereas all patients with cholesterol gallstones form bile containing a relative excess of cholesterol, the mechanisms in *nonobese* and *obese* patients are different. (2) The basic secretory defect in nonobese patients is not excess cholesterol secretion but rather *decreased bile salt and phospholipid secretion.* (3) Conversely, in grossly obese subjects with very adnormal bile, *cholesterol secretion is greatly increased* without any absolute reduction in bile salt or phospholipid secretion. (4) The low bile salt pool previously reported in most gallstone patients is confirmed, but it is found only in nonobese patients. (5) After cholecystectomy, biliary lipid composition distinctly improves. (6) The improvement occurs despite the fact that the bile salt pool remains small because it cycles more frequently around the enterohepatic circulation to increase bile salt secretion. In essence, increased cycling offsets the reduction in pool size. – Ed.] ◄

Changes in Bile Lipids Accompanying Oophorectomy in a Premenopausal Woman. Several observations suggest that ovarian secretions may influence formation of gallstones. Lynn J. Bennion[3] (Natl. Inst. of Arthritis, Metabolism and Digestive Dis., Phoenix, Ariz.) observed changes in bile lipids in a premenopausal woman who underwent bilateral oophorectomy.

Woman, 36, a Pima Indian, was admitted as a volunteer for study of the effects of obesity on biliary lipids. There was a family history of gallstones, but oral cholecystography was negative. The patient was in good health apart from chronic obesity and secondary amenorrhea. The menses had been irregular and scanty since massive weight gain in the middle 20s, and no vaginal bleeding had occurred in the 6 months before admission. An endometrial biopsy showed early adenocarcinoma. A 5-day course of medroxyprogesterone was followed by vaginal bleeding. Radical hysterectomy with bilateral oophorecto-

EFFECT OF CASTRATION ON LIPID COMPOSITION OF GALLBLADDER BILE IN A PREMENOPAUSAL WOMAN

TIME OF STUDY*	LIPID COMPOSITION			CHOLESTEROL SATURATION	
	CHOLESTEROL	BILE ACIDS	PHOSPHOLIPIDS	METHOD I*	METHOD II†
	molar %			%	
Before oophorectomy	7.0	69.9	23.2	100	70
After oophorectomy	4.8	76.4	18.8	81	49

*Method of Hegardt and Dam (1971) and Holzbach et al. (1973).
†Method of Admirand and Small (1968).

(3) N. Engl. J. Med. 297:709–711, Sept. 29, 1977.

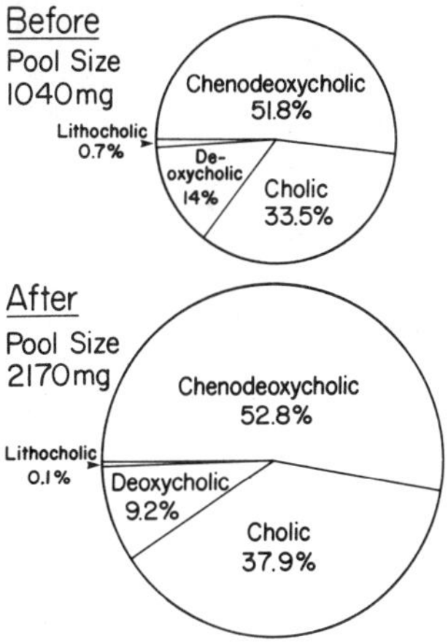

Fig 25.—Expansion of the total pool of bile acids accompanying oophorectomy in a premenopausal woman. (Courtesy of Bennion, L. J.: N. Engl. J. Med. 297:709–711, Sept. 29, 1977.)

my and para-aortic lymph node dissection was carried out. Only early myometrial invasion was reported. Typical menopausal symptoms began postoperatively and lasted several months. There was no evidence of recurrence of malignancy 30 months after operation.

Studies on the bile acid composition and pool size and gallbladder bile lipid composition were done with radiolabeled cholic acid 2 months before and 3 months after oophorectomy. The effects of castration on the lipid composition of gallbladder bile are shown in the table, and changes in bile acid composition and pool size are outlined in Figure 25. The percent saturation of cholesterol in gallbladder bile decreased after oophorectomy. The findings suggest that endogenous ovarian hormones may influence the propensity to gallstone formation in a manner similar to that of exogenous estrogens and progestins. The patient had an abnormal menstrual history and bile cholesterol saturation unusually low for someone so obese. Nevertheless, her response to oophorectomy suggests that ovarian function affects bile acid pool size and bile composition in a way favoring cholesterol gallstone formation.

It appears that presence of functioning ovaries is associated with a smaller bile acid pool and a more lithogenic bile composition. Changes in hormone levels during the normal menstrual cycle may be too rapid and the effects of ovarian hormones on the bile too slow to develop or dissipate for bile composition to reflect the cyclic variations in hormone levels.

► [Women are more likely to develop cholesterol gallstones than men, and there is considerable evidence suggesting that this sex-related difference is partly due to sex hormones. For example, oral contraceptives and pregnancy predispose to gallstones. Blood concentrations of estrogen and progesterone fluctuate considerably during the menstrual cycle. Low-Beer et al. (Br. Med. J. 1:1568, 1977) questioned whether bile cholesterol saturation and consequently the risk of forming gallstones might also fluctuate during the normal menstrual cycle. Accordingly, they measured fasting serum and bile lipid concentrations at three intervals during the normal menstrual cycles of 11 healthy women not taking oral contraceptives. In 9 of them cholesterol saturation of bile was higher 9 days after midcycle than at the end of menstruation; the average saturation index of bile was 18% greater, i.e., 0.83 vs. 0.98. In 4 of 11 women, bile was supersaturated with cholesterol, the saturation index being greater then 1.0. The change in bile cholesterol saturation was preceded by a significant fall in serum lipid concentrations. These changes are presumably due to a direct effect of sex hormones on the liver. In view of these findings, Low-Beer et al. recommend that in any stuides requiring measurements of bile lipid concentrations in women of childbearing age, samples should be taken at standard points in the menstrual cycle. — Ed.] ◄

Gallbladder Disease as Side Effect of Drugs Influencing Lipid Metabolism: Experience in The Coronary Drug Project. The Coronary Drug Project Research Group[4] began a study of gallbladder disease in 1971 when experiments showed that clofibrate elevates biliary cholesterol saturation in postcholecystectomy patients. A total of 8,341 patients were recruited at 53 units over a 3½-year period. All were men aged 30 – 64 years and had had a documented myocardial infarction in the preceding 3 months. Groups of subjects received daily dosages of 2.5 or 5 mg estrogen, 1.8 gm clofibrate, 6.0 gm dextrothyroxine and 3.0 gm nicotinic acid; however, the only ones completing the original protocol were those on placebo, nicotinic acid and clofibrate. A study of aspirin was initiated in 1972 – 74 in 1,529 surviving patients whose treatment had been discontinued.

Incidence rates of cholecystitis and cholelithiasis are given in the table. Rates were highest in the patients given clofibrate and estrogen in both dosages. Nicotinic acid-treated patients had more, and dextrothyroxine-treated patients less, gallbladder disease than the placebo group, but the differences were no significant. The findings for both estrogen groups and the clofibrate group are significant at the 5% level. The only baseline variable that appeared to correlate with the incidence of newly diagnosed gallbladder disease was the serum triglyceride.

The finding that clofibrate predisposes to the appearance of gallbladder disease is consistent with several other studies. It now appears that a medical alternative to cholecystectomy may soon be generally available and that it will be most efficacious in the treatment of patients in whom cholesterol gallstone disease is discovered early. For this reason, the identification of high-risk groups will probably become important. The present inability to identify any baseline risk factors that were important determinants of the subsequent likelihood of the development of manifest gallbladder disease, despite a total of over 39,000 man-years of observation, is disappointing. A search for new, important risk factors in gallbladder disease, at least among men, will apparently have to focus on characteristics not measured in the Coronary Drug Project.

These studies indicate that gallstone formation is a risk whenever clofibrate or estrogen is prescribed.

► [Increasing numbers of drugs have been implicated in the development of cholesterol gallstone disease. For the most part, these drugs cause increased cholesterol saturation in bile and hence increase the "lithogenic index" (1976 YEAR BOOK, pp. 500 – 503). The evidence is fairly convincing for agents such as estrogens, conjugated equine estrogens, oral contraceptives and clofibrate. Grundy et al. (J. Lipid Res. 13: 531, 1972) showed that clofibrate increases the secretion of cholesterol into bile, and Pertsemlidis and his associates (Gastroenterology 66:565, 1974) demonstrated an increased saturation of bile with cholesterol after clofibrate administration and predicted that the drug would be lithogenic. — Ed.] ◄

(4) N. Engl. J. Med. 296:1185 – 1190, May 26, 1977.

Incidence of Definite Cholecystitis or Cholelithiasis

Treatment	Estrogen 2.5 mg	Estrogen 5.0 mg	Clofibrate	Dextro-thyroxine	Nicotinic Acid	Placebo
Total no. at risk of development of new, definite cholecystitis or cholelithiasis	1061	1081	1051	1057	1069	2680
No. of patients with new, definite cholecystitis or cholelithiasis:						
Total for 1st 6 yr of follow-up study (% incidence in parentheses)	46 (4.3)	47 (4.3)	42 (4.0)	23 (2.2)	35 (3.3)	69 (2.6)
No. for each yr of follow-up period (no. of patient-yr of exposure to risk in parentheses):						
Year 1	10 (1024)	12 (1049)	11 (1024)	6 (1024)	9 (1040)	13 (2606)
Year 2	10 (962)	8 (990)	10 (972)	5 (959)	8 (979)	14 (2465)
Year 3	9 (911)	8 (940)	6 (927)	2 (906)	6 (936)	18 (2351)
Year 4	5 (867)	9 (882)	7 (876)	7 (853)	9 (890)	10 (2233)
Year 5	4 (820)	5 (824)	5 (822)	1 (808)	3 (837)	9 (2100)
Year 6	8 (595)	5 (585)	3 (589)	2 (596)	0 (589)	5 (1488)
No. of patients in whom new disease was detected only at autopsy (total no. of autopsies performed in parentheses)	8 (106)	9 (93)	7 (88)	3 (85)	7 (69)	12 (244)

Speed of Change in Biliary Lipids and Bile Acids with Chenodeoxycholic Acid: Is Intermittent Therapy Feasible? Oral chenodeoxycholic acid (CDCA) will dissolve most radiolucent gallstones by reducing the secretion of cholesterol into bile but the time course of unsaturation of the bile with cholesterol is unclear. J. H. Iser, G. M. Murphy and R. Hermon Dowling[5] (Guy's Hosp., London) studied the changes in bile lipid composition occurring in conjunction with CDCA therapy in 5 women and 1 man with lucent gallstones in functioning gallbladders. Their mean age was 56.7. Duodenal fluid was collected after an overnight fast after the intravenous injection of cholecystokinin and during treatment with 13–15 mg CDCA per kg daily. Six women with a mean age of 55.8 whose stones had dissolved after an average of 19 months of treatment with a mean dose of 14.2 mg CDCA/kg daily were studied when the agent was withdrawn.

Bile cholesterol saturation values are given in Figure 26. The mean time needed for the bile to become unsaturated after starting oral CDCA was 12 days, but the pattern varied in individual patients. The mean saturation index increased rapidly after cessation of therapy from 0.74 ± 0.10 to 1.15 ± 0.15 by days 6–8, and the mean time at which the bile became saturated was 12.0 ± 5.5 days (Fig 27). There were statistically significant inverse relationships between saturation indices and percentages of conjugated CDCA in biliary bile acids for patients both starting and stopping CDCA. Generally the bile became unsaturated with cholesterol when the percentage of CDCA exceeded 70%. Significant relationships were also found between saturation indices and the percentages of both cholic and deoxycholic acids.

Fig 26.—Individual results of the biliary cholesterol saturation index in 6 gallstone patients before treatment (day 0) and at frequent intervals during the next 47 days after starting CDCA; 1.0 represents a saturated solution. (Courtesy of Iser, J. H., et al.: Gut 18:7–15, January, 1977.)

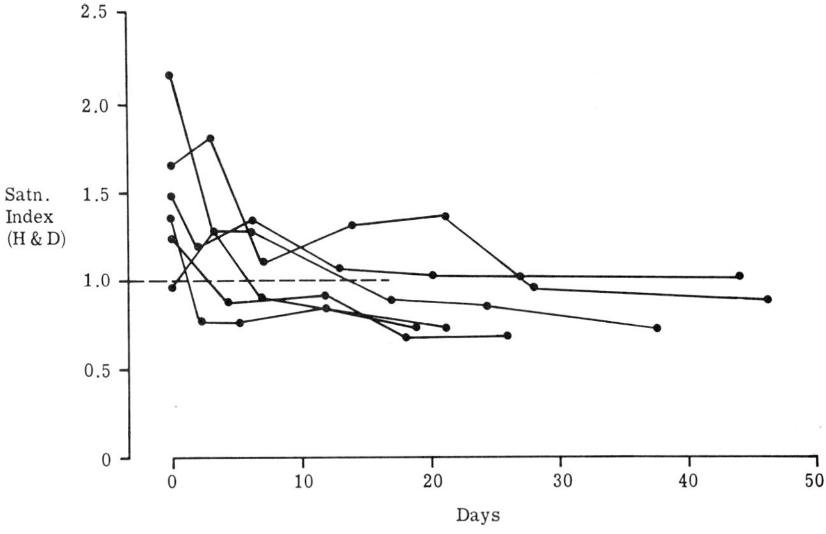

(5) Gut 18:7–15, January, 1977.

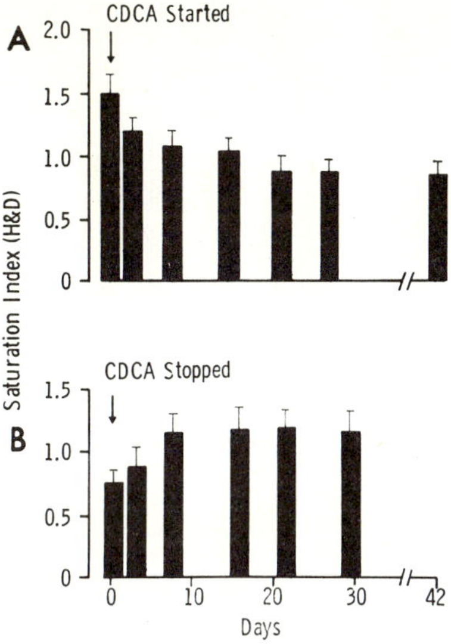

Fig 27.—Overall results of the biliary cholesterol saturation index (means ± SEMs) in patients starting (*A;* data from Fig 26 grouped into different time periods) and stopping (*B*) CDCA. (Courtesy of Iser, J. H., et al.: Gut 18:7–15, January, 1977.)

From 1 to 4 weeks of CDCA therapy are needed to produce an unsaturated bile with the potential for dissolving gallstones. However, on stopping therapy, bile reverts to its supersaturated state in 1–3 weeks. Since the mean time taken for bile to become unsaturated was not shorter than the time taken for bile to revert to its supersaturated state, it seems that intermittent treatment would not be adequate to maintain an unsaturated bile and is, therefore, unlikely to be as effective as continuous treatment in dissolving gallstones.

► [Dowling and his associates have presented additional information on the efficacy of withdrawal from and resistance to chenodeoxycholic acid (CDCA) treatment in patients with gallstones (Gut 18:A976, 1977). Of 135 gallstone patients accepted for treatment, 116 have radiolucent stones and a functioning gallbladder. In those 40 with stones < 15 mm in diameter treated for 1 year with CDCA in a dosage of ≥ 13 mg/kg body weight and who achieved unsaturated bile, complete gallstone dissolution occurred in 65% and complete or partial dissolution in 93%. Of 44 patients stopping CDCA, 9 defaulted in less than 1 month, 14 stopped in less than 1 year, 7 had stones > 15 mm in diameter, 7 took < 13 mg CDCA per kg body weight, 6 developed nonopacifying gallbladders, 4 developed biliary colic or pancreatitis or both, 3 had noncholesterol stones or debris and 1 took clofibrate (which causes supersaturated bile). Thus few patients stopped treatment because of CDCA failure per se. Failure to achieve unsaturated bile despite CDCA treatment in a dosage of 13–15 mg/kg body weight occurred in 19 patients, including 8 obese patients who ultimately achieved unsaturated bile with increased CDCA dosage (18.6 ± 1.4 mg/kg). Two obese and 4 nonobese subjects had supersaturated bile despite 19–22 mg CDCA/kg and > 70% CDCA in biliary bile acids. The mechanism of CDCA "resistance" in these patients is unknown, but results in 1 patient suggest excess hepatic cholesterogenesis.—Ed.] ◄

Dissolution of Cholesterol Gallstones by Ursodeoxycholic Acid. Dissolution of cholesterol gallstones in man by chenodeoxycholic acid (CDCA) has been confirmed, and evidence for the safety of CDCA in man is increasing, Shoichi Nakagawa, Isao Makino, Takashi Ishizaki (Hokkaido Univ.) and Ichiro Dohi[6] (Tokyo) report results of a dou-

(6) Lancet 2:367–369, Aug. 20, 1977.

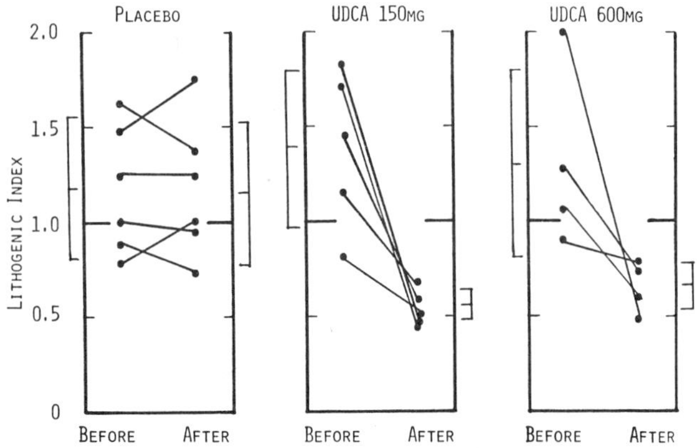

Fig 28. – Changes in lithogenic index in fasting-state bile before and after treatment with UDCA. Statistical evaluation of index: Placebo vs. UDCA, 150 or 600 mg, NS before treatment and P < 0.05 after treatment; UDCA, 150 mg, vs. UDCA, 600 mg, NS both before and after treatment. Ranges alongside vertical scales represent means ±SD. (Courtesy of Nakagawa, S., et al.: Lancet 2:367–369, Aug. 20, 1977.)

ble-blind clinical trial of ursodeoxycholic acid (UDCA), the 7-beta epimer of CDCA, which also has been found to produce gallstone dissolution.

The subjects were 34 women and 21 men with a mean age of 46 years who had radiolucent gallstones. None had had frequent attacks of biliary colic or laboratory findings of obstructive hepatic dysfunction. Patients were assigned to one of three treatment groups: (1) UDCA, 150 mg/day; (2) UDCA, 600 mg/day; (3) a lactose placebo. Medication was taken 3 times a day, orally. Treatment was given for at least 6 months to 44 patients. Gallstone size was assessed by cholecystography.

Gallstones decreased in size in 6 of 16 patients taking 150 mg UDCA daily and in 2 of 15 taking 600 mg daily. No change was noted in the 13 placebo-treated patients. Stones disappeared in 3 patients given the lower dose and in 2 given the higher dose of UDCA. No patient with stones over 10 mm in diameter responded. The minimum dose of UDCA in patients in whom the drug was effective was 2.8 mg/kg/day. Changes in cholesterol saturation of the bile (lithogenic index) in the 15 patients studied are shown in Figure 28. In the UDCA-treated patients no increase in serum enzymes was noted, and blood cholesterol levels were unchanged. The serum triglyceride fell by about 20% in both actively treated groups. No patient had diarrhea during treatment with UDCA.

These findings indicate that UDCA is potent and apparently safe in the dissolution of gallstones. Further studies are needed to compare UDCA with CDCA and to determine the optimal dose; in this study, UDCA appears to be more potent in dissolving gallstones in low doses, and bile became unsaturated in treated patients. It appears that UDCA itself could contribute to the reduced hepatic secretion of cholesterol. While CDCA induces epithelial cell loss, fluid and electrolyte secretion and increased mucosal permeability when perfused into the human colon, these effects have not been observed with UDCA.

► [Ursodeoxycholic acid (UDCA) has been reported to be effective in dissolving gallstones in man. It differs in structure from chenodeoxycholic acid (CDCA) only in the orientation of the hydroxyl group at C-7. There are several theoretical reasons suggesting that UDCA might be a safer gallstone-dissolving agent in man than CDCA.

First, rhesus monkeys treated with UDCA do not develop severe liver damage, whereas treatment with comparable doses of CDCA causes severe hepatoxicity. The absence of hepatoxicity with UDCA can be correlated with low levels of biliary lithocholic acid whereas treatment with CDCA causes high levels of biliary lithocholic acid. It is currently believed that hepatic damage does not occur in human beings after CDCA treatment because the resultant lithocholate formed is sulfated and excreted in the urine. By contrast, monkeys do not effectively sulfate and excrete lithocholate in the urine, and the resultant high biliary lithocholate levels are believed to cause hepatic damage. Although there have been no reports to date of CDCA-associated hepatoxicity in man, there is the possibility that certain subjects will be unable to sulfate the lithocholate and this may lead to increased susceptibility to hepatic toxicity.

The second potential advantage of UDCA concerns the dose administered to man. Presently, 750–1,000 mg CDCA per day is recommended for gallstone dissolution. In part, this high dose of CDCA is necessary because a portion is degraded to lithocholate, thus reducing the circulating pool of CDCA. When UDCA is administered, apparently less bacterial degradation occurs and a smaller dose of this bile may be as effective in maintaining its enterohepatic pool (Gastroenterology 74:81, 1978). Maton et al. (Lancet 2:1297, 1977) administered UDCA to 11 nonobese patients with radiolucent gallstones in dosages of 5 mg, 10 mg and 15 mg/kg body weight for 6 weeks each. It was found that UDCA reduced hepatic hydroxymethylglutaryl-CoA reductase activity, decreased bile cholesterol saturation and dissolved cholesterol gallstones at one half to two thirds the dose of CDCA. This study confirmed other potential advantages of UDCA over CDCA, namely, absence of diarrhea and hypertransaminasemia. – Ed.] ◄

Endoscopic Papillotomy. H. Koch, W. Rösch, O. Schaffner and L. Demling[7] (Erlangen, West Germany) report experience with 267 attempts at endoscopic papillotomy in treatment of patients with common bile duct obstruction. A special cannula was used to divide the sphincter muscles of Vater's segment by electrocautery with a radiofrequency current in order to permit passage or extraction of common duct stones or to open a stenosed distal segment of duct.

In all patients, choledocholithiasis or papillary stenosis was established by previous endoscopic retrograde cholangiopancreatography. In 143 patients, surgical treatment of choledocholithiasis was considered to carry a high risk because of advanced age or associated disease. Sixty-nine other patients had either retained or re-formed common duct calculi after cholecystectomy. Forty-two patients had circumscribed papillary stenosis; 10 also had calculi in the common duct and gallbladder.

Endoscopic papillotomy was accomplished with the high-frequency diathermy probe developed by Demling and Classen. An incision of 1–2 cm was made in the duodenal wall. A Dormia basket was used to extract small calculi. Endoscopic follow-up was carried out after 3–7 days.

Endoscopic papillotomy was successful in 254 patients. Calculi were passed spontaneously by 108 of 122 patients with choledocholithiasis after endoscopic papillotomy. Calculi were extracted in 84 cases, and large calculi were removed surgically in 12 cases. In 18 patients, calcu-

(7) Gastroenterology 73:1393–1396, December, 1977.

li remained in the common bile duct. There were 7 episodes of slight and 2 of severe pancreatitis; all these patients recovered. Five of 7 patients with significant bleeding and 2 with duodenal perforation required operation. One patient with bleeding died 3 days after operation.

None of 107 patients reexamined 1 year after endoscopic papillotomy had evidence of late colangitis. Restenosis was found in 2 patients treated for papillary stenosis. Incomplete endoscopic papillotomy was probably responsible in 1 case; in the other, a papillary carcinoma had been mistaken for adenomyomatosis on biopsy.

The morbidity from endoscopic papillotomy is low, whereas mortality from repeated operations on the common duct is substantial. Endoscopic papillotomy appears to be the procedure of choice for patients at high risk from surgery and those having had previous biliary tract surgery.

► [Endoscopic papillotomy done by experienced operators is an acceptable alternative to surgery in the treatment of retained common bile duct stones in high-risk patients. As experience accumulates, it is anticipated that the complication rate, which is still appreciable, will decrease. In a study comparable to that of Koch et al., Safrany (Gastroenterology 72:338, 1977) attempted duodenoscopic sphincterotomy in 265 patients. The procedure was successful in 243 patients (92%). Indications for sphincterotomy were: 185 patients with choledocholithiasis, 52 patients with papillary stenosis and 6 patients with ampillary carcinoma. The clinical and biochemical evidence of cholestasis resolved in 222 of the 243 patients in whom the procedure was successful. Complications consisting of hemorrhage, perforation, pancreatitis, cholangitis and instrumental injury occurred in 24 patients (10%), resulting in emergency laparotomy in 6 (2.5%) and death in 3 (1.2%). Thus, duodenoscopic sphincterotomy is a fairly safe and effective means of relieving certain types of extrahepatic cholestasis. General anesthesia, laparotomy, duodenotomy, choledocholithotomy and prolonged immobilization are avoided. – Ed.] ◄

The Pancreas

Influence of Amylase Assay Technique on Renal Clearance of Amylase-Creatinine Ratio. The ratio of renal clearance of amylase to creatinine (C_{Am}-C_{Cr}) has been widely used to diagnose acute pancreatitis. Michael D. Levitt, Steven G. Johnson, Carol J. Ellis and Rolf R. Engel[8] (Univ. of Minnesota Hosp., Minneapolis) present evidence that several commonly used amylase assay techniques do not measure amylase activity in serum and urine with equal efficiency and that C_{Am}-C_{Cr} may vary markedly depending on the technique used to measure amylase.

Simultaneously collected serum and urine specimens from 10 normal subjects and 7 patients with typical attacks of acute pancreatitis were analyzed by three techniques: a saccharogenic method, and iodometric technique and a commercial chromogenic method. Recovery of added amylase in serum and urine was measured with use of samples from premature infants.

The C_{Am}-C_{Cr} calculated from the saccharogenic assay was over twice that obtained with the standard chromogenic technique; the iodometric method yielded intermediate values (table). With one exception, each technique distinguished the high ratio of patients with pancreatitis from the normal range for that technique (Fig 29). Recovery studies indicated that the amylase activity measured in urine and saline averaged only about 40% of that in serum with the chromogenic technique. Observed amylase recovery increased with addition of increasing amounts of human serum albumin to urine or saline. Amylase recovery with the iodometric method was also unequal in urine and serum. No significant increase occurred with addition of albumin.

Results of C_{Am}-C_{Cr} measurements in normal subjects vary with the technique used for amylase assay. Erroneous measurements may also result from inaccurate assessment of serum and urine creatinine val-

EFFECT OF AMYLASE ASSAY TECHNIQUE ON CALCULATED C_{Am}-C_{Cr} OF NORMAL SUBJECTS AND OF A PATIENT WITH ACUTE PANCREATITIS

Subjects	Clearance amylase/clearance creatinine (%)		
	Saccharogenic	Chromogenic	Iodometric
		Mean ± *1* SEM	
Normal (10)[a]	2.19 ± 0.18	0.80 ± 0.08	1.52 ± 0.21
Acute pancreatitis (11)	6.57 ± 0.82	2.94 ± 0.23	5.18 ± 0.72

[a]Figures in parentheses indicate number of C_{Am}-C_{Cr} measurements.

(8) Gastroenterology 72:1260–1263, June, 1977.

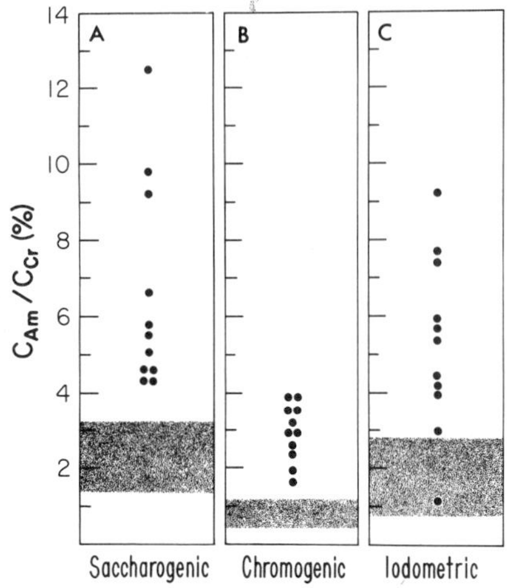

Fig 29.—C_{Am}-C_{Cr} of patients with acute pancreatitis determined by saccharogenic (**A**), chromogenic (**B**) and iodometric (**C**) assays. Shaded area represents mean ±2 SD of normal subjects for each assay technique. (Courtesy of Levitt, M. D., et al.: Gastroenterology 72:1260–1263, June, 1977.)

ues. High levels of ketone bodies falsely elevate the measured creatinine concentration of serum and urine. Accurate clinical interpretation of C_{Am}-C_{Cr} measurements requires knowledge of the amylase assay technique used.

► [These findings provide an explanation for some of the divergent data in the literature on the specificity and sensitivity of the ratio of renal clearance of amylase-creatinine (C_{Am}/C_{Cr}). Levitt et al. clearly demonstrate that C_{Am}/C_{Cr} may vary widely depending on the technique used to measure amylase. Accurate clinical interpretation of the C_{Am}/C_{Cr} measurement requires knowledge of the amylase assay technique used. Such data have not always been included in reports on increased C_{Am}/C_{Cr} in disorders other than acute pancreatitis. In this connection, an elevated C_{Am}/C_{Cr} has been reported in diabetic ketoacidosis, burns, pancreatic tumors, renal failure and alcoholic liver disease. Although it is possible that some of these patients did have occult pancreatitis in addition to their primary problem, the vast majority of the patients apparently did not have pancreatitis. Hence the C_{Am}/C_{Cr} is not specific. Nonetheless, the C_{Am}/C_{Cr} is a simple and sensitive test for the diagnosis of acute pancreatitis. Its nonspecificity does not detract from its clinical usefulness, as the disorders listed above are unlikely to cause confusion by going unnoticed in the clinical situation.

A recent study (Gut 18:703, 1977) examined the mechanism and specificity of increased C_{Am}/C_{Cr} in pancreatitis. The C_{Am}/C_{Cr} was determined in 239 patients. In 87 hospitalized patients without pancreatic disease (controls) the C_{Am}/C_{Cr} ratio was 3.02 ± 0.69 (± 1 SD). The ratio was above the normal range in all 13 patients with acute pancreatitis, but was normal in 30 patients with chronic pancreatitis and 13 patients with carcinoma of the pancreas. In 18 patients with choledocholithiasis a raised ratio distinguished those with pancreatitis, as assessed independently by the surgeon at laparotomy, from those with a macroscopically normal pancreas. Raised C_{Am}/C_{Cr} ratios were also found in 4 diabetics with ketoacidosis and in 3 patients with fulminant alcoholic liver disease. A significant increase in C_{Am}/C_{Cr} ratios was produced in 6 healthy volunteers by intravenous injection of glucagon. However, it is unlikely that glucagon is a major factor in the production of the increased C_{Am}/C_{Cr} as no correlation was found between the clearance ratio and the plasma glucagon concentration.—Ed.] ◄

Isoelectric Focusing Studies of Human Serum and Tissue Isoamylases. Various methods of studying the isoamylases of serum and tissue have yeilded contradictory results. Michael D. Levitt, Carol Ellis and Rolf R. Engel[9] (Univ. of Minnesota Hosp., Minneapolis) investigated isoamylases of human serum and tissues by isoelectric focusing on a column. This method makes possible determination of the isoelectric point of each isoamylase and accurate quantitation of the isoenzymes.

Serum was obtained from 20 healthy subjects and from the following patients: 6 with hyperamylasemia due to typical acute pancreatitis, 4 with hyperamylasemia due to mumps parotitis, 2 with hyperamylasemia and mixed parotid tumors, 1 after subtotal pancreatectomy for chronic pancreatitis, 2 after total pancreatectomy for trauma and duodenal malignancy, 2 with pancreatic insufficiency due to chronic pancreatitis, 3 with Schwachman's syndrome, 2 with cystic fibrosis, 1 with hyperamylasemia and ruptured ectopic pregnancy, 2 with Sjögren's syndrome, 2 with macroamylasemia and 9 who were asymptomatic with unexplained hyperamylasemia and normal urinary amylase excretion. Specimens of saliva, duodenal fluid and sweat were also obtained from normal subjects. Specimens of liver, parotid and submandibular glands, pancreas and fallopian tube were obtained at autopsy or laparotomy.

Normal serum contains three major isoamylases peaks with isoelectric points of pH 6.9–7.1, 6.3–6.6 and 5.9–6.1, respectively. The only serum isoamylase present in elevated concentration in acute pancreatitis and the only one of duodenal drainage or pancreatic homogenates had an isoelectric point of 6.9–7.1. This isoamylase was virtually absent from the serum of patients with pancreatic exocrine insufficiency. Pancreatic isoamylase comprised 32 ± 6% of the serum amylase of normal subjects (Fig 30). The other two major serum isoamylases corresponded to the two major isoamylases of saliva and were the only

Fig 30.—Values of 20 normal subjects for total serum amylase activity, serum pancreatic isoamylase activity and percentage of total serum amylase represented by pancreatic isoamylase. Mean ±1 SD is shown. (Courtesy of Levitt, M. D., et al.: J. Lab. Clin. Med. 90:141–152, July, 1977.)

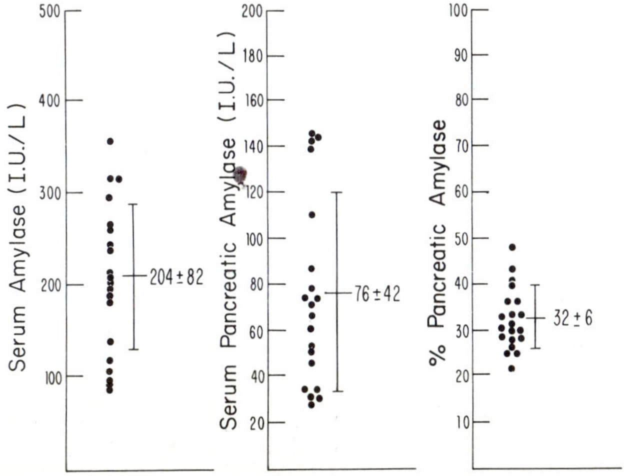

(9) J. Lab. Clin. Med. 90:141–152, July, 1977.

ones of increased concentration in patients with hyperamylasemia secondary to mumps or parotid tumors. Salivary-type amylase was usually increased in concentration in the serum of patients with otherwise unexplained hyperamylasemia. Macroamylase appeared as a broad band with a series of isoelectric points ranging from 4.5 to 6.0. The isoamylase of liver, fallopian tube and sweat generally had a lower isoelectric point than did the bulk of normal serum amylase.

The major disadvantage of isoelectric focusing is that it requires expensive apparatus and takes up to 72 hours. The wide range of normal for serum pancreatic isoamylase concentration limits the value of the measurement in the diagnosis of pancreatitis. The liver, fallopian tube and sweat may not contribute appreciable amylase to the serum.

Enzyme Replacement Therapy of Exocrine Pancreatic Insufficiency in Man: Relation between In Vitro Enzyme Activities and In Vivo Potency in Commercial Pancreatic Extracts. A logical approach to the selection of replacement pancreatic enzymes for individual patients has been hampered by a lack of comparative studies of commercially available extracts in man. David Y. Graham[1] (Baylor College of Medicine) assayed 16 commercially available pancreatic extracts for enzyme activities and evaluated the relationship between in vitro activities and in vivo potency, as measured by decrease in steatorrhea. Six patients (3 men and 3 women) with steatorrhea due to chronic exocrine pancreatic insufficiency were studied on a metabolic ward. Each received a constant diet containing 100 gm fat and 90 gm protein daily. Each test period included 3 days of equilibration and 3 days of collections.

A wide range in all enzyme activities between preparations was found with in vitro tests. Representative findings on the effectiveness

EFFECTIVENESS OF PANCREATIC SUPPLEMENTS ON FAT ABSORPTION IN PATIENTS WITH EXOCRINE PANCREATIC INSUFFICIENCY

CASE NO.	FECAL FAT (G/24 HR)*			
	TREATMENT†			
	none (control)	*tablet (Viokase)*	*capsule (Cotazym)*	*Ent-Tab (Festal)*
1	44.5	7.3	3.4	12.4
2	33.0	21.0	23.1	25.4
3	19.1	5.0	11.8	22.0
4	9.4	4.6	4.6	5.8
5	71.3	23.3	25.6	68.2
6	51.2	38.0	36.0	52.6
Coefficient of absorption	61.6±9‡	83.4±5	80.9±6	68.9±10
% Reduction§	—	56.1±9	48.6±10	20.0±13

*Normal 6.0 gm/24 hours.
†Number of pills administered: Festal, 5; Cotazym, 5; and Viokase, 6.
‡Mean ± SEM.
§In steatorrhea.

(1) N. Engl. J. Med. 296:1314–1317, June 9, 1977.

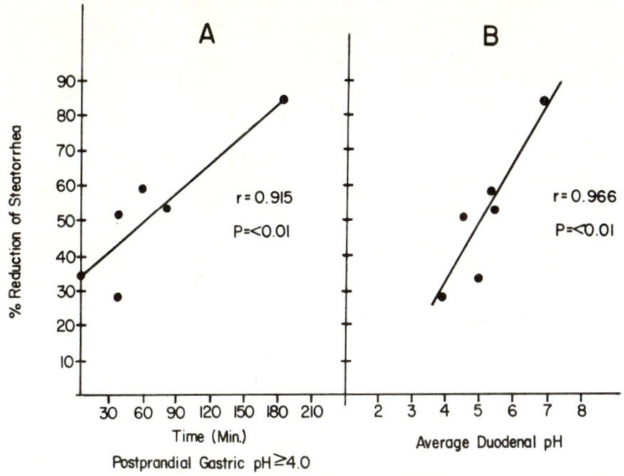

Fig 31. – Correlation between percentage reduction of steatorrhea (mean of tablets and capsules) with the time of postprandial gastric pH ≥ 4 (**A**) and the average duodenal pH (**B**). The line was constructed according to the method of least squares. (Courtesy of Graham, D. Y.: N. Engl. J. Med. 296: 1314–1317, June 9, 1977.)

of pancreatic supplements are given in the table. Steatorrhea was reduced by both tablets and capsules, but enteric-coated tablets were usually less effective. Absorption was best with tablets and capsules. Reduction of steatorrhea is correlated with the time postprandial gastric pH is ≥ 4 and the average duodenal pH, as shown in Figure 31. Fecal chymotrypsin output increased with each of the enzyme preparations, and fecal nitrogen excretion declined with each type of supplement. The reduction in fecal nitrogen excretion correlated with the decrease in steatorrhea.

This study showed a wide range in enzyme activities in commercial pancreatic enzyme preparations. In vitro lipase activity of tablets and capsules can be related to in vivo potency. Enteric coating may reduce the clinical efficacy of pancreatic extracts. Most commercially available supplements contain insufficient levels of lipase activity to be useful for treating exocrine pancreatic insufficiency. A supplement containing relatively large amounts of lipase activity should be prescribed.

► [This article, as well as the following two, deal with the treatment of exocrine pancreatic insufficiency with orally administered pancreatic enzymes. Even when potent pancreatic enzyme preparations are used, correction of the maldigestion and its sequelae may be difficult. The major problem is one of getting enough active enzyme to the duodenum at the time when food is passing into the small bowel. Two fine editorials (N. Engl. J. Med. 296:1347, 1977; and Lancet 2:73, 1977) have addressed this problem and much of the comment that follows regarding this and the following two articles has been extracted from these editorials.

Obviously, the effectiveness of oral enzyme therapy will depend on the activity of the preparation prescribed. Graham has confirmed older observations that commercially available preparations vary widely in enzyme activities. Furthermore, he has provided circumstantial evidence that therapeutic efficiency can be related to in vitro potency. The physical properties of the preparation (enteric coating and ease of dispersion) may determine therapeutic outcome, and enteric coatings may not disintegrate predictably. Meyer (N. Engl. J. Med. 296:1348, 1977) points out that the theory underlying enteric coating of pancreatin may be wrong (the idea is to prevent destruction of orally ingested enzymes in the stomach). His recent studies (Gastroenterology 72:1102, 1977) on gastric emptying of solid materials indicate that the postcibal stomach virtually excludes passage of nondispersed solid material more than a few millimeters in size—for example, plastic spheres are retained, while food is ground up and passed on to the duodenum as a slurry. If these observations are extrapolated to enterically coated capsules, coated pancreatic extract ingested with meals would ultimately arrive in the duodenum after most of the food had already passed. Further, these observations suggest that a therapeutic regimen designed to reproduce appropriate intraluminal conditions in a patient with pancreatic insufficiency would have to assure that adequate amounts of potent pancreatic extract were already present in each aliquot of food as it left the stomach. This brings up the important question as to the lowest enzyme activities compatible with normal digestion and how abnormally low enzyme levels are actually modified by pancreatic enzyme replacement therapy. This is discussed in the following article.—Ed.] ◄

Fate of Orally Ingested Enzymes in Pancreatic Insufficiency: Comparison of Two Dosage Schedules. Rational therapeutic guidelines based on sound physiologic measurements are lacking for oral enzyme replacement in treatment of malabsorption due to chronic pancreatic insufficiency. Inactivation of enzymes before they reach the small bowel may be an important factor.

Eugene P. DiMagno, Juan R. Malagelada, Vay L. W. Go and Charles G. Moertel[2] (Mayo Clinic and Found.) studied the fate of orally ingest-

Fig 32.—Lipase activity delivered to ligament of Treitz postprandially in health *(A)* and in pancreatic insufficiency *(B)*. Bars show mean ± SEM. All values in pancreatic insufficiency are less than those in health ($P < 0.001$). All in pancreatic insufficiency are greater with either treatment schedule of pancreatin (Viokase) than without treatment ($P < 0.05$). Effects of the two schedules are not significantly different. (Courtesy of DiMagno, E. P., et al.: N. Engl. J. Med. 296:1318–1322, June 9, 1977.)

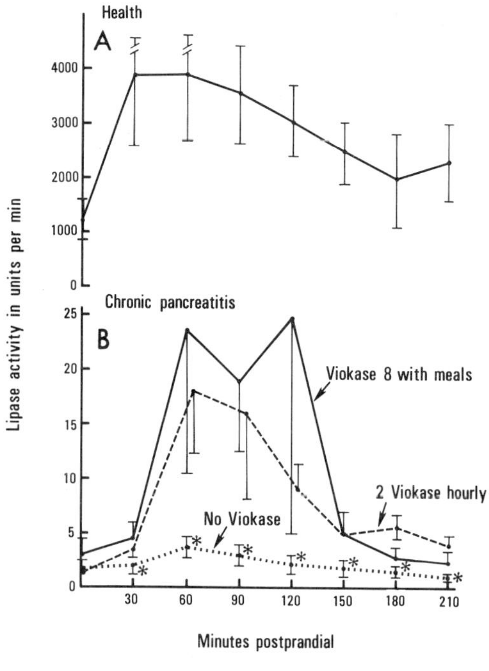

(2) N. Engl. J. Med. 296:1318–1322, June 9, 1977.

ed enzymes in patients with pancreatic insufficiency and the relation of enzyme activity to pH values and correction of malabsorption.

METHOD.—Six patients with pancreatic insufficiency who had steatorrhea and azotorrhea and 6 healthy control subjects matched for sex and age were studied. The average patient age was 56 years. Pancreatin tablets were used in all studies.

In each subject, after an overnight fast, physiologic saline containing the marker ^{14}C-polyethylene glycol was perfused through a duodenal port. Each then had a standard meal with or without pancreatin, 8 tablets given according to two regimens: (1) 2 tablets at the start and the others at intervals during the meal; (2) 2 tablets at the start of the meal followed by 2 every hour for 3 hours. Gastric and duodenal samples were analyzed and fecal balance studies were done.

All patients had severe pancreatic insufficiency, the mean enzyme output being less than 0.2% of normal (Fig 32). Pancreatin treatment increased the cumulative 3-hour active amounts of both trypsin and lipase significantly, although neither exceeded 2% of normal. Delivery in active form was less with hourly tablet administration, but the difference was not significant.

Duodenal pH was consistently lower in the patients than in healthy subjects. Pancreatin ingestion did not significantly affect the gastric or duodenal pH. Fecal weight, fat and nitrogen were significantly reduced by pancreatin in each treatment schedule (Fig 33). However, steatorrhea was corrected only once (with 2 tablets per hour). Azotorrhea was corrected in 5 of 6 patients by tablets with meals, but in only 1 of 4 by 2 tablets per hour.

Since administration of pancreatin with meals is as effective as

Fig 33.—Twenty-four-hour fecal fat (**A**) and nitrogen (**B**). Excretion by 6 patients with pancreatitis, with and without pancreatin (Viokase) treatment. Each rectangle encloses 1 SD above the mean. Values are less with pancreatin by either schedule than without ($P < 0.01$). Effects of the two schedules are not significantly different. Normal ranges of fecal fat (<7 gm/24 hours) and fecal nitrogen (<2.5 gm/24 hours) are shaded. (Courtesy of DiMagno, E. P., et al.: N. Engl. J. Med. 29:1318–1322, June 9, 1977.)

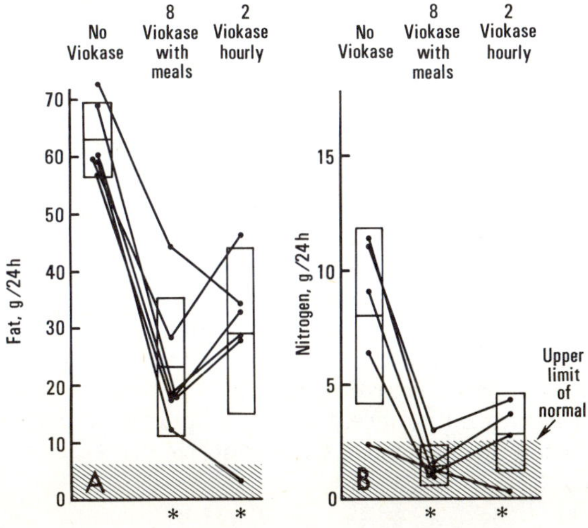

hourly administration in reducing steatorrhea and perhaps more effective in abolishing azotorrhea, and is also more convenient, it is recommended. Enteric coating of tablets and inhibition of gastric acid secretions to protect orally ingested enzymes against acid denaturation require further investigation.

► [Secretion of pancreatic enzymes into the duodenum normally rises to about 70% of maximal (or 4–5 times basal rates) with the arrival of food in the duodenum and is maintained at or near this level as long as food continues to empty from the stomach (Gastroenterology 72:195, 1977; and Mayo Clin. Proc. 49:851, 1974). After a mixed meal of carbohydrate, protein and fat, the pancreas secretes enzymes for 4 hours or more as long as there is food in the stomach (Scand. J. Gastroenterol. 7:489, 1972). Further, there is evidence that digestion by pancreatic enzymes occurs throughout the small intestine during this period (J. Clin. Invest. 52:1586, 1973). The pancreas has an enormous secretory capacity and the amount of enzyme secreted greatly exceeds that needed for normal digestion. This is evident from the studies of DiMagno et al. (N. Engl. J. Med. 288:813, 1973) and Kalser et al. (ibid. 279:570, 1968). DiMagno et al. demonstrated that pancreatic secretory capacity may be reduced to 10% of normal without steatorrhea or azotorrhea; at between 2% and 10% of the normal output, mild to moderate steatorrhea (≤ 25 gm/day) ensues and at 0–2% of the normal capacity to secrete enzymes, steatorrhea is profound (25–80 gm/day). Meyer (ibid. 296:1347, 1977) has theorized that in the patient with pancreatic insufficiency, steatorrhea should be abolished if oral pancreatic extracts could assure the postcibal arrival of exogenous lipase in the duodenum in amounts equivalent to about 10% of normal.

According to the assays of DiMagno et al., 12–16 tablets of pancreatic extract (Viokase) would be required with each meal to provide exogenously 10% of the lipase and trypsin normally secreted in response to their test meal. These investigators gave half this amount, and only 22% of the trypsin and 8% of the lipase administered actually reached the duodenum. This study clearly shows how little orally ingested enzyme actually reaches the duodenum. There are many possible reasons for this, including (1) destruction of orally ingested enzymes in gastric juice, (2) dispersion of the tablets into the meal contents; (3) dilution in the total intragastric volume and (4) delayed entry of enzymes into the duodenum.

It is impressive that such a small amount of ingested enzymes reaching the duodenum produced such a large improvement in fat and nitrogen balance. The explanation would appear to be the steep inverse relation between steatorrhea and azotorrhea and duodenal enzyme content in pancreatic insufficiency cited above. Restoration of enzyme concentration to 0–2% of normal will reduce steatorrhea to about 25 gm/day. However, a much larger input is needed to reduce fecal fat from 25 gm/day to normal levels, and restoration of normal fat balance is not easily achieved by oral enzyme therapy.—Ed.] ◄

► ↓The following article evaluates the effects of neutralizing gastric acid to prevent intragastric destruction of orally ingested enzymes.—Ed. ◄

Comparative Effects of Antacids, Cimetidine and Enteric Coating on Therapeutic Response to Oral Enzymes in Severe Pancreatic Insufficiency. Steatorrhea in patients with pancreatic insufficiency is rarely abolished by oral pancreatic extracts, and some patients remain symptomatic and fail to gain weight. This therapeutic failure appears to be due to inactivation of lipase and trypsin by gastric acid and pepsin. Patrick T. Regan, Juan-R. Malagelada, Eugene P. DiMagno, Scotty L. Glanzman and Vay Liang W. Go[3] (Mayo Clinic and Found.) administered cimetidine, a potent inhibitor of gastric acid secretion, with oral pancreatic enzymes to 6 patients with chronic pancreatitis and advanced pancreatic insufficiency and compared the results with those obtained with a new enteric-coated enzyme prepara-

(3) N. Engl. J. Med. 297:854–858, Oct. 20, 1977.

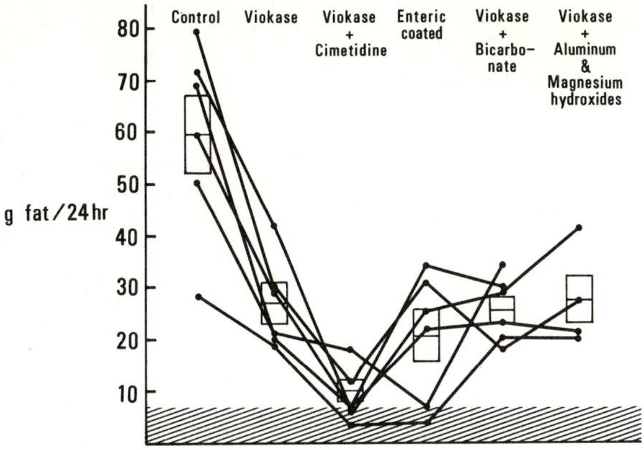

Fig 34.—Effects of different treatments on steatorrhea of pancreatic insufficiency in 6 patients. Regimens were administered in randomized order. Normal values in authors' laboratories for fecal fat excretion (greater than 7 gm/24 hours) are represented by hatched area. Means ± SEM are indicated. (Courtesy of Regan, P. T., et al.: N. Engl. J. Med. 297:854–858, Oct. 20, 1977.)

tion and those obtained with supplemental neutralizing antacids. All patients had alcoholic pancreatitis and 3 had insulin-dependent diabetes. All had previously used 4-8 gm Viokase daily. Both balance studies and perfusion studies were carried out. Cimetidine was given in a dosage of 300 mg 30 minutes before each meal. Bicarbonate was given in a dosage of 2.5 gm 30 minutes after meals and Maalox in a dosage of 30 ml at the same times.

Steatorrhea was reduced significantly by all treatments (Fig 34), but the combination of cimetidine and pancreatin was most effective and was the only treatment that often abolished steatorrhea. Fecal nitrogen excretion was corrected by all treatments in nearly all patients. Only treatment with pancreatin and cimetidine produced sustained increases in lipase concentrations to about 5–10% of normal. Postprandial gastric pH values were significantly higher with this treatment, corresponding to marked inhibition of gastric secretion of acid and pepsin. Steatorrhea was corrected only when the peak postprandial lipase concentrations exceeded 5% of normal. No patient had symptoms attributable to cimetidine.

All patients with exocrine pancreatic insufficiency respond to large intracibal doses of pancreatin with a reduction in steatorrhea and correction of azotorrhea. Adjunctive use of antacids does not further improve fat malabsorption. Acid-resistant, enteric-coated preparations are helpful only in selected cases in which the postprandial intragastric pH is uniformly low. Patients in whom steatorrhea is not corrected by routine enzyme replacement therapy and who remain symptomatic may benefit from the addition of cimetidine.

► [Two other reports have confirmed that cimetidine is a useful adjunct in the treatment of pancreatic insufficiency and improves the efficacy of pancreatic extracts (Br. Med. J. 1:418, 1977; and Lancet 2:878, 1977). The question can be raised as to which patients should receive cimetidine. It bears reemphasizing that relatively simple regimens frequently reduce steatorrhea and eliminate diarrhea in the patient with pancreatic insufficiency. It is not essential to eliminate steatorrhea entirely. A reasonable plan is to start the patient on 3–4 tablets of a potent preparation with meals. If this regimen improves the patient's overall status, the treatment plan may be continued indefinitely. If it does not, further manipulations can be tried. Such manipulations might include: (1) increase the dosage and add a dosage with snacks and at bedtime; (2) change the dosage schedule by administering enzymes every 1–2 hours; (3) give antacids with pancreatic extracts at mealtime; (4) give cimetidine; and (5) reduce dietary fat. Finally, in the patient with pancreatic insufficiency not responding to appropriate enzyme replacement therapy, consideration should be given to excluding occult concurrent disease. In this regard, we and others have encountered a sizable number of patients with exocrine pancreatic insufficiency who also have bacterial overgrowth in the proximal small bowel.

The readers of the preceding three articles may draw the conclusion that hourly administration of pancreatic extracts, as proposed by Jordan and Grossman (Gastroenterology 36:447, 1959), may be less effective than administration of enzymes with meals. As Meyer (N. Engl. J. Med. 296:1348, 1977) emphasized, however, such a conclusion is unjustified. The many variables—preparation of pancreatin, dosage, dosing schedules, gastric acid secretion, size and composition of meals and degree of pancreatic insufficiency—have been poorly controlled or incompletely studied. We are just beginning to understand the complexities of pancreatic insufficiency.—Ed.] ◄

Prospective Comparison of Current Diagnostic Tests for Pancreatic Cancer. The diagnosis of pancreatic cancer is difficult and often is accomplished only at operation or when disease is far advanced. Eugene P. DiMagno, Juan-R. Malagelada, William F. Taylor and Vay Liang W. Go[4] (Mayo Clinic and Found.) compared the results of several diagnostic tests prospectively in 70 patients referred with abdominal pain, weight loss or jaundice who were suspected of having pancreatic cancer. They had otherwise normal physical findings and normal results of routine laboratory tests, cholecystography (if not jaundiced) and barium gastrointestinal roentgenography. All patients were over age 35 years. The final diagnosis was made by laparotomy in 68 cases and by liver biopsy in 2 cases.

Only 4 of the 30 pancreatic cancers found were localized, and in only 4 cases was all malignant tissue resected. Hyperbilirubinemia was present in only 13 of the 30 patients. Pancreatic function testing was with 15 Crick-Harper-Raper units of cholecystokinin/kg/hour. Pancreatic scans were obtained with ^{75}Se-methionine; ^{99m}Tc-sulfur colloid liver scans were recorded simultaneously.

Ultrasonography, pancreatic function testing and the pancreatic scan were all relatively sensitive for pancreatic disease (positive results when the disease is present). Thermography was significantly insensitive. Thermography, ultrasonography and function testing were quite specific (negative results when the disease is absent) in detecting absence of pancreatic disease, whereas the scan was significantly nonspecific. Thermography indicated pancreatic disease in only 2 patients. In cases of pancreatic cancer, endoscopic retrograde pancreatography and arteriography were significantly more sensitive than cytologic study. These tests were also more accurate than cytologic testing in predicting absence of pancreatic cancer. In patients in whom test results disagreed, endoscopic retrograde pancreatography was the best test. The combination of three or four tests was significantly better than a combination of ultrasonography and pancreatic function testing.

---

(4) N. Engl. J. Med. 297:737–742, Oct. 6, 1977.

Testing can definitely eliminate pancreatic cancer in patients with severe, protracted abdominal pain and weight loss. It may obviate surgical exploration in cases of nonneoplastic disease. Use of a combination of tests will narrow the process to the pancreas with almost absolute certainty. Ultrasonography should be done first and, if negative, a pancreatic function test should be performed. Positive results from either or both procedures are an indication for endoscopic retrograde pancreatography (ERP). Arteriography could be substituted for ERP in the event of failure or unavailability of this test. This sequence identified 88% of patients without pancreatic disease and 89% with pancreatic cancer.

► [For a timely review on cancer of the pancreas, see the progress report by Morgan and Wormsley (Gut 18:580, 1977). Cancer of the pancreas is now the fourth most common cancer causing death in the United States, with only cancer of the lung, the colon and rectum, and the breast more frequent. In the United States the incidence of pancreatic carcinoma has increased threefold since 1930 and an annual incidence of 9–10 cases per 100,000 population is now found; the incidence is markedly higher (up to 100 per 100,000) in people over 75 years of age.

Ultrasound is a good test for pancreatic disease, and a brief but authoritative review on ultrasonography of the pancreas has been published (Lancet 2:1212, 1977). In carcinoma of the pancreas, ultrasonic abnormalities are seen in 90% and a carcinoma is specifically diagnosable in between 58% and 83% (ibid). Most tumors are over 2 cm in diameter and lie in the head or body. At present, a small tumor is hard to distinguish from localized chronic pancreatitis. Computerized tomography (CT) of the pancreas is easier to perform and to interpret than pancreatic ultrasonography. Why, then, bother with ultrasound? For one thing, the cost of buying and maintaining a CT scanner is many times the equivalent cost for ultrasound. Though CT scanning gives an inadequate picture of the pancreas in only 7% as against 10–20% with ultrasound, the advantage for CT is slight (ibid). Many authorities feel that ultrasound should be the initial investigation for most patients with suspected pancreatic disease.

Endoscopic retrograde cholangiopancreatography allows a diagnosis of carcinoma to be made in 70–80% of cases (J. Surg. Oncol. 7:107, 1975; Ann. Intern. Med. 84:438, 1976; and Cancer 37:449, 1976), and cytology further increases the diagnostic accuracy. However, cannulation of the pancreatic duct is not always possible, most studies reporting an 80–90% success rate (Gut 13:1014, 1972; Am. J. Surg. 125:432, 1973; and Cancer 37:449, 1976). – Ed.] ◄

Indomethacin-Responsive Pancreatic Cholera. Pancreatic cholera is a rare entity caused by nonbeta islet cell tumors. Neither vasoactive intestinal polypeptide nor human pancreatic polypeptide has been firmly implicated as the diarrheagenic hormone. Elevated plasma prostaglandin E (PGE) levels have been found in several patients with the syndrome and prostaglandin biosynthesis can readily be inhibited with indomethacin. Bernard M. Jaffe, Dan F. Kopen, Katherine DeSchryver-Kecskemeti, Ronald L. Gingerich and Marie Greider[5] (Washington Univ.) obtained improvement with indomethacin in a patient with classic Verner-Morrison syndrome.

Woman, 67, had had diarrhea 9 years previously, with an unremitting, slowly progressive course. There was profuse medication-resistant diarrhea on presentation. She had lost 7 kg in the past 3 months and had marked generalized weakness. A complete workup including celiac axis and mesenteric angiography and pancreatic scanning gave normal results. The diarrhea was profuse (Fig 35). Stool volume and frequency diminished markedly on treatment with 25 mg indomethacin every 8 hours, orally. Intravenous fluid, potassium

(5) N. Engl. J. Med. 297:817–821, Oct. 13, 1977.

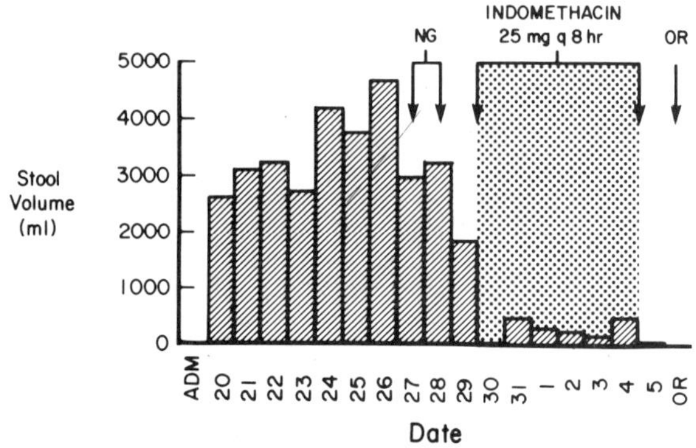

Fig 35.—Fecal output during hospital course. (Courtesy of Jaffe, B. M., et al.: N. Engl. J. Med. 297:817–821, Oct. 13, 1977.)

and bicarbonate requirements were markedly reduced and intravenous supplementation was stopped. A tumor was resected from the tail of the pancreas, along with the distal pancreas and spleen, and normal bowel function resumed 5 days postoperatively. The patient was asymptomatic 3 months postoperatively off medications.

Levels of gastrin, prostaglandin F and vasoactive intestinal polypeptide were normal before operation and did not change substantially during indomethacin therapy or after operation. Levels of human pancreatic polypeptide were elevated at all times. The plasma PGE level was elevated preoperatively and fell to less than a third of the initial level within 24 hours of the start of indomethacin therapy. Plasma PGE levels remained normal without indomethacin after resection of the tumor. Tumor levels of PGE were about 15 times greater than those in the normal pancreas. The tumor resembled a typical islet cell tumor of a nonalpha, nonbeta cell type. Cells with small, round granules and cells containing larger secretory granules were both observed.

Vasoactive intestinal polypeptide was apparently not a factor in the pathogenesis of this patient's symptoms and human pancreatic polypeptide did not appear to be involved. Infusions of PGE can simulate all symptoms of this syndrome and the use of indomethacin rapidly abolished diarrhea and hypercalcemia in the present case.

PART SIX

METABOLISM

PHILIP K. BONDY, M.D.

Introduction

The amount of research published in the field of endocrinology and metabolic diseases increases annually. Moreover, as methods become more specialized, specific and sophisticated, the quality of the research improves. Our discipline was honored this year by the award of the Nobel Prize for research in mechanisms of control of pituitary hormone secretion and for methods of measuring polypeptide and other types of substances by radioimmunoassay. We congratulate Doctors Guillemin, Schally and Yalow for this recognition and mourn the absence of Dr. Solomon Berson's name from the list, because of his premature death. But the successes of our colleagues make life difficult for this editor. Space in the YEAR BOOK does not expand as the volume of research increases. Indeed, because the total size of the volume has remained relatively constant for many years, and because new areas of specialization have been introduced into the book, the amount of space available for my section has become smaller.

I have responded to this problem in two ways. Over the past few years I have reduced the number of articles whose interest is purely theoretical and have tried to select material with a clear practical implication. The reader will find a couple of exceptions to this rule this year, but many less than a decade ago. And, in order to expand the coverage of articles that had to be omitted, I have expanded the comments considerably. The reader will note that, in some instances, the comments about a given disease – e.g., hypothyroidism – range over a fairly wide area and are often not pertinent to the specific article that served as an excuse for the comments. To encompass the entire range of information included in this volume in regard to a particular subject, the reader will have to look at the comments as well as the articles. He should not be discouraged if a particular question is not answered in the index, since the material in the comments is not indexed.

PHILIP K. BONDY

Hypothalamus and Anterior Pituitary Gland

► The hypothalamus is the region in which stimulation and inhibition of pituitary function is induced in response to signals from the upper central nervous system. The effectors involved appear to be small polypeptide-releasing and release-inhibiting hormones. The release of these agents is controlled by neurohumors released from nerve endings in the hypothalamus. Dopamine and serotonin are two of the most important of these and appear to have opposite types of effects. The subject has been reviewed in some detail by Smythe (Clin. Endocrinol. (Oxf.) 7:325, 1977). To oversimplify a complex discussion, I can summarize by quoting: "The broad conclusions which emerge from this review are that hypothalamic serotonergic pathways predominantly stimulate pituitary hormone release, while dopaminergic pathways are predominantly inhibitory." In line with this argument, Lamberts et al. suggest that dopamine depletion may be a factor in the pathogenesis of Cushing's disease (ibid., p. 185). Smythe's synthesis would suggest that dopamine depletion reduces the inhibitory potency of the hypothalamus for release of corticotropin-releasing hormone. Cyproheptadine, a serotonin antagonist, suppresses secretion of growth hormone, according to Delitala et al. (Metabolism 26:931, 1977), a finding which is in accord with Smythe's presentation. The pattern is not so simple as this, however. For example, Samarthji and his colleagues (J. Clin. Endocrinol. Metab. 44:766, 1977) point out that in normal human beings the dopamine agonist, apomorphine, which should reduce secretion, according to theory, actually stimulates growth hormone secretion. Thus, although this is a useful rule of thumb, it may not always work.

When a stimulus is applied to the hypothalamus, releasing or inhibiting hormones are secreted. One would therefore expect to find a reduction of the content of these polypeptides in the stimulated hypothalamus, but this is not necessarily so. Yasuda and Greer (Neuroendocrinology 22:48, 1976) found no reduction of rat hypothalamic corticotropin-releasing potency despite acute or chronic changes in ACTH secretion; and Kardon et al. (Endocrinology 100:1604, 1977) found a similar stability of the content of thyrotropin-releasing hormone (TRH) in the hypothalamus after hypophysectomy, thyroidectomy or administration of thyroxine. Insulin (which I, at least, would not have expected to alter hypothalamic TRH content) caused a fall in the hormone concentration. These data suggest that the release of hypothalamic regulating hormones is closely adjusted to synthesis. When secretion depletes the hormone content, it is immediately made up by synthesis of new hormone. Of course, another possibility is that the methods available to the researchers were too inaccurate to pick up the small changes of hormone concentration which actually occurred.

Although a great deal is known about the chemical nature of the pituitary hormones extracted from the gland or found in the plasma, the sequence of changes that occurs as the proteins are evolved from their parent polypeptide is not clear. A good example is the protein β-lipotropin. Within its amino acid sequence this protein includes ACTH, β-MSH and a group of peptides which bind to morphine receptors in the brain and are called "endorphins" (See review by Goldstein: Science 193:1081, 1976). These polypeptides produce behavioral changes when they are injected into the brain of experimental animals. Thus ACTH, MSH and behavior-modifying substances all come from the same parent molecule. To have an effect, the endorphins and their close relatives the enkephalins must be secreted from the pituitary "backward" into the brain. This is discussed later in an article. But there is also the interesting question of whether any of the polypeptides whose activity we think we understand—ACTH, for example, or MSH, have effects on brain function (separate from the effects resulting from stimulation of peripheral effectors such as the adrenal cortex). They probably do—or, at least, Sandman et al. (J. Clin. Endocrinol. Metab. 44:884, 1977) found that the amino acids 4–10 in the MSH/ACTH sequence caused changes in the ability of human volunteers to perform certain perceptual tests. A considerable literature exists indicating that these substances have an effect on learning, avoidance behavior and memory in rats. Although these effects are seen when the hormone is given systemically, the effects in animals are more striking when the substances are given intraventricularly. Since MSH is a fragment of lipotropin, one might expect the larger molecule to have melanocyte-stimulating activity, and this turns out to be the case. What one might not have expected is the recent report (from many sources) that "MSH" in the plasma and pituitary is, in fact, an artifact of chemical manipulation. There is now general agreement that the actual MSH is β-lipotropin. The concentration of lipotropin increases after adrenalectomy or blockage of adrenal cortical hormone synthesis and falls after administration of corticosteroids (see, for example, Bachelot et al.: ibid., p. 939).

The general pattern of hormone synthesis is for large molecules to be trimmed down to the smaller, effective hormone form. The exact location of this conversion is not always clear. Lowenstein and colleagues (Endocrinology 101:651, 1977) found that in the pituitary, growth hormone is formed from the larger molecule, progrowth hormone, while the latter is still attached to the ribosomes which are synthesizing it. Probably the active form of growth hormone is the polypeptide which has been isolated from the pituitary and characterized as to size, amino acid sequence, etc. When this material is permitted to stand in plasma or is injected into human beings, however, some of it becomes larger, until it is the same size as "big" growth hormone which is usually considered to be the prohormone. It is not entirely clear what happens—whether the hormone forms dimers with itself or whether it associates with a carrier protein—and what the significance of this change may be (Beitins et al.: ibid., p. 350). It is also somewhat unexpected to find—as Gorden and colleagues did (J. Clin. Endocrinol. Metab. 43:364, 1976)—that in acromegalic plasma the proportion of little growth hormone compared with the big form is higher than it is in normal plasma. The usual pattern, typified by proinsulin in insulinomas, is for tumors to release excess amounts of prohormone into the plasma.

Finally, a glimpse into the probable future is provided by the report that *Escherichia coli* have been induced to synthesize somatostatin by insertion of the appropriate gene (Itakura et al.: Science 198:1056, 1977). This is a tremendous achievement of molecular biology, but it is not merely an exercise of scientific interest. Somatostatin is a small enough molecule that it could be synthesized for clinical use, but other polypeptide hormones are so large that at present it seems hopeless to attempt a commercially practical synthesis. These hormones include some which are already in very short supply, such as growth hormone, and some which are now available from animal sources, but which would be better if the human molecule were available. Insulin is an example. Moreover, with an increasing population of diabetics and a limited availability of animal sources, even insulin may become scarce in the near future. It is of particular interest, therefore, that research is in progress in preparation for performing the same trick with these more difficult hormones. For example, Ullrich et al. (Science 196:1313, 1977) have constructed the DNA for rat insulin and inserted it into plasmids of *E. coli.* The sequences are complete for one form of rat insulin prohormone, but translation has not occurred, probably because initiator sequences were not included. At any rate, the ability to cause bacteria to make insulin and probably other useful hormonal peptides is within reach, it seems.

A brief comment about somatostatin: In studies undertaken a few years ago, this substance seemed likely to be of clinical significance. Then reports appeared that it interfered with the coagulation mechanism in experimental apes. This problem has been studied by Rasche and co-workers, who found that intravenous infusions lasting as long as 5 days did not induce significant alterations of blood clotting. Indeed, 1 patient with a bleeding peptic ulcer stopped bleeding within an hour after infusion was started, possibly because of inhibition of gastrin production. At any rate, if there is a use for chronically administered somatostatin, the risk of trying it is probably acceptable, at least for the period which has already been studied (Klin. Wochenschr. 54:977, 1976).—Ed. ◄

Pituitary Secretes to Brain: Experiments in Sheep are reported by Richard M. Bergland, Steven L. Davis and Robert B. Page[1] Ana-

(1) Lancet 2:276–278, Aug. 6, 1977.

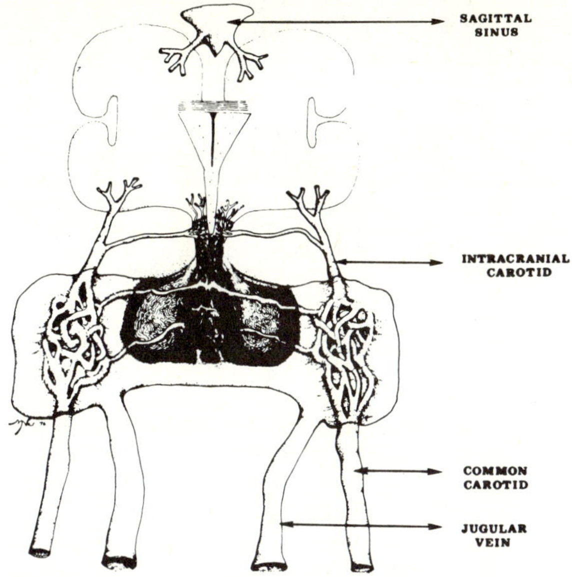

Fig 1.—Vascular relations in sheep pituitary. Neurohypophysis receives three sets of arteries (inferior hypophyseal, middle hypophyseal and superior hypophyseal). Capillaries that are confluent between median eminence and hypothalamus are shown. Four sites of sampling are indicated; intracranial carotid artery was sampled above origin of middle hypophyseal artery and below origin of superior hypophyseal artery. (Courtesy of Bergland, R. M., et al.: Lancet 2:276–278, Aug. 6, 1977.)

tomical studies suggest that the vascular route of both hypothalamic and adenohypophyseal secretions may be controlled by events within the capillary bed of the neurohypophysis. The sheep has a large middle hypophyseal artery that anastomoses between the right and left portions of the rete mirabile (Fig 1). Blood was sampled from the cervical common carotid artery, intracranial internal carotid artery, sagittal sinus and internal jugular vein of 9 female Hampshire sheep to determine whether the middle hypophyseal vessel serves as an efferent route from the neurohypophysis to the carotid rete mirabile and hence to the brain. Plasma samples were analyzed for prolactin and growth hormone by radioimmunoassay.

Three sheep had slightly increased prolactin concentrations in jugular venous samples but normal growth hormone values. Two had the highest levels of both hormones within the sagittal sinus, but intracranial carotid levels were not elevated. Four sheep had the highest concentrations of both hormones in samples from the intracranial internal carotid artery above the pituitary.

The findings imply that the neurohypophyseal capillary bed can direct blood to the adenohypophysis, the systemic circulation or the brain. The efferent routes from the neurohypophysis include the inferior hypophyseal veins, portal vessels extending from the median eminence to the adenohypophysis, confluent capillaries extending from the median eminence to the hypothalamus and ependymal tanycytes stretched between internal plexus vessels of the median eminence and the 3d ventricle. Pituitary secretions are carried directly to the brain to modify many, if not all, cerebral functions.

► [Oliver et al. performed a more direct experiment (Endocrinology 101:598, 1977). They cannulated the portal system which runs between the anterior pituitary and the hypothalamus in rats and found that the concentrations of LH, TSH, ACTH, prolactin, melanocyte-stimulating hormone and vasopressin were at least 100 times higher (all except TSH, which was only 68 times) in the portal vein plasma than in the peripheral arteries. Other experiments have shown that the brain contains high amounts of pituitary hormones and that these are not derived from peripheral plasma sources. So the pituitary is capable of secreting into the brain. The hypothalamus, of course, is also capable of secreting into the pituitary. Thus there is a circulatory short loop feedback system which probably plays a critical role in adjusting the secretory pattern. But, more important perhaps even than this, the high levels of pituitary hormones in the brain raise a question about what they may do to cerebral function. In the Introduction to this section, I have commented on the behavior-modifying effects of ACTH and other fragments of β-lipotropin. The possible role of the other pituitary hormones is not known at present.—Ed.] ◄

Endocrine Morbidity in Adults Treated with Cerebral Irradiation for Brain Tumors during Childhood. Short stature and growth hormone (GH) deficiency may complicate the treatment of intracranial tumors and acute leukemia in childhood. S. M. Shalet, C. G. Beardwell, I. A. MacFarlane, P. H. Morris Jones and D. Pearson[2] (Manchester, England) evaluated pituitary function in 20 adults who had received cerebral irradiation for brain tumors in childhood. The 12 women and 8 men had a mean age of 24.2 years and were studied a mean of 14.2 years after cerebral irradiation. Ten had had gliomas and 8, medulloblastomas. All tumors were anatomically distant from the hypothalamic-pituitary region. Thirteen patients had had partial or total surgical removal of the tumor. Tumor doses of 2,000–5,000 rad had been given over 9–31 days. Seven patients also received spinal irradiation. None received cytotoxic drugs.

Eight subjects are below the 3d height centile and 4 others are between the 3d and 10th centiles for standing height. Six of these 12 subjects had spinal irradiation. Peak GH responses to hypoglycemia were impaired in 9 subjects; 7 of these were below the 3d height centile. Peak cortisol responses to hypoglycemia were normal in all cases. Three subjects had elevated basal serum thyrotropin values, but none was clinically hypothyroid. All women had normal menstrual histories. Six of 7 men had elevated plasma testosterone values, but age-corrected values were probably normal. Gonadotropin levels were normal in all men but 1, who had a minor elevation in serum FSH. No patient had a history suggestive of diabetes insipidus.

The high rates of short stature and GH deficiency in these adults confirm the findings in children who were studied much sooner after cranial irradiation. No significant damage to the hypothalamic-pituitary-gonadal axis was evident. No patient had overt depression of ACTH production. Multiple pituitary hormone deficiencies are not found when the radiation dose is below a critical level. Radiation damage to the hypothalamic-pituitary axis is dependent mainly on the dose given, rather than on the interval after radiotherapy.

---

(2) Acta Endocrinol. (Kbh.) 84:673–680, April, 1977.

► [It is important to remember that the general practice of radiotherapists is to irradiate the entire brain no matter where the major bulk of tumor is located. Thus these patients had radiation to the hypothalamus and pituitary areas. Recognizing the late deleterious effects of brain radiation in children is the first step. Obviously, one would not want to withhold radiation in situations where it might cure a brain tumor (and results in patients such as these are often excellent). But the physician alert to the possibility that growth hormone secretion may be inhibited by previous radiotherapy will want to consider the possible advantages of treatment with growth hormone to minimize the growth defect.

These changes, following radiation by many years, must be differentiated from the acute degeneration of pituitary adenomas which results in hemorrhagic, cystic or necrotic changes after radiation. The clinical syndrome is one of pituitary apoplexy, with acute deterioration of visual and cerebral function. The problem was described in 14 of 300 patients with pituitary adenoma treated by radiation by Weisberg (Am. J. Med. 63: 109, 1977).

A curious situation was described by Hoffenberg et al. (Clin. Endocrinol. (Oxf.) 6:443, 1977) in which excessive growth and, in one instance, acromegaly, developed in 2 patients with elevated plasma concentrations of somatomedin, but with normal concentrations of growth hormone. Moreover, the growth hormone concentration was normally suppressible by glucose. It seems unlikely that this is a pituitary disease. More probably, it represents a disorder of control of somatomedin production. – Ed.] ◄

Combined Test of Anterior Pituitary Reserve. Determination of the functional reserve of the anterior pituitary requires serial measurements of hormones released from the pituitary by specific stimuli. S. J. Judd and L. Lazarus[3] (Sydney) evaluated the simultaneous use of insulin, thyrotropin-releasing hormone (TRH) and gonadotropin-releasing hormone (GnRH) as a means of assessing pituitary reserves of growth hormone (GH), ACTH, gonadotropins, thyrotropin and prolactin. Studies were done in 6 normal subjects and 54 patients. Hormone therapy was discontinued 24 hours before testing. Insulin was given intravenously in a dose of 0.1 unit neutral porcine insulin per kg; a dose of 0.15 unit/kg was given to acromegalic patients. Thyrotropin-releasing hormone was given in an oral dose of 20 mg or an intravenous injection of 400 μg. Gonadotropin-releasing hormone was given intravenously in a dose of 100 μg.

Symptoms of hypoglycemia occurred in all subjects, as well as flushing and nausea from TRH. The test never had to be terminated. Responses of normal subjects are given in the table. Maximum responses usually appear within an hour. Intravenous TRH produces a more rapid rise in TSH; measurement of triiodothyronine provides assessment of thyroid response to endogenously generated TSH. The test was most useful in estimating residual pituitary reserve after hypophysectomy. In 5 patients tested before and after hypophysectomy, maximum incremental hormone responses were less after operation except for prolactin reserve. The test was useful in investigating boys with short stature and delayed puberty. Although the test did not distinguish hypothalamic from pituitary lesions, response patterns may suggest a diagnosis. An isolated deficiency of gonadotropin release in amenorrheic patients strongly suggested a hypothalamic site of the lesion. A total isolated deficiency of gonadotropins was not found in any patient with pituitary tumor or even after hypophysectomy.

---

(3) Aust. N. Z. J. Med. 6:30–36, February, 1976.

Pituitary Hormone Responses in Six Normal Subjects after Combined Stimulus

Hormone	Units	Mean basal ±SEM	Mean max Δ ±SEM
Growth hormone	μU/ml WHO standard	4·2±2	83·0±10·6
Cortisol	μg/100 ml	13·7±1·3	12·4±2·6
FSH			
Males	ng/ml LER 907	74·6±29·1	300±40
Females		108±13·5	321±57
LH			
Males	ng/ml LER 907	28±10·8	215±61
Females		31·5±11·7	237±45
TSH	μU/ml MRC 38/68	2±0·3	25·5±2·5
T_3	ng/100 ml	130±12·7	63·7±20·3
Prolactin	ng/ml VLS # 1	13·2±0·9	56±10·2

The combined test is a convenient one, permitting most patients to be evaluated without their having to be admitted to hospital. The sensitivity and convenience of the test allow accurate monitoring of pituitary reserve, as, for instance, after hypophysectomy or pituitary irradiation or in the investigation of pituitary tumors. With the increasing availability of the hypothalamic-releasing hormones, the combined test is likely to become the standard means of assessing pituitary function.

► [We started using this method when I was in England, after the publication by Besser et al. (J. Endocrinol. 51:699, 1971). It is a very convenient method and safely applicable to children as well as adults. We usually hospitalized patients overnight for the procedure, but I doubt that this is really necessary if they can be watched closely for 2 or 3 hours. The saving in time, effort and inconvenience to the patient is gratifying, and the accuracy of diagnosis seems entirely as good as when the stimulating hormones are given separately. — Ed.] ◄

Prevalence of Severe Growth Hormone Deficiency. G. V. Vimpani, A. F. Vimpani, G. P. Lidgard, E. H. D. Cameron and J. W. Farquhar[4] (Univ. of Edinburgh) reviewed the findings in a Scottish survey of short stature that involved the screening for height of 48,221 children aged 6–9 years in three cities. Severe growth hormone deficiency (GHD) was defined as a height more than 2.5 SD below the mean for age, a height velocity less than the 25th percentile for chronological age and a maximum growth hormone (GH) value of 9 mU/L or less in two or more tests. The series included 24,670 boys. A total of 449 children had heights 2.5 SD or more below the mean height for age. Initial screening for GHD was by an exercise test in most cases. Growth hormone was radioimmunoassayed.

(4) Br. Med. J. 2:427–430, Aug. 13, 1977.

Nine children had maximum GH responses to insulin-induced hypoglycemia of 9 mU/L or less. Four children were already known to have GHD, but only 1 was receiving GH at initial height screening. When the 3 children whose short stature may have been genetic were omitted, the prevalence of severe GHD was 14.5 – 20.7/100,000. Ninety-six children had GH levels of 10 – 20 mU/L on screening. The diagnostic status of 25 children is unclear.

The prevalence of severe GHD in this sample may have been as high as 1 in 4,018, much higher than previously reported. The findings suggest that present referral patterns may account for delayed or missed diagnoses of GHD in girls or in children with less severe short stature. There appear to be some children in the community who could benefit from GH treatment but in whom diagnosis is delayed longer than necessary. Some children with isolated GHD or less severe growth retardation may be missed altogether. The findings support the recommendations of others who have urged early referral of children with short stature.

► [Growth hormone deficiency may sometimes be transitory. Trygstad (Acta Endocrinol. (Kbh.) 84:11, 1977) reports that 8 of 13 children with extremely short stature and low plasma growth hormone concentration returned to normal after puberty, whereas the others remained refractory to all sorts of stimuli of growth hormone secretion. All patients responded well to treatment with growth hormone prepuberally, achieving normal or even supernormal height. He also mentions a girl with severe anorexia nervosa and growth hormone deficiency whose growth pattern was improved by treatment with the hormone. The endocrine abnormalities in anorexia nervosa are discussed later in this section. – Ed.] ◄

Treatment of Acromegaly by Transsphenoidal Microsurgery. Massimo A. Giovanelli, Enrico D. F. Motti, Alessandra Paracchi, Paolo Beck-Peccoz, Bruno Ambrosi and Giovanni Faglia[5] (Univ. of Milan) report the results of transsphenoidal microsurgery in 29 consecutive acromegalic patients. The 14 men and 15 women, aged 23 – 71, were seen in 1970 – 74 with active acromegaly. Seven patients had enlargement of the pituitary fossa with destructive changes limited to part of the sellar floor and 2 had extensive sellar destruction. Seven patients had previously had conventional radiotherapy. Selective removal of a microadenoma was possible in 3 patients. There were 24 eosinophilic and 5 mixed adenomas.

Serum growth hormone (GH) levels are shown in Figure 2. Serum GH levels fell below 10 ng/ml in 10 patients, to below 50% of basal levels in 10 patients with a further drop to below 20 ng/ml after radiotherapy, and did not fall below 30 ng/ml after either surgery or radiotherapy in 7 patients. Operation, sometimes repeated, and radiotherapy gave satisfactory results in 4 of 6 patients with suprasellar extension of the tumor. Transitory diabetes insipidus occurred in 5 patients and regressed spontaneously. Postoperative rhinorrhea resolved in 3 patients after repeated lumbar punctures.

These results clearly favor selective microsurgery in early diagnosed and surgically treated tumors or microadenomas. A less than radical approach does not hold out much promise of functional normalization

(5) J. Neurosurg. 44:677 – 686, June, 1976.

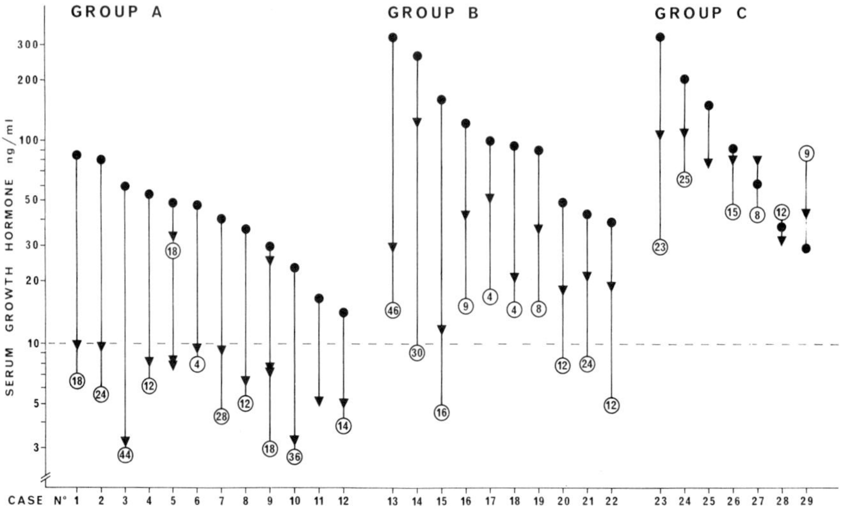

Fig 2.—Serum GH levels before surgery *(closed circles)*, after surgery *(closed triangles;* double triangles indicate a second operation) and after conventional radiotherapy *(open circles)*. Figures enclosed in the circles indicate the time interval in months between surgery and the latest GH determinations. (Courtesy of Giovanelli, M. A., et al.: J. Neurosurg. 44:677–686, June, 1976.)

in patients with larger adenomas. Radiotherapy may be effective in nonnormalized cases. Results of thyrotropin-releasing hormone tests are a good indication for radiotherapy even where the GH becomes normal by common assay methods after surgery. Transsphenoidal microsurgery resulted in improved visual acuity and visual fields in all but 1 of the present patients. No death or long-lasting complications have been reported in connection with this approach.

► [Note in Figure 2 that although all of the patients in Group A achieved growth hormones within normal levels after surgery, 2 required second operations and all except 1 had radiotherapy in addition to surgery. The best results are probably achieved when an isolated adenoma can be removed completely. In the others, these authors removed as much of the tumor as they could, but the results were not as good as they were when the tumors were small and completely resectable.

Nielson et al. (World J. Surg. 1:79, 1977) also describe 29 patients treated in this way for a variety of pituitary tumors, including Nelson's syndrome. They emphasize that this approach is safe and useful even in certain tumors producing visual symptoms and, therefore, extending above the diaphragma sellae.

After hypophysectomy for acromegaly, other pituitary hormone production may be deranged. Lamberg and colleagues (Acta Endocrinol. (Kbh.) 82:254, 1976) reported that neither a subnormal nor a low-normal response of TSH to testing with thyrotropin-releasing hormone necessarily indicates that there is an increased risk of developing secondary hypothyroidism postoperatively. They remark that the pituitary remnant seems to have a powerful potential for regenerating.

Radiotherapy is probably the most commonly used method of treating acromegaly. The criterion of good response is usually return of plasma growth hormone concentration to normal. This criterion may be deceptive, since sometimes the improvement is only temporary and the growth hormone concentration may rise again to abnormal levels (Grayzel: Arch Intern Med. 137:808, 1977.—Ed.] ◄

► ↓ There is no totally satisfactory method of treating acromegaly, although in a given instance, either surgery or radiation or both combined may be beneficial. The development of a third modality—medical treatment with bromocriptine—is therefore welcome. The following article discusses this form of therapy.—Ed. ◄

Long-Term Treatment of Acromegaly with Bromocriptine. Bromocriptine is a long-acting dopamine agonist that raises serum growth hormone (GH) levels in normal subjects but reduces them in acromegalic patients. J. A. H. Wass, M. O. Thorner, D. V. Morris, Lesley H. Rees, A. Stuart Mason, A. E. Jones and G. M. Besser[6] (London) treated 73 patients with bromocriptine for a mean of 12.8 months; 45 were treated for a year or longer. The series included 48 men; the age range was 18–72. Active acromegaly was confirmed by lack of suppression of circulating GH to below 2 μg/L during a 50-gm oral glucose tolerance test. Forty-two patients had had pituitary tumors treated by irradiation; 5 had had partial hypophysectomy and 1, yttrium implantation. The dose of bromocriptine was increased from 2.5 mg at bedtime to 2.5 mg every 12 hours after 72 hours, and further 2.5-mg increments were then added every 48–72 hours up to a daily dose of 20 mg. Growth hormone was determined by radioimmunoassay.

Mean serum GH fell by 7 μg/L or more in 57 of 73 patients and became undetectable in another patient (Fig 3). Growth hormone levels fell in 36 of the 45 patients treated for a year or longer. Maximum GH suppression was reached at doses ranging from 20 to 60 mg daily. Glucose tolerance improved in 20 of 23 diabetic patients and became normal in 15. Prolactin levels became undetectable during treatment in all 23 patients with initially elevated levels. Symptomatic improvement was noted by 71 of the 73 patients. Growth hormone increases and symptomatic changes followed the cessation of bromocriptine therapy but were less than pretreatment values and symptoms. Early side effects were not a major problem when the dose was increased gradually. Four patients acquired peptic ulcers, 1 died of hematemesis from an ulcer and another died of septicemia after surgical treatment.

Bromocriptine produced considerable subjective and objective clinical improvement, reduced circulating GH levels and improved glucose tolerance in acromegalic patients in this trial. The benefit was maintained during treatment for up to 2 years. Only rarely were GH levels reduced to normal. Hyperprolactinemic patients have been safely treated with a lower dose of bromocriptine for up to 6 years but it is too soon to determine whether serious side effects will occur when higher doses are used for a prolonged period in acromegalic patients.

Fig 3.—Change in mean serum GH before *(closed circle)* and during *(open circle)* bromocriptine treatment in 73 patients. Asterisks indicate nonresponders. Growth hormone was plotted on logarithmic scale for convenience. (Courtesy of Wass, J. A. H., et al.: Br. Med. J. 1:875–878, Apr. 2, 1977.)

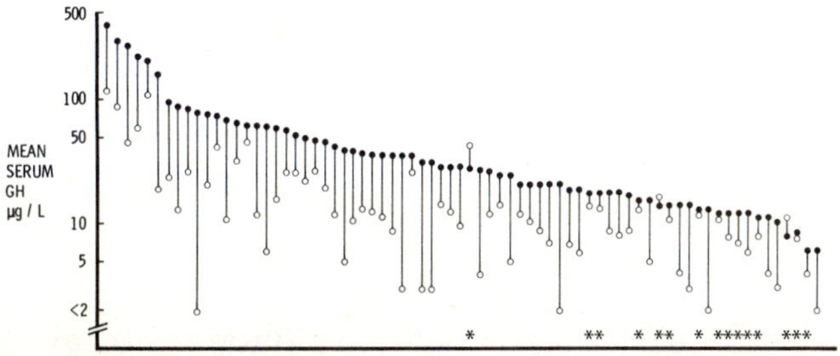

(6) Br. Med. J. 1:875–878, Apr. 2, 1977.

► [Belforte and colleagues (Acta Endocrinol. (Kbh.) 85:235, 1977) report observations on 30 acromegalic patients and confirm in all respects the findings reported in this article. They feel that the probability of a successful result from bromocriptine treatment can be predicted by a preliminary test consisting of giving 2.5 mg bromocriptine by mouth between 8:30 and 9 A.M. and following the plasma GH concentration at 30-minute intervals for 4 hours. Responders show a fall of GH of more than 50% from control value. Failure to have such a response was associated in their series with a minor or absent response of plasma GH concentration during chronic treatment, whereas 18 of 21 responders to the acute test had a good plasma GH response. In 12, the GH concentration returned entirely to normal. Like Wass et al., they mention that a good clinical response can be seen in patients whose plasma GH concentration remains somewhat abnormal. I have also seen this in my limited experience with this treatment.

Dunn et al. (Clin. Endocrinol. (Oxf.) 7:273, 1977) report that response to bromocriptine treatment is unusual in patients who have not responded to previous external radiation or surgical treatment, but neither Wass et al. nor Belfort et al. confirm this in their series.

Wass et al. make a point of the difficulty of assessing accurately the GH secretion by single determinations of the hormone's concentration in plasma. He recommends multiple sampling during the day. It is possible that failure to remember that GH is secreted in spurts and that multiple samples are needed to determine overall secretory patterns explains the apparent discrepancy between clinical response and persistent elevation of plasma GH concentration in some patients. It is also possible, however, that bromocriptine, in addition to its effect on pituitary GH secretion, affects the peripheral effects of GH on metabolism. And, of course, the drug suppresses powerfully the secretion of certain other pituitary hormones, especially prolactin.

The fact that bromocriptine can suppress GH production by a pituitary adenoma implies that the adenoma is under hypothalamic control. This consideration has received attention from a number of authors. Nakagawa and Obara (ibid. 5:713, 1976), for example, have studied the responses of patients with acromegaly to glucose. When the blood glucose concentration was raised to 500 mg/dl or more, patients with basal GH levels of 20 mu/L suppressed, but those with levels over 80 mu/L did not. This concentration of glucose is much higher than can be obtained with the standard 100-gm oral glucose tolerance test, and they feel that the oral test is less useful than the large intravenous load in separating subgroups of patients.

Bromocriptine does not necessarily inactivate normal control mechanisms in acromegalics treated with it. For example, acromegalics responding to the drug still have a rise of plasma GH concentration during sleep (Chihara et al.: J. Clin. Endocrinol. Metab. 44:78, 1977). Dopamine, like bromocriptine, suppresses GH secretion in acromegalics (though it has no effect in normal subjects). Camanni et al. (ibid., p. 465) suggest that the pituitary tumor probably lacks the normal blood-brain barrier to passage of dopamine, since this substance does not get into the normal brain or its appendages from the peripheral blood. Finally, Delitala et al. (ibid. 43:1382, 1976) report that metergoline, an antiserotonin agent, suppresses release of GH and prolactin in patients with acromegaly. The effect was comparable to that seen with bromocriptine in the 6 patients studied and could be maintained for the entire 6 days of the treatment course. Thus metergoline may prove a useful partner to bromocriptine in treating this disease.

It should be emphasized that medical treatment must be maintained steadily. It does not produce a cure—only a form of control. When the medication is stopped the abnormal GH pattern returns. Moreover, despite observation of a large number of patients treated with the drug, it is not yet certain that tumor growth (with associated dangerous pressure on adjacent structures) or long-term damage to the small blood vessels from this ergotamine derivative can be eliminated as risks of prolonged treatment. The patients need careful follow-up.—Ed.] ◄

Hypothalamic Endocrine Dysfunction in Anorexia Nervosa. Patients with anorexia nervosa have many signs indicating possible disturbances in endocrine function, including amenorrhea, signs of hypothyroidism and hirsutism. Antti Aro, B. -A. Lamberg and Risto Pelkonen[7] (Univ. of Helsinki) examined pituitary-adrenal and thyroid

(7) Acta Endocrinol. (Kbh.) 85:673–683, August, 1977.

function and growth hormone secretion in 21 consecutive young women with anorexia nervosa. All had lost over 20% of body weight, had had amenorrhea for at least 3 months, were under age 35 at onset of symptoms and had no medical illness or major psychiatric disorder explaining the weight loss. Mean age was 22 years and mean body weight, 37 kg. Mean loss of weight was 33%. Two patients had primary amenorrhea, and the rest had had secondary amenorrhea for a mean of 23 months.

The free thyroxine index of 19 patients was significantly below the normal mean, and 4 patients had abnormally low indices. Three of these had clinical signs of hypothyroidism. Mean protein-bound iodine and thyroxine concentrations were also significantly below control means. All but 3 patients had a delayed thyrotropin response to thyrotropin-releasing hormone (TRH). Fasting serum growth hormone (GH) values were increased in 9 of 17 patients, and 7 of 14 had an absent or subnormal GH response to insulin-induced hypoglycemia. The morning plasma cortisol value was increased in 9 patients. Diurnal variation was inadequate in 6 patients, 3 of whom had an increased morning cortisol level. Four patients had subnormal plasma cortisol responses to insulin-induced hypoglycemia. Two of 5 patients tested failed to show adequate plasma cortisol suppression after dexamethasone administration.

The results clearly indicate a frequent occurrence of hypothalamic-pituitary dysfunction in anorexia nervosa. The most consistent finding was a delayed thyrotropin response to TRH stimulation. Clinical hypothalamic hypothyroidism may be evident in some patients. The abnormalities of endocrine function found in anorexia nervosa are apparently of hypothalamic origin. The findings can be explained by dietary factors, primary hypothalamic damage or both. The similarities to kwashiorkor and the prompt effect of feeding on many of the findings suggest that dietary factors probably play a major role.

► [Croxon and Ibbertson (J. Clin. Endocrinol. Metab. 44:167, 1977) confirm the low levels of thyroxine and also find low concentrations of triiodothyronine in the plasma of similar patients. On the other hand, neither they nor Beumont et al. (ibid. 43:487, 1976) confirmed an abnormality of TSH release after administration of thyrotropin-releasing hormone. Beumont et al. also emphasize the reduced concentration of gonadotropic hormones in the plasma of patients with anorexia nervosa and remark on the poor response to gonadotropin-releasing hormone. As the patients regained weight, these abnormalities returned toward normal.

What is going on in the hypothalamus in these patients? It is possible that the observed abnormalities in endocrine control are entirely secondary manifestations of weight loss, as has usually been maintained in the past. It is also possible that the primary lesion in anorexia nervosa is in the appetite control centers of the hypothalamus and the observed disturbances reflect secondary changes within the hypothalamus as a result of the primary damage to the appetite control centers. A third possibility is that some influence—perhaps a substance which normally suppresses the appetite—is secreted in excess and has an effect both on the appetite centers and on other hypothalamic units. This last possibility occurs to me because of the profound anorexia and endocrine disturbances sometimes seen in patients with cancer. They are usually associated with specific cancers, such as the pulmonary oat cell carcinoma, and bear no relationship to the size or location of the tumor. If such distant effects on appetite can be produced by a tumor, perhaps a similar kind of appetite suppressant may play a part in normal appetite regulation. Anorexia nervosa may then represent excessive activity of this hypothetical anorexigenic material. And what about the undoubted psychologic disturbances in this disease? Possibly they are secondary to the anorexia, or possibly they are a secondary effect of the hypothetical hormone. Of course, this possibility is absolutely unsupported by data. But I can't help remembering the cachectic tumor patients. – Ed.] ◄

Prevalence and Presentation of Hyperprolactinemia in Patients with "Functionless" Pituitary Tumors. S. Franks, J. D. N. Nabarro and H. S. Jacobs[8] (London) measured prolactin in 57 female patients, aged 18–76, and 54 male patients, aged 16–70, with radiologic enlargement of the pituitary fossa. The patients were seen at the Middlesex Hospital between 1973 and 1976. No patient had evidence of acromegaly, Cushing's syndrome or Nelson's syndrome. Sixty-four patients were assessed before treatment and 47 only after pituitary surgery for adenoma. An adenoma was confirmed in 29 of the patients assessed before treatment. Serum prolactin was measured by specific radioimmunoassay.

Prolactin was elevated in 45 of 64 untreated patients and in 15 of 47 postoperative patients. Galactorrhea occurred in 11 patients studied before treatment and in 1 postoperative patient. Reproductive disorders predominated in the hyperprolactinemic group. Amenorrhea or impotence was present in 32 of these patients and in 2 with normal prolactin levels. All but 5 of 39 hyperprolactinemic women presented with amenorrhea. Eight of 21 men presented with impotence and 6 with a visual field defect. In only 1 impotent man was pituitary tumor recognized at an early stage. Six amenorrheic women were not found to have a pituitary tumor until a visual field defect occurred. Galactorrhea occurred in 1 patient with primary amenorrhea and in 10 with secondary amenorrhea. Gonadotropin deficiency occurred in only 2 hyperprolactinemic patients before treatment and in a third of those patients studied after pituitary surgery.

Serum prolactin should be determined in all patients with impotence and primary or secondary amenorrhea. Only if the level is elevated should detailed radiology of the pituitary fossa be performed. Persistent reproductive difficulties after hypophysectomy are more often attributable to hyperprolactinemia than to gonadotropin deficiency and, in suitable cases, are reversible by secondary treatment with bromocriptine.

► [Please go back and reread the last sentence of this article. It is terribly important! – Ed.] ◄

Galactorrhea: Study of 235 Cases, Including 48 with Pituitary Tumors. David L. Kleinberg, Gordon L. Noel and Andrew G. Frantz[9] (New York) analyzed data on 235 patients seen in 1969–75 with galactorrhea. Prolactin was measured initially by mouse breast bioassay and later by radioimmunoassay. Several pharmacologic agents were used to stimulate or suppress prolactin secretion in efforts to localize functional abnormalities within the central nervous system. Mean patient age was 30.9 years.

Pituitary tumors were radiologically evident in 20% of all patients and in 34% of women with amenorrhea. Amenorrhea was present in 34

(8) Lancet 1:778–780, Apr. 9, 1977.
(9) N. Engl. J. Med. 296:589–600, Mar. 17, 1977.

of 42 women with pituitary tumors and was primary in 5. These patients had the highest serum prolactin concentrations (Fig 4). Chlorpromazine did not produce positive prolactin responses in any of 9 tumor patients studied. Responses to thyrotropin-releasing hormone (TRH) were markedly blunted. L-Dopa suppressed prolactin in 4 of 9 patients. Eight patients had clinical acromegaly. Six had hypothyroidism and 1 had hypoadrenocorticism.

Idiopathic galactorrhea with menses was diagnosed in 32% of patients. Serum prolactin concentrations were normal in 65 of these 76 patients. Over half the patients tested had subnormal responses to chlorpromazine. Twenty patients (8.5%) had idiopathic galactorrhea with amenorrhea. Prolactin concentrations were markedly elevated in these patients. Eighteen patients had Chiari-Frommel syndrome. Twenty-three patients had galactorrhea apparently related to oral contraceptive use, and 16 patients had an association with drug therapy, usually tranquilizers. Ten patients had primary hypothyroidism. Five had the empty sella syndrome. Thirteen men, 6 of whom had pituitary tumors, had galactorrhea. Four of the 7 men without tumors had drug-associated galactorrhea.

If fertility is not desired, galactorrhea is often not troublesome enough to warrant specific treatment in idiopathic cases with amenorrhea. Ergot derivatives are indicated if treatment is to be given. Both surgery and radiotherapy are used for treatment of pituitary tumors. Lergotrile mesylate has produced a functional response in a few tumor patients that was as good as that obtained by operation or radiotherapy.

► [This article confirms the preceding one, but approaches the problem from a dif-

Fig 4.—Plasma prolactin concentrations in 235 patients with galactorrhea of various causes. Among patients with tumor, triangles denote those with acromegaly. Open symbols denote patients studied only after radiotherapy or operation. (Courtesy of Kleinberg, D. L., et al.: N. Engl. J. Med. 296:589–600, Mar. 17, 1977.)

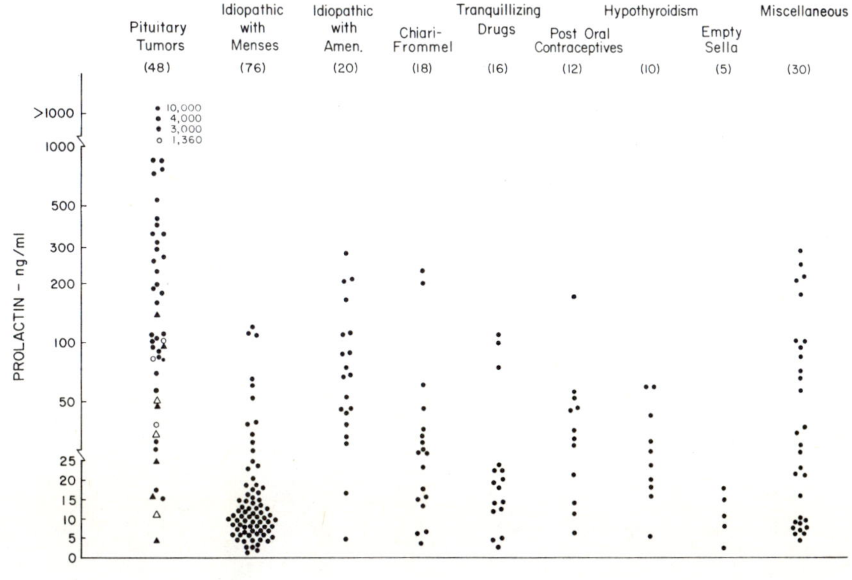

ferent angle, since all of these patients were defined by the presence of galactorrhea. Boyd et al. also found high levels of prolactin in the plasma of patients with galactorrhea-amenorrhea and pituitary tumors, but found that the hormone was also elevated in patients with normal pituitary fossae (Ann. Intern. Med. 87:165, 1977). Thus it appears that hyperprolactinemia must be sought in two types of patients: those with "functionless tumors" and those with galactorrhea combined with sexual hypofunction. In women this usually means amenorrhea, but in men it may mean impotence. It is easy to miss minimal galactorrhea on physical examination unless a specific effort is made to massage the mammary glands and look for even a drop of secretion. The diagnosis is more likely to occur to the physician when he is evaluating a woman than when he has a male patient; but impotence is often associated with hyperprolactinemia and may be a major problem to the patient. This type of impotence is not of psychogenic origin.

Schaison and Metzger studied 12 patients with the empty sella syndrome (Acta Endocrinol. (Kbh.) 83:483, 1976). Five had no endocrine disturbance; 2 had panhypopituitarism, in 1 caused by meningoencephalitis and in the other by cranial trauma, and 5 had the amenorrhea-galactorrhea syndrome. In 2 of these serum prolactin was elevated, but it was normal in the others. The authors point out that the empty sella is a neuroanatomical diagnosis and that it can be associated with several different endocrine syndromes or with none.—Ed.] ◄

The Adrenal Gland

► The ability of ACTH to stimulate synthesis and release of corticosteroids is well recognized, and the fact that chronic exposure of the adrenal cortex to ACTH causes hyperplasia of the gland is also commonplace. What is perhaps not so clearly recognized is that ACTH does not cause an increase in mass of the adrenal cortex when given over a brief period. Indeed, some observers have suggested that there are two factors controlling the adrenal cortex—ACTH for secretion and something else for growth. Hornsby and Gill (J. Clin. Invest 60:342, 1977) investigated this problem and found that a concentration of ACTH in tissue culture medium which stimulated adrenal cortical cells to increased production of corticosteroids simultaneously inhibited incorporation of thymidine into DNA. This inhibition of DNA synthesis disappeared and cell growth resumed if ACTH was continuously applied over periods of several days. Another factor, called "fibroblast growth factor," also stimulated growth of adrenal cortical cells in tissue culture. Its stimulating effect was independent of the ACTH effect. The exact nature of this growth factor is not known.

The relationship of the adrenal cortex to essential hypertension has been studied for many years, but the connection remains confusing. The form of adrenogenital syndrome in which 11-hydroxylation is defective is associated with excessive production of deoxycorticosterone and deoxycortisol ("compound S"). Hypertension is the usual finding in patients with this disease. Honda and colleagues (J. Clin. Endocrinol. Metab. 44:264, 1977) find the same secretory pattern in patients with essential hypertension. They also found evidence of defective 17-hydroxylation and raise the question of whether an important element in producing essential hypertension may be a mild defect in steroid biosynthesis.

It has become commonplace for patients receiving steroid treatment to carry cards with them indicating the nature and dosage of steroids that they are receiving. In case of accident, it is hoped that the card will protect the patient against inadvertent discontinuation of treatment. But how careful are patients about carrying the cards, and how well do they understand their importance? A brief but disturbingly convincing study by Downie and collaborators (Br. Med. J. 1:428, 1977) suggests that about 20% of patients did not know why it was important to carry a card, 24% were not carrying one and 12% denied ever receiving one. Moreover, when the cards were reviewed, 33% carried erroneous information. If we believe that the steroid cards are important, we should check up at intervals to make sure our patients are still using them. The study did not include evaluation of identifying jewelry like Medicalert, but it would be useful to check this form of identification as well.

Certain forms of topical steroids are advertised as being so poorly absorbed through the skin that they present no risk of systemic overdose. May et al. (Arch Intern. Med. 136:612, 1976) describe a patient who developed Cushing's syndrome from percutaneous absorption of triamcinolone acetonide. This is a step worse than the pituitary suppression which has often been described in the past.—Ed. ◄

Plasma ACTH and Cortisol Responses to TRF, Vasopressin or Hypoglycemia in Cushing's Disease and Nelson's Syndrome. Dorothy T. Krieger and Martin Luria[1] (Mount Sinai School of Medicine) sought to distinguish between a hypothalamic and a primary pituitary etiology of Nelson's syndrome. Responses of plasma ACTH or cortisol or both to thyrotropin-releasing factor (TRF), vasopressin and insulin were determined in 5 patients with Nelson's syndrome and 12 with untreated Cushing's disease. Minimal to moderate sellar enlarge-

(1) J. Clin. Endocrinol. Metab. 44:361–368, February, 1977.

ment was present in 3 patients with Nelson's syndrome. All the patients with Nelson's syndrome had received pituitary irradiation. Studies were also done in 36 normal subjects.

No increase in plasma cortisol concentration was found after TRF in normal subjects. Plasma ACTH concentration rose after TRF in all patients, and those with Cushing's disease also showed a rise in plasma cortisol concentration. No rise in serum thyrotropin concentration followed TRF in patients with Cushing's disease. Patients with Nelson's syndrome showed an increment of 3.9 IU/ml, significantly less than that seen in normal subjects. Patients and normal subjects had similar prolactin responses. Plasma ACTH concentration rose markedly after insulin-induced hypoglycemia in patients with Nelson's syndrome, whereas those with Cushing's disease showed a lesser increase than normal subjects. Neither patient group showed a significant increase in growth hormone values. Increments in plasma ACTH concentrations after vasopressin were significantly greater in both patient groups than in normal subjects, although percentage changes were similar. Increments in plasma cortisol concentrations were greater in patients with Cushing's disease than in normal subjects.

Pituitary secretory function in patients with Nelson's syndrome is not autonomous since ACTH secretion can be stimulated by hypothalamic agents. This may suggest that the associated tumors are not of primary pituitary origin but arise from altered hypothalamic or central nervous system function; however, spontaneous tumors may lack autonomous function—e.g., some primary adrenal adenomas which respond to ACTH and are suppressed by dexamethasone. The mechanism responsible for the effect of TRF in eliciting ACTH and cortisol release in patients with Nelson's syndrome or Cushing's disease, in contrast to the absence of such a response in normal subjects, is unknown.

► [In Cushing's disease, as in acromegaly discussed earlier, the mechanisms controlling pituitary secretion are abnormal. Although ACTH secretion is the most obviously deranged function, other hormones are also released under abnormal circumstances. In the case of ACTH, its secretion is not suppressed by corticosteroids; indeed, its secretion may be stimulated (Fehm et al.: N. Engl. J. Med. 297:904, 1977). The secretion of growth hormone after hypoglycemia is impaired, especially when a pituitary tumor is present, but this returns to normal when the disease becomes inactive (Tyrrell et al.: J. Clin. Endocrinol. Metab. 44:218, 1977).

The nature of normal pituitary ACTH is well known, and its amino acid sequence has been determined. Do pituitary tumors produce the same kind of ACTH as the normal pituitary? Krieger and her colleagues (Clin Endocrinol. (Oxf.) 5:455, 1976) cultured a basophilic pituitary tumor which had caused Cushing's disease and studied the ACTH it produced. The amount of hormone per gram of tumor was much lower than that found in normal pituitary, and there was much more "big" ACTH as well as fragments too small to have biologic effect. The pattern is reminiscent of that seen in tumors producing ectopic ACTH. As Krieger points out, however, the tumor had previously been irradiated, and the influence of this treatment cannot be evaluated.

It is sometimes difficult to distinguish Cushing's syndrome arising from pituitary hyperactivity from that caused by ectopic hormone production. Gilkes and colleagues (Br. Med. J. 1:996, 1977) measured both ACTH and lipotropin in the plasma of patients with pituitary and ectopic Cushing's syndrome. When the source of these hormones was pituitary, the concentration of ACTH in plasma was higher than that of lipotropin, but when an ectopic source was involved, lipotropin predominated. Two different types of lipotropin were studied. That produced by the pituitary was predominantly of the beta form, whereas that from ectopic sources was predominantly gamma. The authors feel that predominance of lipotropin—especially the gamma form—might be a valuable indicator of an ectopic form of Cushing's syndrome.—Ed.] ◄

Nelson's Syndrome: Frequency, Prognosis and Effect of Prior Pituitary Irradiation. Thomas J. Moore, Robert G. Dluhy, Gordon H. Williams and John P. Cain[2] (Harvard Med. School) reviewed 120 cases of Cushing's disease, in 9 of which pituitary tumors appeared after adrenalectomy. Bilateral adrenal hyperplasia was confirmed in all cases. Mean follow-up is 8 years. The 9 patients displayed radiographic evidence of a pituitary tumor and progressive cutaneous melanosis after adrenalectomy. Three patients had radiographic evidence of pituitary tumors before adrenalectomy.

The female-male ratio was 11:1, compared with 4:1 in Cushing's disease alone. Fifty-six percent of adrenalectomized patients developed cutaneous hyperpigmentation. Two patients each presented with headache and visual field disturbances. Four tumors did not appear until more than 9 years after adrenalectomy. Pigmentation decreased after surgery or pituitary irradiation in half the patients with Nelson's syndrome. Two of the 3 patients with evidence of pituitary tumor when Cushing's disease was initially diagnosed were asymptomatic. All 3 had cutaneous melanosis. Tumors causing compressive symptoms were generally operated on and then irradiated. Five patients had pituitary surgery. Two of the 3 patients with preadrenalectomy pituitary tumors are well; the third died suddenly 2 years after the tumor was irradiated. Seven patients with Nelson's syndrome are living. Only 1 died of the pituitary tumor. Two patients have stable visual field defects and 1 developed a 3d nerve palsy after pituitary irradiation. Three patients required thyroid supplements for secondary hypothyroidism.

All patients should be followed indefinitely by sellar x-rays after adrenalectomy for bilateral adrenal hyperplasia, regardless of previous pituitary irradiation, for the possible occurrence of Nelson's syndrome. Pathogenic differences may exist between tumors present at the time Cushing's disease is diagnosed and those that appear after adrenalectomy.

► [The abstracter did not bother to put in the most important conclusion! There was *no advantage* to radiation treatment in preventing growth of the tumor! Thus the idea that Nelson's syndrome can be prevented by prophylactic radiotherapy is not supported by these studies.

The other major lesson is that once a pituitary tumor is demonstrated to be present, or when the characteristic pattern of Nelson's syndrome develops, it is important to initiate treatment to the pituitary. Surgery is a possibility, and radiation to an established tumor may also help, as Moore's group showed. Another possibility is discussed in the following article.—Ed.] ◄

Treatment of Nelson's Syndrome by Pituitary Implantation of Yttrium-90 or Gold-198. J. Cassar, F. H. Doyle, P. D. Lewis, K. Mashiter, S. Van Noorden and G. F. Joplin[3] (Postgrad. Med. School, London) report experience with 8 patients who had Nelson's syndrome and who were treated with a pituitary implant of ^{90}Y or ^{198}Au or both. Nelson's

(2) Ann. Intern. Med. 85:731–734, December, 1976.
(3) Br. Med. J. 2:269–272, July 31, 1976.

syndrome was defined as gross pigmentation, with or without a radiologically evident pituitary tumor, developing after previous effective adrenalectomy and despite adequate replacement therapy. In 3 patients with initial partial adrenalectomy the remnant was removed because of recurrent Cushing's disease. Adrenal hyperplasia was found in all patients. Mean age at diagnosis was 35 years, and a mean of 6 years had elapsed after the last adrenal operation. All patients showed considerable pigmentation. Only 1 patient had had treatment directed to the pituitary. Six patients underwent implantation with ^{90}Y, 1 with ^{198}Au and 1 with a combination. Mean follow-up was 5 years.

Skin pigmentation became normal in 6 patients and nearly normal in 1. No patient developed new cranial nerve disease or showed further expansion of the pituitary fossa. All patients but 3 had normal plasma ACTH values at follow-up; 2 of those with elevations remained abnormally pigmented. One patient had a temporary 3d nerve paresis after surgery, and another had a cerebrospinal fluid leak that was plugged successfully. One patient developed clinical gonadal deficiency, and 1 was considered to be hypothyroid. All 6 patients who underwent biopsy showed the presence of a basophil mucoid adenoma.

The effect of pituitary implantation of ^{90}Y or ^{198}Au in Nelson's syndrome appears to be long lasting. None of these patients relapsed, and 1 was still in clinical remission with normal plasma ACTH values 13 years after the implantation. The series was too small to indicate which type of radionuclide gives the best results.

► [This form of treatment, in experienced hands, seems to work very well indeed. The group at the Hammersmith Hospital has more experience with this particular form of treatment than anyone else in the world, I believe. They can get good results in patients most other surgeons would insist on exploring transfrontally.

How often is the pituitary fossa abnormal in patients with pituitary Cushing's disease? MacErlean and Doyle carefully examined the pituitary fossa retrospectively in 93 patients and found radiologic evidence of a pituitary tumor in 23%. In over half, the diagnosis was based on evaluation of lateral tomograms of the fossa. Of 7 patients with extrapituitary Cushing's syndrome, none had abnormal pituitary fossae (Br. J. Radiol. 49:820, 1976).—Ed.] ◄

Overnight Urinary 11-Hydroxycorticosteroid Estimations in Diagnosis of Cushing's syndrome. Estimation of 11-hydroxycorticoids in a 24-hour urine specimen is extremely useful in identifying patients who require further study to confirm Cushing's syndrome, but accurate collection of such specimens by outpatients is not easy. D. Mattingly and Christine Tyler[4] (Univ. of Exeter) determined whether an overnight collection is sufficient to identify patients who are secreting excessive amounts of cortisol. Studies were done in 29 healthy women and convalescent inpatients, 49 obese women, 38 women with considerable hirsutism, 20 of whom were also obese and 11 women with Cushing's syndrome due to bilateral adrenal hyperplasia. The diagnosis of Cushing's syndrome was confirmed surgically in 9 patients. In all cases the normal circadian variation of plasma 11-hydroxycorticoids was impaired or absent and the plasma and urinary 11-hydroxycorticoid levels were elevated and failed to fall normally during

(4) Br. Med. J. 2:668–669, Sept. 18, 1976.

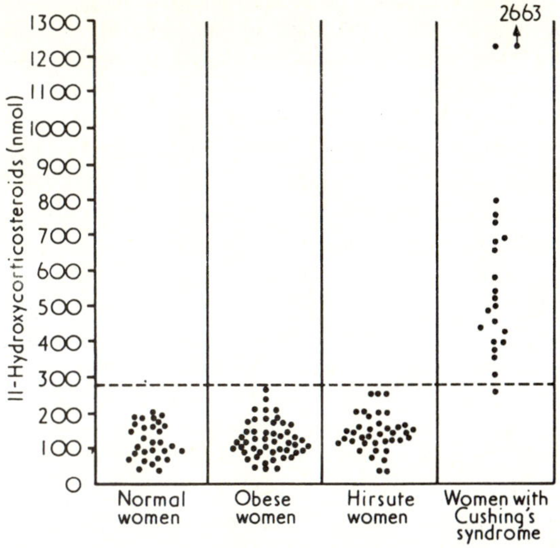

Fig 5.—Overnight urine values in all subjects; 22 specimens were collected from the 11 women with Cushing's syndrome. Conversion to traditional units—11-hydroxycorticosteroids: 1 nmol ≈ 0.36 μg. (Courtesy of Mattingly, D., and Tyler, C.: Br. Med. J. 2:668–669, Sept. 18, 1976.)

dexamethasone administration. Urine was collected over 24 hours in 3 patients with Cushing's syndrome and 7 control subjects.

A strong circadian rhythm in urinary 11-hydroxycorticoids was confirmed in normal subjects; the smallest percentage of the 24-hour excretion occurred during the night. No similar pattern was apparent in patients with Cushing's syndrome and the overnight excretion was much higher than in control subjects. Results in overnight specimens are shown in Figure 5. Only 1 patient with Cushing's syndrome had a value less than 276 nmol (100 μg) during the night, whereas the highest value in the other groups was 271 nmol in an obese patient. The highest overnight value in the group with Cushing's syndrome was 2,663 nmol (965 μg).

Patients with adrenocortical overactivity can be identified by their higher overnight urinary excretion of 11-hydroxycorticoids. This simple screening test is useful in selecting those women with obesity and hirsutism, hypertension or diabetes who require more extensive investigation. Overnight levels exceeding 276 nmol are highly indicative of adrenocortical overactivity and call for further action. The diagnosis cannot be entirely excluded by one normal result but, if doubt persists, the test can easily be repeated.

► [It is a good deal easier to collect an overnight urine sample than it is to collect a 24-hour sample, The test relies for its validity on the fact that the plasma cortisol level is reduced at night and that the clearance of cortisol by the kidney is rapid, so what is excreted in the urine reflects quite accurately what is present in the plasma.

Cushing's syndrome is often diagnosed on the basis of plasma cortisol concentration. Tan and colleagues point out that the apparent concentration of cortisol may be elevated in patients with the adrenogenital syndrome when plasma concentrations of progesterone, 17-hydroxyprogesterone and 21-deoxycortisol may be 10–100 times the normal concentration. Under these circumstances there may be sufficient cross-reactivity in the plasma assay to give an appearance of elevated cortisol levels. The error is roughly equal by competitive protein binding or by fluorogenic assay methods. The true answer can be obtained after chromatography (J. Lab. Clin. Med. 89:735, 1977). —Ed.] ◄

Drug Control of Cushing's Syndrome: Combined Aminoglutethimide and Metyrapone Therapy. Drug control of Cushing's syndrome is often necessary to prevent surgery on a weak, potassium-depleted patient and to reduce postoperative respiratory complications secondary to muscle weakness of the chest and obesity. D. F. Child, C. W. Burke, D. M. Burley, Lesley H. Rees and T. Russell Fraser[5] evaluated combined aminoglutethimide and metyrapone therapy in 18 consecutive patients with Cushing's syndrome. Sixteen patients had pituitary-dependent Cushing's disease, 1 had a primary adrenal adenoma and 1 had ectopic ACTH production from a pancreatic carcinoid tumor. Patients were treated for 2 weeks, but 4 with Cushing's disease were treated for longer periods when their definitive management was delayed.

All 12 patients given 1 or 2 gm aminoglutethimide and 2–4.2 gm metyrapone daily, as well as dexamethasone and fludrocortisone, had a fall of cortisol levels into the normal range by day 5. One patient showed escape of the plasma cortisol on day 11. Severe myopathy resolved nearly completely in 2 patients. Diabetes improved in all 4 affected patients, and 7 patients showed general clinical improvement. Three patients developed a rash in the 2d week of treatment and 3 had severe drowsiness. One patient had slurred speech and ataxia. Only 3 patients had elevated plasma compound S levels during treatment. Six patients received 750 mg aminoglutethimide and 2 gm metyrapone daily for 2 weeks. All 5 studied had a fall of urinary free cortisol to normal by day 3 and of plasma cortisol by day 1. Four patients showed general clinical improvement. Severe myopathy resolved in 1 patient and diabetes improved in 2. Two patients developed a rash. Plasma compound S levels remained elevated in 3 of 5 patients. Four patients were treated for 26 days to 1 year. Steroid values became normal and remained so. Two patients showed marked symptomatic improvement and 1 showed general clinical improvement. No side effects occurred in these patients, who received 500 or 750 mg aminoglutethimide daily.

A satisfactory fall in cortisol levels can be achieved with 0.75 gm aminoglutethimide daily. Glucocorticoid replacement is necessary from the start of drug therapy. Patients are given 2 gm metyrapone daily, 0.5 mg dexamethasone twice daily and 0.1 mg fludrocortisone daily, besides aminoglutethimide. This regimen is useful in preparing patients for surgery and may be used as long-term treatment in milder cases.

► [The important point is that no significant toxicity occurred when the dose of aminoglutethimide was restricted to 0.75 gm daily, though rashes and other toxic manifestations occurred at higher doses. The low dose controlled both the symptoms and the biochemical abnormalities when it was combined with metyrapone, though alone it was insufficient. The decision to use dexamethasone to protect against adrenal hypofunction may not be entirely appropriate. Not only does this steroid have negligible

(5) Acta Endocrinol. (Kbh.) 82:330–341, June, 1976.

salt-active potency, but its half-life is affected by the medication, so maintaining good control of adrenal function may be difficult. Santen and colleagues found cortisol replacement to be preferable (Cancer 39:2948, 1977).

Other forms of medical treatment have also been proposed. Jeffcoate et al. (Br. Med. J. 2:215, 1977) report good results in the long-term management of 13 patients with pituitary Cushing's syndrome with metyrapone alone or in combination with pituitary irradiation (8 patients) or transfrontal hypophysectomy (1 patient). The dose required varied from 0.25 gm twice daily to 1 gm 4 times daily. The dose was decided on the basis of its ability to maintain the plasma 11-hydroxycorticosteroid concentration between 11 and 14.5 μg/dl throughout the day. The authors do not consider this definitive treatment, but consider it a nontoxic and successful adjuvant to more specific treatment. In this respect it is worth noting that Jennings et al. (N. Engl. J. Med. 297:957, 1977) report cure of pituitary Cushing's syndrome within 18 months of external radiation of the pituitary with from 3,500 to 4,950 rad in 12 of 15 children. In 10, control was complete within 9 months. There were no complications and the authors recommend this form of treatment for childhood Cushing's disease. – Ed.] ◄

Failure of Cyproheptadine to Inhibit Vasopressin-Stimulated Cortisol Release in a Patient with Cushing's Disease. Cyproheptadine reduces ACTH secretion in normal subjects and patients with Cushing's disease, presumably through its antiserotonin properties, but the level at which this effect occurs is undefined. W. F. George, M. Husain, J. P. Lock and F. H. Katz[6] (Univ. of Colorado) evaluated cyproheptadine in a woman, aged 21, with Cushing's disease due to a pituitary tumor. She presented with a blood pressure of 150/100 mm Hg and amenorrhea. High-dose but not low-dose dexamethasone suppressed urinary 17-ketogenic steroid secretion. The pituitary was irradiated and cyproheptadine was then given in a dosage of 4 mg 3 times a day orally, which was increased to 20 mg daily over 4 weeks. Tests were repeated 2 weeks after the end of cyproheptadine therapy.

Hypertension and elevated ketogenic steroids were unchanged during cyproheptadine therapy, and adrenal responsiveness to ACTH was unaltered. Cyproheptadine failed to modify vasopressin-stimulated cortisol release. The serum cortisol response to insulin-induced hypoglycemia was markedly blunted during and after cyproheptadine therapy. Adequate hypoglycemia was obtained during both tests. Basal serum cortisol concentration was reduced after cyproheptadine.

This study showed no efficacy of cyproheptadine therapy in a patient with Cushing's disease. The reduction in basal serum cortisol concentration after therapy was probably due to the pituitary irradiation.

► [Allgrove et al. (Br. Med. J. 1:686, 1977) also describe a 13-year-old boy whose Cushing's disease failed to respond to cyproheptadine in doses up to 24 mg daily for 2 months. Although he became less irritable and his sleep pattern improved, there was no alteration of the overactive adrenal function and he was considered a failure on this form of treatment. He responded well to bilateral adrenalectomy. In both of these patients the reported failures are important as indicators that the treatment proposed by Krieger and colleagues (N. Engl. J. Med. 293:893, 1975) sometimes fails, but Krieger has stated informally that response is slow and may not appear until after a considerable period of treatment. Perhaps a response would have occurred if treatment had been continued longer. In the case presented by George et al., a month of treatment is not very long; 2 months in the patient described by Allgrove et al. seems a long enough trial. The failure of cyproheptadine to produce amelioration of the abnormal steroid metabolism 2 weeks after completion of treatment in the case presented by George et al. is, of course, nonsense! Nobody has suggested that the effects of cyproheptadine continue for more than a day or less after it is discontinued.

(6) Horm. Res. 7:308–312, 1976.

Thus, one must continue to be skeptical of cyproheptadine treatment, but the cases cited are not sufficient evidence to justify rejecting further tests.

In designing treatment of patients with adrenocortical hyperfunction, it is essential to be certain whether the disease is of pituitary origin or whether it originates in an adrenal tumor. One attempt to differentiate the two was based on demonstration of the fluctuating nature of the plasma cortisol concentration. It was hoped that pituitary hyperfunction would be associated with fluctuations whereas tumors would not. The test provided Vetter and his colleagues with no useful differentiation. Other methods are needed. The application of physical techniques to this problem is discussed in the following article. – Ed.] ◄

Comparative Study of Ultrasound, ^{131}I-19-Iodocholesterol Scintigraphy and Aortography in Localizing Adrenal Lesions. H. Kehlet, M. Blichert-Toft, S. Hancke, J. Fog Pedersen, J. Kvist Kristensen, F. Efsen, H. Dige-Petersen, J. Fogh, K. Lockwood and E. Hasner[7] (Copenhagen) compared the diagnostic value of ultrasound, iodocholesterol scintigraphy and renal angiography in a prospective study of 27 consecutive patients who underwent adrenal surgery in 1973–76. Nine patients had pituitary-dependent Cushing's syndrome, 5 had pituitary-independent Cushing's syndrome, 4 had adrenocortical androgenic excess and 9 had a preoperative diagnosis of pheochromocytoma. Ultrasound study was performed on all patients and renal angiography in all but 1. Adrenocortical scintigraphy was performed with ^{131}I-19-iodocholesterol and a rectilinear scanner in 23 patients.

Ultrasound study correctly identified 13 of the 16 unilateral adrenal lesions but gave false negative results in 3 cases. Angiography gave true positive results in 10 cases and was falsely negative in 5. Scintigraphy correctly localized the lesion in 10 of 12 patients. Ultrasound study was normal in all 11 patients with bilaterally normal or hyperplastic adrenals. Angiography was falsely positive in 2 cases. Scintigraphy gave normal findings in all 11 cases. A correct scintigraphic diagnosis was made in all 14 patients with Cushing's syndrome, 5 of whom had a glucocorticoid-secreting adenoma. Five of 7 cases of androgen excess or pheochromocytoma were correctly diagnosed by scintigraphy. Scintigraphy was more valuable than angiography for investigation of patients with Cushing's syndrome, but it was no more useful than ultrasound study. The three techniques were of comparable value in diagnosis of androgen-secreting tumors and pheochromocytomas.

The diagnostic accuracy of adrenal ultrasound imaging in adrenal lesions is similar to that of renal angiography and adrenocortical scintigraphy. Scintigraphy has high diagnostic accuracy in Cushing's syndrome. Ultrasound is the first study used. Scintigraphy may be preferable for diagnosis of small glucocorticoid-secreting adenomas. Aortography should be reserved for inconclusive cases and suspected extra-adrenal pheochromocytomas.

► [It appears that there is not much to chose betwen ultrasound and scintigraphy as far as accuracy is concerned. Both methods are still in their infancy and will probably give still better results in the future. On the other hand, renal aortography (which is the angiographic method used) is clearly a poor choice. Not only does it require intra-arterial catheterization, but it is not as reliable as the other two. Although the authors did not do venography (probably a preferable diagnostic method to arteriography) this method also has drawbacks, the chief one being the occasional development of adre-

(7) Br. Med. J. 2:665–667, Sept. 18, 1976.

nal thrombosis and infarction. Thus it seems that noninvasive methods probably should be encouraged and catheterization with contrast studies relied on only when the other methods leave doubt as to the answer.

But scintigraphy is not without difficulties. Byck and Pauwels (Radiol. Clin. (Basel) 45:302, 1976) describe a patient in whom the gallbladder accumulated and retained so much ^{131}I-iodocholesterol that it gave a "hot spot" on the reading, suggestive of an adrenal hot area. A right lateral scan showed the hot spot to be anterior and thus to be different from the right adrenal. Ordinarily the gallbladder would not retain the radioactive steroid long enough to show up after the delay of several days required for the adrenal to concentrate the radioactivity. In a patient whose gallbladder retains the iodinated cholesterol for a week or more, considerable radiation could be delivered to the mucosa.

Troncone and colleagues (Br. J. Radiol. 50:340, 1977) report scintigraphic studies of 38 patients, with a high rate of success in patients with adrenocortical hyperactivity. They found the studies less useful in characterizing tumors which were not hyperfunctioning. Thus scintigraphy would be helpful in clarifying the problem of Cushing's syndrome but not very helpful with pheochromocytomas, most malignant tumors and many benign tumors with a low level of function. Part of the problem with the tumors of low functional capacity may be that ^{131}I-19-iodocholesterol, the original isotopic compound used in adrenal scanning, may not be the ideal compound to use. The following article discusses another compound, which may be better. – Ed.] ◄

Scintigraphic Detection of Hepatic Metastases with ^{131}I-Labeled Steroid in Recurrent Adrenal Carcinoma: Case Report. When symptoms of adrenocortical hormone overproduction from adrenocortical carcinoma are present, the diagnostic value of adrenal scintigraphy with ^{131}I-iodocholesterol is thought to be low, since the uptake in foci of disease is small. K. Watanabe, I. Kamoi, C. Nakayama, I. Koga and K. Matsuura[8] (Kyoshu Univ.) visualized hepatic metastases in a postoperative patient with adrenocortical carcinoma and Cushing's syndrome by imaging with ^{131}I-6-NCL (iodine-131-6β-iodomethyl-19-norcholest-5(10)-en-3β-ol), a new steroidal agent with a much higher adrenal uptake than ^{131}I-iodocholesterol.

Woman, 40, had had palpitations, headache and exertional dizziness for 5 years. Characteristic findings of Cushing's syndrome and high blood pressure had been noted and evidence was suggestive of autonomous hormone production. Pneumoperitoneum and adrenal venography showed a left adrenal tumor, and total left adrenectomy, left partial nephrectomy and splenectomy were carried out. The 1,450-gm tumor was an adrenocortical carcinoma. Cobalt therapy was given postoperatively. The patient was readmitted about 1½ years later with abdominal distention, anorexia and right upper quadrant pain. The cushingoid symptoms were aggravated. The levels of blood cortisol and urinary steroids were markedly elevated and the liver was enlarged. Hepatic scintigraphy with ^{99m}Tc-sulfur colloid showed numerous defects, and scintigraphy done 8 days after the injection of 700 μCi ^{131}I-6-NCL showed multifocal abnormal accumulation at sites corresponding with the defects noted on technetium scanning (Fig 6). Methotrexate was given, but the patient died 22 months after surgery, with general prostration and cardiac insufficiency.

Autopsy showed metastases in the liver, lumbar vertebrae and nodes near the left renal artery. The right adrenal was markedly atrophied. The markedly enlarged liver contained many nodular metastatic foci 4 – 10 cm in diameter. The centers of the larger nodules were necrotic. The foci resembled adrenocortical cells.

Hepatic metastases of adrenocortical carcinoma were detected by

(8) J. Nucl. Med. 17:904 – 906, October, 1976.

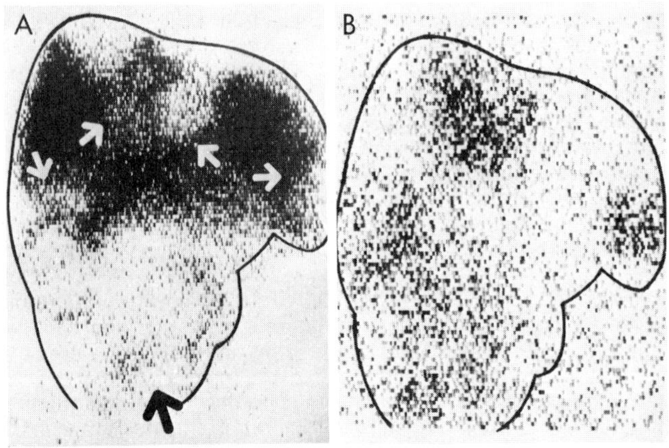

Fig 6.—**A,** anterior liver scan, made with ^{99m}Tc-sulfur colloid, shows numerous large and small defects *(arrows)*. **B,** liver scan, made 8 days after intravenous injection of ^{131}I-6-NCL, shows activity accumulations corresponding to defects in scan **A**. (Courtesy of Watanabe, K., et al.: J. Nucl. Med. 17:904–906, October, 1976.)

scintigraphy with ^{131}I-6-NCL in this case. In a large defect, the uptake of this nuclide is better around the periphery and weak in the center. Accumulation of the nuclide in the adrenal cortex compared with that in liver is about 10 times the ratio for ^{131}I-iodocholesterol.

► [The new compound is a contaminant in the usual preparation of ^{131}I-19-iodocholesterol. Couch and Williams (J. Nucl. Med. 18:724, 1977) synthesized preparations of each of these substances that were more than 98% pure. With these preparations they showed in rats that the uptake of isotope was at least 18 times greater in the adrenal at 24 hours and 50 times greater at 72 hours when 6-iodomethyl-19-norcholesterol is used than when the 19-iodocholesterol preparation is tested. This increased uptake undoubtedly accounts for the success of Watanabe and his colleagues in demonstrating the presence of metastases in the liver. There are other practical advantages to the new compound. Because a high uptake is achieved rapidly, the delay between administration of the test substance and imaging can be reduced from several days to only a few days or even less. In demonstrating the metastasis the Japanese group waited 8 days, but this delay might not be necessary in ordinary adrenal scanning. Probably the 6-iodomethyl preparation is not the best possible one, but it seems a considerable advance over the 19-iodo compound.—Ed.] ◄

Alcohol-Induced Pseudo-Cushing's Syndrome. L. H. Rees, G. M. Besser, W. J. Jeffcoate, D. J. Goldie and V. Marks[9] describe 4 patients in whom Cushing's syndrome was strongly suspected but subsequently disproved and in whom the initial biochemical abnormalities appear to have been caused by alcohol abuse.

Man, 30, a known alcoholic for 13 years, had some features suggestive of Cushing's syndrome, including plethoric facies, easy bruising and truncal obesity. The 9 A.M. plasma fluorogenic corticosteroid levels were elevated on 2 consecutive days. On several subsequent admissions over 3 years, the plasma corticosteroid levels ranged from 840 to 1,260 nmol/L (30–45 μg/dl). Urinary 17-oxosteroids and 17-oxogenic steroids were high on a number of occasions. The plasma corticosteroid levels fell progressively over 5 days during one admission, from 1,260 to 364 nmol/L (45–13 μg/dl). An overnight dexamethasone

(9) Lancet 1:726–728, Apr. 2, 1977.

suppression test with 2 mg reduced the plasma cortisol level to 84 nmol/L (3 μg/dl) excluding true Cushing's syndrome. There was no clinical evidence of liver disease, and tests of liver function gave normal or only slightly abnormal results.

Cushing's syndrome was diagnosed or seriously considered from the biochemical findings in 2 of these patients and on both clinical and biochemical grounds in 2. All the patients drank excessively, and in all instances the biochemical abnormalities resolved during admissions and presumed alcohol abstinence. Corticotropin secretion was deranged in 1 of the 3 patients in whom it was evaluated. None of the patients exhibited more than slight liver damage, and urinary steroid excretion was increased, not decreased.

Great care is needed to avoid confusion of pseudo-Cushing's syndrome with true Cushing's syndrome. Alcohol ingestion may cause severe hyperlipemia that interferes with the fluorogenic corticosteroid assay. A history of alcohol intake should always be sought in a patient in whom Cushing's syndrome is considered.

► [Smals et al. report an additional 3 cases from Holland (Br. Med. J. 2:1298, 1976). The British patients consumed most of their alcohol in the form of beer, although they also took wine and whiskey. The Dutch patients indulged in Dutch gin. The source of alcohol is less important than the quantity. The suggestion that alcoholism should be considered as a cause of Cushing's syndrome deserves strong support, but the problem is more complex than it may seem on the surface. Many patients with hyperadrenocorticism become depressed and may therefore turn to the bottle for solace. Thus alcoholism could be a result of Cushing's syndrome rather than a cause. The differentiation is not difficult in theory. If alcohol is withheld, those in whom it is a cause of the clinical picture will recover quite promptly, whereas those in whom alcohol abuse is a result of the adrenal disease will continue to have abnormal adrenal function. – Ed.] ◄

The Thyroid Gland

► It seems increasingly clear that autoimmune processes play an important part in the pathogenesis of both hyperthyroidism and thyroid deficiency. Robert Volpé has reviewed the role of autoimmunity in endocrine disease, covering many different organs but cutting closest to the clinical area in discussing the thyroid (Ann. Intern. Med. 87: 86, 1977). His review is highly recommended, but it does not lend itself to abstracting.

In most instances, hyperthyroidism is in some way associated with an abnormality of the immune mechanism. One of the immunoglobulins (long-acting thyroid stimulator (LATS) or LATS-protector) is usually increased in the plasma, and the concentration of thyroid-stimulating hormone (TSH) is too low to measure. It is interesting, therefore, that a patient with primary pituitary hyperthyroidism has been described by Reschini et al. (J. Clin. Endocrinol. Metab. 43:924, 1976). This patient had a pituitary tumor, a high level of plasma TSH and an elevated basal metabolic rate, thyroidal iodine uptake and serum thyroxine level. The elevated plasma TSH concentration could not be suppressed with triiodothyronine or somatostatin, though there was a modest decline with the latter. Thyrotropin-releasing hormone did not increase the plasma concentration of TSH. The situation seems entirely analogous to Cushing's disease of the adrenal, where a functioning tumor of the pituitary is often the cause of excessive inappropriate secretion of ACTH by the pituitary. Probably this case will not be duplicated for a long time, but it is possible that with modern methods for measuring TSH easily, this syndrome will prove to be a little less rare than it now seems. Still—hyperthyroidism is not caused by hypersecretion of TSH in any but the most unusual patient.—Ed. ◄

Concentration of Thyroxine-Binding Globulin: Value of Direct Assay. The possibility that triiodothyronine (T_3) uptake may not be an accurate measure of high levels of thyroxine-binding globulin (TBG) was suggested by the finding of an elevated free thyroxine index (FTI) in pregnancy and during oral contraception. W. A. Burr, D. B. Ramsden, S. E. Evans, T. Hogan and R. Hoffenberg[1] (Univ. of Birmingham) examined the relationship between the results of a T_3 uptake test, the Thyopac-3, and TBG concentrations in healthy euthyroid subjects with widely differing levels of TBG. Also, the ability of the FTI and the thyroxine-TBG ratio to distinguish between thyrotoxic, myxedematous and euthyroid states was compared. Studies were done in 29 men and 13 women euthyroid subjects aged 18–50, 10 pregnant women, 9 women taking oral contraceptives, 16 patients with inherited high serum TBG levels and 5 men with inherited absence of TBG. Serums were also obtained from 21 patients with proved thyrotoxicosis and 10 with myxedema. Serum TBG was measured by immunoelectrophoresis.

Mean ±SEM serum level of TBG was 11.2±0.5 mg/L in normal men and 12.5±0.8 mg/L in normal women. Women on oral contraceptives had a mean value of 16.1±0.7 mg/L and pregnant women, a mean of 24.9±1.0 mg/L, both significantly above normal. Thyrotoxic patients had a mean of 10.4±0.5 mg/L and myxedematous patients, a mean of 14.9±1.0 mg/L. Extremely high levels were found in patients with hereditary high TBG levels, the mean for men being 43.9±2.1 mg/L.

(1) Br. Med. J. 1:485–488, Feb. 19, 1977.

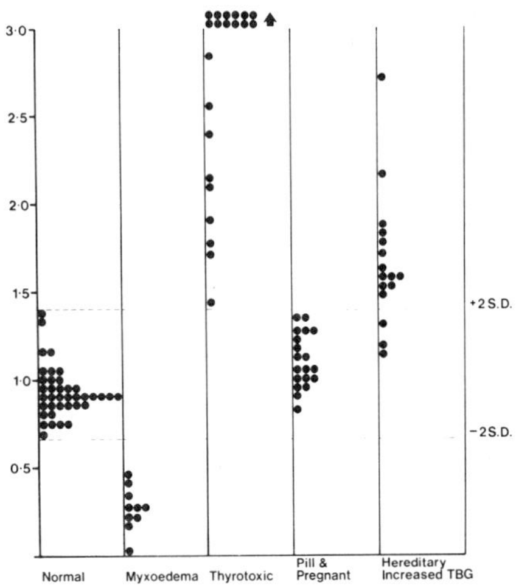

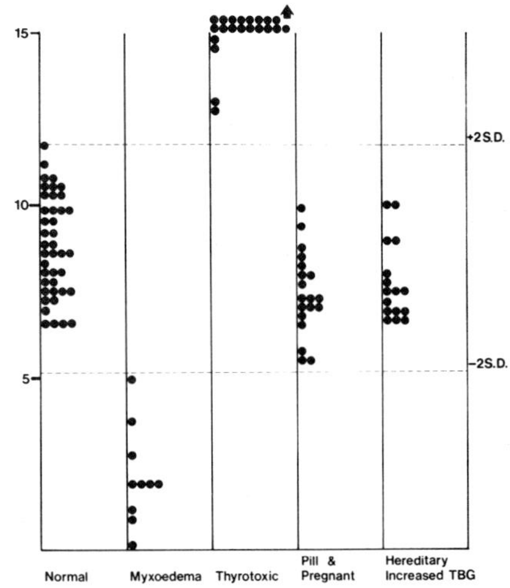

Fig 7 (left).—Free thyroxine index in abnormalities of thyroid function and TBG concentration.
Fig 8 (right).—The T_4-TBG ratio in abnormalities of thyroid function and TBG concentration.
(Courtesy of Burr, W. A., et al.: Br. Med. J. 1:485–488, Feb. 19, 1977.)

These patients also had elevated levels of total serum thyroxine. Patients with undetectable TBG had a mean serum thyroxine of 20 nmol/L (1.6 μg/dl). The Thyopac-3 curve plateaued at about 130, above which little or no rise occurred despite a doubling of the TBG level from 25 to 50 mg/L. Serum thyroxine and TBG values distinguished between the euthyroid, thyrotoxic and myxedematous states when graphed. The free thyroxine indices and thyroxine-TBG ratios are shown in Figures 7 and 8.

Direct measurement of serum TBG will probably soon be available as a routine diagnostic aid. Correlation between total thyroxine and TBG levels in euthyroid subjects is excellent. The conflicting results obtained with conventional thryoid function tests in patients with inherited abnormalities of TBG concentration are readily resolved by directly measuring TBG. Such abnormalities are not rare.

► [Direct measurement of thyroxine-binding globulin makes sense. I must confess that measurement of T_3 binding has seldom been useful to me in the clinic. Total T_4 can be misleading because of the binding effect. It is interesting that the total T_3 in plasma seems the most reliable single test. Partly this may be because thyroxine-binding globulin has only a low affinity for T_3 so its concentration is not so much affected by differences in the level of the binding protein as is T_4. It is also probable that the effective form of the hormone is T_3 and not T_4. For example, Horwitz and Refetoff (J. Clin. Endocrinol. Metab. 44:242, 1977) report data on 5 patients with Graves' disease associated with low concentrations of thyroxine-binding globulin. As might have been predicted, the total plasma T_4 was not elevated. The free T_4 was very high, but this test is tricky and not available to all physicians. The total T_3, unlike the total T_4, was elevated. Thus, if only a single test is to be used, total T_3 is probably the best. Of course, this also is a difficult test, but it is becoming more widely available through radioimmunoassay. If I have access to the total plasma T_3 concentration, I do not need other information to diagnose hyperthyroidism. Especially, I do not need still another index, this one incorporating T_3 resin uptake, total T_3 and total T_4 (Demers et al.: Am. J. Clin. Pathol. 65:356, 1976). It is a pretty safe guess that if you have to use three factors to derive a ratio, you are measuring the wrong thing.—Ed.] ◄

Extrathyroidal Conversion of Thyroxine to 3,3′, 5′-Triiodothyronine (Reverse T_3) and to 3,5,3′-Triiodothyronine (T_3) in Humans. L. Gavin, J. Castle, F. McMahon, P. Martin, M. Hammond and R. R. Cavalieri[2] (Univ. of California, San Francisco) assessed the relative contributions of thyroidal secretion and peripheral deiodination of thyroxine in the production of reverse T_3 (rT_3) by determining turnover rates of T_3 and rT_3, through use of tracer doses given simultaneously to adults with intact thyroids and to hypothyroid patients on replacement doses of L-thyroxine. Studies were done in 6 men without endocrine or hepatic dysfunction or other serious systemic illness and in 5 patients who had been receiving replacement doses of L-thyroxine for at least 2 years for established hypothyroidism, either spontaneous or after thyroidectomy. The mean daily dose of L-thyroxine was 0.19 mg. A euthyroid male with an idiopathic increase in serum thyroxine-binding globulin was also studied. Studies used ^{131}I-T_3 and ^{125}I-labeled thyroxine and rT_3. Subjects were on a metabolic ward during the study. Serum thyroid hormones were radioimmunoassayed. Metabolic clearance rate (MCR) was computed by a noncompartmental method of analysis.

In hypothyroid patients the MCR of rT_3 averaged 97.1 L/day and the production rate (PR) of rT_3, 34.3 μg/day. The MCR of T_3 was 28.7 L/day, and the PR of T_3, 20.3 μg/day. (All these values are corrected to 70 kg body weight.) The results were not significantly different from those in controls. The proportion of total triiodothyronine (rT_3 + T_3) production accounted for by rT_3 averaged 62% in hypothyroid patients and 57% in controls.

The findings indicate that production of rT_3 is a major route of thyroxine metabolism, equal to or exceeding that of T_3. Most if not all of the rT_3 produced in normal human beings appears to be derived by extrathyroidal conversion from thyroxine. The recognition that rT_3 is a major product of thyroxine metabolism in human extrathyroidal tissues raises questions regarding the organs responsible for this inactivating pathway, the regulatory controls over its activity and the effects of various pathologic states. Production rates of T_3 and rT_3 are being determined in patients with thyroidal and nonthyroidal systemic illness.

► [Chopra (Endocrinology 101:453, 1977) has studied the conversion of T_4 to T_3 and rT_3 in an in vitro system. The most active tissue homogenate was kidney, with liver next. Conversion was unaffected by high concentrations of methimazole, hydrocortisone, iodide, iodotyrosines, 3,5-diiodothyronine, thyronine and analogues of rT_3 in which the iodine was replaced with other halogens. Formation of T_3 was inhibited by rT_3, however. Thus the presence of rT_3 would tend to inhibit formation of the biologically effective mono-deiodinated derivative of T_4.

Although the thyroid may itself release some T_3 and rT_3, the major source of these compounds is peripheral metabolism of T_4, which is apparently the thyroid's major secretory product. Moreover, it is not necessary for the thyroid gland to be present in order for the distribution of rT_3/T_3 to be normal. Kaplan et al. (J. Clin. Endocrinol. Metab. 45:447, 1977) studied patients similar to those of Gavin et al. and found the same pattern as Gavin et al. did in hypothyroid patients. In addition, they reported a number of factors affecting the relative amounts of rT_3 and T_3 formed by the peripheral tissues. In hyperthyroidism both compounds are increased, but rT_3 is increased more than T_3. In "T_3 hyperthyroidism," the elevation of T_3 occurs even though the T_4 concentration

(2) J. Clin. Endocrinol. Metab. 44:733–742, April, 1977.

remains normal. In the serum of pregnant women and in cord blood, both are increased and the concentration of rT_3 is disproportionately high. Propylthiouracil diverts some of the T_4 to rT_3 at the expense of T_3. This finding does not agree with Chopra's finding in vitro that the ratio was unaffected by methimazole (see above). In the intact human being, however, if rT_3 is favored by propylthiouracil, the lower activity of rT_3 as compared with T_3 would help to explain previous reports of a "peripheral" action of the thiourea antithyroid drugs. The effect of propylthiouracil on preferential formation of rT_3 has also been reported by Westgren et al. (Acta Endocrinol. (Kbh.) 85:345, 1977).

Although peripheral conversion of T_4 to T_3 is an important factor in Graves' disease, it is probably not the only way in which excess T_3 is formed. Izumi and Larsen (J. Clin. Invest. 59:1105, 1977) report that the thyroglobulin of patients with Graves' disease contains about 50% more T_3 per molecule of thyroglobulin than does normal thyroglobulin. The content of T_4 per mole was the same in thyroglobulin from patients with Graves' disease and in that from control subjects. Thus it appears that the thyroid forms more T_3 in this disease, complementing the increased peripheral conversion. It is uncertain why T_3 is preferred both by the thyroid gland and the periphery in Graves' disease. One possibility might be that the hyperstimulated thyroid tends to make T_3 preferentially; however, Laurberg has shown that hyperstimulation of the dog thyroid (at least over a period of several hours) does not alter the ratio of T_3/T_4 released by the gland. This experiment does not shed light on the effects of stimulation lasting for months, as is probably the situation in human beings with thyroid disease (Endocrinology 100:656, 1977).

The sympathetic system is involved in regulating this reaction, since propranolol diverts T_4 from T_3 to rT_3 in hyperthyroid patients (Vernoeven et al.: J. Clin. Endocrinol. Metab. 44:1002, 1977), and dexamethasone also shifts the metabolic pathway toward rT_3. Both of these therapeutic maneuvers improve the clinical picture in hyperthyroidism, and it has usually been supposed in the past that their action occurs through peripheral changes in responsiveness to the thyroid hormone. The mechanism of this peripheral change may be explained in part by the shift of T_4 metabolism.

These observations point up the limitations of measuring T_4 as an indicator of thyroid function. Even when the serum T_4 level is corrected for differences in thyroxine-binding globulin content, as discussed previously, and for high levels of plasma free fatty acids, which can spuriously alter the apparent T_4 concentration (Pannall et al.: Clin. Chem. 23:990, 1977), the results may not give useful information. For example, Birkhäuser et al. (Lancet 1:53, 1977) describe high serum T_4 and free T_4 concentrations in 31 patients with acute disease of nonthyroidal type. The serum T_3 was normal, and all of the patients had normal thyroid function after recovering from their initial disease. Serum T_4, T_3 and free T_4 may often be elevated in patients with hydatid mole and yet hyperthyroidism rarely occurs. Nagataki and colleagues suggest (J. Clin. Endocrinol. Metab. 44:254, 1977) that this may reflect relatively low T_3/T_4 ratios—i.e., slow conversion from the inactive precursor to the active form. These authors did not measure rT_3, but an excessive production of the inactive metabolic product is an additional possible explanation for the absence of clinical symptoms, especially if their method for measuring T_3 cross-reacted with rT_3. The increased thyroid function of patients with molar pregnancies is a reflection of the very high concentrations of chorionic gonadotropin, which has some thyroid-stimulating effect as well as its more widely recognized actions on the reproductive system.

Livadas and colleagues (Clin. Endocrinol. (Oxf.) 7:121, 1977) report that autonomously functioning thyroid nodules are especially likely to increase the concentration of both T_4 and T_3 in the serum when iodine is given. This is in contrast to the situation in nontoxic goiter, where iodine causes a rise of T_4 and a decrease of T_3.

This was confirmed by Sobrinho et al. (J. Clin. Endocrinol. Metab. 45:25, 1977.) They found that iodine caused a disproportionate increase of T_3 as compared with T_4 in the serum of patients with Graves' disease or toxic nodular goiter, but when iodine induced hyperthyroidism ("jodbasedow"), both $T_3$and T_4 increased in a parallel manner. Jubiz and colleagues studied patients with normal thyroid function receiving large amounts of iodides for treatment of chronic obstructive pulmonary disease and found that the serum T_4 tended to be low and the T_3 normal (ibid. 44:379, 1977).

To make matters more complicated, Smals et al. (ibid., p. 998) report that both the T_3 and T_4 concentration in the plasma fluctuate with the seasons, being lowest in summer. Perhaps this is a reflection of diminished need for caloric expenditure to maintain the body heat in that season. – Ed.] ◄

Changes of Circulating Thyroxine, Triiodothyronine and Reverse Triiodothyronine after Radiographic Contrast Agents. Radiographic contrast agents depress thyroid radioiodine uptake and elevate plasma protein-bound iodine, but thyroid hormone secretion is assumed to remain constant. Hans Bürgi, Claus Wimpfheimer, Albert Burger, Wolfgang Zaunbauer, Helmut Rösler and Thérèse Lemarchand-Béraud[3] found that oral cholecystography with sodium iopanoate consistently leads to changes in circulating thyroid hormones due to alterations in peripheral hormone metabolism. Thyroid function was studied for 42 days in 58 patients, 28 of them with euthyroid goiter, after urography with diatrizoic acid, cholangiography with ioglycamic acid and cholecystography with sodium iopanoate. Four women with severe idiopathic myxedema who were on L-thyroxine therapy and appeared to be euthyroid were also studied, as were 4 healthy men who received L-thyroxine for 21 days and took 2 gm sodium iopanoate orally on day 17.

Short-lived increases in serum thyroxine concentration occurred in a few patients after urography and cholangiography, but the mean thyroxine and triiodothyronine (T_3) concentrations were unchanged. The serum thyroxine concentration rose by 22% a week after oral cholecystography, with a concomitant rise in free thyroxine concentration. The T_3 value fell by 15% and the reverse T_3 concentration rose by 50%. The mean serum thyrotropin concentration doubled. Values for thyroxine and T_3 were normal after 42 days. None of the 58 patients developed clinical hyperthyroidism. Iopanoate produced similar changes in patients with myxedema, except for the rise in serum thyroxine concentration. In normal subjects given thyroxine, T_3 concentration fell and reverse T_3 concentration in serum rose after sodium iopanoate. The thyroxine and free thyroxine values rose insignificantly.

Cholecystography consistently produces changes in circulating thyroid hormones. The primary event after sodium iopanoate is probably a fall in serum T_3 concentration, leading to T_3 deficiency of the peripheral tissues, a rise in thyrotropin and stimulation of thyroxine secretion by the thyroid. It is unclear whether the reduction in serum T_3 concentration is due to decreased production or enhanced degradation of the hormone. A larger and longer study is needed to assess the risk of hyperthyroidism after use of radiographic contrast agents.

► [Such hyperthyroidism would be transient and clinically insignificant unless the patient had congestive heart disease. Indeed, I am not aware that such a syndrome has been described. I suppose it is possible that the iodine released during metabolism of contrast mediums might trigger production of true Graves' disease – ("jodbasedow"). The mechanism of this change is uncertain but probably not related to the suggestion made in this article.

There is so much iodine in the environment now, especially from antiseptic solutions and from iodination of salt, bread and other substances, that the radioiodine uptake is becoming relatively useless diagnostically. Hooper and Caplan, for example, point out that the range of uptakes in patients with Graves' disease dropped from 20–90% in 1970–72 to 10–80% in 1975–76 and that for nodular toxic goiter from

(3) J. Clin. Endocrinol. Metab. 43:1203–1210, December, 1976.

12–70% in the early series to 4–40% in the later series. Indeed, considering their "normal" range, set in 1972, to be 0–24%, 6 of 9 toxic nodular goiters fell within the "normal" range. Of course, when the lower limit of "normal" is zero, the test is totally useless in diagnosing hypothyroidism (J.A.M.A. 238:411, 1977). Perhaps the place of radioiodine uptake is now restricted to calculating therapeutic doses of radioactive iodine (and I'm skeptical that this calculation is valid) and performing scans.

One of the troubles with scans is the need for the patient to stay around (or return) for a late session on the scanner. If the rate of uptake or the intensity of radiation could be improved, the test could be made more convenient. With this in mind, Rosenthal et al. (J. Nucl. Med. 17:1050, 1976) studied the use of ^{123}I rather than the conventional isotopes, ^{125}I and ^{131}I. The half-life of ^{123}I is short (13 hours); the emission is a convenient gamma form of energy, without the beta radiation that makes ^{131}I damaging to tissues; and the dose absorbed by the thyroid is only about 1%, and by the whole body 10%, of that delivered by an equal dose of ^{131}I. The scans obtained with this isotope are superior to those for the other iodines, and a satisfactory picture can be obtained after only 4 hours. This is comparable to technetium, but since technetium is metabolized differently from iodine, it should avoid some of the discrepancies between scans and function recognized when ^{99m}Tc is used.—Ed.] ◄

Changes in Serum Triiodothyronine, Thyroxine and Thyrotropin during Treatment with Thyroxine in Severe Primary Hypothyroidism. Thyroxine (T_4) has been recommended as replacement therapy for hypothyroid patients but it is not clear whether it plays a physiologic role as an active thyroid hormone. Michiko Maeda, Nobuaki Kuzuya, Yuko Masuyama, Yasuo Imai, Hitoshi Ikeda, Hidemasa Uchimura, Fukashi Matsuzaki, Lindy F. Kumagai and Shigenobu Nagataki[4] (Univ. of Tokyo) studied the reactions of 40 patients with severe primary hypothyroidism during treatment with varying doses of T_4. Ten untreated patients received 50 μg T_4 daily for at least 2 months, followed by sequential increases in dosage of 25 μg T_4 daily at 2-month intervals until the serum thyrotropin (TSH) was below 10 $\mu U/ml$. Thirty patients who had taken thyroid hormones had previous dosages stopped and received 50 or 75 μg T_4 daily until the serum TSH was well elevated.

The rate of decrease in serum TSH in response to T_4 treatment was very gradual. Most serum T_4 levels were in the normal range even when some patients were receiving only 50 μg T_4 daily, but over half the samples had subnormal triiodothyronine (T_3) levels. Half the samples had elevated TSH levels despite normal T_4 levels. Most patients with elevated TSH were those with subnormal T_3 levels. A few patients with normal T_3 and T_4 levels had slightly elevated TSH levels. Several subnormal T_3 values were associated with TSH levels below 10 $\mu U/ml$. Patients with subnormal serum T_3 levels and normal T_4 values showed hyperresponsiveness to TSH-releasing hormone (TRH) testing, whereas responses in patients with normal T_3 and T_4 levels were normal. The calculated maintenance dose of T_4 associated with normal TRH responses was 115 μg daily or 2.08$\mu g/kg$ daily.

During the treatment of hypothyroidism with T_4, normal basal TSH correlates better with normal serum T_4 and T_3 than with normal T_4 alone. These results show that normal T_4 levels are insufficient to sustain normal basal TSH levels. However, they support the thesis that T_4 plays an important role in regulating serum TSH levels. The same

(4) J. Clin. Endocrinol. Metab. 43:10–17, July, 1976.

dose of T_4 should be given for at least 2 months after the serum TSH approaches the normal range or when both serum T_4 and T_3 approach normal, to determine the ideal maintenance dose of T_4. The ideal maintenance dose is that dose which normalizes the TRH test.

► [Note once again that the best prediction of a rise of plasma TSH (i.e., of undertreatment) is the level of T_3 in the plasma.

Several interesting papers have discussed aspects of hypothyroidism which are not pertinent to this article by Maeda et al., but seem worth mentioning. Adler et al. (Johns Hopkins Med. J. 138:180, 1976) review the literature concerning development of hypothyroidism after irradiation of the neck and present 3 cases. The radiation was administered for treatment of tumors in the cervical region. Two patients received 6,000 rad but 1 (with Hodgkin's disease) received only 3600 rad. The other patients gleaned from the literature had received 3,000 rad or more, except in 1 instance when the radiation was directed to the thyroid but was only 2,625 rad. Undoubtedly this syndrome is sufficiently frequent in patients receiving neck radiation that it should be sought actively. For example, in a group of 166 patients receiving cervical radiation for Hodgkin's disease, Rosenberg and Kaplan found 6 who developed hypothyroidism (quoted by Adler et al.). As radiotherapy of cervical malignancy becomes more common, we can expect to see this pattern more often.

Patients with severe hypothyroidism often have muscular aching, arthralgias, clumsiness and even joint effusions. Kabadi et al. (N.Y. State J. Med. 77:1489, 1977) studied a family in which spontaneous hypothyroidism was associated with acute arthritic manifestations. These symptoms were completely cured by thyroid replacement. — Ed.]

Age-Related Change in Pituitary Threshold for TSH Release during Thyroxine Replacement Therapy for Cretinism. Several indices of thyroid function indicate greater thyroid activity in children and adolescents than in adults, and age-related changes in thyroid activity are probably associated with altered activity of the hypothalamic-pituitary-thyroid axis. Tamotu Sato, Yukichi Suzuki, Tokuo Taketani, Kazumasa Ishiguro and Hironori Nakajima[5] (Kanazawa Univ.) used sequential thyrotropin-releasing hormone (TRH) testing after alterations in thyroxine dosage to study patients of various ages with cretinism who were receiving exogenous thyroxine. Nine patients aged 6 months to 17 years with athyrotic or ectopic cretinism were investigated. All but 1 had endogenous thyroxine concentrations below 1 μg/100 ml before treatment. All patients were considered to be euthyroid or slightly hyperthyroid at the time of study. The thyroxine dosage was increased or reduced by 25 or 50 μg at 2–12-month intervals, according to the thyrotropin response to TRH. The dose was considered to be inadequate if the basal thyrotropin concentration remained above 10 μU/ml for 2 months or longer or if the response to TRH was exaggerated. The overall observation periods were 13–24 months.

The thyroxine dosages associated with normal thyrotropin responsiveness to TRH are shown as a function of age in Figure 9. The dosage declined from 10 μg/kg per day in infancy to 3 or 4 μg/kg per day at puberty. The correlation with age was significant. At ages 4–12 years the adequate thyroxine dosage was 4–6 μg/kg per day. Serum triiodothyronine concentrations were elevated in the youngest patients and declined with age. The serum thyroxine iodine values associated with normal thyrotropin responsiveness to TRH were significantly higher in patients under age 5 years than in older patients. Thyroxine iodine

(5) J. Clin. Endocrinol. Metab. 44:553–559, March, 1977.

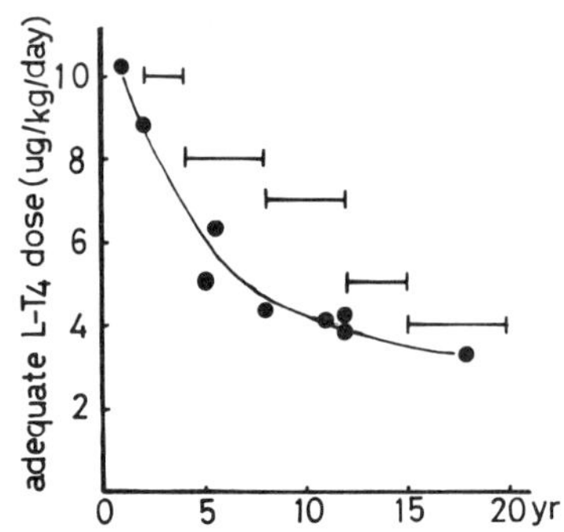

Fig 9. – Adequate levothyroxine (L-T_4) dosage, plotted individually as function of age, shows curvilinear relation from infancy to adolescence (correlation coefficient r = –0.820, P < 0.01). Horizontal bars indicate replacement dosages of L-T_4 during childhood and adolescence recommended by Fisher, which are substantially higher than adequate L-T_4 dosages of corresponding ages, particularly between 4 and 12 years. (Courtesy of Sato, T., et al.: J. Clin. Endocrinol. Metab. 44:553–559, March, 1977.)

concentrations of 9 μg/100 ml and triiodothyronine concentrations of 250 ng/100 ml or less were associated with complete thyrotropin inhibition by TRH in all older patients but not in young patients.

The findings suggest that the pituitary threshold for feedback regulation of thyrotropin secretion by thyroxine decreases with age in children with cretinism. The usually recommended replacement doses of L-thyroxine for patients aged 4–12 years are probably overestimated. Direct estimates of free thyroxine and triiodothyronine levels in a larger number of children with cretinism are needed.

► [This article and the preceding one base their evaluation of thyroid replacement treatment on the concentration of TSH in the plasma, either unstimulated or after TRH. A paper similar to this also was presented by Rezvani and DiGeorge (J. Pediatr. 90:291, 1977). Curiously, they found no variation with the required dose of T_4 with age, when expressed as μg/kg. The dose they determined to be correct – 3.8 ± 0.6 μg/kg/day – is the same as that found by Sato and his colleagues for patients aged 10 years or more. Rezvani and DiGeorge studied 11 children, so both estimates are based on small populations. I must say that I am surprised at the suggestion that the dose required is independent of the age, and I am inclined to believe the data of Sato et al., but further information is needed.

Thyrotropin measurements may also be useful in evaluating the opposite problem. There are situations in which it is desirable to suppress TSH secretion completely. Nontoxic goiter and disseminated thyroid cancer are examples. But measuring the TSH in plasma is not very useful because the lower limit of normal is too low to measure. Moreover, since TSH is secreted episodically, a single specimen might be misleadingly low. There could be no such thing as a misleadingly high level in this situation, since the presence of detectable TSH would indicate incomplete suppression. To improve the specificity of the test, Hoffman and colleagues (J. Clin. Endocrinol. Metab. 44:892, 1977) first confirmed the episodic secretion of TSH and then demonstrated that totally suppressed patients failed to secrete TSH even when stimulated with TRH. With this test they could identify patients who were inadequately suppressed and could produce complete suppression – and complete failure to respond to TRH – by increasing the dose of T_4.

The problem of recognizing hypothyroidism in infants as early as possible remains a serious one. Any delay in treatment reduces the chance of maintaining normal brain function, so screening of newborns is potentially useful. A committee of the American Thyroid Association has reported its recommendations in this regard (Am. J. Med. 61:

932, 1976). They point out that cord blood has been obtained for screening in about 121,000 infants in a group of pilot studies. Twenty-one infants with congenital hypothyroidism were identified. The plasma T_4 concentration in all was less than 7 μg/dl. Thyrotropin was measured in 16 of the hypothyroid infants and was over 50 μU/ml in 12 either in cord blood or in reassessment plasma obtained 2-4 weeks after birth. One other infant had a level which was modestly elevated (32 μU/ml), and another was hypopituitary. The last was, in fact, euthyroid with a normal T_3 though the T_4 was low. The procedure is time consuming, and each test costs money—60¢ for the T_4 and $1.50 for the TSH. Nevertheless, by conservative estimate, the number of cretins picked up early and prevented from becoming public charges would make the routine use of this screening method financially as well as medically profitable. The most important item is to make the test easy for the obstetrician or pediatrician to do at the time of delivery. This is accomplished by collecting the cord blood on filter paper, in a fashion analogous to the screening method for phenylketonuria. In view of the trouble of recalling for follow-up TSH tests those infants who are suspected of hypothyroidism, it has been suggested that TSH might be tested directly, and a method has been developed for measuring this hormone from filter paper disks with cord blood, as part of an automated system (Foley et al.: J. Lab. Clin. Med. 90:11, 1977).—Ed.] ◄

Hypothyroidism due to Thyroid Hormone-Binding Antibodies. A familial syndrome of hypothyroidism with "peripheral resistance" to thyroid hormones has been reported. F. Anders Karlsson, Lars Wibell and Leif Wide[6] (Univ. of Uppsala) describe a hypothyroid patient with normal thyroid tissue function in whom the hypothyroid state was probably due to abnormal binding of triiodothyronine (T_3) to circulating antibodies of high amount and affinity.

Woman, 26, had low serum thyroxine and resin uptake test values and had long preferred warmth. Cold intolerance had increased recently, and impaired memory and concentrating ability and a weight increase had occurred. She had a history of atopic allergy. Myxedematous swelling of the face and limbs was seen, with a slightly enlarged thyroid and cool, dry skin. Slight blood eosinophilia was observed. The serum thyrotropin concentration was 18 mU/L, and a low T_3 resin test value was obtained. Total thyroxine was normal. The serum T_3 value exceeded 50 nmol/L. Thyroid ^{131}I uptake was normal. Repeated thyroid biopsies gave normal findings. Immunofluorescence against cytoplasmic thyroid antigen was found. The serum contained hormone-binding antibodies, and the patient was given 20 μg T_3 4 times daily until euthyroidism returned. When the serum thyroid-stimulating hormone was normal, the ^{131}I uptake was 6% at 4 hours and 18% at 24 hours.

Serum electrophoresis showed the existence of polyclonal immunoglobulins with binding capacity for T_3 and thyroxine. Total binding of antibody capacities in the serum corresponded to 14 mg T_3 antibodies per L and 130 mg thyroxine antibodies per L. The free T_3 concentration was calculated as 85-90%, declining to 30-40% of the value at the time of euthyroidism.

The high concentration of T_3 antibodies in this patient was probably clinically important. The patient had a normal thyroid gland. The mechanism of development of thyroid hormone antibodies is obscure. The patient may have passed through a state of subclinical thyroiditis, during which intracellular material, including immunogenic amounts of thyroglobulin, was released. There is experimental evidence that antibody formation against hormones may have clinical effects, with

(6) N. Engl. J. Med. 296:1146-1148, May 19, 1977.

symptoms of hormone deficiency despite a high plasma hormone concentration.

► [Hypothyroidism is a common final point in the course of Graves' disease. This has been recognized in the past, before there was any effective treatment for the disease, and recently has been rediscovered after treatment with radioactive iodine, where all of the hypothyroidism after treatment has been (erroneously) blamed on the radiation. Surgery also produces hypothyroidism—or, at least, surgical patients develop hypothyroidism. Is this a result of the thyroidectomy or is it also a manifestation of the usual course of the disease? If the cause is excessive removal of the thyroid mass, one might expect the incidence of hypothyroidism to be greater in patients who had had a larger proportion of the gland removed. Tweedle and colleagues reviewed this problem in 122 patients who had had partial thyroidectomy 1–7 years previously by two surgeons, one of whom routinely removed substantially more of the gland than the other. There was no difference in the incidence of hypothyroidism in the two groups of patients. This suggests that most of the patients who became hypothyroid could blame it on the natural course of the disease, not on excessive enthusiasm on the part of the surgeon (Br. J. Surg. 64:445, 1977).—Ed.] ◄

^{125}I Therapy in Graves' Disease: Long-Term Results in 355 Patients. Treatment of hyperthyroidism with ^{131}I is effective and safe, but posttreatment hypothyroidism limits its usefulness. I. R. McDougall and W. R. Greig[7] (Glasgow) undertook a trial of ^{125}I as the therapeutic nuclide in 367 patients (312 women and 55 men), 355 of whom were evaluable. Hyperthyroidism was confirmed in all cases before treatment. The patients had small diffusely enlarged thyroids. Only 8.7% were under age 40 at the time of initial treatment. Second or subsequent doses of radioiodine were not prescribed until at least 3 months had elapsed from the previous dose.

After an average follow-up of 49.4 months, 63.4% of patients are euthyroid, 33.5% are hypothyroid and 3.1% are hyperthyroid. The dose range was 4–56 mCi. Hypothyroid patients received a slightly greater average dose than those who are euthyroid, whereas hyperthyroid patients received smaller doses. Nearly two thirds of patients given over 20 mCi initially are hypothyroid, and none remains hyperthyroid. The apparent high incidence of hypothyroidism in patients given the lowest doses was due to the frequent need by these patients of multiple doses to produce symptomatic control. Fourteen patients have died, 4 with metastatic tumor of the lung or stomach, 2 of cerebrovascular accidents and 3 of myocardial infarction.

Because of the high rate of posttreatment hypothyroidism in this series and because ^{131}I has stood the test of time, ^{131}I is considered the nuclide of choice for the routine treatment of hyperthyroidism. Iodine-125 does not prevent posttreatment hypothyroidism, and, although no long-term complications have arisen, it should not be used for routine treatment of hyperthyroidism.

► [The problem of hypothyroidism after treatment was discussed briefly in the comment on the preceding article. I am not aware of any evidence that reducing the dose of radiation reduces the incidence of hypothyroidism after treatment. Perhaps there is a higher incidence of posttreatment hypothyroidism in isotope-treated Graves' disease than in patients treated with medical or surgical methods. For example, in the article by Tweedle et al., quoted previously, only 15% of the patients operated on had developed hypothyroidism in the follow-up period of 1–7 years, whereas in this group the incidence was twice as high over a comparable period of observation. Perhaps radiation

(7) Ann. Intern. Med. 85:720–723, December, 1976.

synergizes with hyperthyroidism to produce a joint incidence of thyroid failure higher than what would be expected from the natural course of the disease, but proof of this is lacking. The two studies mentioned are not sufficiently parallel to permit comparing them statistically.

The authors have tried to improve results of isotope treatment by using the somewhat unconventional isotope ^{125}I rather than the usual ^{131}I. They seem not to have improved matters. There is a good deal of popular fear of the effects of ^{131}I radiation on the gonads when therapeutic doses are administered. Robertson and Gorman (J. Nucl. Med. 17:826, 1976) studied this carefully and concluded that the radiation to the ovaries or testes after 10 mCi ^{131}I is only about 3 rad. This is a good deal less than the dose delivered by such common diagnostic methods as barium meal, urography (intravenous or retrograde), barium enema or radiogram of the upper femur. On genetic grounds, they feel, there is no justification for denying ^{131}I treatment of Graves' disease if it is otherwise justified.

It is worth commenting on some of the medical methods of treating hyperthyroidism. The standard for many years has been the thiourea drugs, and for almost 25 years it has generally been accepted that treatment should be continued for at least a year after euthyroidism was achieved, in which case about 50% of patients would remain in remission for 5 years or more after treatment was withdrawn (Solomon et al.: J.A.M.A. 152:201, 1953). The bother of continuing treatment for so long, in contrast to the relatively acute pattern in surgical or radioactive isotope treatment, has tended to make medical treatment less attractive in recent years than it was when it was first introduced. Now Greer et al. report (N. Engl. J. Med. 297:173, 1977) that 12 of 31 patients given a single daily dose of methimazole or propylthiouracil, which was discontinued as soon as the patients were clearly euthyroid, had remissions lasting an average of 29 months. The course of treatment lasted only 4.5 months on the average. This form of treatment is easier than the conventional on two grounds—(1) the fact that only one dose a day was used rather than the conventional "around-the-clock" treatment and (2) the short duration. If the remission rate continues to be maintained, medical treatment would look much more attractive. The authors found that patients with T_3 toxicosis and with small goiters had a better outlook with this form of treatment than the rest of the hyperthyroid patients.

Propranolol has an important place in treating hyperthyroidism. Toft et al. (Clin. Endocrinol. (Oxf.) 5:195, 1976) point out that the major effect on heart rate achieved with this medication can be observed within 24 hours of starting treatment. They feel that the drug need be given only 3–4 days in preparation for surgery. If it is continued longer, there may be a problem in evaluating the patient's status. For example, Eriksson et al. (N. Engl. J. Med. 296:263, 1977) report data on 2 patients considered to be well controlled on propranolol who developed acute thyroid storm despite the drug. Another problem may also arise. Shenkman et al. (J.A.M.A. 238:237, 1977) describe 3 patients who had been receiving propranolol in treatment of angina pectoris. None of the patients had a previous history of hyperthyroidism, but they all developed the clinical picture when propranolol was discontinued or decreased abruptly. In these patients, propranolol probably hid the thyroid disease as long as the drug was continued, and hyperthyroidism was able to emerge when it was discontinued.—Ed.] ◄

Identification of Subgroups of Euthyroid Graves' Ophthalmopathy. David H. Solomon, Inder J. Chopra, Usha Chopra and Francoise J. Smith[8] (Univ. of California, Los Angeles) attempted to determine if euthyroid Graves' ophthalmopathy is a single entity or a heterogeneous group of disorders by seeking defining characteristics of Graves' thyroid disease, Hashimoto's disease and Graves' ophthalmopathy in 22 patients thought to have euthyroid Graves' disease. Five patients proved to have definite elevations of serum free triiodothyronine (T_3) and, in some cases, free thyroxine as well. The other 17 were truly euthyroid. Serums also were obtained from 33 patients with untreated Graves' hyperthyroidism.

---

(8) N. Engl. J. Med. 296:181–186, Jan. 27, 1977.

Positive assays for long-acting thyroid stimulator (LATS) and antithyroglobulin antibodies were similarly frequent in the two patient groups, excluding the patients found to be mildly hyperthyroid. Antimicrosomal antibodies were considerably more frequent in Graves' hyperthyroidism than in euthyroid Graves' ophthalmopathy and LATS protector (LPA) was far more common in the former state. Half the cases of ophthalmopathy showed nonsuppressibility of T_3. Six patients had positive LPA and thyroid nonsuppressibility (group 1), 3 had positive LPA and normal suppressibility (group 2), 5 had undetectable LPA and normal suppressibility (group 3) and 3 had undetectable LPA and nonsuppressibility (group 4). Five study patients who proved to have hyperthyroidism were classified in group H. Four of these patients showed thyroid nonsuppressibility and all 5 had LPA in their serums. In group 1, as in group H, all but 1 patient had high titers of at least one antithyroid antibody and the thyroid was enlarged or abnormally firm. Thyroid antibodies were insignificant in group 3 cases and the thyroid was usually normal in size and consistency. Ophthalmology was milder than in groups 1 and H. No distinguishing features were found in groups 2 and 4.

Group 1 patients appeared to have three autoimmune disorders: Graves' ophthalmopathy, Graves' thyroid disease and Hashimoto's thyroiditis; group H is very similar to group I. Group 3 patients may have had a single autoimmune disease, "isolated" Graves' ophthalmopathy. Further study is needed of the nonconforming groups 2 and 4. In group 2 this should include study of the possibility that the serums of some patients with Graves' disease contain IgGs that are poor thyroid stimulators and allow thyrotropin, but not LATS, to bind to receptors. In group 4, further study is needed of the possibility that insensitivity of the LPA assay system or the presence of non-IgG factors in thyroid nonsuppressibility explains the dissociation of findings.

► [Teng and Yeo (Br. Med. J. 1:273, 1977) reviewed data on a similar group of patients and obtained figures roughly similar to those of Solomon et al. The combination of a normal (or even elevated) level of thyroid hormones in the plasma and reduced or absent TSH and TSH response to TSH is a paradox which impressed Teng and Yeo. It seems that in these patients, at least, the usual ideas about feedback control of TSH secretion are inapplicable.

Mullin and co-workers (Endocrinology 100:351, 1977) studied the effects of extracts of thyroid gland and retro-orbital tissues from patients with ophthalmic complications of Graves' disease on migration of their own T-cells. Migration was inhibited. The inhibiting material has been partially purified and found to be similar in its properties to thyroglobulin. This implies that at least one element in the exophthalmos is related to the immune system.

There is considerable interest in the application of gray-scale ultrasound to diagnosis of thyroid disease. Frank and Zollikofer (Fortschr. Roentgenstr. 124:456, 1976) used the method on 315 patients over a period of 2 years. In 166 instances the data could be compared with other methods of evaluation. Ultrasound is particularly useful in the differentiation of nodules which are "cold" on scintiscan, since a distinction between cysts and solid masses is easy. The method is not useful in retrosternal problems because the bones and gas in the thorax interfere, and retrotracheal regions are also difficult to examine. – Ed.] ◄

Successful Treatment of Thyrotoxic Crisis by Continuous Plasmapheresis with Blood Cell Separator is described by K.

Horn, G. Brehm, J. Habermann, C. R. Pickardt and P. C. Scriba[9] (Univ. of Munich). Confirming the clinical diagnosis of "thyroid storm" 13 hours after thyroid surgery, this man, aged 26, showed an increased serum thyroid hormone level at time of admission. Progressively deepening coma led to the decision to use continuous plasmapheresis with an IBM blood cell separator in an attempt to eliminate circulating thyroid hormone.

Five liters of plasma was exchanged, removing 633 μg thyroxine (T_4) and 13.6 μg triiodothyronine (T_3). The patient regained consciousness during the procedure. Because the replacement plasma contained 280 μg T_4 and 5.7 μg T_3, the actual amounts of hormone removed were 353 μg T_4 and 7.9 μg T_3. No fall in total T_4 and T_3 levels in the serum was observed, most likely due to the rapid reflux of thyroid hormones from the tissue into the intravascular space. The T_3-uptake test result, and thus the index of free thyroid hormone, fell as proof of diminished circulation of free thyroid hormone. This decrease of free serum T_4 and T_3 was particularly evident in the diminished urinary excretion of both

Fig 10. – Thyroid hormone levels in serum and thyroid hormone excretion in urine before, during and after plasmapheresis in patient with thyrotoxic crisis. Horizontal striated lines represent upper and lower limits of normal region for all recorded parameters. Striated column represents time of plasmapheresis. On ordinate are indicated: total serum T_4 *(T_4, closed circles);* total serum T_3 *(T_3, open circles);* T_3 uptake *(RT_3U, open triangles);* and urinary excretion of T_4 *(U_{T_4}, open squares)* and T_3 *(U_{T_3}, closed squares).* (Courtesy of Horn, K., et al.: Klin. Wochenschr. 54:983–986, Oct. 15, 1976; Berlin-Heidelberg-New York: Springer.)

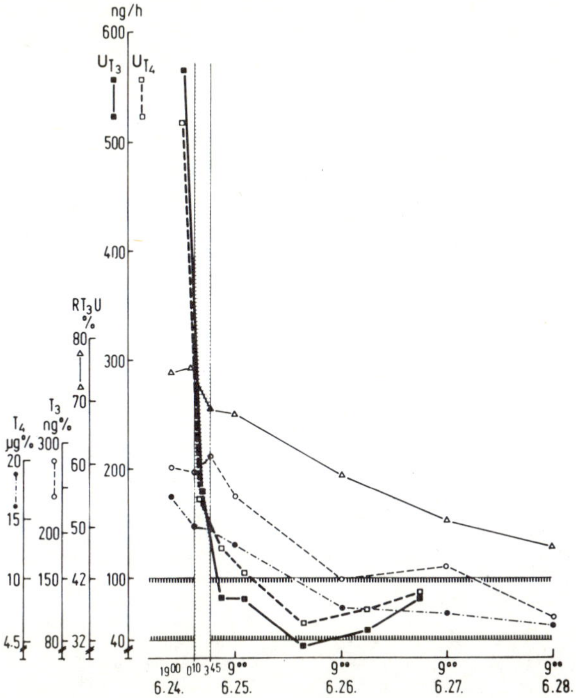

(9) Klin. Wochenschr. 54:983–986, Oct. 15, 1976.

hormones during the plasmapheresis (Fig 10). These findings are explained on the basis of a new supply of binding sites for thyroid hormone with the donor plasma and the increased serum level of the T_4-binding globulin. With continued antithyroid treatment total thyroid hormones in the serum diminished surprisingly rapidly during the next 24 hours.

The present observation confirms the value of plasmapheresis with a cell separator for management of a thyrotoxic crisis. Practical advantages include the easy and nontraumatic technique; the only disadvantage is the immediate need for large amounts of fresh plasma and the risk of hepatitis. The present findings indicate that the increased supply of thyroid hormone binding sites is even more important for management of the crisis than is the removal of thyroid hormones.

► [The amount of hormone removed by this maneuver was negligible, so the good effect was probably, as suggested, a result of tying up hormone with T_4-binding globulin (TBG). Could the same beneficial result be obtained by simply injecting purified TBG? I don't believe the protein is available for therapeutic trial, but perhaps someday this method of removing the hormone from the metabolic arena will prove practical. – Ed.] ◄

Fine-Needle Aspiration Cytology in Preoperative Diagnosis of Thyroid Nodules. Fine-needle aspiration biopsy has been used for preoperative diagnosis of abnormalities in a number of organs. Marvin C. Gershengorn, Michael R. McClung, Elizabeth W. Chu, Thomas A. S. Hanson, Bruce D. Weintraub and Jacob Robbins[1] (Natl. Inst. of

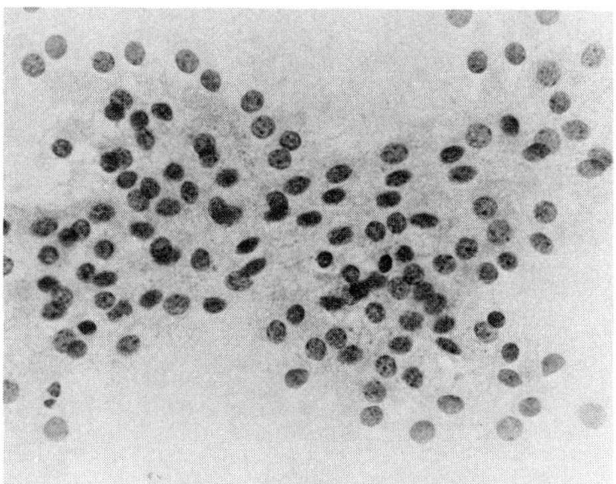

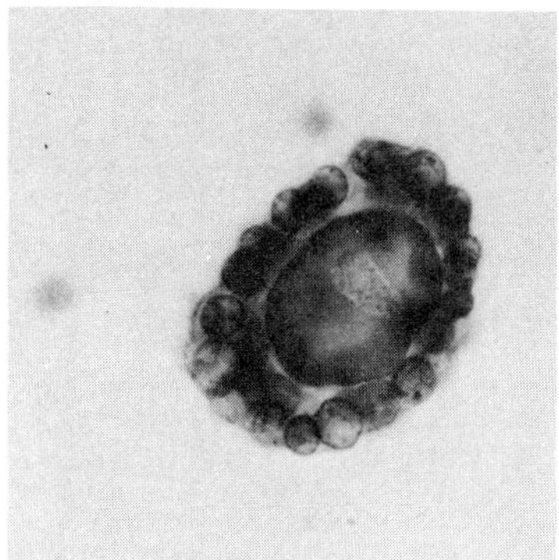

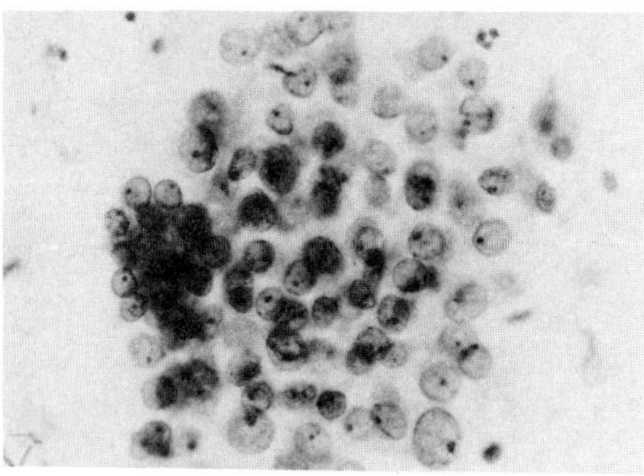

Fig 11 (above left). – Benign follicular cells. Note uniformity of size and shape; reduced from ×500.

Fig 12 (above). – Normal thyroid follicle; reduced from ×600.

Fig 13 (left). – Follicular carcinoma. Note noncohesive cells varying in size; reduced from ×600.

(Courtesy of Gershengorn, M. C., et al.: Ann. Intern. Med. 87:265–269, September, 1977.)

(1) Ann. Intern. Med. 87:265–269, September, 1977.

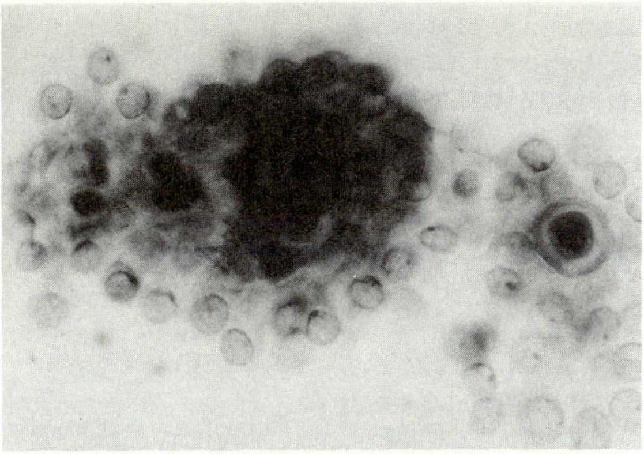

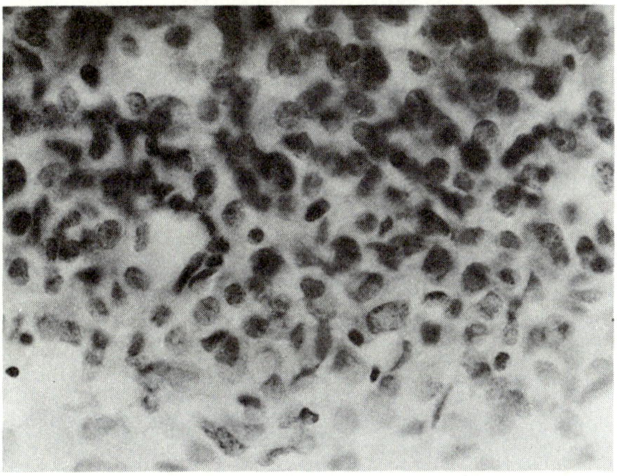

Fig 14 (top).—Papillary carcinoma with psamomma body; reduced from ×600.

Fig 15 (bottom).—Medullary carcinoma. Note abundance of round and fusiform cells: reduced from ×600.

(Courtesy of Gershengorn, M. C., et al.: Ann. Intern. Med. 87:265–269, September, 1977.)

Health) assessed the utility of aspiration cytology in a study of consecutive adults seen in 2½ years with thyroid nodules. Fifty consecutive patients with discrete, usually single nodules were studied. None had hyperfunctioning nodules. Fine-needle aspiration was performed in the outpatient clinic with intradermal anesthesia. Each nodule was aspirated twice. No bleeding into the thyroid or surrounding tissues occurred except in 2 patients. The classification of smears is illustrated in Figures 11–13 and the findings of malignancy in Figures 14 and 15.

Serous fluid was aspirated from 2 patients with echograms compatible with totally cystic lesions. Thirty-three patients had excision biopsy; 5 of them had 2 nodules. One patient had a "warm" nodule on technetium scanning. Ultrasound study showed 15 solid and 4 mixed cystic and solid lesions; 2 lesions were not demonstrable. Five of 25 patients given L-thyroxine showed a reduction in nodule size; 2 showed regrowth during continued therapy. A satisfactory aspiration specimen was obtained in 32 cases (97%). Malignancy was diagnosed in 9 cases and was confirmed by histologic study in 7. There was 1 false positive diagnosis and 1 occult carcinoma. Three of 5 lesions interpreted as suspicious for malignancy proved to be malignant. Seventeen of 18 interpretations of benignancy were correct.

Fine-needle aspiration cytology is of definite value in preoperative evaluation of thyroid nodules. A definite cytologic diagnosis of malignancy warrants excision biopsy, and a positive or suspicious cytologic diagnosis should increase the index of suspicion for malignancy. A negative cytologic diagnosis should not at present preclude excision biopsy. The procedure can help evaluate the need for excision biopsy in aged and ill patients and those with multinodular goiter and it can help in selection of patients for a long-term trial of thyroid suppression therapy.

► [Other series have also been published recently. Walfish et al. (Ann. Intern. Med. 87: 270, 1977) studied 150 patients of whom 90 had surgical follow-up, and 60 of these had tumors other than colloid nodules. Suitable cytologic preparations were obtained in 83 of the 90. Of 66 solid lesions, 63 (95%) were correctly diagnosed as malignant. With cystic lesions, 88% were correctly diagnosed. In this series, although there were false negative results for malignancy there were no false positive results. Diagnosis was most reliable with solid papillary and metastatic tumors.

A much larger series was reported by Galvan et al. (Schweiz. Med. Wochenschr. 106: 1247. 1976). These authors examined thyroid nodules in 4,555 patients over a period of 8 years. Surgical confirmation could be obtained in 1,076 instances. In 715 patients with normal or nontumorous degenerative disease, the diagnosis was correct in 95%. Malignancy was suspected in 322 and confirmed in 129, for a rate of only 40%. Most of the errors were atypical adenomas such as Hürthle cell adenomas or Hashimoto's thyroiditis, which could only be identified with security in the advanced stages.

These three articles lead to certain clear conclusions. The probability of missing a tumor—and, especially, a cancer—is at least 5% unless, as in the article of Galvan et al., one includes as "suspicious" a very large group of patients who turn out not to have tumors. A clear-cut diagnosis of tumor using the criteria of Gershengorn et al. or Walfish et al. is almost certain to be correct and should be accepted as indication for surgery, but a questionable diagnosis by aspiration is not so secure. My own experience watching cytologists at work, especially on breast cancer, leads me to believe that critical evaluation and increasing experience will improve the performance of the American groups, but never to the point of complete reliability. But then, what examination of any type is completely reliable? Needle puncture seems to have a useful place in diagnosis, provided the examiner is experienced in cytologic technique.

At this point, some surgeon always complains about the danger of seeding cancer cells along the needle track. A very extensive experience with breast cancer indicates that there is no such danger, *provided* a small needle is used. The largest suitable needle is a 21-gauge needle. With this, seeding along the track is not a significant risk.

Another point is the nature of thyroid cancer. It is well recognized that the differentiated tumors such as follicular and, especially, the papillary types tend to grow slowly and be amenable to treatment. Indeed, a good many of the cancers diagnosed by the pathologist are biologically so unaggressive that they seem to be a form of carcinoma in situ. Thus the risk of using fine-needle aspiration for diagnosis is a good deal less than it might be in a more aggressive sort of tumor. — Ed.] ◄

Functioning Thyroid Masses in Childhood and Adolescence: Clinical, Surgical and Pathologic Correlations. Solitary or multiple thyroid nodules as the only palpable thyroid tissue are rare in childhood and are suggestive of autonomous units. Nancy J. Hopwood, Robert G. Carroll, Frederic M. Kenny and Thomas P. Foley, Jr.[2] (Univ. of Pittsburgh) describe 6 girls who presented with thyroid masses and in whom no other thyroid tissue could be palpated. The girls, aged

(2) J. Pediatr. 89:710–718, November, 1976.

5 – 15 years, had normal serum thyroxine levels. Scintiscanning with thyroid-stimulating hormone stimulation confirmed autonomous nodules in the 4 adolescents, 2 of whom had elevated triiodothyronine levels. Surgery showed adenomatous thyroid hyperplasia in 3 of these girls and papillary adenocarcinoma in the other. The fifth girl proved to have agenesis of the left lobe with an enlarged right lobe due to lymphocytic thyroiditis. The sixth had an ectopic thyroid with chronic inflammation.

Thyroid nodules are unusual in children and adolescents, and when they occur they are frequently malignant. Thorough diagnostic evaluation of single or multiple functioning thyroid masses in such subjects is essential. Scintiscanning with an iodine radionuclide is indicated to determine the functional status of thyroid nodules. Most patients with autonomous nodules are clinically euthyroid, although the appearance of toxic symptoms at some time is not uncommon. Surgery should be considered for hyperfunctioning autonomous nodules when there is significant morbidity due to toxicity or the opportunity for long-term follow-up is limited. Excision of a nodule is preferred where adequate surgical facilities are available, because carcinoma may be present.

► [Several more papers have appeared commenting on the danger of inducing cancer in the thyroid by exposure to radiation. Greenspan (J.A.M.A. 237:2089, 1977) reviewed the literature and pointed out that there is an increased incidence of cancer even when the dose to the thyroid was only 6.5 rad, after irradiation of the scalp. The probability of cancer rises as the thyroid radiation dose increases until very high levels are achieved, for instance with ^{131}I radiation for hyperthyroidism. At this point, tumors become less common and hypothyroidism becomes a risk. The relationship between radiation and hypothyroidism has been commented on earlier in these pages. Various excuses were found in the past for exposing children to radiation to the chest, neck and head. Pertussis, for example, was treated by radiation and some of these children developed thyroid cancer later (Ann. Intern. Med. 86:449, 1977). The scalp has been irradiated for treatment of tinea. In a group of such patients followed parallel with control groups, the incidence of thyroid cancer was increased sixfold (Modan et al.: Radiology 123: 741, 1977). Shalet and colleagues (Clin. Radiol. 28:511, 1977) followed 32 patients who had received radiation to the head and neck for Hodgkin's disease in childhood. The dose to the thyroid was from 2,500 to 3,000 rad. All patients were clinically euthyroid but 16% had a low free thyroxine index and 53% had a high serum TSH concentration. Only 9% had tests which were entirely normal. There were no tumors in this group, suggesting that it fits into the high-dose group of Greenspan, where hypothyroidism is more likely to occur than tumor. Incidentally, there is probably no such thing as a "safe period" after exposure to radiation, since Greenspan's summary showed that an increased incidence of thyroid cancer could be observed as late as 40 years after exposure! – Ed.]

Thyroid Carcinoma and Concurrent Hyperthyroidism: Study of 10 Patients. B. W. Hancock, R. F. Bing, Susan M. Dirmikis, D. S. Munro and F. E. Neal[3] (Univ. of Sheffield) studied 10 patients in whom thyroid carcinoma and thyrotoxicosis coexisted and in 6 of whom the neoplasm was suspected clinically before thyroidectomy. A total of 549 thyroidectomies were done for thyrotoxicosis at the authors' institution in 1960 – 72. The thyroid was nodular in 92 cases. Carcinoma was diagnosed in 110 of 936 other patients who underwent thyroidectomy in the same period.

Nine women and 1 man, aged 19 – 80 years, comprised the study group. Three patients presented with symptoms of thyrotoxicosis alone,

(3) Cancer 39:298 – 302, January, 1977.

5 with a progressively enlarging goiter as well and 2 with rapid goiter enlargement only. All were thyrotoxic on initial assessment. One developed florid thyrotoxicosis after surgery. Malignancy was suspected from palpable thyroid abnormalities in 6 patients. Five of six radionuclide scans showed abnormalities of uptake in areas where carcinoma was later found. In 3 cases, low uptake corresponded to the tumor. Papillary carcinoma was present in 4 patients, follicular carcinoma in 4 and mixed papillary-follicular carcinoma in 2. All carcinomas but 1 were well differentiated. Three patients in whom neoplasia had been unsuspected had extremely small, localized intrathyroid papillary tumors. Four patients received ablative doses of radioiodine postoperatively. Two patients have died after progressive spread of carcinoma; 8 have shown no recurrence after follow-up for 18 months to 12 years. No long-acting thyroid stimulator (LATS) activity was found in the 8 patients in whom it was sought, and only 1 patient had significant LATS protector activity.

None of these patients showed evidence that the thyroid carcinoma itself produced the hyperthyroid state, although this has been reported. All patients had evidence of toxic hyperplasia in residual thyroid tissue. In a region where palpable thyroid abnormalities are common, surgery is not routinely recommended. In most of these 10 cases, the history, physical findings and thyroid scan provided justification for thyroid exploration.

► [Lesson: Presence of hyperthyroidism does not *guarantee* absence of cancer—but when cancer is present, usually the physical examination or scan provides evidence of suspicious regions that should alert the clinician.—Ed.] ◄

Serum Thyroglobulin and Recurrent Thyroid Cancer. Patients who have had total thyroidectomy for malignancy should have no circulating thyroglobulin and the presence of peripheral thyroglobulin could provide a simple and specific indicator of recurrence. P. Lo Gerfo, T. Stillman, D. Colacchio and C. Feind[4] (Columbia Univ.) determined serum thyroglobulin levels in 30 patients who had total thyroidectomy for malignancy; 10 had known recurrences at the time of study. Serum thyroglobulin was determined by a double antibody disequilibrium radioimmunoassay procedure with use of ^{125}I-labeled thyroglobulin. Twenty patients were disease free 10 years or more after surgery, whereas 10 had known residual or metastatic disease. All 10 had mixed papillary carcinoma. Controls included 46 healthy subjects aged 20–40.

The disease-free patients had thyroglobulin levels below 10 ng/ml. Seven of 10 patients with known active metastatic disease had levels above 450 ng/ml, whereas 3 had moderately elevated levels of 100–260 ng/ml. The control subjects had serum thyroglobulin levels of 10–60 ng/ml. The serum thyroglobulin levels in cancer patients all had immunologic features identical to those of standard thyroglobulin, as demonstrated by parallel dilution curves.

It is possible that highly specific immunotherapy, with use of thyroglobulin-producing cells as the target and hapten-associated thyroglob-

(4) Lancet 1:881–882, Apr. 23, 1977.

ulin as the immunizing agent, will soon be available to patients with differentiated metastatic thyroid malignancy. This therapy would be especially useful in patients in whom radioiodine therapy has reached the limits of its usefulness. The serum thyroglobulin assay should prove to be of value in following patients who have had total thyroidectomy for recurrent thyroid malignancy.

► [The demonstration by Van Herle and Uller that thyroid cancers can release thyroglobulin into the blood (J. Clin. Invest. 56:272, 1975) suggested that measurement of this protein might provide a marker for the presence of active disease and thus help in treatment. This hope has been clearly fulfilled by the data produced by P. Lo Gerfo and his colleagues. There are not so many specific markers for cancer that we can afford to be blasé about this development, even though thyroid cancer is not one of the major killers. The need for intensive search for other markers of equal specificity suitable for studying other diseases of higher prevalence is obvious. The question is pursued further in the following chapter. – Ed.] ◄

Ectopic Endocrinopathies

► One obvious possibility as a marker for cancer is the ectopic hormones secreted by certain tumors. I have personally chased this will-o'-the-wisp for the past 5 years and can assure you that it is not a simple problem. One reason for this is the difference between the ability of a tumor to make a particular polypeptide and its ability to release the substance into the plasma. Extracts of tumors often contain many substances that have not been released in detectable quantities into the blood. It is uncertain exactly what controls this release, but Matsukura and colleagues (J. Clin. Endocrinol. Metab. 44:392, 1977) have made an important contribution by demonstrating that the adenylate cyclase of two ectopic ACTH-producing tumors was activated by a considerable group of physiologically active substances such as thyrotropin-releasing hormone, gonadotropin-releasing hormone, norepinephrine, epinephrine, serotonin, prostaglandin E_1 and extract of rat median eminence. The normal pituitary gland would respond to many of these stimuli, but would not release ACTH except when exposed to median eminence extract and perhaps serotonin. So the tumor was more catholic in its taste than the pituitary. More studies of this type are needed to define the regulating factors in "secretion" by such tumors. Until we can reproducibly cause release of a marker—or count on its spontaneous release—the marker is of little value.—Ed. ◄

Ectopic Production of Chorionic Gonadotropin and Its Subunits by Islet Cell Tumors: Specific Marker for Malignancy. C. Ronald Kahn, Saul W. Rosen, Bruce D. Weintraub, Stefan S. Fajans and Phillip Gorden[5] found that the subunits of human chorionic gonadotropin (hCG), hCG-α and hCG-β, are present in a high proportion of patients with functioning islet cell carcinomas and are specific indicators for malignancy. Serum was obtained from 76 patients with islet cell tumors, 33 of which were malignant. Two patients with Zollinger-Ellison syndrome but no tumor were also evaluated. Serum concentrations of hCG, hCG-α and hCG-β were determined by independent radioimmunoassays.

The findings are shown in Figure 16. An elevated hCG-α level was the most frequent finding. Eight of 14 patients with malignant insulinoma had increased serum hCG-α concentrations, whereas only 3 had elevated hCG-β values. Immunoreactive hCG was elevated in 2 of the 8 patients in whom it was measured. Results were similar in patients with other types of malignant functioning islet cell tumor, including malignant gastrinoma. None of 41 patients with benign insulinoma and neither of the 2 with benign Zollinger-Ellison syndrome had elevated concentrations of hCG or the subunits. Six patients with nonfunctional malignant islet cell tumors also had normal subunit values. In most patients with malignant islet cell tumors the secretion of hCG-α and hCG-β was discordant. All 4 malignant tumors examined contained hCG subunits. Subunit levels correlated with clinical course during streptozocin therapy in the 2 patients studied. Placental lactogen was detected in the extract of 1 malignant insulinoma. Carcinoem-

(5) N. Engl. J. Med. 297:565–569, Sept. 15, 1977.

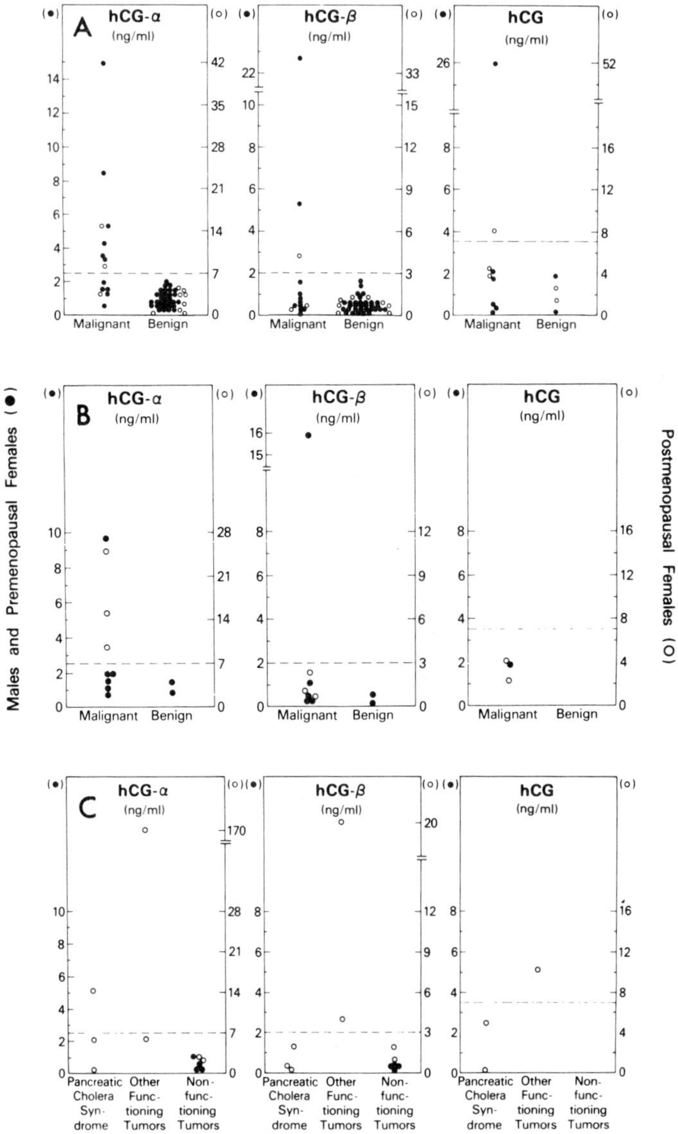

Fig 16.—Plasma concentrations of hCG and hCG subunits in patients with insulinomas (**A**), gastrinomas (**B**) and other malignant islet cell tumors (**C**). Solid circles indicate male and premenopausal female patients and should be read from scale at left of each panel. Open circles indicate postmenopausal female patients and should be read from scale at right of each panel. Broken lines represent highest values ever observed for serums of patients without neoplastic disease in authors' assay. (Courtesy of Kahn, C. R., et al.: N. Engl. J. Med. 297:565–569, Sept. 15, 1977.)

bryonic antigen was minimally elevated in 3 of 5 serums from patients with islet cell carcinoma. α-Fetoprotein was elevated in 2 of 8 serums from patients with islet cell carcinoma.

Human chorionic gonadotropin and its subunits are specific and prevalent markers for islet cell carcinoma. Ectopic secretion does not occur in the same tumor types when they are benign, supporting the derepression hypothesis of ectopic polypeptide production, rather than the "cell rest" concept.

► [In other words, if hCG or its subunits are increased in the plasma, malignancy is likely, but if levels are normal no conclusions can be drawn. – Ed.] ◄

Human Chorionic Gonadotropin-like Substance in Nonendocrine Tissues of Normal Subjects. Yoshio Yoshimoto, Ada R. Wolfsen and William D. Odell[6] (Univ. of California, Torrance) postulated that ectopic peptide elaboration is a universal concomitant of cancer and represents activation of repressed genetic data during the process of neoplasia. Chorionic gonadotropin (CG) has been described in extracts of normal human testis. Extracts from cancer patients have now been examined to determine whether activation of the genome for CG synthesis is specific for cancer or, alternatively, also occurs during replication of other, normal, cells. Normal liver and colon were taken at autopsy from 3 male patients who died of nonneoplastic disorders. Rat testicular homogenates were obtained for a radioreceptor assay. Chorionic gonadotropin was measured by a double-antibody radioimmunoassay.

The two assay systems demonstrated a CG-like substance in extracts of liver and colon from subjects without neoplasia. In contrast to placental CG, it was not bound to concanavalin A-Sepharose columns, indicating the presence of little or no carbohydrate. Previous studies have shown that desialylated human CG possesses little or no bioactivity in vivo but retains full radioreceptor and radioimmunoassay activity in vitro.

The findings suggest that the genome responsible for human CG production is not completely suppressed in adult nonendocrine tissues and that the CG produced by colon and liver has little or no bioactivity in vivo because of its low carbohydrate content. Since many normal tissues produce CG, bioactivity may be modulated by regulation of its carbohydrate content. Recently Chen et al. showed the presence of CG-like material in pituitary and urinary extracts of a patient with Klinefelter's syndrome, supporting the concept that normal tissues produce the peptide structure of CG.

► [This information complicates incredibly the concept of "ectopic hormones." How can a substance be "ectopic" if it is present normally in tissues which are not considered to be endocrine in nature? Of course, what Yoshimoto et al. found was not the hormone – just the protein skeleton which is inactive until it is supplied with carbohydrate side chains. Not only are these carbohydrate moieties needed for biologic activity, they are also needed to protect the protein skeleton from rapid excretion or metabolism once it enters the blood. Thus the presence of these immunoreactive polypeptides in plasma is unlikely, at least in concentrations high enough to be useful.

If chorionic gonadotropin-like polypeptides are so widely distributed, one cannot help wondering whether other proteins generally considered to be "specific" for certain organs are also found widely distributed throughout the body. In recent years, the lung has become a happy hunting ground for several biologically active polypeptides previously considered to be of gastrointestinal origin, and the gut has provided a number of hormones believed originally to originate elsewhere, such as glucagon and somatostatin. The entire concept of endocrine specificity needs reexamination. – Ed.]

---

(6) Science 197:575–577, Aug. 5, 1977.

Medullary Thyroid Carcinoma: Ectopic Production of Peptides with ACTH-like, Corticotropin-Releasing Factor-like and Prolactin Production-Stimulating Activities. Medullary thyroid carcinoma is often associated with pheochromocytoma and hyperparathyroidism and less commonly with the ectopic ACTH syndrome. Jan C. Birkenhäger, G. Virginia Upton, H. Jaqueline Seldenrath, Dorothy T. Krieger and Armen H. Tashjian Jr.[7] studied a patient with medullary thyroid carcinoma, galactorrhea and Cushing's syndrome, who had laboratory findings of pituitary-dependent Cushing's syndrome rather than the classic type of ectopic ACTH syndrome.

Woman, 45, presented with a round, red face, darkened skin and increased body hair of 1 year's duration and breast enlargement and galactorrhea for 3 months. Moon face, proptosis, truncal obesity, slight galactorrhea and a nodule in the left lobe of the thyroid were observed. An oral glucose tolerance curve was diabetic. Blood pressure was 160/100 mm Hg. A cold nodule was found on thyroid scanning. The plasma calcitonin concentration was 32 ng/ml and increased with intravenous calcium but not with glucagon infusion. The plasma calcitonin concentration was 10.4 ng/ml 2 weeks after total thyroidectomy. The cortisol secretion rate was 65 mg/24 hours. Dexamethasone reduced urinary steroid excretion. Lysine vasopressin increased the plasma cortisol concentration by 17 μg/100 ml. The plasma immunoreactive ACTH concentration fell from 320 to 200 pg/ml with intravenous dexamethasone. The signs of cortisol excess and the galactorrhea abated rapidly after operation, and steroid data returned to normal. The tumor was a histologically typical medullary thyroid carcinoma. A papillary carcinoma was present in the right thyroid lobe, and lymph nodes contained medullary thyroid carcinoma. The hormonally active substances found in the carcinoma are shown in Figure 17.

Fig 17.—Thyroid tumor-neuroendocrine interactions. *CRF,* corticotropin-releasing factor; *PRL-SA,* prolactin production-stimulating activity—1 unit *(U)* is amount required to double rate of prolactin production per 24 hours by pituitary cells in culture. All values for ACTH were determined by bioassay; tumor content was measured after trypsin treatment. (Courtesy of Birkenhäger, J. C., et al.: Acta Endocrinol. (Kbh.) 83:280–292, October, 1976.)

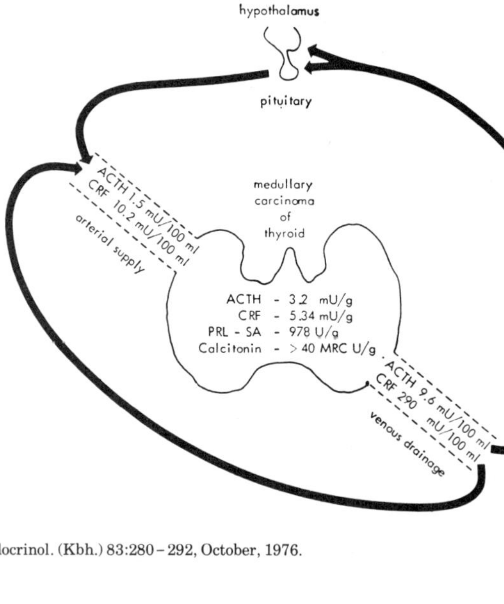

(7) Acta Endocrinol. (Kbh.) 83:280–292, October, 1976.

The findings in this case explain the Cushing's syndrome and the galactorrhea. The galactorrhea was presumably due to stimulation of prolactin synthesis and its release from the pituitary induced by material from the carcinoma. The tumor material did not affect growth hormone production.

► [In Figure 17, "CRF" refers to corticotropin-releasing factor. The most notable feature of this tumor was the huge amount of this activity found in the venous drainage and tumor extract. The tumor also (independently?) produced ACTH, but the pituitary was probably the major source of the excessive ACTH found clinically, and the stimulus to pituitary secretion was CRF from the tumor. This pattern has now been described on a number of occasions in oat cell carcinoma of the lung and carcinoid of the bronchus (e.g., Upton and Amatruda: N. Engl. J. Med. 285:419, 1971; Yamamoto et al.: Acta Endocrinol. (Kbh.) 82:183, 1976; and Suda et al.: J. Clin. Endocrinol. Metab. 44:440, 1977). The pattern is not confined to lung tumors, since the observations of Suda et al. concerned a human colonic cancer and a rat mammary tumor.

It is not always easy to differentiate hyperadrenocorticism caused by excessive secretion of ACTH by the pituitary from the caused when a tumor releases ACTH ectopically. Corrigan and colleagues (N. Engl. J. Med. 296:861, 1977) used selective venous sampling by catheter to demonstrate a region of increased ACTH activity in the pituitary drainage. If the source of ACTH had been ectopic (but of unknown location), the pituitary would not have been secreting ACTH and the venous effluent from the pituitary region would have had a concentration of the hormone equal to that of the mixed venous blood. – Ed.] ◄

Pancreatic Somatostatinoma: Clinical Features and Physiologic Implications. All identified islet cell types seem able to give rise to tumors, producing distinct clinical symptoms. L.-I. Larsson, M. A. Hirsch, J. J. Holst, S. Ingemansson, C. Kühl, S. Lindkaer Jensen, G. Lundqvist, J. F. Rehfeld and T. W. Schwartz[8] report the first recorded case of a pure somatostatin-producing tumor.

Woman, 55, with a history of abdominal pains, nontoxic goiter and diarrhea, had hypochlorhydria and steatorrhea. Episodes of headache and tachycardia ensued. A pancreatic tumor and liver metastases were noted at cholecystectomy. Review of x-rays made 2 years before showed the tumor to have been present at that time. The patient's condition deteriorated rapidly postoperatively and she died. Autopsy showed central hepatic necrosis without evidence of residual tumor. The tumor cells were ultrastructurally characteristic of D cells. Nearly all tumor cells showed granular cytoplasmic staining intensely with somatostatin antiserum. Marked hyperplasia of extrainsular pancreatic polypeptide cells was observed. Radioimmunoassay showed the tumor to contain large amounts of somatostatin immunoreactivity. The material inhibited insulin and glucagon secretion in isolated perfused porcine pancreas; polypeptide secretion was only slightly affected. Blood samples from the pancreatic and hepatic veins contained up to 107 ng/ml somatostatin equivalents of immunoreactivity. Peripheral blood samples showed low to normal levels of insulin, pancreatic polypeptide and gastrin, and glucagon levels significantly below normal.

This patient very likely had a pancreatic somatostatin-producing tumor. The somatostatin-immunoreactive material produced by the normal pancreatic D cell is likely to inhibit the release of insulin and glucagon. Quite high somatostatin levels were found in the venous effluent from the tumor. Neoplastic D cells, at least, seem to deliver their products to the bloodstream. It is of interest that hypersecretion

(8) Lancet 1:666–668, Mar. 26, 1977.

of this strongly inhibitory peptide does not give rise to more severe symptoms than were noted in the present patient.

► [This is an interesting report, but it is not clear to me that all—or even most—of the symptoms were caused by somatostatin. The patient also had extensive liver involvement, and malnutrition as a consequence of her diarrhea could have been a problem. We shall have to keep an eye out for other examples of this pattern to see whether it proves consistent.—Ed.] ◄

Carbohydrate Metabolism

► An excellent book, of 244 pages, has been published by *Acta Medica Scandinavica* as its Supplementum 601 (1977). It is edited by Rolf Luft and is concerned with the chemistry, biology and pathophysiology of insulin.

Progress is gradually being made in understanding the pathogenesis of diabetes in human beings. A good many of the fragments involved in the story have already been mentioned or abstracted in this section of the YEAR BOOK in previous years. The story starts with the demonstration that certain strains of mice, when infected with the M variant of the virus of encephalomyocarditis, develop diabetes (Yoon et al.: Nature 264: 178, 1976; and Buschard et al.: Acta Pathol. Microbiol. Scand. [C] 84:299, 1976). In nude mice, which lack a thymus-mediated immune mechanism, diabetes does not develop. Thus it is not a matter of lack of immunity, but rather of genetic susceptibility. Presumably, a difference in the cell surface antigens determines the ability of the virus to attack the beta cells, or, alternatively, to initiate an antibody-directed attack on the islet cells. A study of human diabetic patients (Lendrum et al.: Lancet 2:1273, 1976) showed that antibodies directed against the cytoplasmic components of islet cells could be demonstrated in the plasma of 38% of patients with insulin-dependent diabetes, but in only 5% of patients with diabetes not requiring insulin. Such antibodies were present in 1.7% of the normal population. The close relationship between the insulin-dependent type of diabetes and the presence of human leukocyte antigens (HLA) BW15 and B8, has been discussed previously in these pages. This has led to proposals that diabetics be classified in two general groups, based on the immune characteristics of their disease. One classification, proposed by Irvine (ibid. 1:638, 1977), breaks them down into type I (juvenile-onset diabetics who require insulin, adult insulin-dependent diabetics and patients who fail after 3 months or more of oral diabetic treatment, but have antibodies against islet cells) and type II (adult-onset diabetics who do not require insulin and a small number of juvenile-onset diabetics who do not require insulin and lack antibodies against islet cells). Ganda and Soeldner (Arch. Intern. Med. 137:461, 1977) come up with an almost identical classification, except that they use type A and type B rather than type I and type II. In both classifications, type I (or A) is considered to have an inherited pattern (cell surface or HLA antigen) which makes the islet cells sensitive to outside influences (virus infection, probably). The cell-virus interaction changes the cell surface pattern so that it is recognized as a foreign cell and antibodies against it arise which damage or destroy the cell. In type B (or II) there is also a genetic component, not yet clearly understood, but the precipitating factor is not a virus. It is probably a metabolic insult, perhaps associated with advancing age. Both of these papers are worth study, but that by Ganda and Soeldner marshalls the evidence and criticizes the implications of the theory more extensively than does the one by Irvine. Of course, these classifications oversimplify the matter. For example, they do not explain the high incidence of diabetes in certain populations like the Pima Indians, who should have type I (or A) diabetes because of the population and age pattern but whose disease is insulin independent. "Ordinary" juvenile diabetes (type A or I) is common in the West Indies but it is almost always mild and nonaggressive. Although the theory is not entirely satisfactory, it is a good start. Aged readers like myself will recognize a certain similarity between the classifications derived from immunologic considerations and those developed by clinical observation in the 1920's!

Other types of diabetes can occur, though they are rare. For example, Blackard et al. describe a patient with insulin-resistant diabetes whose serum contained an IgG that reacts with insulin receptors. This blocks the ability of insulin to control cellular metabolism. It is the opposite of anti-insulin antibodies and, apparently, a very rare condition (Ann. Intern. Med. 86:584, 1977). Chromium deficiency can cause diabetes in experimental animals and has been suggested as a cause of adult-onset diabetes in some human patients. Jeejeebhoy and colleagues (Am. J. Clin. Nutr. 30:531, 1977) describe a patient aged 40 who developed diabetes after receiving total parenteral nutrition for 5 years. When chromium was measured in the plasma it was very low, and when the ion was added the diabetes disappeared. The patient no longer required insulin, gained weight and recovered from a peripheral neuropathy. This pattern may become a common problem if patients with prolonged total intravenous alimentation become more numerous. But one also wonders whether there is an element of chromium deficiency in some adult-onset (type II or B) diabetics without evident explanation.

The role of glucagon and somatostatin in the pathogenesis of human diabetes remains a matter of debate. Felig et al. (Diabetes 25:1091, 1976) reviewed the problem in their Lilly lecture. They conclude that the improvement of hyperglycemia produced by somatostatin in diabetics is largely a reflection of its ability to inhibit carbohydrate absorption by the gastrointestinal tract. Diabetes is a disease of insulin deficiency and not of glucagon hypersecretion. Although glucagon may worsen diabetes, it is in itself neither sufficient nor necessary for the development of the disease. The data on which these conclusions are based are set forth in some detail in a paper from the same laboratory, by Tamborlane et al. (N. Engl. J. Med. 297:181, 1977). They also point out that administration of somatostatin to patients with maturity-onset diabetes (type II or B) accentuates hyperglycemia, hyperketonemia and hyperaminoacidemia (probably by suppressing insulin secretion) and therefore that the polypeptide should not be given to this type of patient. Barnes et al., who studied the role of glucagon in ketoacidosis, came to the same conclusion—i.e., that glucagon is not necessary for development of ketosis, but that it may accelerate its onset in the presence of insulin deficiency (ibid. 296:1250, 1977). The only dissenter—and perhaps with only a mild dissent at that—is Gerich (Arch. Intern. Med. 137:659, 1977), who suggests that somatostatin might be a useful therapeutic agent in slowing down the development of ketoacidosis. In view of the very short half-life of somatostatin, however, it is not practical to use it at present.

The problem of maternal diabetes and its effects on the infant is still under study. Cassady and colleagues (Am. J. Obstet. Gynecol. 127:21, 1977) studied the relationship among maternal diabetes, fetal age and amniotic fluid glucose content. The glucose concentration in amniotic fluid fell with increasing fetal age (because the fetus puts out more insulin as it gets older?) and the concentration of amniotic fluid glucose was higher in more severely diabetic mothers. The ability of the fetus to regulate its amniotic fluid glucose concentration suggests that higher concentrations of maternal glucose, calling forth a greater fetal insulin response, would be associated with a higher incidence of postpartum hypoglycemia in the infants of women with high blood glucose concentrations. This was confirmed by Haworth and Dilling (J. Pediatr. 89:810, 1976). There was a direct relationship between the maternal fasting blood glucose concentration and the rate at which the infant cleared glucose from the blood. If an oral glucose tolerance test was done on the mother, the likelihood of infantile hypoglycemia could be predicted from the maternal glucose concentration 2 hours after the glucose load. For example, half of the newborns would develop hypoglycemia (less than 30 mg glucose per dl blood) if the maternal 2-hour concentration was 180 mg/dl, and 90% would develop it if the mother's 2-hour concentration was 220 mg/dl. Obviously, the baby will benefit in this respect (as in many others) by careful control of the maternal glucose metabolism and rigorous postnatal care.

Diabetes is a disease treated by patients under the supervision of their doctors. Since it is a chronic condition requiring continuing daily treatment, and since the physician or nurse cannot provide this sort of supervision except under unusual circumstances, the quality of the diabetic care depends to a great degree on the ability of the patient to understand his disease and carry out his treatment. Two interesting studies have addressed themselves to this problem. Simon and Stewart (Mt. Sinai J. Med. N.Y. 43:189, 1976) administered a multiple choice quiz to 99 patients at the diabetic clinic of the City Hospital in Elmhurst, New York. The diabetics, on average, answered about half of the questions correctly. Lack of understanding was higher among older patients, those with less education, those who had had treatment for 3 years or less, those relying on the clinic as their only source of information and those speaking Spanish as their first language. Patients who used insulin and those who had had major complications did better in the examination than those with mild disease. Several obvious conclusions could be drawn: that special instruction should be provided for Spanish (or other foreign) patients, that more intensive instruction should be provided by the clinic early in the patient's course and that the material being taught should be structured for poorly educated patients. But even if this type of improved instruction is provided, and the patients show improved understanding of the disease on retesting after classes, there may not be any improvement in the quality of care. At least, this is what Grabner and colleagues discovered when routine teaching exercises were used. When intensive education was provided, with emphasis on integration of the patient into the health care system, rather than merely on care of diabetes, both the rate of hospitalization and the incidence of complications improved (Diabetes 26:61, 1977). – Ed. ◄

Three-Year Controlled Follow-up Study of Persons Identified in a Mass Screening Program for Diabetes. Harold B. Houser, Wilma Mackay, Narendra Verma and Saul Genuth[9] matched each of 529 persons identified as positive in a diabetes mass screening industrial program, conducted in Cleveland since 1964, with a negative screenee of the same sex, race, age and place of employment. A glucose tolerance test confirmed positivity in 204 cases and failed to confirm it in 141; 184 subjects were given the test. The screening test was a capillary blood glucose measurement, made 2 hours after 75 gm glucose was ingested. A 3-year follow-up used a mail questionnaire.

Deaths were more frequent in confirmed positives; the rate was 7%. The self-perceived current health state was poorer in this group than in the controls. A positive screening test resulted in increased early contact with physicians, but only confirmed positives had evidence of continuing increased contact. Oral antidiabetes medications were being used by 28% of confirmed positives, 17% of those not tested and 1% of not-confirmed subjects.

With no clear evidence of modification of behavior toward continued medical care, and considering the potential harm of improper or early exhibition or oral drugs or the incorrect labeling of persons as diabetic, the possible benefits of early physician intervention and weight loss do not appear to offset the potential nonbenefit of mass screening. The Cleveland program has now been modified to one of discriminate screening, rather than indiscriminate mass screening.

► [Its about time someone took a good look at the diabetic screening program! In my experience, it seldom picks up patients with diabetes that could benefit from treatment, it generates an immense amount of extra unnecessary work to sort out the erroneous laboratory values and it produces unnecessary and damaging anxiety in the subjects, and for what? To find some patients with minimal deviations of glucose tolerance who can't be treated effectively by present methods anyway! Sometimes the most important step to take is a backward one. If this article helps reduce the fruitless effort previously put into screening, it will be a step backward that is a great step forward. – Ed.] ◄

Regulation of Brittle Diabetics by a Preplanned Insulin Infusion Program. The poor prognosis of juvenile diabetics is due to development of nephropathy and cardiovascular disease, which appear to be dependent on the quality of metabolic control during the preceding years. Inadequate adjustment of plasma levels of pancreatic islet hormones leads to unphysiologic fluctuations in blood glucose in brittle diabetics. Fluctuations in plasma insulin are important in glucose homeostasis, since constant insulin infusion in brittle diabetics results in marked elevations of blood glucose after meals (Fig 18). T. Deckert and B. Lørup[1] (Gentofte, Denmark) developed a program of infusing

(9) Diabetes 26:619–627, July, 1977.
(1) Diabetologia 12:573–579, December, 1976.

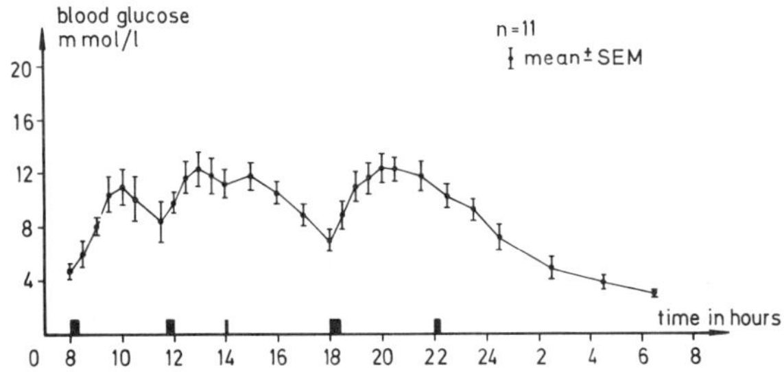

Fig 18.—Capillary blood glucose during intravenous insulin infusion at a constant rate (0.26–0.53, mean 0.39 mU/kg/minute) in 4 insulin-treated, normal-weight diabetics. Three patients were of the juvenile brittle type and 1 patient, of the more stable type. Mean ± SEM of 11 infusion days. (Courtesy of Deckert, T., and Lørup, B.: Diabetologia 12:573–579, December, 1976; Berlin-Heidelberg-New York: Springer.)

soluble insulin at rates simulating physiologic plasma insulin variations in nondiabetics in everyday life. Eleven consecutive brittle diabetics, 7 male and 4 female patients with diabetes for a mean of 11.5 years, while ambulatory received intravenous insulin infusion for 2 days after unsuccessful regulation on twice-daily NPH insulin and subcutaneous injection of regular insulin 4 times daily based on determination of blood glucose level. Seven patients had late diabetic manifestations. An electric precision pump (Infusomat) was used. Infusion rates varied from 7 to 30 ml per hour. Regular porcine insulin was used.

All the patients felt well. Three required interruption of the infusion. Fluctuations in blood glucose were much less marked during the infusion period. Only 1.3% of blood glucose values were below 2.5 mmol/L (45 mg/dl) on infusion days after the 7-hour equilibrium period, and 2.9% of values exceeded 10 mmol/L (180 mg/dl). Hypoglycemic reactions were about as frequent as on the NPH day but less frequent than on days when regular insulin was given 4 times daily, subcutaneously. Daily insulin doses did not differ significantly. The mean blood glucose and mean amplitude of glucose excursions were greatly reduced on infusion days, as was glucosuria.

This infusion program provides significantly better blood glucose control in brittle diabetics than does treatment with NPH insulin or short-acting insulin 4 times daily. Unpredictable absorption from subcutaneous insulin depots can be avoided and probably so can immunologic side effects. A fairly good estimate of the daily insulin requirement is necessary for successful insulin infusion therapy.

► [A very similar system was described by Genuth and Martin (Diabetes 26:571, 1977). Both systems used a pump assembly so large it had to be pushed about on a cart, so it would not have been appropriate for ordinary activities, but it permitted the patients to be ambulatory during the infusion. Both systems were programed to inject different amounts of insulin at different times of the day, but neither required feedback information about the patient's blood glucose to adjust the rate of insulin injection. Although these systems are bulky and probably less precise than the computer-controlled systems we have discussed in these pages in past years, they seem to work a great deal better than intermittent subcutaneous injection of insulin. The trick now will be to miniaturize them, but the methods are already available. Although one could not call these systems "artificial pancreata" one might call them "artifical carbohydrate pacemakers."

The general problem of the artificial endocrine pancreas is discussed by Albisser et al. (Arch. Intern. Med. 137:639, 1977). They point out that with the computer-controlled systems now available it is possible to return the blood glucose concentration to normal after a glucose load or to maintain it during moderate physical exercise. The chief problem is the sensitivity and stability of a glucose sensor, which is an essential part of a feedback control system. Still, a great deal of progress has been made.

In view of the limitations of the artificial endocrine pancreas, there is continuing interest in islet cell transplantation. This has been notably unsuccessful in human beings (Groth et al.: Surg. Gynecol. Obstet. 143:933, 1976), but interesting experiments are in progress in rats. If it were possible to implant islet cells in such a way that they had free access to small diffusible molecules and ions, but were inaccessible to the destructive effects of T lymphocytes, it might be practical to implant cells from an incompatible donor without immune suppression of the host. Conceivably, one could even use islets from a different species. The trick would be to put the cells in a millipore container or in a vessel traversed by semipermeable plastic tubing which would let glucose and insulin through but would hold back defensive cells. Such experiments have been tried in rats by Tze et al. (Nature 264:466, 1976), but they found that clotting occurred unless the recipients were anticoagulated. Survival of the recipients was poor because of bleeding or clotting. Still, the idea is a good one, requiring mainly the development of suitable plastics that can be tolerated by the patient. The advantage of this system would be the automatic incorporation of a biofeedback control built into the cells. This area is exciting and will undoubtedly see great advances in the next few years.

It is important to remind ourselves of the medications which can aggravate diabetes. Zumoff and Hellman (J.A.M.A. 237:1960, 1977) report an insulin-dependent diabetic whose disease was aggravated by chlordiazepoxide. They review the psychoactive drugs and comment that almost all of them affect diabetes. Most tranquilizers aggravate it and most antidepressants ameliorate it.

There is a good deal of agreement now that physiologic control of diabetes is likely to improve or abolish the vascular complications. Unfortunately, ordinary methods of treatment do not provide adequate control in most cases. Evaluating the excellence of control is difficult because chemical tests are episodic and patients are often unreliable witnesses. What is needed is a sort of indicator of the average blood glucose elevation. Exactly this may be available, according to Gabbay et al. (J. Clin. Endocrinol. Metab. 44:859, 1977), in the form of glycosylated hemoglobins A_{1a+b} and A_{1c}. These minor deviants of hemoglobin A are formed when glucose is transferred to normal hemoglobin A. This reaction is similar to the glycosylation of basement membrane proteins that has been described by many observers, but especially by Spiro, and discussed in previous years in these pages. If hemoglobin A acts as a model system reflecting glycosylation of membranes, it could be a good indicator of the degree of aberration introduced by poor control of the blood glucose. The glycosylation of membranes is reviewed by Williamson and Kilo (Diabetes 26:65, 1977), who agree that this chemical reaction, which is related to the level of blood glucose, is an important factor in producing the initial abnormality of many blood vessels attacked by the disease. These include the glomerular and retinal capillaries.—Ed.] ◄

Metabolic Response to Moderate Exercise in Diabetic Man Receiving Intravenous and Subcutaneous Insulin. Insulin is a key regulator of metabolic adjustments during exercise, and a variety of abnormalities in such responses has been recognized in human diabetics. Frederick T. Murray, Bernard Zinman, Patricia A. McClean, Araceli Denoga, A. Michael Albisser, Bernard S. Leibel, Azima F. Nakhooda, Elaine F. Stokes and Errol B. Marliss[2] (Univ. of Toronto) examined metabolic responses to exercise in two groups of diabetics, one given insulin subcutaneously an hour before exercise and one given a continuous intravenous infusion of insulin starting 10–12 hours

(2) J. Clin. Endocrinol. Metab. 44:708–720, April, 1977.

before and continuing throughout exercise at a constant rate. Twelve insulin-dependent diabetics and 7 controls were studied. The diabetics were active, nonobese and in good nutritional balance. Moderate (50% maximum) bicycle ergometer exercise was carried out for 45-minute periods. The subcutaneous dose of insulin was one third of the usual daily dosage. Seven subjects received 8–20 mU of insulin per minute during exercise.

The diabetics given subcutaneous insulin showed a sharp fall in glycemia from elevated resting levels, whereas controls showed no change. Further, a rise in insulin was noted, whereas a fall occurred in the controls. In these diabetics exercise induced a further rise in glucagon from elevated concentrations. Free fatty acid values failed to increase on exercise, as in the controls. The respiratory quotient in-

Fig 19.—Glucose, insulin *(IRI)* and glucagon *(IRG)* in patients given insulin subcutaneously *(squares),* those given insulin intravenously *(triangles)* and controls *(circles)* during rest, exercise and recovery. Open symbols signify significant change ($P < 0.05$) from mean resting values for that variable. Asterisks indicate points in subjects treated subcutaneously or intravenously that are significantly different ($P < 0.05$) from value in controls at that time. Number of observations is given in parentheses. (Courtesy of Murray, F. T., et al.: J. Clin. Endocrinol. Metab. 44:708–720, April, 1977.)

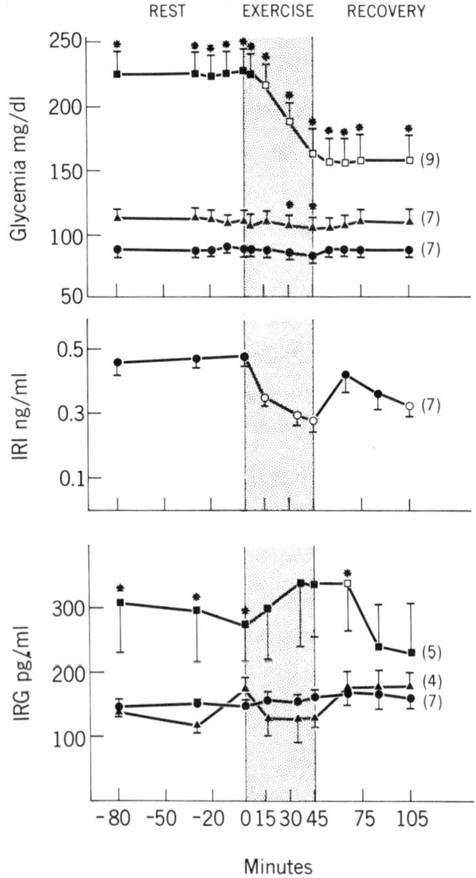

creased and remained elevated. The diabetics given insulin by infusion showed no glycemic change with exercise (Fig 19). Fourfold rises in lactate and pyruvate were seen. The significantly elevated free fatty acid values increased even during recovery. Glycerol and ketone body increments tended to be greater than in controls.

Intravenous insulin sustained euglycemia in diabetics during exercise in this study, obviating the fall in glycemia seen with subcutaneous insulin. The responses of other metabolites were abnormal and consistent with a subtle degree of underinsulinization. Intravascular insulin delivery by the "artificial pancreas" can maintain glycemia and normalize the glycemic response to meals, and no new control parameters would appear to be required during exercise under the conditions of this study. On the other hand, increased absorption of the subcutaneous insulin limits the availability of fat-derived substrates and suppresses the normal rise in glucose production during exercise. It may be logical to augment the carbohydrate supply just before exercise by consuming rapidly absorbed carbohydrates, rather than by decreasing the insulin dose in anticipation of exercise.

► [The same authors have published a companion article (Zinman et al.: J. Clin. Endocrinol. Metab. 45:641, 1977) elaborating on these experiments by determining the glucose turnover by isotopic methods. Glucose entry into the plasma is reduced in the group given subcutaneous insulin, whereas in both the control and the infusion group the rate of glucose production increased. In all three groups, the rate of glucose utilization increased, but the subcutaneous group could not keep up with increased utilization and therefore suffered a fall of blood glucose concentration.

In interpreting these experiments, two considerations must be kept in mind. The insulin was given subcutaneously into the thigh of subjects exercising on a stationary bicycle. These subjects had an increase of plasma insulin during exercise which was not observed in the group getting intravenous insulin infusions or the normal group. This increase of insulin occurred despite falling blood glucose concentrations. So the first conclusion is that if you massage the area in which the insulin is injected, it will be absorbed more rapidly! The second conclusion—and much more important—is that if enough insulin is supplied, the demands of exercise are handled by regulatory processes without demanding alteration of the rate of insulin entry into the blood. This set of experiments therefore confirms in more detailed fashion the advantages of using constant insulin infusions rather than depot administration which were discussed in the preceding article in more general clinical terms.—Ed.] ◄

Efficacy of Low-Dose versus Conventional Therapy of Insulin for Treatment of Diabetic Ketoacidosis. There is little consensus on the optimal means of treating diabetic ketoacidosis with respect to the amount of insulin and its route of administration. Abbas E. Kitabchi, Ventachalam Ayyagari, Sonia M. O. Guerra (Univ. of Tennessee) and Medical House Staff of the City of Memphis Hospitals[3] (Memphis, Tenn.) prospectively evaluated low-dose intramuscular insulin therapy and conventional high-dose intravenous and subcutaneous therapy in a randomized manner in adults with diabetic ketoacidosis. The initial insulin dose was based on plasma glucose in the high-dose group and on body weight in the low-dose group, subsequent doses were based on plasma glucose in both groups. Supportive therapy was similar in the two groups.

The average age of 24 low-dose patients was 38.7 years and of 24

(3) Ann. Intern. Med. 84:633–638, June, 1976.

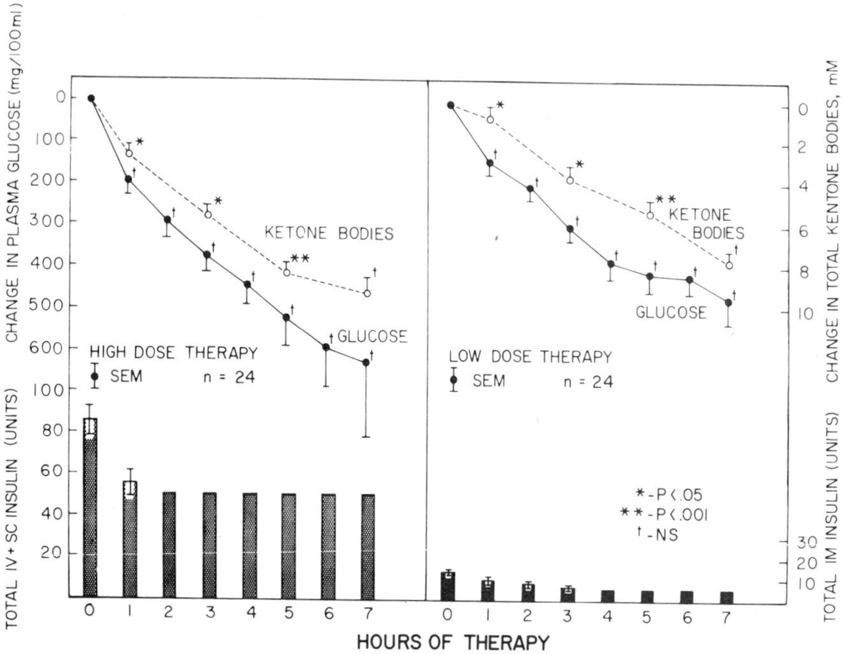

Fig 20.—Effect of insulin and fall in glucose and ketone bodies in ketoacidotic patients treated with high- and low-dose insulin. (Courtesy of Kitabchi, A. E., et al.: Ann. Intern. Med. 84:633–638, June, 1976.)

high-dose patients, 40.3 years. Seven patients in each group were new diabetics. Biochemical profiles for the two groups were similar. Initial effects of insulin are shown in Figure 20. Ketone bodies fell more rapidly in the high-dose group at early intervals. The initial insulin dose was 86 units per hour in the high-dose group and 13.5 units per hour in the low-dose group. There was no difference in the rates of glucose fall at any interval. Hypokalemia was noted in 1 low-dose patient and 7 high-dose patients. Six high-dose patients had hypoglycemia. A supraphysiologic level of plasma insulin persisted at 6 hours in the high-dose group. A total of 232.9 units of insulin was used in this group in a 6-hour period.

The presence of infection, severe dehydration or hypotension did not appear to affect the responsiveness of patients to low doses of insulin in this study. Intramuscular insulin administration may have contributed to the success of low-dose treatment. Treatment of diabetic ketoacidosis by low-dose intramuscular insulin injection is simple, effective and free of the risk of hypoglycemia observed in conventional high-dose therapy. Contrary to long-standing opinion, diabetic ketoacidosis does not cause "insulin resistance."

► [A good deal of fuss was raised several years ago about the loss of insulin by adsorption to container and tubing if small amounts were added to infusions. This was the reason that originally those recommending low-dose insulin treatment of diabetic ketoacidosis used small volumes of relatively concentrated insulin solutions injected by electric pumps. It appears that this precaution is unnecessary. Clarke and colleagues (Br. Med. J. 2:1395, 1977) found that as little as 6 units added to a liter of saline produced the desired metabolic effect. This leaves us with several variables worth considering: the dose, the method of administration and the schedule. George and Alberti reviewed this problem (Arch. Intern. Med. 137:1367, 1977) and found that doses ranging from 4 to 10 units per hour worked about equally well if given by infusion. A loading dose of 20 units followed by 5 units per hour intramuscularly was also satisfactory. Piters et al. (Diabetologia 13:317, 1977), studying children, found that 50 units by intravenous push repeated after 2 hours worked about as well as 10 units by continuous infusion every hour, but 2 units per hour by infusion was inadequate. Menzel et al. (Endokrinologie 67:230, 1976) comment that the use of 4–10 units by infusion each hour has been a successful method of treatment in their Karlsburg clinic since 1946! So what is the excitement, except that it has taken a long time for the English-speaking world to shake off the influence of Joslin's aggressive approach? If you prefer to give insulin by intravenous bolus, Clumeck et al. (Br. Med. J. 2:394, 1976) will support you by observing that hourly intravenous boluses of 5 units work well. Despite the short half-life of insulin in plasma, the metabolic effect of the bolus lasts about 60 minutes. If you are old-fashioned and prefer to give insulin subcutaneously, Heber et al. (Arch. Intern. Med. 137:1377, 1977) give you support, in that 6 units per hour by infusion or subcutaneously produced the same rate of fall of blood glucose. To summarize: Insulin in small doses can be given with good therapeutic effect in treating diabetic ketosis of adults or children. The minimum effective dose is probably 4 units per hour. In children the minimum is probably about 0.25 units/kg/hour (Veeser et al.: Am. J. Dis. Child. 313:308, 1977). The most reliable method, most people agree, is by intravenous infusion, and the insulin can be added to the infusion solution. It is probably wise to use 6–10 units if it is decided to add the insulin to the bottle of fluid. On the other hand, good results can be obtained by intramuscular injection. Indeed, in most hands the results are not different when the same dose is given intramuscularly hourly as when it is given by intravenous infusion. Pulse doses by intravenous are also acceptable. Even subcutaneous administration will work, though the dose may have to be a little higher. All methods mentioned avoid the requirement of using an electric infusion pump, and most are suitable for use in clinics or hospitals not blessed with an elaborate support system. For the doctor who sees a patient in ketoacidosis outside the hospital, it is probably best to start treatment with intramuscular insulin in small dose while awaiting transportation of the patient to the medical center. – Ed.] ◄

Treatment of Insulin-Induced Lipoatrophy. The cause of insulin-induced lipoatrophy remains unknown. Therapeutic trials have been rather successful, especially since the introduction of highly purified insulins. S. G. Th. Hulst[4] (Utrecht, The Netherlands) reports the results of treatment of 20 children having lipoatrophy with monocomponent and less purified insulins. The 20 patients were among 167 diabetic children (12%) and 14 of the group were girls. The mean age was 11.2 and the mean duration of diabetes and insulin therapy was 4.1 years. Ten children received monocomponent insulins and 10 received the insulins they had previously used. The monocomponent products were Monotard, Actrapid MC and Semilente MC. Insulin was injected with size 18 needles in both groups. Reinspection of the atrophic areas was made after 2 and 6 months of treatment.

The 10 children given monocomponent insulins showed marked disappearance of the lipoatrophy after 2 months of treatment. No abnormality was apparent after 6 months of treatment. The 10 children given their previous insulins showed essentially the same mode of recovery, but some lipoatrophy was still noted after 2 months of treatment. The lipoatrophy had disappeared completely after 6 months of treatment (Fig 21).

---

(4) Diabetes 25:1052–1054, November, 1976.

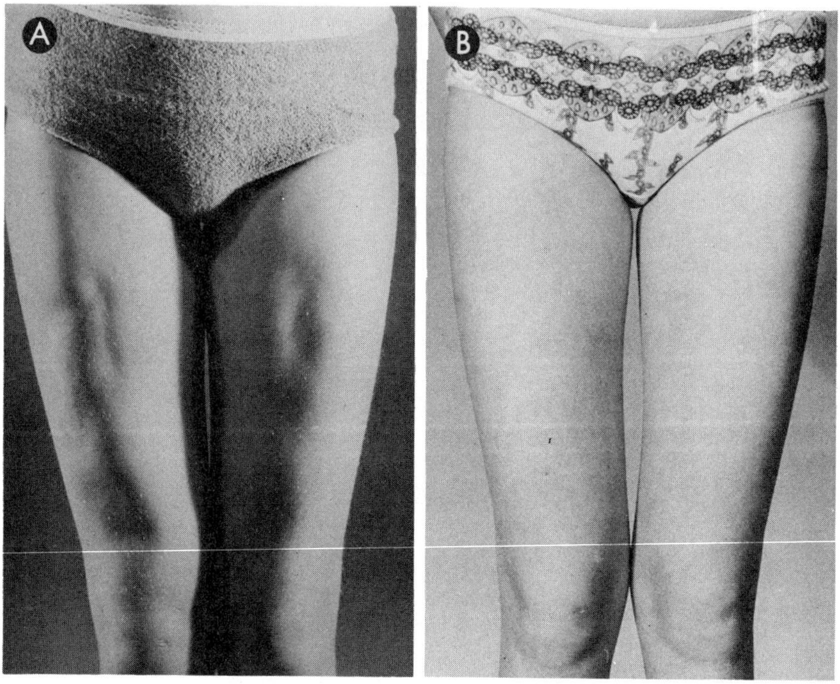

Fig 21.—Insulin-induced lipoatrophy before (**A**) and after (**B**) 6 months of treatment with Monotard and Actrapid MC. (Courtesy of Hulst, S. G. Th.: Diabetes 25:1052–1054, November, 1976.)

The primary factor in treatment of insulin-induced lipoatrophy appears to be careful injection of insulin into the atrophic area. There are several reasons for using purified insulins in young diabetics, including less antigenicity, but it hardly seems worthwhile to change the regimen in a well-controlled subject in order to treat insulin-induced lipoatrophy. Since no lipoatrophy has been reported in patients treated with monocomponent insulins, it may be advisable to begin insulin treatment in young diabetics with monocomponent insulins.

► [Monocomponent insulin has been suggested as an alternative to ordinary insulin in treating patients with insulin allergies. This does not always work. Leslie (Br. Med. J. 2:736, 1977) describes a woman with an urticarial reaction to ordinary insulin. When she was switched to monocomponent insulin she had an identical reaction. After desensitization over 4 weeks, she was able to tolerate monocomponent insulin without further reactions.

Can one predict whether monocomponent insulin will improve resistance of certain diabetic patients to the hormone? Mustaffa et al. (Diabetologia 13:311, 1977) found that if the plasma binds 40 μU or more of insulin per ml, changing from ordinary to monocomponent insulin is highly likely to be useful, but when the binding capacity is less, it is unlikely that purified insulin will improve matters.—Ed.] ◄

Diabetic Vascular Changes in Children. Diabetic retinopathy has rarely been studied by physicians caring for diabetic children. The microvascular complications of diabetes are demonstrated in the eye at an early stage by retinal fluorescein angiography. John I. Malone, Thomas C. Van Cader and William C. Edwards[5] (Univ. of South Flori-

(5) Diabetes 26:673–679, July, 1977.

da) performed fluorescein angiography in 154 children who had had diabetes for 1 month to 18 years. Age range was 5–18 years.

Vascular defects were seen on retinal photographs in children who had had clinical diabetes for 4 months to 18 years, but the more advanced stages were seen only in those who had had diabetes for 6 years or longer. Twelve of the 21 children with retinopathy were aged 8–15 years. Angiography showed more disease than did color photographs; a total of 77% of the children showed vascular abnormalities. Fifteen children (10%) had evidence of growth failure, but this finding was not associated with retinopathy. The degree of retinopathy was the same in children with and in those without proteinuria. No child was hypertensive. The more advanced stages of vascular abnormalities, as seen on fluorescein study, were associated with a longer duration of clinical diabetes.

Vascular defects were found on fluorescein angiography in 75% of children with normal retinal color photographs in this study. Diabetes-associated vascular changes can be observed clinically much earlier in the eye than in the kidney. All children in the study who took two doses of insulin daily had vascular abnormalities. The findings support the ideas that the vascular changes associated with diabetes occur soon after recognition of the disorder in some children and that the vascular abnormalities may precede the clinical onset of diabetes. There may be two types of clinical diabetes, one with and one without associated vascular changes.

► [This suggestion needs more study. Certainly it is common to find patients who have had diabetes for only a short time and have never been grossly uncontrolled who have major involvement of the small blood vessels. Much less common—but not unknown—are patients who have had diabetes for many years, often poorly controlled, who appear to have minimal or absent microvascular disease. The differences in susceptibility to vascular changes may indeed reflect different types of disease, but defining the difference early in the course of the disease is, so far, impossible.

Maternal diabetes carries some risk of damage to the fetus. Day and Insley (Arch. Dis. Child. 51:935, 1976) studied 205 babies born to diabetic mothers and a control group of matched mothers of equal parity whose hospital registration number was closest to that of the diabetic. Of the diabetic group, 12% had malformed infants, as compared with 6% in the control group. Malformation was most common among women who needed insulin at the time of conception (17 of 117, or 15%). There was no correlation between major malformations and age of onset, duration of diabetes, progressive vascular complications, maternal age or parity. The most important and most common complications were cardiovascular.—Ed.] ◄

Relationship of Clinical Findings and Therapeutic Measures to Course of Diabetic Retinopathy was investigated by A. Teuscher[6] (Univ. of Bern). It has been suggested that simple insulin deficiency may lead to typical retinal complications even in the absence of genetic influences. The present study was designed to uncover the possible relationship between diabetic retinopathy and other factors simultaneously operating in these diabetic patients. The results of hypophysectomy in 15 diabetics with progressive retinopathy are also reported (observation period, 16 years).

Available methods do not effectively control the natural course of diabetic retinopathy. Griffith et al. examined 49 patients with hemo-

(6) Schweiz. Med. Wochenschr. 106:1041–1045, July 31, 1976.

chromatosis, 32 of whom were diabetic, 21 requiring insulin. Among these 21, 9 had diabetic retinopathy (6 had diabetes for more than 10 years). In animal experiments Engerman was able to forestall a retinopathy by giving insulin for a 10-year period. More recent studies question the exclusive role of insulin; it is possible that hormonal imbalance with deficient blockage of the GH by somatostatin, as well as too much glucagon, may lead to insufficient insulin concentration. In the present study 1 patient underwent GH treatment as a means of improving renal function; the diabetic retinopathy remained unaffected.

Lipid metabolism has been examined with relation to retinopathy. Clofibrate was useful in combating retinal lipid deposits, although this does not influence the development of further exudation or hemorrhage. There is at present no medication which could influence the course of diabetic retinopathy on a long-term basis nor does hypophysectomy bring significant improvement. In the 15 patients observed, mean survival after transsphenoidal hypophysectomy was 4⅓ years and no clear evidence emerged that impending blindness could be arrested, although a temporary stabilization was achieved in individual diabetics. "Scatter photocoagulation" has had some favorable effect on certain forms of retinopathy.

► [The data provided in this article are not of great value, but I selected it as representing one point of view about the treatment of diabetic retinopathy. The following article gives a contrasting one, which is more optimistic from the ophthalmologic viewpoint, although the mortality data are not much different. This article implies that control of diabetes is important, but says—correctly—that present methods of treatment do not provide sufficiently physiologic control to permit judgments of what might happen if it were possible to normalize carbohydrate metabolism entirely. The comment about somatostatin is purely speculative. Growth hormone may be important, but there is no evidence at present to prove it.

The most substantial question is what one could expect improved metabolic control to do. Some scattered data are available in animal experiments with islet cell transplants; these have been discussed in this section in previous years. True controlled experiments are impossible in human patients and difficult in animals. Quite a good experiment was reported by Engerman et al. (Diabetes 26:760, 1977), in which alloxan-diabetic dogs were randomly distributed into two groups, one of which was given inadequate amounts of insulin and the other was given amounts of insulin planned to provide the best possible diabetic control. The well-controlled group had considerable improvement in their metabolic patterns as compared with the poorly controlled group. They had glucosuria only about 67% of days, whereas the poor group had it 100% of days. The concentration of plasma free fatty acids was normal, whereas it was elevated in the poor group. The same was true of serum cholesterol, but triglycerides were not entirely normal (though better than in the poorly controlled group). Thus the experiment mimics pretty accurately what can be accomplished by modern clinical control in human patients. Retinopathy developed with increasing frequency and intensity in the poorly controlled group over the first 5 years, by which time all of the animals had retinal deterioration. At this time only 9 of the 20 eyes of the well-controlled group had any aneurysms and none had retinal hemorrhages, varicose capillaries, patches of atrophic capillaries or fatty vessels seen in the poorly controlled group. Insofar as this experiment reflects the human problem, it supports the notion that careful control improves prognosis and implies that complete normalization might prevent complications entirely.

With respect to other types of microvascular disease, the basic pathogenesis is probably similar, but clinical implications may be different. Fuller et al. (Br. Med. J. 2: 861, 1977) point out that the predominant risk for cardiovascular mortality and morbidity is from hypertension. They feel that in protecting diabetics against heart trouble, more would be achieved by treating the blood pressure than by tinkering (my word) with the carbohydrate metabolism. They agree that hypolipemic treatment would probably be useful as well. The patients had minimal diabetes. I agree with this evaluation from two points of view. Firstly, in patients with borderline diabetes present methods of treatment do not produce much, if any, improvement in the metabolic pattern. Indeed, Fuller and colleagues found no advantage in giving phenformin together with carbohydrate restriction either with respect to metabolic control or cardiac deterioration. Secondly, it is folly to blame all of the ills of a diabetic on his diabetes. Surely such patients will benefit by treating as well as possible all of the other abnormalities which age, diet, social patterns or previous stresses may have imposed on the patient.

With all its limitations, metabolic control still is useful. The blind patient has a particularly difficult task in performing simple tasks such as checking his urine glucose. A new instrument has been described by May et al. which monitors the color evolved by a dip-strip technique and translates it into an audible signal. The article gives the electronic diagram and describes Mr. May's own experience in using the machine. It could be built for about $150 for parts and about 24 hours of work by an electronic technician (Diabetes 26:192, 1977).—Ed.] ◄

Prolonged Follow-up in Diabetic Retinopathy Treated by Sectioning the Pituitary Stalk. Bruce R. Zimmerman and George D. Molnar[7] reviewed the records of all 40 patients who underwent section of the pituitary stalk for diabetic retinopathy at the Mayo Clinic in 1961–68. Reliable information was available on all patients but 1. No patient had more than minimal renal impairment at the time of surgery. About half the patients had manifestations of other diabetic complications, most often mild peripheral neuropathy. The 24 men and 16 women had a mean age of 35 years. Mean duration of diabetes was 20 years. Only 1 patient was not insulin dependent at the time of surgery. The first patient died postoperatively. Optic nerve section was necessary in three eyes that had some useful vision and three that had minimal vision. Diabetes insipidus lasted many months in 14 patients but was always mild and easily controlled. All patients received cortisone preoperatively.

Two thirds of the 38 patients followed after the postoperative period have died after a mean follow-up of 63 months, whereas 11 are alive after a mean of 117 months. Only 2 of 13 patients aged 40 or over at operation are alive. Four deaths may have been related to pituitary or adrenal insufficiency or to hypoglycemia. Pituitary ablation succeeded in 85% of cases. Four patients may have had return of some pituitary function. Three patients had partial ablation and 2 had unsuccessful ablation. Visual acuity was stable or improved at 1 year in 79% of patients and retinopathy was stable or improved in 68%. At last follow-up, acuity was stable or improved in 77% and retinopathy in 62% of the patients who died. Seven of 11 survivors had stable or improved acuity and retinopathy when most recently evaluated. Nine of the 13 patients aged 40 or over had stable or improved acuity when last evaluated. Of 9 patients who had unsuccessful or only partial ablation or return of pituitary function, 5 had stable or improved visual acuity when last seen.

Young, well-motivated diabetics with florid retinopathy appear to have the best chance of improved or stabilized vision when pituitary ablation is done before fibrosis begins. The operation is a reasonable

(7) Mayo Clin. Proc. 52:233–237, April, 1977.

recommendation for these relatively uncommon patients, despite the currently favorable report on the effectiveness of photocoagulation.

► [There are three methods used at present for preventing and treating diabetic retinopathy. Metabolic control (discussed in the preceding article and my comments thereon) is a failure. This article discusses hypophysectomy or induced hypopituitarism and is more optimistic than the preceding article, though the indications for the operation are restricted. With proper selection of patients, a fairly high probability exists of producing improvement or, at least, of postponing progression. The third method, photocoagulation, is discussed in the following article. – Ed.] ◄

Proliferative Diabetic Retinopathy: Treatment with Xenon Arc Photocoagulation: Interim Report of Multicenter Randomized Controlled Trial. In the British Multicenter Photocoagulation Trial, coordinated and conducted by D. W. Hill, R. K. Blach, H. Cheng, E. M. Kohner, H. Keen, P. Armitage, J. Bailey, A. M. Hamilton, Magnus Odland, G. Lovatt, E. W. G. Davies, G. Paterson, D. A. Pyke, P. J. Watkins, A. Chignell, T. J. Ffytche, C. Lowy, P. H. Sonksen, N. R. Galloway, M. V. Wells and D. S. J. Maw,[8] 100 patients with symmetric proliferative diabetic retinopathy had one eye treated by xenon arc photocoagulation, whereas the other was left untreated as a control. Patients unlikely to live 1 year and those with intercurrent ocular disease or more than a wisp of fibrous retinitis proliferans in the fundus were excluded, as were those with macular scarring or detachment or retinoschisis in the temporal half of the fundus. Most patients were treated under retrobulbar anesthesia. The Zeiss or O'Malley light coagulator was used. An attempt was made to coagulate all flat retinal vessels except those too near the macula or over the papillomacular bundle. More recently, large areas of nonperfused retina were treated diffusely in eyes that had new vessels on the disc. Treatment was given as often as new vessels were detected.

Fifty-eight patients were followed for 2 years or longer and 23 for at least 3 years. Most patients had been insulin dependent from the onset of diabetes; mean duration of diabetes was 16.3 years. The difference in deterioration between treated and untreated eyes was significant after 3 years in patients with new vessels on the disc but not in those with peripheral new vessels only. Eighteen patients became blind in one or both eyes during follow-up. Four were blind in both eyes, 1 in the treated eye only and 13 in the untreated eye only. Blindness was most commonly due to vitreous hemorrhage. When eyes were classed according to whether new disc vessels increased, were unchanged or decreased, more treated than untreated eyes showed an improvement in grade. New vessels disappeared completely in 10 treated eyes and in 2 untreated eyes. Of 45 patients, with peripheral new vessels only, who were followed for 1 year, 3 developed new vessels on both discs, 3 in the treated eye and 6 in the untreated eye only.

Vision deteriorated less in treated eyes in patients in this trial with new disc vessels. New vessels on the disc regressed more in treated than in untreated eyes. Early diagnosis of diabetic retinopathy is essential, as are systematic follow-up and further treatment where necessary. Inadequate treatment or delay in its application may prejudice

(8) Br. Med. J. 1:739–741, Mar. 19, 1977.

the prognosis for an eye that may pass rapidly from a treatable to an irreversible phase of retinopathy.

► [When the patients are divided into two groups according to whether there were new vessels on either optic disc (or both) at the time of initial evaluation, or whether such vessels were absent, it turns out that photocoagulation clearly prevented deterioration of the treated eye when vessels were present, but had no statistically significant effect when they were absent. One conclusion therefore might be that only patients with vascularization of the disc should be treated by this method. This conclusion might be incorrect, since treated eyes in the group initially lacking disc vascularization were less likely to develop disc vessels later than were untreated eyes. Since new vessels on the disc indicate a bad prognosis for vision, this probably means that further observation of these patients will show benefit in prevention of progression in the initially nonvascularized group as well as in the more severely affected group. These conclusions are based on a very carefully controlled randomized study in which the degree of retinitis was equivalent in both eyes at the start of the study. The large number of patients which fitted this criterion is unusual and means that many others had to be rejected for the study. Deckert et al. (Diabetes 11:728, 1967) came to very similar conclusions 10 years ago, studying patients whose eye lesions were not so well matched. This is not an indictment of the British study, but suggests that sometimes correct results can be obtained even with experimental designs which are less than optimal.

For curious internists, I can recommend an article by Little and colleagues on techniques of photocoagulation (Am. J. Ophthalmol. 82:675, 1976). It is unlikely that most readers of this book will need to use the methods themselves, but it is useful to know what our surgical colleagues are talking about when they use such picturesque terms as "feeder-frond photocoagulation."

Another factor has been suggested as important in progression of diabetic retinopathy. Paetkau et al. (Diabetes 16:46, 1977) investigated the smoking habits of a group of patients with this complication and found that the prevalence of proliferative retinitis was significantly increased in smokers. Moreover, the incidence of proliferation increased with increased duration of diabetes in the smokers, but not in the nonsmokers. The difference was all the more striking because the age of the smokers was significantly lower than that of the nonsmokers. – Ed.] ◄

Renal Transplantation in Patients with Insulin-Dependent Diabetes Mellitus. Horst Zincke, John E. Woods, P. J. Palumbo, Frank J. Leary and William J. Johnson[9] (Mayo Clinic and Found.) reviewed experience with renal transplantation in 40 patients with insulin-dependent diabetes treated in 1970–75. Living related donors were preferentially used. Eighteen of 28 such donors were siblings. Nine kidneys from cadaver donors pretreated with cyclophosphamide and methylprednisolone were used since 1973. The 25 men and 15 women treated had an average age of 36.1 years at transplantation. Average duration of diabetes was 22 years. All but 3 patients had juvenile diabetes. Nine patients were blind and all had moderate to severe neuropathy. Ten had histories of myocardial infarction, angina or both. All patients but 1 had bilateral nephrectomy and splenectomy before renal transplantation. Average follow-up was 29 months.

Thirty patients were alive 6–72 months after transplantation. Four patients died of sepsis and 3 of myocardial infarction. Nine of 10 deaths occurred within 9 months after transplantation. Twenty-nine of the 42 renal allografts were functioning at follow-up, including 21 of 28 from living related donors and 7 of 9 from pretreated cadaver donors. No wound infections occurred in recipients of living related donor kidneys. Complications included 2 cystic lymphangiomas and 2 cases of venous

(9) J.A.M.A. 237:1101–1103, Mar. 14, 1977.

iliofemoral thrombosis with evidence of pulmonary embolism. Diabetic management was not a particular problem. Of 29 living patients with a functioning kidney, 3 have not been rehabilitated and 7 have been partially rehabilitated. Nine survivors had peripheral vascular problems necessitating amputations of fingers or toes or below-knee amputations.

Renal transplantation is justified because of the poor results of hemodialysis in diabetics with renal failure. The use of pretreated cadaver kidneys seems to be attractive.

Abdominal Pain Caused by Diabetic Radiculopathy. Abdominal pain secondary to radiculopathy has been recognized in diabetic patients, but the relationship is poorly documented in the literature. George F. Longstreth and Albert D. Newcomer[1] (Mayo Clinic and Found.) encountered 4 diabetics with significant abdominal pain secondary to radiculopathy in the past few years. In no case was the diagnosis considered until after an extensive negative investigation for malignancy, often including invasive procedures, was carried out.

Woman, 51, an insulin-requiring diabetic, had had abdominal pain for 1 year after an episode of right thigh pain that lasted 2–3 months. A bilateral "beltlike" constriction was described, which woke the patient at night. Early during the course of the pain there were upper abdominal paresthesias. The patient reported anorexia and had a weight loss of 18 kg. Extensive studies, including endoscopic pancreatography and abdominal arteriography, were negative. There were no abnormal physical findings. Ankle reflexes were symmetrically reduced. The fasting blood sugar was 136 mg/dl. Roentgenograms showed extensive retained gastric secretions, and small bowel studies showed dilatation and reduced jejunal motility. Electromyography showed extensive denervation of paraspinal muscle with a relative paucity of fibrillation in the lower paraspinal muscles. Mild diffuse neuropathy was evident. Pain began to subside during hospitalization, and the patient's appetite rapidly improved. Eight months after presentation the patient's pain had disappeared, and there was a weight gain of 9 kg.

One patient underwent laparotomy before the cause of pain was ascertained. All 4 patients had adult-onset diabetes. The pain began gradually and was initially intermittent. Neurologic clues to radiculopathy were subtle in the 2 patients who manifested them. Only 1 patient had symptomatic peripheral neuropathy; 2 had evidence of autonomic dysfunction. No patient had retinopathy or nephropathy. Two patients had lower-limb discomfort with features suggestive of lumbar radiculopathy. Electromyographic examination showed involvement of many thoracic and/or lumbar nerve roots in all cases.

Significant abdominal pain due to thoracic radiculopathy can develop in the diabetic patient. Radiculopathy should be considered in the diabetic with abdominal pain of obscure origin, and, if the condition is suspected, electromyography should be performed.

► [In addition to the abdominal pain caused by sensory nerve involvement, abdominal symptoms may occur because of lesions in the autonomic nervous system. Fraser et al. (Diabetes 26:546, 1977) evaluated autonomic function in 10 newly diagnosed male diabetics and followed them closely over 6 months. All patients had impared peroneal

(1) Ann. Intern. Med. 86:166–168, February, 1977.

nerve conduction, indicating peripheral neuropathy, and 6 had abnormal control of the resting heart rate, which resulted in a fluctuation of the r-r interval on the ECG. One also had an abnormal response to the Valsalva maneuver. The group of 6 treated with insulin all had improvement, but the sulfonylurea-treated group had none. None had postural hypotension.

Autonomic neuropathy may manifest itself in prolonged gastrointestinal transit time. Delayed small intestinal transit was observed in all diabetics with autonomic neuropathy studied by Scarpello et al. (Br. Med. J. 2:1225, 1976). The authors blame this on vagal neuropathy and point out that the slow transit would permit bacterial proliferation which might cause diarrhea once the ileal contents arrived in the colon. Thus delayed transit above could cause increased movement below.

Patients with autonomic neuropathy also fail to release glucagon in response to hypoglycemia (Maher et al.: Diabetes 26:196, 1977). This may help explain the increased metabolic lability of some advanced diabetics, who may become subject to hypoglycemic attacks after years during which this was not a problem.

Gastroparesis is a problem in diabetics with autonomic neuropathy. Longstreth et al. (Ann. Intern. Med. 86:195, 1977) describe 1 patient in whom metoclopramide improved gastric motility.

Impotence in male diabetics is another manifestation of autonomic neuropathy. It has sometimes been suggested that this impotence could be a manifestation of endocrine disease, but Wright et al. (Diabetes 25:975, 1976) found that the release of luteinizing hormone after testing with gonadotropin-releasing hormone was entirely comparable in impotent and in nonimpotent diabetic men. The same was true for serum testosterone concentration, sex hormone-binding globulin capacity and basal serum LH concentration. The response of FSH to gonadotropin-releasing hormone was marginally higher in impotent than nonimpotent diabetics. None of these data lends support to the idea that impotence is caused by gonadal hypofunction in these patients. Still, diabetic gonadal function was not entirely normal, since the rise of LH on stimulation was significantly lower in all diabetics than in nondiabetic controls. – Ed.] ◄

Nonclostridial Gas Gangrene in the Diabetic Lower Limb. The susceptibility of diabetics to nonclostridial gas-forming infection is sometimes overlooked, and diagnostic delay often occurs while attempts are made to isolate clostridia. The diagnosis is essentially clinical, and urgent operation is necessary to avoid death. D. Bird, A. E. B. Giddings and S. M. Jones[2] report 3 cases of nonclostridial gas gangrene in diabetic lower limbs. The condition occurs only in diabetics with peripheral neuropathy and is always fatal unless treated surgically.

Woman, 61, with maturity-onset diabetes for 21 years, had been well controlled by diet and chlorpropamide. A verruca was removed from the right sole 3 weeks before admission, and cellulitis and a necrotic ulcer developed. The infection progressed rapidly despite oral ampicillin therapy and the diabetes became uncontrolled. The patient was febrile and exhibited diabetic retinopathy and sensory impairment below the midcalf levels bilaterally, with absent ankle jerks and sluggish knee jerks. The right dorsalis pedis and posterior tibial pulses were impalpable. Extensive cellulitis and edema of the right food and ankle were seen, with a clean plantar wound. Interstitial gas was seen on x-rays (Fig 22). Swabs from the ulcer grew *Streptococcus faecalis, Escherichia coli* and *Bacteroides* species. Gentamicin was given and the diabetes was controlled with soluble insulin. Extensive necrosis and cellulitis extended to the knee and a midthigh amputation was performed a week after admission. Muscle necrosis had extended to the knee and multilocular gas-containing abscess cavities were present in the muscle and under the skin. The patient recovered well. The diabetes was controlled with oral agents at the time of discharge.

The slow development of nonclostridial gas gangrene in the diabetic

(2) Diabetologia 13:373–376, 1976.

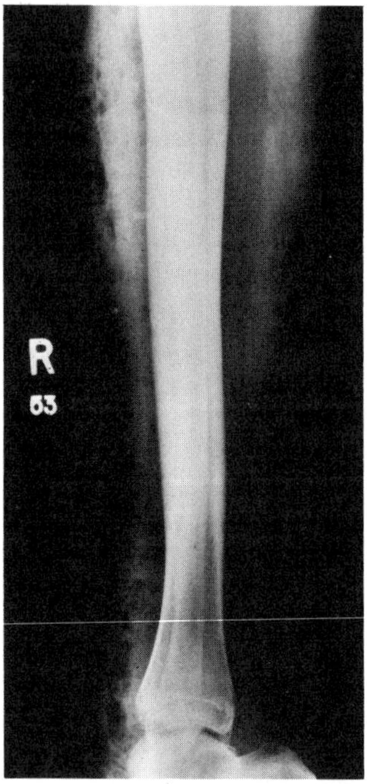

Fig 22.—Extensive interstitial gas. (Courtesy of Bird, D., et al.: Diabetologia 13:373–376, 1976; Berlin-Heidelberg-New York: Springer.)

lower limb contrasts with the acute onset and profound toxemia of clostridial gas gangrene. The absence of pain in the affected limb may be due to the peripheral neuropathy, which, with the associated microangiopathy and the elevated tissue glucose content, favors extension of bacterial colonization. The clinical presentation may be extremely misleading. If there is any doubt whether a lesion is clostridial gas gangrene, it almost certainly is not. Antibiotic therapy will not control the infection, and a decision to amputate must be made urgently and on clinical grounds alone.

Hypoglycemic Coma due to Chlorpropamide: Observations on 22 Patients. Chlorpropamide has undoubted advantages, but an insidious danger of protracted, sometimes fatal, hypoglycemia exists, to which the elderly are especially prone. R. J. Schen and Y. Benaroya[3] (Hadassah Municipal Hosp., Tel-Aviv) found that hypoglycemic coma is not uncommon when chlorpropamide is widely prescribed in a population with a large proportion of old people. Review was made of data on patients seen in 1968–74 with hypoglycemic coma due to chlorpropamide, with a blood glucose below 50 mg/100 ml and a history of chlorpropamide therapy as the sole hypoglycemic drug.

Twenty-three episodes of hypoglycemic coma occurred in 22 patients in the 7-year review period. All patients but 2 were admitted in a state of coma, somnolence or confusion. All received intravenous glucose for up to 4 days, and 2 also received steroid treatment. Four patients died,

(3) Age Ageing 5:31–36, February, 1976.

3 in direct relation to hypoglycemia. One patient had a myocardial infarction after recovering from hypoglycemia. The median patient age was 72 years. Two patients were hypoglycemic postoperatively. Two other instances of hypoglycemic coma occurred in patients given both chlorpropamide and insulin. Contraindications to the use of chlorpropamide existed in 5 of 8 patients under age 70 in this series and in 4 of the 14 older patients. If full precautions had been taken in prescribing the drug and if old age had been considered a contraindication, hypoglycemia might have been avoided in 19 of the 22 patients. Factors predisposing to hypoglycemia in patients given chlorpropamide include old age, hepatic, renal or adrenal insufficiency, impaired food intake and the potentiating effect of other drugs. Old age appeared to be the main predisposing factor in the present series. Impaired renal function was present in 4 patients, alcoholism in 2 and impaired food intake in 3. Deliberate overdosage was discovered in 1 patient. Other possible factors were respiratory infection in 2 patients and congestive heart failure in 3.

Chlorpropamide can be given safely if due care is used and no contraindications are present. A short-acting drug is preferred in the elderly if a sulfonylurea is really needed.

► [The authors consider old age to be a contraindication to using chlorpropamide, but they do not reject the use of oral hypoglycemic agents entirely, despite the clear-cut risks. Others are less charitable. Shen and Bressler (N. Engl. J. Med. 296:493, 1977; ibid., p. 78) review the physiology and practical uses of all of the hypoglycemic agents and come to the following conclusions: "Diabetes is a chronic condition requiring long-term treatment. The long-term effectiveness of controlling blood glucose by oral hypoglycemic agents (tolbutamide and phenformin) is minimal. . . .Since neither agent caused a sustained lowering of the blood sugar of the populations studied, no question of gain versus risk can be raised. Even the safest drug is of no value if it has no efficacy. . . . .Maturity-onset diabetes can probably be controlled in many patients with diet alone. Those whose disease is not controlled by diet should be treated with insulin. *At present oral hypoglycemic agents have no demonstrated useful role in the management of maturity-onset diabetes mellitus, asymptomatic or symptomatic*" (emphasis added).

To my mind, there has never been evidence that the hypoglycemic agents were beneficial, and I have always taught, "No one could be accused of malpractice for failure to use the oral agents." This statement could not be made with regard to insulin, where there are many absolute indications. The UGDP findings some years ago came to the same conclusions, in the limited area which was studied. These conclusions caused anguish in many clinics, but the burden of proof still rests on people who claim that these medicines are useful. Anecdotal arguments such as those of clinicians who criticized the UGDP are not scientifically acceptable and therefore are suspect. The statistical criticisms of the study are another matter, which I am not qualified to discuss. Doubts about the clinical usefulness of oral diabetic agents are spreading. From the Joslin Clinic, for example, comes an article by Tan et al. (Diabetes 26:561, 1977) which finds no significant difference among patients treated with chlorpropamide, tolbutamide, phenformin, acetohexiraide and placebo in respect to improvement of glucose tolerance, insulin secretion dynamics or triglyceride and cholesterol levels—in other words, no demonstrable benefit!

To quote Chen and Bressler again: if there are no benefits, there can be no calculation of the risk-benefit ratio. But there can be an infinite risk, under these circumstances, if there is any risk at all. The article mentions one—hypoglycemia. This may be more than a passing inconvenience. Turkington describes 3 patients with severe hypoglycemic encephalopathy after treatment with chlorpropamide (2) and phenformin (1). Two of these patients had disabling residual damage (Arch. Intern. Med. 137:1082, 1977). Nattrass et al. (Diabetologia 13:145, 1977) followed the 12-hour metabolic rhythms of 6 maturity-onset diabetics and found multiple metabolic abnormalities when the patients were exposed to phenformin, metformin (not available in the United States) and glibenclamide. The biguanides, in particular, caused impressive increase of the plasma lactate concentration. Berger et al. (Schweiz. Med. Wochenschr. 106: 1830, 1976) describe 10 cases of lactic acidosis in patients being treated with biguanides—only one of many such reports over the past decade. Glibenclamide is known to produce diuresis, possibly by antagonism to the effects of the antidiuretic hormone. This is probably not the mechanism, however, since the medicine did not counteract the effects of vasopressin released in a patient with the syndrome of inappropriate antidiuretic hormone secretion (Yap et al.: Br. Med. J. 1:1137, 1977).—Ed.] ◄

Hypoglycemia in Man: Pathologic and Physiologic Variants. Thomas J. Merimee and John E. Tyson[4] conducted 72-hour fasts in 60 normal-weight women and 20 men, 16 obese subjects and 6 of 11 patients with proved insulinomas, to determine if an effective means exists to distinguish the physiologic hypoglycemia of fasting from pathologic hypoglycemia. Subjects fasted for 72 hours after receiving a diet of 150 – 200 gm carbohydrate daily for 2 weeks. The 6 insulinoma patients studied tolerated periods of fasting ranging from 10 to 36 hours. Two of the 6 patients were 10 – 20% over ideal body weight.

The mean lowest plasma glucose in normal women during fasting was 42.5 mg/dl and in men, 66.8 mg/dl. No subject had an insulin level of 10 μU/ml or above when the prevailing glucose level was 40 mg/dl or below. No obese subject had a glucose level below 55 mg/dl during the 72-hour fast. The mean lowest glucose level was 65 mg/dl in obese men and 60 mg/dl in women. Only 4 subjects had insulin values of 10 μU/ml or less during fasting. In both sexes, insulin-to-glucose ratios (I/G ratios) during fasting were less than the prefast value. The mean ratio in obese subjects was 0.29 and in insulinoma patients, 0.31. Changes in ratios during fasting in obese subjects were slight. Three patients with insulinoma maintained insulin levels above 15 μU/ml during fasting. The I/G ratios increased dramatically in all insulinoma patients, but declined in all 12 control subjects evaluated.

The best distinctions between insulinoma patients and women with a normal tendency toward low glucose levels in fasting are (1) a tendency for hypoglycemia to occur early during fasting in insulinoma patients and (2) an inappropriate change of insulin relative to glucose during fasting, i.e., I/G ratios increase rather than decrease. When I/G ratios increase during fasting, hypoglycemia secondary to an insulin-producing tumor can be predicted. A consistent increase in the I/G ratio rather than an arbitrary, absolute figure for the basal I/G ratio is the primary diagnostic feature.

► [This is a new wrinkle in the well-established fasting test, which should improve its specificity. Several causes of hypoglycemia are more common than insulinoma and should be mentioned. The effects of oral hypoglycemic agents were discussed in the preceding article. Alcoholic hypoglycemic reactions are the most common form of low blood glucose seen in emergency rooms and probably rival so-called reactive hypoglycemia even among the prosperous population with private physicians. Perhaps the two are not entirely separable. O'Keefe and Marks (Lancet 1:1286, 1977) showed that drinking gin to the point of drunkeness (50 gm alcohol) did not produce hypoglycemia if taken with a sugar-free mixer. Ordinary mixer, with carbohydrate, did not cause hypoglycemia either; but when gin and tonic were taken together, there was a rise of insulin

(4) Diabetes 26:161 – 165, March, 1977.

and a fall of glucose. This combination, which is considered the equivalent of 3 drinks in Great Britain—but which would be about 5 ounces of American gin or less than two standard bar equivalents—would certainly make driving difficult and doing business irresponsible, to say the least. Perhaps the 2-martini business lunch can be justified, but a 2-gin-and-tonic lunch would be hazardous—that is, assuming that the tonic was sweetened with carbohydrate rather than saccharin.

There is a good deal of experience to suggest that vagal blockade reduces the frequency of reactive hypoglycemic attacks. Permutt et al. (Diabetes 26:121, 1977) studied the effects of propantheline, 30 mg, 45 minutes before a standard glucose tolerance test. The overall glucose response was flattened, although insulin secretion was unaffected. In patients subject to hypoglycemia, the mean blood glucose nadir was raised from 44 to 84 mg/dl (highly significant). Excessive vagal stimulation may contribute to the hypoglycemia seen in patients with reactive hypoglycemia, but the effect is probably predominantly on the gastrointestinal tract rather than on insulin secretion. In any case, anticholinergic drugs should be included among treatments for reactive hypoglycemia.

Certain tumors are associated with hypoglycemia. The obvious one is insulinoma, but massive retroperitoneal or mediastinal sarcomas also can produce the syndrome. The importance of hepatomas has been emphasized in the past and has been mentioned in these pages. However, metastatic tumors of other types invading the liver rarely cause hypoglycemia. Presumably their mechanism of action would be replacement of the liver parenchyma to such an extent that inadequate glucose secretion could occur. One such case is described by Younus and colleagues (Gastroenterology 72:334, 1977). The primary tumor was consistent with prostatic carcinoma, since this tumor had been recognized 4 years previously and biopsy fitted the picture. Treatment with cyclophosphamide and fluorouracil, in doses I would have predicted would be ineffective, caused some reduction in the glucose requirement of 500 gm/24 hours and some shrinkage of the liver defects on scan.—Ed.] ◄

Clinical Correlations of Serum Proinsulin-like Material in Islet Cell Tumors. A high proportion of patients with islet cell tumors have elevated circulating levels of proinsulin-like material (PLM). Some may have relatively normal insulin levels. Changes in the level of endogenous PLM might be an important indicator of the response to treatment. R. N. Alsever, M. R. Stjernholm, K. E. Sussman, M. E. Mako and A. H. Rubenstein[5] correlated PLM concentrations with changes in plasma glucose and hypoglycemic symptoms in 1 man and 2 women with islet cell tumors before and after treatment.

A woman aged 80 with a single islet cell adenoma had no significant change in insulin concentration postoperatively, but a threefold fall in PLM was observed as she became asymptomatic. In a man aged 56 with two islet cell adenomas, insulin levels were not different after surgery, but PLM was reduced by nearly 15% as symptoms resolved. In a woman aged 78 with an unresectable islet cell carcinoma who was treated with streptozotocin, the time of fasting resulting in hypoglycemia increased sixfold after streptozotocin therapy. The insulin fraction was unchanged, but the percentage PLM decreased. Symptoms returned to the pretreatment level in 19 weeks after treatment, as the serum PLM increased and the time of fasting to the onset of hypoglycemic symptoms decreased.

These findings support the concept that the serum PLM concentration is a useful indicator of the activity of islet cell tumors in some patients. Insulin release may be appropriately inhibited by a falling circulating glucose concentration. The failure of PLM secretion to cease

(5) Diabetologia 12:527–530, October, 1976.

may indicate a potentially important role for this material in the production of hypoglycemia by enhancing the effect of the falling serum insulin concentrations.

► [The definition of "proinsulin-like" material is simply material that reacts with antibody against insulin and is eluted early in a chromatographic system, indicating that it is larger in molecular weight than insulin. If the large fraction is studied more closely, two subfractions can be identified – one of about 9,000 molecular weight, representing true proinsulin, and the rest much larger – 50,000 – 100,000 molecular weight. Permutt et al. (J. Clin. Endocrinol. Metab. 44:536, 1977) studied the large fraction and were able to show that the very large material was not a precursor of proinsulin or insulin but, rather, that it is an aggregate of proinsulin and/or insulin either with one another or with larger carrier molecules. These conclusions concern only the material in plasma. In rat tumors, there is a proproinsulin which is larger than proinsulin. Such a material may also occur in some human tumors, but if so, it did not appear in the plasma of the 2 patients studied. – Ed.] ◄

Treatment of Malignant Metastatic Pancreatic Insulinoma with Streptozotocin: Review of 21 Cases Described in Detail in the Literature and Report of Complete Remission of a New Case are presented by Georg Herbai and Åsa Lundin[6] (Univ. of Uppsala). The 21 reported cases of malignant metastatic insulinoma were in patients treated with streptozotocin in 1968 – 75. Mean patient age was 56 years. The modes of streptozotocin administration differed widely. The daily dose ranged from 1 to 17 gm and the total dose from 4 to 30 gm. Durations and lengths of remissions also varied considerably. No remission occurred in extremely advanced, severe malignancy. Average length of remission in all cases was about 7 months. Ten patients had varying degrees of acute tubular necrosis, but in several it was reversible. Four deaths may have been accelerated by large drug doses and 2 by severe diabetes insipidus related to high doses. A new patient with liver metastases was treated with 14 gm streptozotocin in seven injections at increasing intervals, and marked amelioration of disease was observed, without serious side effects. The patient has been well for 22 months since the start of treatment.

Streptozotocin therapy should be started immediately after early diagnosis, before widely dispersed metastases have developed. Intraarterial administration to the celiac axis via the aorta must be avoided to prevent acute tubular necrosis from spillover into the renal artery. Optimal effects of the drug can be obtained by rather slow intravenous injection in daily doses of 1 or 2 gm. One or 2 weeks should intervene between injections. Severe nephrotoxicity occurs if streptozotocin is given daily for several days.

► [This is the optimistic side of the picture, because most patients who did not respond to streptozotocin treatment are probably not described. From casual conversations with some of my colleagues at the National Institutes of Health, I get the impression that they do not consider streptozotocin regularly useful. Indeed, they have described 2 patients refractory to streptozotocin who responded well to Adriamycin. One did well with 4 divided doses over 10 weeks, receiving a total dose of 270 mg/sq m body surface area. The hypoglycemia ceased, plasma insulin fell to normal, the mass of tumor shrank and the patient had a remission for 5 months. The recurrence was treated with 2 further doses, to bring the final total dose to 410 mg/sq m, but these were ineffective, as was L-asparaginase. Ligation of the hepatic artery was temporarily helpful. This works because metastases are directly hooked into the hepatic arterial blood sup-

(6) Acta Med. Scand. 200:447 – 452, 1976.

ply and derive little of their circulation from the portal vein. The second patient received 15 mg 5-fluorouracil per kg per week with good temporary response. At recurrence, Adriamycin, 60 mg/sq m every 3 weeks, produced a response lasting 6 months. (Eastman et al.: J. Clin. Endocrinol. Metab. 44:142, 1977). So insulinomas should be treated aggressively with chemotherapy of other types if streptozotocin fails. One might even consider combining streptozotocin and Adriamycin, with due respect for the bone marrow. – Ed.] ◄

Inborn Errors of Metabolism

Massive Extraglandular Aromatization of Plasma Androstenedione Resulting in Feminization of a Prepubertal Boy. Feminization of prepubertal boys is extremely uncommon. David L. Hemsell, Clare D. Edman, James F. Marks, Pentti K. Siiteri and Paul C. MacDonald[7] (Univ. of Texas Southwestern Med. School) studied a prepubertal boy with advanced feminization but no masculinization, which was associated with the formation of large amounts of estrone sulfate through extraglandular aromatization of plasma androstenedione to estrone. Sulfurylation of the estrone occurred within the tissue site(s) of aromatization before entry of the product estrogen into the blood. The boy was studied at age 10½ years, when progressive gynecomastia had been present for 2 years. Growth had been accelerated and the voice was high pitched. There was no accentuation of male pubertal characteristics. A 46 XY karyotype was documented. The adrenals were normal at exploration.

The hyperestrogenism was found to result from massive extraglandular conversion of plasma androstenedione to estrone. Plasma androstenedione production rates were 1.2–1.6 mg daily. Over 55% was metabolized by aromatization to estrone, which was extensively sulfurylated before its entry into the blood. The plasma production rate of estrone sulfate from plasma androstenedione was 782 μg/24 hours. The extent of extraglandular conversion was 50 times that found in 2 normal prepubertal boys, and 94% of the aromatization occurred in extraheptic sites. The metabolic clearance rate of plasma androstenedione was 2,380 L per day per sq m. The fractional conversion of testosterone to estradiol, 0.16, was 50 times greater than in normal young adult men. Aromatization of 16-hydroxycorticosteroids resulted in estriol formation independent of estrone formation.

The advanced feminization in this prepubertal boy resulted from extensive aromatization of plasma androstenedione in extraglandular sites. The excessive estrogen production became clinically evident at age 8 years, perhaps at adrenarche, a time when plasma androstenedione availability begins to increase in the prepubertal years.

► [Formation of estrogen by aromatization of testosterone occurs mainly in the adipose tissue, and it is believed to be the explanation of hyperestrogenism and the high incidence of endometrial carcinoma in obese postmenopausal women. It may also play a part in the increased incidence of mammary cancer in obese women of all ages, but this is not proved. In this unusual patient, obesity was not present, and the increased estrogen formation probably reflected an inborn error, though the nature of this error is not clarified as yet.

Another problem which is probably genetic is congenital excessive growth of girls. This can present a serious social and emotional problem. Attempts have been made to

(7) J. Clin. Invest. 60:455–464, August, 1977.

restrict growth during puberty by administration of estrogen. Puttkamer and colleagues (Dtsch. Med. Wochenschr. 102:983, 1977) report results in 41 girls with constitutionally tall stature treated with conjugated estrogen over an average period of 22 months. Progestogens were given orally during the last 5 days of each menstrual cycle. The actual final height was 7 cm less than predicted, and the effect was more pronounced by 2 cm if treatment was started before menarche. There were no uncomfortable side effects. The authors suggest that this treatment should not be undertaken unless the predicted height is over 183 cm (6 ft). In an editorial review in the same issue of *Deutsche Medizinische Wochenschrift* (p. 1002), Stolecke discusses a number of risks of this treatment which cannot yet be evaluated. These include possible long-term disorders of ovarian control in patients treated with estrogens at or before puberty, histologic changes in the ovary (which have frequently been described in such patients) and the possibility of hormone-induced neoplasia, especially in view of the observed association between maternal diethylstilbestrol treatment and vaginal carcinoma in daughters. He concludes that the treatment can be given with due regard to the psychologic indications and in children with a clear pattern of excessive height, but the dangers must be discussed openly with the family and long-term observation must be undertaken. It is also essential that studies be undertaken to clarify the best time to start treatment. – Ed.] ◄

Partial Androgen Insensitivity: Reifenstein's Syndrome Revisited. Reifenstein described a clinical phenotype of hereditary male pseudohermaphroditism consisting of hypospadias, gynecomastia with incomplete virilization at puberty and infertility. Reduced urinary testosterone excretion was found in some patients, but recent studies indicated lowered end-organ sensitivity to androgen, rather than decreased androgen production. James A. Amrhein, Georgeanna Jones Klingensmith, Patrick C. Walsh, Victor A. McKusick and Claude J. Migeon[8] (Johns Hopkins Univ.) reinvestigated 1 member of each of two original families with Reifenstein's syndrome and 6 other patients with the syndrome. Plasma androgens and serum gonadotropins were studied and androgen metabolism and binding by skin fibroblasts were evaluated. Fibroblast strains were established from explants of genital or pubic skin from 5 of the 8 patients and from 22 normal subjects for dihydrotestosterone receptor and 5 α-reductase assays. The patients, aged 16 – 64 years, were from eight families. All had reduced penile size, small testes and various genital abnormalities. Sex assignment had been inappropriate or delayed in 4, but all the patients were ultimately reared as males.

Five patients received testosterone enanthate intramuscularly for 12 weeks, in a final dosage of 400 mg weekly. All patients had basal plasma testosterone values within or above the normal adult male range. Levels of dihydrotestosterone and androstenedione indicated no abnormality in androgen production. All patients had serum luteinizing hormone (LH) values more than 2 SD above the mean for normal adult males. In the 3 patients studied, blood production rates of testosterone and dihydrotestosterone were essentially normal. The metabolic clearance rate of testosterone was normal in 1 patient but definitely low in 2 patients. The 5 α-reductase activity of fibroblasts was normal, as was the whole cell dihydrotestosterone-binding capacity of fibroblasts. Pubic skin fibroblasts from 1 patient showed extremely low dihydrotestosterone binding. Responses to treatment are shown in

(8) N. Engl. J. Med. 297:350 – 356, Aug. 18, 1977.

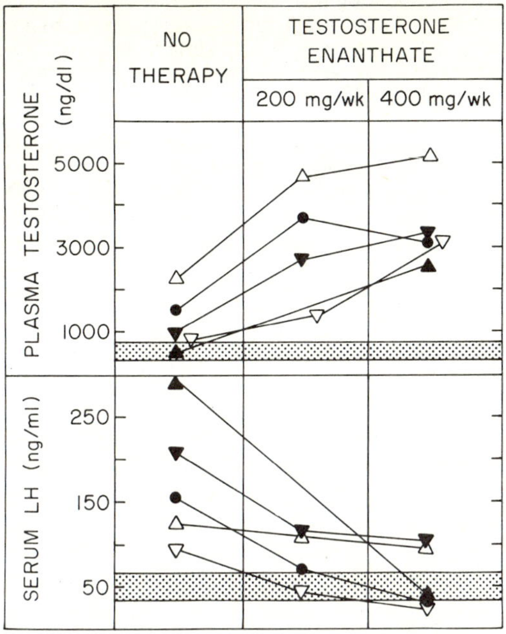

Fig 23.—Response of plasma testosterone and serum LH concentrations to testosterone enanthate therapy in 5 patients with partial androgen insensitivity. Stippled areas represent mean ± SD in normal men. (Courtesy of Amrhein, J. A., et al.: N. Engl. J. Med. 297:350–356, Aug. 18, 1977.)

Figure 23. All patients noticed a slight clinical response. The 2 patients with elevated LH values did not respond until a dose of 400 mg testosterone enanthate weekly was given, but the others responded maximally to 200 mg weekly.

There appear to be at least two distinct genetic variants within the syndrome of complete androgen insensitivity. In one, deficient cytoplasmic androgen binding results from a mutation of the X-linked gene specifying the dihydrotestosterone receptor. In the second variant, androgen insensitivity is due to a defect in steroid hormone action after the binding of dihydrotestosterone to its cytoplasmic receptor and translocation of the steroid-receptor complex to the nucleus. Either X-linked recessive or autosomal dominant, male-limited transmission is a possibility. Routine testosterone therapy is not recommended for partial androgen insensitivity until more is known of the long-term effects of such therapy.

► [There are three general forms of androgen insensitivity. In one, 5α-reductase defect, or "pseudovaginal perineoscrotal hypospadias," failure to reduce testosterone to the active form, dihydrotestosterone, interferes with differentiation of the external genitalia, producing hypospadias, a blind vagina without a uterus, and an increased concentration of testosterone, estrogens and usually of LH in plasma. In this type, somatic masculinization occurs more or less normally at puberty. The children are sometimes raised as females if the difficulty is not recognized until puberty. Ideally, they should be accepted socially as males from infancy.

The second and third types involve absent or reduced sensitivity to androgens. When there is a complete absence of the intracellular cytoplasmic androgen receptor, the patient looks feminine in all respects, except for reduced pubic hair, but lacks a uterus. The gonads are intra-abdominal testes and the patient has the syndrome of testicular feminization. Plasma concentration of testosterone is normal for a man, and the estrogen level is normal for a woman. Follicle-stimulating horome and LH are increased. A few patients with this syndrome have normal cytoplasmic testosterone receptors but are totally resistant to androgens for some other, presently undetermined, reason.

The third type, which this article discusses, has reduced but not absent cytoplasmic androgen receptors or, in a few cases, has normal receptors but reduced sensitivity to androgens for an unknown reason. The clinical picture may be only mild hypospadias or an enlarged clitoris. Plasma testosterone concentration is usually at the normal masculine level and estrogen, at the normal adult female concentration. Both testicular feminization and Reifenstein's syndrome are transmitted as X-linked recessive traits, and the patients are infertile. In contrast, the 5α-reductase-deficient patients are usually fertile and the trait is transmitted as an autosomal recessive. – Ed.] ◄

Normal Insulin Binding to Cultured Fibroblasts from Patients with Lipoatrophic Diabetes. Lipoatrophic diabetes (LD) is characterized by loss of subcutaneous fat, large increases in circulating insulin levels and marked resistance to the effects of exogenous insulin. When diabetes develops, ketosis is unusual and insulin requirements are high. Arlan L. Rosenbloom, Samuel Goldstein and Cecil C. Yip[9] studied insulin binding to fibroblasts from skin biopsy specimens of 3 LD patients to determine whether their insulin resistance might reflect a basic abnormality in formation of the critical insulin-receptor complex. The patients had generalized lipoatrophy, accelerated growth, hypermetabolism, virilization and insulin resistance with non-ketosis-prone diabetes. Punch biopsy specimens of the anterior forearm were cultured, and a binding assay that used ^{125}I-insulin was performed.

In the physiologic range of insulin there were no significant differences in number of insulin molecules bound specifically or nonspecifically per cell between control and LD cells. Cell density was not significantly different in the two groups.

The findings indicate that a basic defect in insulin receptors does not exist in LD patients. A secondary disruption of binding, such as by a circulating factor, is a possibility. Serum factors from insulin-resistant patients can impair the binding of insulin to receptors on normal leukocytes. Whether this is the action of the "diabetogenic peptide" found in the urine of LD patients deserves study.

Hereditary Hemochromatosis: Diagnosis in Siblings and Children. The mode of inheritance of idiopathic hemochromatosis is unresolved. Corwin Q. Edwards, Michael Carroll, Paul Bray and George E. Cartwright[1] (Univ. of Utah) report the findings in 5 patients with clinically manifest disease and 19 of their siblings and children. Children of an iron-loaded mother and grandchildren of a patient with clinical disease were among those studied. Nineteen subjects were members of one pedigree and 4 were members of another. The family of 1 patient with latent disease was unavailable for study. None of the subjects was alcoholic or had ever received oral or parenteral iron or blood transfusions. Routine hematologic studies were normal in all subjects, except 1 with a persistent, unexplained anemia.

(9) J. Clin. Endocrinol. Metab. 44:803–806, April, 1977.
(1) N. Engl. J. Med. 297:7–13, July 7, 1977.

Clinically manifest disease was present in 5 male patients. Two presented with symptoms related to liver disease and 1 each with cardiac disease, arthropathy and hypogonadism. Biopsy showed advanced cirrhosis in 4 patients. Hepatic iron concentration exceeded 450 μg/100 mg wet tissue in the 2 patients in whom it was measured. All 5 patients had a serum iron concentration above 170 μg/100 ml and transferrin saturation exceeding 90%. Five patients had latent disease, with grade 3 or grade 4 stainable hepatic parenchymal cell iron but normal clinical findings. The liver histologic pattern was normal except for excessive iron deposit. Liver function was generally normal. Increased hepatic cell iron was seen in 6 patients, all children of patients with manifest or latent disease. All were clinically well and had normal liver histologic appearances except for excessive iron deposit. Hepatic iron concentration exceeded 40 μg/100 mg wet tissue in 5 patients and 2 had a serum iron concentration above 170 μg/100 ml. All 6 had a transferrin saturation greater than 50%. "Normal" hepatic cell iron was found in 8 children of patients with manifest or latent disease. Hepatic iron concentration exceeded 40 μg/100 mg wet tissue in 3 of these children. Transferrin saturation exceeded 50% in 2. All 8 had normal serum ferritin concentrations.

The earliest changes detected were increases in stainable iron, hepatic and serum iron concentrations, and transferrin saturation. All iron-loading tests were distinctly abnormal in all patients with latent and clinically manifest disease, except for a normal serum ferritin concentration in 1 subject. The disease is defined as a hepatic cell stainable iron of grade 3 or grade 4; a hepatic iron concentration above 250 μg/100 mg wet tissue; a serum iron over concentration 170 μg/100 ml; transferrin saturation greater than 70%; urinary iron excretion after deferoxamine of more than 2.2 mg/24 hours; and an increased serum ferritin concentration. The frequency of hemochromatosis in the population is unquestionably underestimated.

► [One might expect to see an article about hemochromatosis in the sections on hematology or gastroenterology in this book, rather than in the metabolism section; even then, it would be expected to be in the chapter on carbohydrate. However, the important point about this article is that hemochromatosis is, in fact, a hereditary disease. The University of Utah group is exploring its population ramifications by metabolic methods. An interesting sidelight, however, is the observation by Simon and colleagues at the Pontchaillou Hospital in Rennes, France, that the disease is associated with a particular pattern of cell surface transplantation antigens (HLA A3 and B14). They suggest that, since two genes are involved (one for each HLA locus), the disease must be recessive. It should be possible, therefore, to identify members of a family known to be susceptible to the disease by performing HLA typing at an early age. This would make preventive treatment possible.—Ed.] ◄

PART SEVEN

KIDNEY, WATER AND ELECTROLYTES

FRANKLIN H. EPSTEIN, M.D.

Glomerulonephritis and the Nephrotic Syndrome

Clinical Course of IgA Nephropathy in Adults. J. van der Peet, L. Arisz, J. R. H. Brentjens, J. Marrink and Ph. J. Hoedemaeker[1] (Univ. of Groningen) reviewed the findings in 27 patients in whom IgA nephropathy was diagnosed since 1967, when routine immunofluorescence study of renal biopsy specimens was started in their hospital. The 23 male and 4 female patients had a mean age of 27.5 years. The diagnosis was based on a diffuse granular deposit of IgA in the mesangium and the absence of Henoch-Schönlein purpura and systemic lupus erythematosus.

No patient had signs of nephrotic syndrome at the time of diagnosis, but 8 were hypertensive and 24 had proteinuria. Protein excretion never exceeded 4.5 gm/24 hours. All patients had microscopic hematuria, but in 10 it was only intermittent. Ten patients had had attacks of gross hematuria associated with signs of upper respiratory tract infection. The mean serum IgA concentration was increased, and 7 patients had values above the upper limit of normal. All patients had an increase in mesangial matrix, and all but 1 showed mesangial cell proliferation. The basement membranes were essentially unchanged. Glomerular scarring or hyalinization was seen in 14 cases and tubular degeneration and interstitial fibrosis in 13. All four repeat renal biopsies, done in patients in whom renal function had deteriorated, showed more severe glomerular and tubular involvement. Thirteen of the 27 patients had evidence of recurrent upper respiratory tract disease at follow-up. Renal function remained normal in 10 patients but decreased in 15, necessitating regular dialysis in 5. The patients with reduced renal function were older than the others, had had the disease longer and had higher frequencies of hyalinized glomeruli, tubular degeneration and interstitial fibrosis.

Immunoglobulin A nephropathy in adults not infrequently slowly progresses. Studies of qualitative changes in serum IgA may provide more insight into the pathogenesis of IgA nephropathy.

► [Immunoglobulin A nephropathy, described by Berger, has been associated with the clinical syndrome of benign recurrent hematuria of young adults, with little or no proteinuria. But it is now apparent that the association is not absolute. Most patients with idiopathic hematuria and normal renal function do not, in fact, have IgA nephritis (1976 YEAR BOOK, p. 612). Furthermore, in most patients in this series with IgA glomerular deposits, the disease was slowly progressive and proteinuria was present in excess of 1 gm per day. The significance of the elevated levels of IgA in the serum of a minority of patients is still uncertain. – Ed.] ◄

---

(1) Clin. Nephrol. 8:335–340, August, 1977.

Membranoproliferative Glomerulonephritis: One or Many Diseases? David B. Jones[2] (State Univ. of New York, Syracuse) believes that membranoproliferative glomerulonephritis (MPGN) is a pathologic lesion of diverse causes, associated with several clinicopathologic entities. Type 1 MPGN with subendothelial deposits of IgG and IgM is distinct from type 2 MPGN with intramembranous dense deposits. The light microscopic appearance of type 2 MPGN may resemble that of type 1 disease, but splitting of the capillary basement

Fig 1 (top).—Membranoproliferative glomerulonephritis (type 1) with subendothelial deposits. Note red blood cells *(R)* in lumen, extension of mesangial matrix around capillary *(arrow)* and deposits *(D)* underneath capillary basement membrane; original magnification ×3800.

Fig 2 (bottom).—Membranoproliferative glomerulonephritis (type 2) with intramembranous dense deposits *(arrows)*. Note electron-dense deposits thickening capillary basement membrane; original magnification ×1700.

(Courtesy of Jones, D. B.: Arch. Pathol. Lab. Med. 101:457–461, September, 1977; copyright 1977, American Medical Association.)

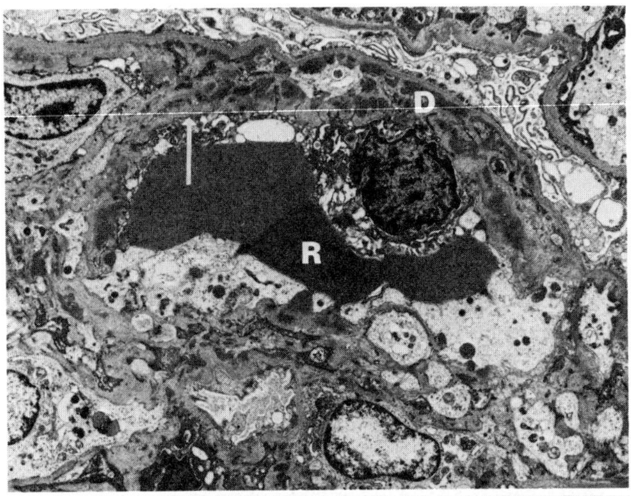

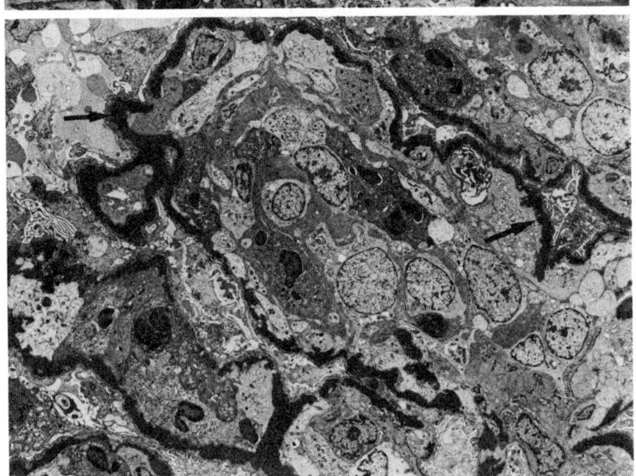

(2) Arch. Pathol. Lab. Med. 101:457–461, September, 1977.

membrane is often less striking, and the basement membrane is thicker and more refractile with hematoxylin-eosin staining (Figs 1 and 2). The intramembranous dense deposits are structureless, electron-dense material present in a ribbon-like or segmented distribution within the peripheral capillary basement membrane lamina densa. The nature of the material in these deposits is unclear.

Much of the confusion about MPGN results from the diverse clinical states that may be associated with it, especially if it is seen late in the course or at autopsy. Chronic antigenemia is suggested as a pathogenic mechanism in cases associated with chronic bacteremia, chronic hepatitis, parasitic infections, certain blood dyscrasias and partial lipodystrophy. Both the classical and the alternate paths of complement activation may be important. Activation of the alternate pathway appears to be important in formation of the dense intramembranous deposits in type 2 MPGN. Type 1 MPGN appears to be an immune complex disease resulting from chronic antigenemia of unknown or known causes; type 2 remains an enigma.

► [Membranoproliferative (mesangiocapillary) glomerulonephritis is a diagnosis made strictly on anatomicopathologic criteria. I include this article and the following one to keep us straight on the terms our friends the pathologists are using. The light microscopic picture of mesangial proliferation and "lobular" glomerulonephritis, often superficially resembling Kimmelstiel-Wilson disease, can be seen by electron microscopy to be characterized by electron-dense glomerular deposits. If these are subendothelial, the pathologist calls them "type 1"; if they are very dark and ribbon-like, "type 2"; and if the intramembranous deposits are less dense, small and irregular, "type 3." It is not possible to distinguish the forms on clinical grounds. Chronic antigenemia is sometimes, but certainly not always, identifiable. It is more often seen in type 1. The serum complement is usually, but not always, low. Patients most often present with the nephrotic syndrome plus hematuria, but sometimes with insidious renal failure or a picture resembling acute nephritis. While progression is the rule, the following article illustrates that remissions occur and patients sometimes have a mild course and get completely better. – Ed.] ◄

Mesangial Proliferative Glomerulonephritis with Irregular Intramembranous Deposits: Another Variant of Hypocomplementemic Nephritis. Alvin E. Davis, Eveline E. Schneeberger, Robert T. McCluskey and Warren E. Grupe[3] (Boston), in the course of reviewing material from 27 patients classified as having membranoproliferative glomerulonephritis (MPGN), found 2 patients whose disease did not conform morphologically or clinically to any of the variants described. Both exhibited mild mesangial proliferation and irregular intramembranous deposits, and both had had reduced serum C3 levels for several years, persistent nephritis with a mild course and persistently normal renal function. Both have shown morphological improvement without treatment of the renal lesion.

The clinical course of these patients is shown in Figure 3. Initial renal biopsies showed mild, diffuse increases in mesangial cellularity and mesangial matrix. Granular staining of capillary walls and the mesangium for C3, IgM and fibrin was observed. Electron microscopic examination showed numerous, irregular, intramembranous electron-dense deposits (Figs 4 and 5), occurring primarily within the lamina

(3) Am. J. Med. 63:481–487, September, 1977.

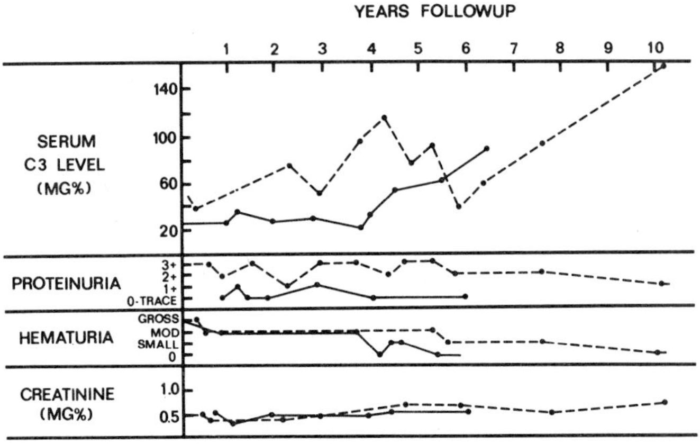

Fig 3.—Clinical courses of Patient 1 *(broken line)* and Patient 2 *(solid line)*, showing serum C3 levels, urinalyses and serum creatinine levels. Proteinuria and hematuria conform to semiquantitative results obtained with Labstix brand reagent strips. (Courtesy of Davis, A. E., et al.: Am. J. Med. 63:481–487, September, 1977.)

Fig 4.—Glomerular peripheral capillary loop from most recent biopsy specimen from Patient 2. Irregular, finely granular, electron-dense deposits are present within glomerular basement membrane *(arrows)*. Several irregular, electron-lucent areas containing membrane-bound vacuoles *(asterisk)* are also present. Central, collapsed capillary is lined by endothelial cell *(E)*. Few foot processes show moderate spreading; reduced 37% from ×17,000. (Courtesy of Davis, A. E., et al.: Am. J. Med. 63:481–487, September, 1977.)

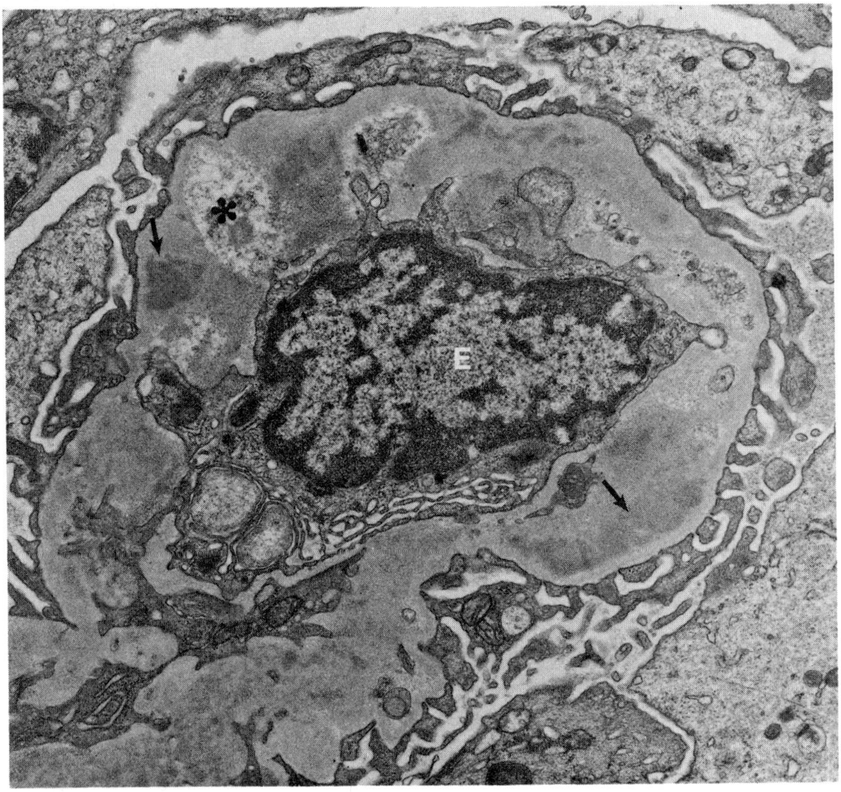

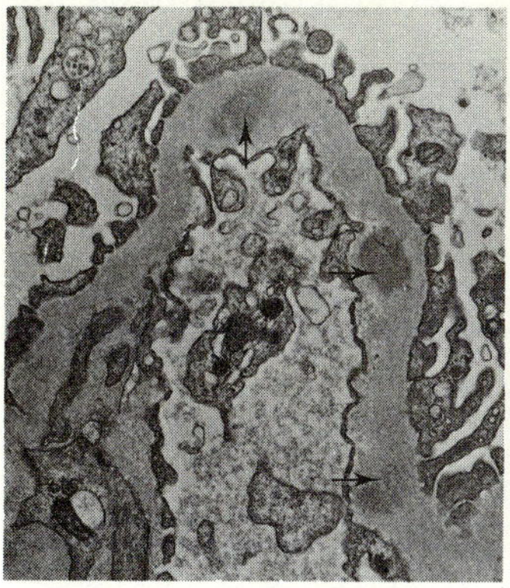

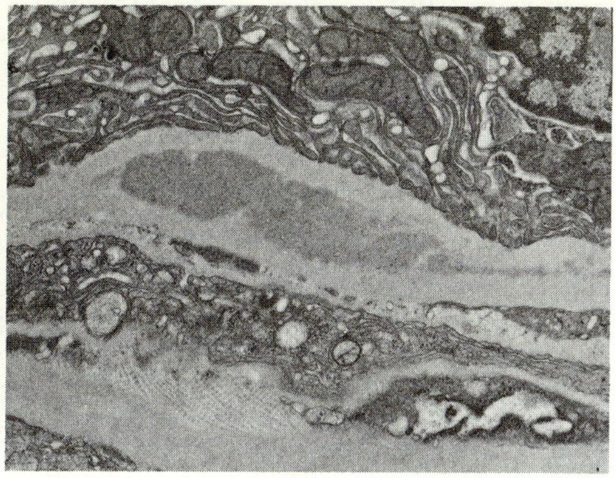

Fig 5 (left).—Peripheral capillary loop from same specimen as in Figure 4 shows three rounded deposits *(arrows)* in glomerular basement membrane; reduced from ×12,240.

Fig 6 (right).—Tubular basement membrane from same specimen as in Figures 4 and 5 shows elongated, electron-dense deposit; reduced 37% from × 14,760.

(Courtesy of Davis, A. E., et al.: Am. J. Med. 63:481–487, September, 1977.)

densa. Intramembranous deposits were also present in Bowman's capsule and in tubular basement membranes (Fig 6). There were no linear bandlike deposits within the basement membrane or subendothelial deposits. Both intramembranous and subendothelial electron-lucent areas containing vesicles were observed; these appeared to be residua of cellular debris.

These cases may represent a new disease, but the entity is clinically indistinguishable at presentation from reported variants of MPGN. The mild course and gradual resolution without treatment appear to distinguish the condition from both dense deposit disease and pure MPGN. The possibility of a persistently hypocomplementemic nephritis variant of MPGN with spontaneous morphological improvement is important in assessing treatment in this disease group.

► [Further experience will be necessary to substantiate or refute the validity of type 3 and other milder atypical forms of membranoproliferative glomerulonephritis. Of greater practical importance is the differentiation from poststreptococcal glomerulonephritis, which any form of membranoproliferative nephritis can resemble on histologic section. Electron microscopy can help by showing the characteristic subepithelial bumps of poststreptococcal disease, which, of course, has a very good prognosis.

Human β lymphocytes have been shown recently to possess a unique set of surface antigens, some of which are strongly associated with specific diseases. P. S. Friend et al. reported on a "β cell alloantigen associated with chronic mesangiocapillary glomerulonephritis" (Lancet 1:562, 1977).—Ed.] ◄

Prognosis of Henoch-Schönlein Nephritis in Children was examined by R. Counahan, M. H. Winterborn, R. H. R. White, J. M. Heaton, S. R. Meadow, N. H. Bluett, H. Swetschin, J. S. Cameron and C. Chantler.[4] In 1972, Meadow et al. reported the follow-up after 2 years or longer of 62 of a series of 88 children with Henoch-Schönlein nephritis. All survivors have now been traced, and their outcomes have been assessed 6½–21 years after presentation. Mean follow-up has been 9.9 years.

---

(4) Br. Med. J. 2:11–14, July 2, 1977.

Sixty-one of the 88 patients were normal, 6 had minor urinary abnormalities, 9 had evidence of active renal disease and 12 were in chronic renal failure or were dead. Patients with a nephritic-nephrotic presentation did worse than the others, but over 40% of this group were normal. The proportion of patients with a poor outcome rose with age at presentation, but the clinical state at follow-up was not apparently related to age at presentation. Six of 21 patients whose rash recurred and 15 of 67 without a recurrence had poor outcomes. All patients with minimal renal biopsy changes were normal or nearly so at follow-up, whereas all those with over 75% crescents had persistent renal disease or had died. Evidence of preexistent streptococcal infection, as reflected by antistreptolysin O titers, was unrelated to outcome. No significant differences in outcome were related to treatment with corticosteroids alone, immunosuppressive agents alone or combination therapy. The patients with the most extensive renal lesions were likelier to have received active treatment.

Presentation of Henoch-Schönlein nephritis with a nephritic and nephrotic picture combined is associated with a poor prognosis, as is an increased proportion of crescents on renal biopsy. Neither the clinical presentation nor the renal morphology, however, is a clear discriminant of outcome. Significant changes in outcome may occur more than 2 years after presentation. An annual blood pressure check and urine testing for protein and blood would effectively identify patients for whom specialist follow-up is unnecessary. All patients should be followed for at least 5 years.

► [The value of renal biopsy in determining prognosis in this generalized vasculitic disease is underlined by this long-term study. Widespread epithelial crescents early in the course were a guarantee of progressive renal disease. On the other hand, focal or minimal involvement had a good prognosis. Clinical features at the onset of the illness were less accurate in forecasting the course. Sixty percent of those children who presented with nephrotic syndrome, hypertension and hematuria (nephritis-nephrosis)—a combination traditionally associated with a gloomy prognosis—had persistent renal disease. However, 40% were normal on follow-up. The role of steroids and immunosuppressives in Henoch-Schönlein purpura is still undetermined, but if these agents do anything, it is certainly not dramatic.—Ed.] ◄

Lupus Nephritis: Clinical Course as Related to Morphological Forms and Their Transitions. David S. Baldwin, Melvin C. Gluck, Jerome Lowenstein and Gloria R. Gallo[5] (New York Univ.) undertook an intensive study of the course of lupus nephritis in 88 patients in whom strict morphological criteria were used in classification. All patients received steroids and 17 also received cytotoxic drugs. A total of 135 specimens of renal tissue were obtained at biopsy or autopsy. Serial pathologic observations were made in 31 patients. Transition from one form of lupus nephritis to another was observed in 16 patients. The renal lesions were categorized as focal proliferative lupus nephritis in 12 cases, diffuse proliferative lupus nephritis in 44, membranous lupus nephritis in 24, mesangial lupus nephritis in 12 and glomerular sclerosis in 6.

Focal proliferative lupus nephritis generally followed a benign course, except occasionally where transition to the diffuse proliferative

(5) Am. J. Med. 62:12–30, January, 1977.

or membranous form occurred. Membranous lupus nephritis, when characterized by persistent nephrotic syndrome, led slowly to renal failure, but this course was aborted in the one third of cases in which remission of nephrotic syndrome was achieved. Most patients with diffuse proliferative lupus nephritis and nephrotic syndrome died within 5 years, often in association with necrotizing renal vasculitis, severe hypertension and accelerated renal failure. A small number of patients with diffuse proliferative disease underwent remission and then showed only mesangial changes usually, however, with the appearance of glomerular sclerosis. Mesangial immune deposits with or without proliferation, sometimes without clinical renal disease, were seen early in the course of systemic lupus erythematosus (SLE) and could proceed to the diffuse proliferative or membranous forms.

These observations emphasize the importance of strict morphological classification when different treatments of lupus nephritis are compared. Early treatment may be the key to the management of lupus nephritis, in view of the grave prognosis of established diffuse proliferative lupus nephritis, which probably evolves from a mesangial involvement common to all patients with SLE from its onset. A prophylactic approach to lupus nephritis based on early treatment of all patients warrants serious consideration.

► [Perhaps because of the selection of cases referred to a renal service, Doctor Baldwin, like most nephrologists, feels that immunosuppressive agents have the edge over prednisone alone in patients with diffuse proliferative lupus nephritis. That disease has a gloomy prognosis, especially if it is associated with an unremitting nephrotic syndrome that resists therapy.

It is interesting that 2 of 12 patients with focal proliferative disease went on to develop diffuse proliferative glomerulonephritis and 1, membranous nephritis. In previous articles, transition from one form of lupus nephritis to another was considered rare. An abrupt change for the worse in lupus patients was often associated with the appearance of necrotizing vasculitis, frequently associated with encephalopathy, retinopathy or heart failure. – Ed.] ◄

Prognosis in Steroid-Treated Idiopathic Nephrotic Syndrome in Adults: Analysis of Major Predictive Factors after 10-Year Follow-up. Beldon A. Idelson, Neil Smithline, Gordon W. Smith and John T. Harrington[6] (Boston) report long-term findings in 68 adults seen in 1953 – 67 with idiopathic nephrotic syndrome (INS) who were treated with steroids. The patients were aged 16 – 65 years and their protein excretion exceeded 5 gm daily. They had hypoalbuminemia. No severe impairment of renal function was present. They had not previously received steroid therapy. One patient died of cerebral infarction shortly after treatment began. Renal tissue was obtained by biopsy before treatment in 49 cases and at autopsy in 3 others. Mean follow-up was 9 years. It was 11 years for survivors.

Sixteen patients had a steroid-complete or steroid-dependent response, and 7 had a partial remission during steroid therapy. All 16 patients who progressed to renal failure failed to respond to steroid therapy (Fig 7). Fourteen of 22 patients who showed no reduction in urinary protein excretion to below 2 gm daily during or after steroid therapy progressed to end-stage renal failure in a mean of 5½ years. None of 41

(6) Arch. Intern. Med. 137:891 – 896, July, 1977.

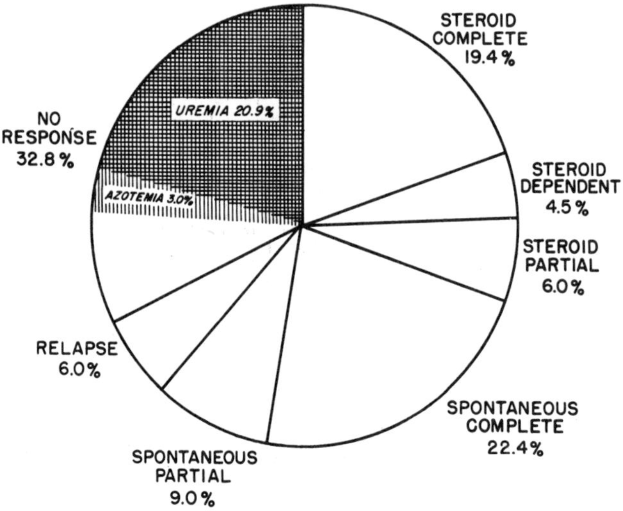

Fig 7.—Clinical status at end of study. Open sectors indicate patients with normal renal function; hatched sectors, those with azotemia (serum creatinine concentration less than 2 mg/100 ml); and crosshatched sector, patients with uremia (renal death or dialysis). Note that all azotemic and uremic patients are in group with no reduction in proteinuria below 2 gm per day (no response). (Courtesy of Idelson, B. A., et al.: Arch. Intern. Med. 137:891–896, July, 1977; copyright 1977, American Medical Association.)

responders developed renal insufficiency. The period of greatest risk was the first 3 years; the likelihood of loss of renal function thereafter was minimal. The degree of histologic damage was closely correlated with renal function at follow-up. Only 2 of 22 patients with minimal or mild abnormalities had a serum creatinine concentration above 1.5 mg/100 ml at any time.

Partial or complete remission during steroid therapy, reduction in protein excretion to below 2 gm daily, persistence of normal renal function beyond 3 years and the presence of mild histologic abnormalities auger a favorable long-term outcome in patients with INS. Few patients in this series with mild to minimal histologic changes or with normal renal function 3 years after onset progressed to renal failure, and no patient with a fall in urinary protein excretion to below 2 gm daily developed renal insufficiency.

► [The patients included in this study had proliferative or membranous glomerulonephritis as well as minimal-change disease (lipoid nephrosis). Regardless of the histologic type of disease, substantial improvement in proteinuria and the failure of renal function to decline within the first 3 years augured well for the future. I think this is useful information to keep in mind when counseling patients. Even in the 12 patients with "severely abnormal" glomeruli, 4 had a serum creatinine level below 1.5 mg/100 ml on long-term follow-up.—Ed.] ◄

Glomerulopathies of Neoplasia are discussed by Jeremiah W. Eagen and Edmund J. Lewis[7] (Chicago). Proteinuria, often sufficient to cause nephrotic syndrome, is a recognized manifestation of various neoplastic diseases, and variable glomerular lesions have been asso-

(7) Kidney Int. 11:297–306, May, 1977.

Renal Morphological Findings in Patients with Neoplasia and Nephrotic Syndrome[a]

Neoplastic lesion	No. of patients	No. with renal pathology	Minimal change[b]	Membranous glomerulopathy[c]	Membrano-proliferative glomerulo-nephritis[d]	Amyloidosis[e]	Other[f]
Carcinoma	67	48	3	33	4	2	6
Hodgkin's disease	63[g]	52	26	4	0	18	4
Malignant lymphoma (non-Hodgkin's)	7	6	2	2	1	0	1
Leukemia	9[h]	9	1	4	1	1	2
Benign solid tumors	6	3	0	2	1	0	0
Embryonal tumors	12	9	1	1	0	0	7
Waldenström's macro-globulinemia and multiple myeloma	7[i]	7	0	0	1	6	0
Totals	171	134	33	46	8	27	20

[a]To be acceptable as nephrotic syndrome, patients must have had heavy proteinuria (excretion usually more than 3.5 gm/24 hr in adults) with hypoalbuminemia and edema or have been stated to have nephrotic syndrome when these data were not reported.

[b]Minimal change glomerular lesion: glomeruli appeared normal or only slightly modified at light microscopy.

[c]Membranous glomerulopathy: glomeruli showed diffuse, homogeneous thickening of capillary walls without significant hypercellularity.

[d]Membranoproliferative glomerulonephritis: glomeruli showed accentuation of lobular pattern with mesangial cell proliferation and increased mesangial matrix and thickening of capillary walls.

[e]Amyloidosis: glomeruli showed tinctorial staining of amyloid.

[f]Other: this group includes extracapillary glomerulonephritis (5), proliferative sclerosing glomerulonephritis (4), proliferative glomerulonephritis (4), unclassified glomerulonephritis (4), renal dysplasia (2) and thrombotic microangiopathy (1).

[g]Hodgkin's disease: case reports without renal pathology from literature.

[h]Leukemia: 1 patient had both hypernephroma and monocytic leukemia and is included in carcinoma group.

[i]Waldenström's macroglobulinemia and multiple myeloma: case reports in literature.

ciated with these tumors. About 70% of cases exhibit immune complex membranous glomerulopathy in association with carcinoma (table). Recently several cases of extracapillary glomerulonephritis with nephrotic syndrome have been related to malignancy. It seems plausible that some patients with neoplasms are susceptible to glomerular deposit of tumor-associated antigen-antibody complexes, with subsequent induction of significant glomerular injury. An alternative possibility is involvement of a viral antigen. The possibility that immune complex glomerulopathy in patients with neoplasia is an expression of autoimmunity directed against normal antigens also deserves consideration. The clinical course has been grave.

Amyloid disease in patients with Hodgkin's disease is now less frequent. Most patients with this condition and nephrotic syndrome have minimal-change glomerulopathy, or, less frequently, membranous glomerulopathy or proliferative glomerulonephritis. Onset of nephrotic syndrome is early in this setting. Effective treatment of the neoplastic process almost uniformly causes remission of the nephrotic syndrome. Relapses of nephrotic syndrome coincident with periods of reactivation of Hodgkin's disease have been described. A third of the remissions reported were associated with radiotherapy only. Glomerulopathies are also associated with miscellaneous benign and malignant neoplasms, including embryonal tumors.

► [How important is it to undertake a search for malignancy in a patient who presents with the nephrotic syndrome? Five years ago I would have said, "Not very." In most patients with Hodgkin's disease, the diagnosis of lymphoma is apparent when the nephrotic syndrome is recognized. Nevertheless, particularly with carcinoma, the tumor is often occult when the patient presents with edema. Almost half of the patients with carcinoma (19 of 42) developed proteinuria and edema a month to a year before the tumor became manifest. Lung carcinoma is the most common solid tumor associated with glomerulopathy, but almost every kind of carcinoma has been reported. – Ed.] ◄

Other Diseases of the Kidney

Acute Renal Insufficiency due to Lymphomatous Infiltration of the Kidneys: Report of Six Cases. Massive bilateral neoplastic infiltration of the renal parenchyma has rarely been held to be responsible for uremia but is important to recognize, since radiotherapy or chemotherapy has been shown to improve renal function. Alain Kanfer, Alain Vandewalle, Liliane Morel-Maroger, Marie-José Feintuch, Jean-Daniel Sraer and Jean Roland[8] (Paris) describe 6 patients with acute renal insufficiency due to lymphomatous renal involvement. Renal symptoms were relieved in the 2 young men who were treated. The patients were admitted to a renal intensive care unit in a 6-year period.

Woman, 60, was admitted with acute renal insufficiency about 4 months after an episode of lumbar pain with fever and vomiting. She had become oliguric the month before admission, and a left lower abdominal mass was found, as well as hepatomegaly and a right-sided pleural effusion containing neoplastic cells. Urine output was 400 ml/24 hours, with protein excretion of 0.7 gm/24 hours. The blood urea nitrogen was 122 mg/100 ml. Pyelography showed marked enlargement of the left kidney and moderate enlargement of the right; the ureters were normal. Bilateral ureteral catheterization did not produce diuresis and hemodialysis was performed. A surgical renal biopsy specimen showed complete replacement of the renal tissue by lymphomatous cells. Poorly differentiated lymphocytic-type malignant lymphoma was diagnosed. The glomeruli were normal. The patient died 8 days after admission of retroperitoneal hemorrhage, probably caused by the renal biopsy.

Only 16 cases of rapidly progressive or acute renal insufficiency due to lymphomatous infiltration of the renal parenchyma have been reported. Hyperuricemia was present in 5 of the authors' 6 patients, but it probably was not responsible for the oliguria. The renal failure must be pathogenically related to the massive replacement of renal parenchyma by tumor cells. Acute renal insufficiency developed in 4 patients with known disseminated lymphoma, whereas 2 presented with oliguria. Percutaneous renal biopsy may lead to a correct diagnosis and to appropriate treatment by local irradiation or administration of antimitotic drugs. If biopsy is unsuccessful or is impossible because of hemostatic problems or severe hypertension, therapeutic trials should be undertaken before lumbotomy is considered.

► [Parenchymal infiltration of both kidneys by lymphoma is an unusual cause of uremia, but is important because it is reversible with treatment. The key to the diagnosis is that the kidneys are enlarged, while proteinuria is mild. More common is partial or complete obstruction to both ureters by retroperitoneal lymph nodes. Hypercalcemic nephropathy and multiple urate deposits should also be considered in the differential diagnosis. In the glomerulonephritis associated with lymphoma, proteinuria is heavy, with the nephrotic syndrome usually overshadowing azotemia, and oliguria is uncommon.

(8) Cancer 38:2588–2592, December, 1976.

An excellent editorial review, "Electrolyte and Acid-Base Disturbances in the Management of Leukemia," by S. O'Regan et al., appeared recently (Blood 49:345, 1977). —Ed.] ◄

Resolution of Renal Amyloidosis. Regression of nephrotic syndrome consequent to renal amyloidosis has occasionally been recorded after improvement of the underlying disease, but only 1 previous report indicating that amyloid deposits may decrease in the kidney has appeared. Steven H. Dikman, Thomas Kahn, Donald Gribetz and Jacob Churg[9] (Mount Sinai School of Medicine) documented clinical and morphological regression of renal amyloid in four renal biopsies of a child with amyloidosis after extensive infected burns.

Boy, 10, was admitted, 11 months after incurring 30–40% burns of the skin, with contractures and generalized edema that had developed in the past 2 weeks. Urinalysis showed granular hyaline casts and protein. Liver and renal biopsies showed amyloidosis. Further biopsies were performed at 8 months and 3 and 6 years after burn injury. The urine was protein free on the last two occa-

Fig 8 (top).—First renal biopsy specimen (obtained 16 months after burn), showing extensive glomerular amyloid deposits. Periodic acid-Schiff; reduced from ×150.

Fig 9 (bottom).—Fourth renal biopsy specimen (obtained 6 years after burn), showing marked resolution of amyloid deposits. Periodic acid-Schiff; reduced 34% from ×150.

(Courtesy of Dikman, S. H., et al.: Am. J. Med. 63:430–433, September, 1977.)

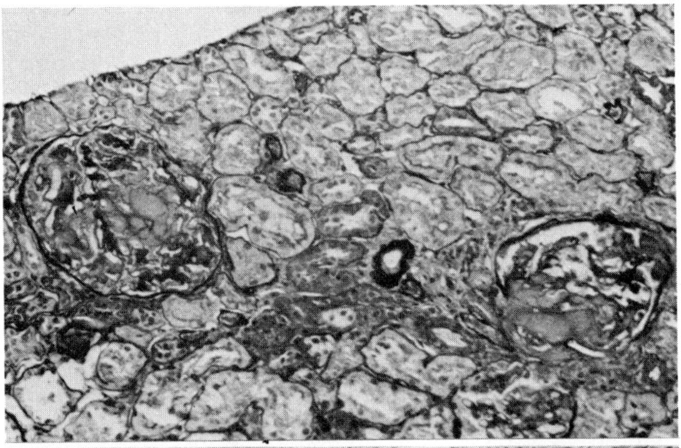

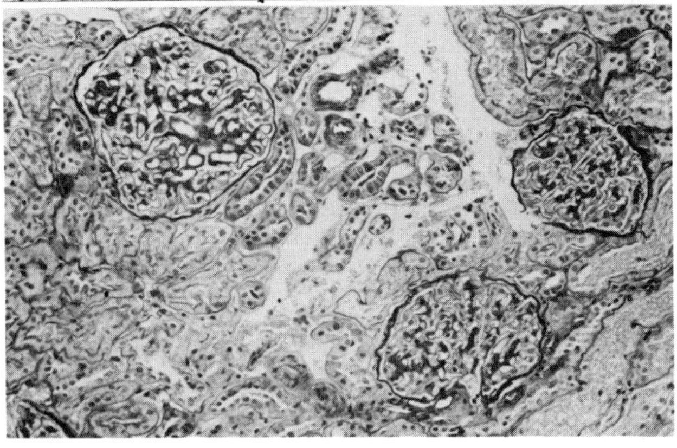

(9) Am. J. Med. 63:430–433, September, 1977.

sions. The patient is an active man with no physical abnormalities other than scars about 14 years after injury. He is normotensive.

The first biopsy, 16 months after injury and 10 months after onset of nephrotic syndrome, showed prominent segmental glomerular amyloid deposits replacing an average of over half the glomerular tuft (Fig 8). Marked deposit of amyloid in glomerular capillary walls was also seen. Biopsy 2 years after injury showed quantitatively similar amyloid deposits and the third biopsy showed marked deposits. The fourth biopsy, 6 years after injury, showed small, segmental amyloid deposits and no amyloid in one glomerulus (Fig 9). Ultrastructural studies showed more extensive subepithelial basement membrane-like material in the later specimens and smaller amounts of such material on the subendothelial aspects. Liver biopsy 13 months after burn injury showed minute amyloid deposits in the sinusoids.

The findings in this case indicate that renal amyloid deposits may regress. Basement membrane thickening and double capillary wall contours may represent a form of scarring similar to that found with other processes that affect the glomerular capillary wall.

► [Previous reports of secondary renal amyloidosis had suggested that when the inciting stimulus was removed, the nephrotic syndrome might reverse itself, but renal deposits of amyloid remained stable or progressed. This article (together with one by Triger, D. R., and Jackes, A. M.: Q. J. Med. 42:15, 1973) establishes that renal deposits of amyloid may actually regress. This provides more encouragement for the aggressive treatment of such patients directed at the primary underlying disease. – Ed.] ◄

Mechanism of Increased Renal Clearance of Amylase-Creatinine in Acute Pancreatitis. Possible mechanisms of elevation of the amylase-creatinine clearance ratio in pancreatitis include an increased serum concentration of an extremely rapidly cleared isoamylase, increased glomerular permeability to amylase and decreased renal tubular reabsorption of filtered amylase. Steven G. Johnson, Carol J. Ellis and Michael D. Levitt[1] (Univ. of Minnesota) investigated each of these mechanisms in patients with a serum amylase level over 300 Somogyi units, urinary amylase excretion over 300 Somogyi units per hour and an amylase-creatinine clearance ratio over 4.5%. Clearances of pancreatic and salivary isoamylases were determined in 10 patients with acute pancreatitis and 20 normal subjects.

Serum and urine from patients with acute pancreatitis showed a preponderance of pancreatic isoamylase and no anomalous isoamylase peaks. The amylase-creatinine clearance ratio was 9.2% in patients with pancreatitis (normal, 2.4 ± 0.2%). The clearances of both isoamylases were significantly more rapid than in normal subjects. There was no significant difference between patients and normal subjects in renal clearance of dextrans of any size relative to creatinine, suggesting that glomerular permeability is normal in acute pancreatitis. The ratio of renal clearances of β_2-microglobulin and creatinine was markedly elevated in all patients during the acute phase of pancreatitis and returned toward normal during recovery from acute pancreatitis, paralleling the decline in the amylase-creatinine clearance ratio with recovery.

---

(1) N. Engl. J. Med. 295:1214–1217, Nov. 25, 1976.

The reversible renal tubular defect demonstrated in these studies presumably reduces amylase reabsorption and explains the elevated renal clearance of amylase-creatinine observed in acute pancreatitis. Apparently some "tubular dysfunction factor" comes into play in pancreatitis, which inhibits tubular handling of amylase and other low molecular weight proteins. Whether this "factor" is operative in conditions other than acute pancreatitis is unknown.

► [What this key article shows is that the increased clearance of amylase in pancreatitis is not specific for that protein, but is a more general phenomenon. The β-microglobulin excretion is also increased, suggesting a defect in the reabsorption of medium molecular weight proteins normally reabsorbed by the proximal tubule. You might predict that the amylase-creatinine clearance ratio would be elevated as well in patients with chronic renal insufficiency, since in that circumstance proximal tubular reabsorption also tends to be depressed. Sure enough, that is the case (see article by Morton et al.: 1977 YEAR BOOK, p. 424; and Schiffer, C. F., et al.: Amylase-creatinine clearance fractions in patients on chronic hemodialysis, Ann. Intern. Med. 86:65, 1977). The same situation obtains after cardiopulmonary bypass, even without renal failure (Travers, L. W., et al.: Am. J. Surg. 133:298, 1977). An increased secretion of parathyroid hormone (PTH) would be an attractive way to explain things, since PTH decreases absorption in the proximal tubule. Unfortunately, PTH levels in the plasma of patients with pancreatitis do not seem to be elevated, despite hypocalcemia. It would be interesting to see what the clearance of lysozyme is in pancreatitis, since it is increased in other disorders of tubular function.

Speaking of pancreatitis, D. A. Goldstein et al. called attention to the frequency of acute oliguric renal failure complicating acute pancreatitis, even without obvious circulatory shock (Arch. Intern. Med. 136:1363, 1976). Crescentic glomerulonephritis with immune deposits was an unusual cause of reversible renal failure in a patient with chronic relapsing pancreatitis described by J. P. Dickmeyer (ibid. 137:1065, 1977). – Ed.]

Uremia and Renal Failure

Simple Method of Estimating Progression of Chronic Renal Failure. As chronic renal failure develops the serum creatinine should rise with increasing rapidity and, if this were so, the reciprocal serum creatinine might fall linearly with time. W. E. Mitch, M. Walser (Johns Hopkins Univ.), G. A. Buffington and J. Lemann, Jr.[2] (Med. College of Wisconsin) examined this hypothesis in 34 patients with chronic renal failure of varying causes who had been followed for at least a year and in whom seven or more creatinine determinations had been performed. All had had at least a threefold increase in creatinine determination.

In 3 of the 34 patients the plot of reciprocal serum creatinine against

Fig 10.—Composite plot of reciprocal serum creatine concentration (in mg/dl) versus months of observation in 6 patients with chronic renal failure. Final value for reciprocal of serum creatine concentration is shown for each patient. Ordinate has uniform divisions of 0.1 dl/mg. (Courtesy of Mitch, W. E., et al.: Lancet 2:1326–1328, Dec. 18, 1976.)

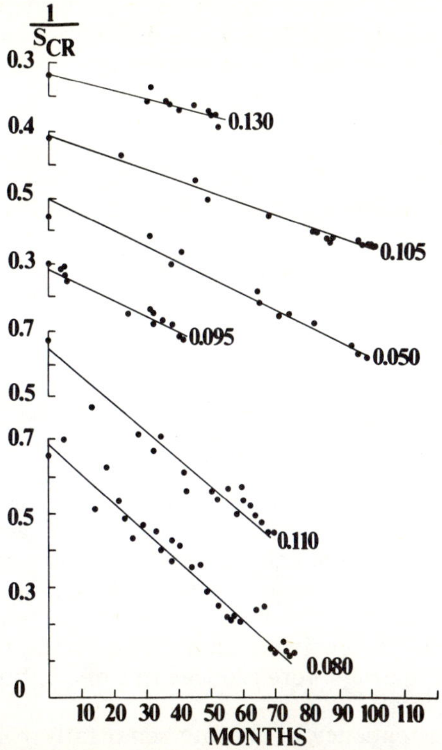

(2) Lancet 2:1326–1328, Dec. 18, 1976.

time was clearly nonlinear by inspection. The linear fall in reciprocal serum creatinine with time in 6 representative patients is shown in Figure 10. Two patients each had glomerulonephritis, pyelonephritis and medullary cystic disease. The average correlation coefficient in all patients, excluding those with a nonlinear fall in reciprocal serum creatinine, was 0.954. The 95% confidence limits of the slopes averaged 17.1% of the individual slopes, with a range of 5.6 – 32%.

In most patients, reciprocal serum creatinine concentration falls linearly as chronic renal failure progresses. It may be possible in this way to predict when dialysis will be required. The simplest explanation of the relationship observed is that clearance of endogenous creatinine declines linearly as renal failure progresses. Reciprocal serum creatinine falls linearly even as renal failure becomes terminal. Since creatinine excretion is said to decline in severe renal failure, the rate of decline in creatinine clearance must accelerate in the end stages of chronic renal failure, but this remains to be tested.

► [In most patients with slowly progressive disease of the kidneys, the glomerular filtration rate declines by roughly the same number of milliliters per minute each year, producing a straight line when the reciprocal of the serum creatinine is plotted against time. The method outlined here should be useful in prospective studies of therapeutic interventions in chronic nephritis, especially when an adequate control period can be obtained to establish the rate of progression. – Ed.] ◄

Reversibility of "Salt-Losing" Tendency of Chronic Renal Failure. Gabriel M. Danovitch, Jacques Bourgoignie and Neal S. Bricker[3] (Albert Einstein College of Medicine) propose that the obligatory excretion of sodium in chronic renal disease could result from the adaptive processes that lead to a progressive increase in sodium excretion per nephron that is required to maintain sodium balance in the face of a falling glomerular filtration rate and constant salt intake. The adaptive natriuresis would be slowly suppressible, and an inappropriate natriuresis would ensue when salt intake was suddenly reduced. A slow, stepwise reduction in dietary sodium intake might reverse the adaptation, allowing patients with far-advanced chronic renal failure to regain their capacity to reduce urinary sodium excretion to extremely low levels. This hypothesis was examined in 5 patients with advanced chronic renal failure and glomerular filtration rates of 5.2 – 16 ml per minute. Patients were initially in sodium balance on metabolic diets containing 58 – 342 mEq sodium daily. The sodium content of the diet was reduced at intervals of at least 1 week over 4 – 14 weeks.

Four patients exhibited a salt-losing tendency, and 2 temporarily required intravenous salt replacement. All the patients remained in sodium balance after the studies when they were ingesting a mean of 5 mEq sodium daily. No change in renal function was observed, and there was no consistent change in plasma volume in the 4 patients in whom it was measured. A small loss of body weight of 0.44 kg was observed. There were no consistent changes in blood pressure, but doses of antihypertensive drugs were reduced in 2 of 3 patients who received them from the outset.

The salt-losing tendency of chronic renal failure is reversible and

(3) N. Engl. J. Med. 296:14 – 19, Jan. 6, 1977.

appears to be a manifestation of the long-term adaptation for sodium excretion. When a salt-retaining stimulus exists over a long period, the mechanism providing for salt excretion can be overcome or become inoperative. The present protocol required patient cooperation in a difficult regimen and prolonged hospitalization on a metabolic ward. Performance of the sodium-reducing protocol in any other circumstances is fraught with danger. The salt-reducing protocol might have clinical value in patients whose quality of life is affected adversely by massive, inappropriate salt loss.

► [The physiologic impact of these studies is that they support the idea of a chronic natriuretic influence (hormone?), as yet undefined, that operates on remaining nephrons in patients with renal insufficiency who eat a diet unrestricted in salt and enables a higher fraction of the filtered load of sodium to be excreted so as to avoid salt retention. A possible alternative explanation for the remarkable ability of these salt-wasting patients to learn to retain sodium (and one that bypasses "natriuretic hormone") is that their sodium reabsorptive mechanism (e.g., distal tubular Na-K-ATPase) slowly got revved up under the chronic stimulus of increased aldosterone secretion. – Ed.] ◄

Glucagon and Insulin Binding to Liver Membranes in Partially Nephrectomized Uremic Rat Model. Chronic renal failure is commonly associated with glucose intolerance. The findings suggest insulin resistance. Hyperglucagonemia also is observed. Hypersensitivity to glucagon is reversible after dialysis. Vijay Soman and Philip Felig[4] (Yale Univ.) determined whether increased glucagon sensitivity and insulin resistance in uremia might be mediated by alterations in the binding of the peptide hormones to their specific liver plasma membrane receptors. Insulin and glucagon binding to hepatic plasma membranes was examined in uremic rat models produced by 70% nephrectomy and 90% nephrectomy. The respective creatinine concentrations 4 weeks after surgery were 2.2 and 4.2 mg/100 ml.

The 90% nephrectomized rats had significantly higher levels of plasma glucose, insulin and glucagon than controls. Similar but less marked elevations were seen in the 70% nephrectomized rats. In liver plasma membranes from nephrectomized rats, specific binding of ^{125}I-glucagon was increased by 80 – 120%, and glucagon-stimulated adenylate cyclase activity was twofold higher than in controls. Fluoride-stimulated adenylate cyclase activity was similar in the experimental and control rats. Specific binding of ^{125}I-insulin to liver membranes was reduced by 40 – 50% in nephrectomized rats. Data analysis suggested that the changes in glucagon and insulin binding resulted from alterations in binding capacity rather than from changes in affinity. Liver plasma membranes from nephrectomized rats degraded ^{125}I-glucagon and ^{125}I-insulin to the same extent as those from control rats.

Nephrectomized rats simulate the hyperglycemia, hyperinsulinemia and hyperglucagonemia observed in clinical uremia. Specific binding of glucagon to liver membranes is increased in these rats and specific binding of insulin is reduced. These changes may explain glucagon hypersensitivity and may contribute to the resistance to insulin observed in the glucose intolerance of uremia.

► [These elegant experiments provide a neat explanation for the mild tendency to

(4) J. Clin. Invest. 60:224 – 232, July, 1977.

carbohydrate intolerance that characterizes the uremic state. Peptide hormones act on specific organs by virtue of hormone receptors in the cell membrane. In uremia, insulin receptors on liver cells are reduced while receptors for glucagon are increased. It is not yet clear whether this is just a by-product of the uremic state or a secondary consequence of the increase in circulating insulin and glucagon that occurs because the renal sink for disposal of these polypeptides is removed. See the following article. – Ed.]

Degradation of Parathyroid Hormone and Fragment Production by Isolated Perfused Dog Kidney: Effect of Glomerular Filtration Rate and Perfusate Ca^{2+} Concentrations. The heterogeneous nature of circulating parathyroid hormone (PTH) is recognized, but the origin and biologic significance of the various hormone fragments found in the circulation are unclear. Keith A. Hruska, Kevin Martin, Paul Mennes, Allen Greenwalt, Charles Anderson, Saulo Klahr and Eduardo Slatopolsky[5] (Washington Univ.) performed studies in the isolated perfused dog kidney to assess directly the role of the kidney in the degradation of intact bovine PTH (b-PTH 1-84) and the production of PTH fragments and to evaluate the effects of calcium concentration on the renal degradation of PTH. Column eluates were radioimmunoassayed for both COOH- and NH_2-terminal immunoreactive PTH (iPTH).

Disappearance of b-PTH 1-84 from the perfusate occurred concomitantly with the appearance of smaller molecular weight forms of iPTH, including both COOH- and NH_2-terminal regions of the PTH peptide. Perfusates from kidneys with lower glomerular filtration rates (GFRs) contained b-PTH 1-84 for longer periods than those with higher rates and showed greater accumulation of COOH-terminal PTH fragments. Perfusates containing high Ca^{2+} concentrations retarded and those with low Ca^{2+} concentrations accelerated the rate of degradation of b-PTH 1-84 by the kidney.

These studies documented the production of PTH fragments in the course of intact hormone degradation by the dog kidney and demonstrated renal clearance of the PTH fragments. The findings do not exclude the possibility that circulating PTH fragments in vivo can originate from direct secretion by the parathyroids. The finding that COOH-terminal fragments depend on glomerular filtration and tubular reabsorption for their degradation may explain the marked retention of COOH-terminal fragments observed in chronic renal failure as the GFR falls.

► [The impact of this article (see also, by the same authors, J. Clin. Invest. 60:808, 1977) is that (1) the kidney is a major avenue for removal of parathyroid hormone (PTH) from the circulation, as it is for insulin, gastrin and glucagon, and (2) fragments of peptide hormones – like the carboxy-terminal fragment of PTH – that may be immunologically but not biologically active – are also filtered and excreted or destroyed by normal kidneys. This means that (1) the concentrations of peptide hormones will tend to be elevated in the plasma of patients with renal insufficiency and (2) the plasma concentration of immunoreactive hormone products will also be high and differ from normal in their pattern. For example, the enormously elevated immunoreactive PTH levels reported in chronic uremia may give a false impression of true parathyroid activity, since they may be due in part to a high level of immunoreactive but biologically less potent fragments. That this is a general phenomenon is suggested by two other articles, "Abnormalities in Circulating Beta Cell Peptides in Chronic Renal Failure: Comparison of

(5) J. Clin. Invest. 60:501–510, September, 1977.

C Peptide, Proinsulin and Insulin," by J. B. Jaspan et al. (J. Clin. Endocrinol. Metab. 45: 441, 1977), and "Immunochemical Heterogeneity of Calcitonin in Renal Failure," by J. C. Lee et al. (ibid., p. 528). —Ed.] ◄

Relief of Uremic Pruritus with Ultraviolet Phototherapy. Data suggesting that ultraviolet irradiation may be an effective treatment of generalized uremic pruritus have been reported. Barbara A. Gilchrest, John W. Rowe, Robert S. Brown, Theodore I. Steinman and Kenneth A. Arndt[6] (Harvard Med. School) undertook a randomized, controlled study of the effect of ultraviolet light on severe pruritus in 24 adults with chronic renal failure requiring hemodialysis. All had had pruritus for at least 2 months, which was unresponsive to routine oral and topical medications and was severe enough to disturb sleep and interfere with daytime activities. All patients had been on hemodialysis for at least 4 months. Eighteen patients completed the course of therapy. Midrange or sunburn-spectrum ultraviolet light (UVB) was used. Initial treatment times were 75% of the estimated minimal erythema dose (MED), and subsequent treatments were lengthened by 25% of the MED. Placebo phototherapy consisted of long-wave ultraviolet light (UVA). Patients received eight ultraviolet light exposures twice weekly before or after dialysis.

Nine of 10 patients responded to UVB and 2 of 8 to UVA. Improvement followed an average of 5.2 UVB exposures. One of the 3 control patients who were subsequently treated with UVB responded. Three responders had recurrent pruritus after 1–3 weeks, and all again responded promptly to a second course of UVB. In all, 13 of 16 UVB treatments were successful. The response to phototherapy was not related to the complexion. Slight tanning occurred, which also was unrelated to relief from pruritus. The occurrence or severity of hyperparathyroidism was unrelated to the response to phototherapy, and therapy had no effects on the serum calcium or phosphorus levels.

This study shows the efficacy of ultraviolet phototherapy against uremic pruritus in patients on hemodialysis. Ultraviolet phototherapy is a practical modality. Conventional light boxes are a convenient source of artificial UVB light. The efficacy and safety of ultraviolet phototherapy call for further study of its use in uremic pruritus.

► [Intravenous lidocaine is said to relieve itching for about a day in many uremic patients (N. Engl. J. Med. 296:261, 1977). Oral cholestyramine, 5 gm twice daily, was also effective in 4 of 5 patients (Br. Med. J. 1:752, 1977). Ultraviolet suntanning, as described here, has obvious advantages over drugs. Why is it that some uremic patients itch and others don't? My impression is that at least a few of those who do itch have unrecognized hypersensitive skin reactions to drugs or drug products that are present in abnormally high concentration because of impaired excretion. —Ed.] ◄

(6) N. Engl. J. Med. 297:136–138, July 21, 1977.

Transplantation and Dialysis

End-Stage Renal Failure in Juvenile Diabetes Mellitus: Five-Year Follow-up of Treatment. John C. Mitchell[8] followed 43 juvenile diabetic patients for up to 5 years after they were accepted for renal transplantation. The 26 men and 17 women had an average age of 36 years when they presented in terminal renal failure and had had clinical diabetes for an average of 21 years. Onset of diabetes was at or before age 30 years in all. Most patients had neuropathy, retinopathy, symptomatic ischemic heart disease and hypertension at onset of dialysis before transplantation. Thirty-four patients received renal transplants; 1 of them received two grafts at different times. Six patients died while awaiting transplantation and 3 were still on dialysis at the end of the study.

After 5 years, 8 patients had died while on dialysis. Six of 20 men undergoing transplantation died, all but 1 within 8 months. One woman died 2 weeks after transplantation. Cardiovascular and cerebrovascular events accounted for over half the deaths. Four of the 15 deaths followed nephrectomy. The rate of death from infection was 27%. The overall cumulative survivals were 66% at 1 year, 61% at 2 years and 58% at 5 years. Cumulative survival for patients given living related donor kidneys was nearly 82%. Diabetic blindness appeared to stabilize after transplantation. Neuropathy improved in several patients. Only 3 of 16 surviving men were working at follow-up and only 6 of 12 women could function at work or as housewives.

Half the patients in this study who survived transplantation for a year or more required amputation of one or more extremities. Only a fourth of 1-year survivors were without blindness, severe peripheral vascular problems or both. Rehabilitative efforts should be increased for patients who have useful vision, neurologic stability and relatively little peripheral vascular disease.

► [A major problem of diabetic patients after transplantation is the relentless progression of vascular disease. Virtually all patients in this series with significant diminution in arterial pulsations suffered major sequelae—chronic painful ischemic ulcerations or amputation, or both. Neuropathy was another difficulty. Whereas some patients improved after transplantation (suggesting that uremic neuropathy contributed to the picture), about half of the patients with diabetic neuritis became worse. Cardiovascular and cerebrovascular events accounted for over half (56%) of the deaths. Obviously, transplantation does nothing to modify the natural history of diabetic vascular disease in organs other than the kidney. What is surprising is the cumulative survival—almost 60% at 5 years after the transplant.—Ed.] ◄

Risks of Vesicoureteral Reflux in the Transplanted Kidney. Vesicoureteral reflux has been described in from 4% to 64% of patients undergoing renal transplantation. Timothy H. Mathew, Priscilla Kin-

(8) Mayo Clin. Proc. 52:281–288, May, 1977.

caid-Smith and Poroor Vikraman[9] (Melbourne) reviewed experience with vesicoureteral reflux among 150 consecutive primary cadaver kidney transplants performed in 1965–75, in which the kidney functioned for over 3 months. A micturating cystogram was obtained at least once in 119 patients, and reflux was detected in 24% of these studies. The sodium iodide test was considered to be positive if any contrast was seen entering the transplanted ureter. The test was done without prior dehydration.

The initial cystogram was made a mean of 19.9 months after operation in refluxing patients and at a mean of 20.6 months in those without reflux. Urinary tract infection appeared to result from the examination in 6 of 167 procedures. The prevalence of reflux did not decline in recent years but was higher when only implantations of the simple type with no intramural tunnel were performed. Patients with reflux resembled the others in age and sex. Five refluxing patients died, all at least partly of graft failure. Two of 6 deaths in nonrefluxing patients were associated with graft failure. Grafts failed in 14 of 29 refluxing and 14 of 90 nonrefluxing patients, a significant difference. Whereas the typical focal scarring of reflux neuropathy was seen only occasionally, most failed refluxing grafts had macroscopic evidence consistent with high pelvic pressure. Rates of urinary tract infection were comparable in the groups with and without reflux. There was no increase in the rate of any of the common causes of renal failure in the group with reflux. Once detected, reflux did not disappear and tended to remain at the same radiologic grade. A urine leak occurred shortly after operation in 10 of the 29 patients with and 7 of the 90 without reflux.

The link between glomerular changes and vesicoureteral reflux after renal transplantation is unclear. The association of urine leak with long-term reflux stresses the need for care regarding the viability of the lower ureter. Once reinsertion of a shortened ureter has been necessary, future correction of reflux is usually technically impossible.

► [Late graft failures, ascribed to chronic rejection, were impressively more frequent in patients with ureteral reflux. The point the Melbourne nephrologists make is a good one; could some of these kidneys have been saved by a more careful ureteral implantation procedure in the initial operation? The clinical course of refluxing patients and the morphological appearance of the failed refluxing kidneys resembled chronic rejection, rather than obstructive nephropathy; infection was not present or did not play a major role. One is tempted to ascribe the association to chance or to turn it around; perhaps rejecting kidneys (and ureters) are more susceptible to reflux. Yet there is much we do not know about the local factors that make a transplanted kidney more or less susceptible to the complex immunologic and vascular changes of rejection (see, for example, the report by Nishikawa et al. that prostaglandin release is enhanced by ureteral obstruction, in the chapter Prostaglandins, in this YEAR BOOK). So, I would pay close attention to the recommendations of Doctor Kincaid-Smith and her colleagues.—Ed.]

Effect of Antilymphocyte Globulin Potency on Survival of Cadaver Renal Transplants: Prospective Randomized Double-Blind Trial. Several clinical studies have confirmed the efficacy of antilymphocyte globulin (ALG) in renal transplantation, but enthusiasm for its use has been tempered by inconsistent and negative clinical results and difficulty in standardizing individual batches of ALG for po-

(9) N. Engl. J. Med. 297:414–418, Aug. 25, 1977.

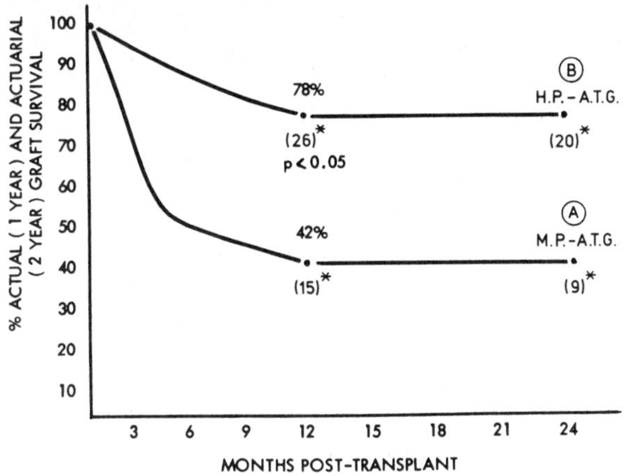

Fig 11.—Actual (1-year) and actuarial (2-year) cadaver graft survivals in randomized, double-blind ALG study. Asterisks indicate number of patients followed for interval shown and still having graft function. (Courtesy of Thomas, F., et al.: Lancet 2:671–674, Oct. 1, 1977.)

tency and toxicity. F. Thomas, G. Mendez-Picon, J. Thomas, K. Peace, R. Flora and H. M. Lee[1] (Med. College of Virginia) determined whether preclinical primate testing is a valid means of assessing the clinical efficacy of ALG preparations. A prospective, double-blind study compared the clinical results in two groups of cadaver kidney recipients, aged 14–55 years, each given one of two standard ALG preparations of different potencies as defined by primate skin graft testing. Group A patients received moderate-potency (MP) ALG and group B, high-potency (HP) ALG. The MP preparation gave 17–20 days of graft survival in rhesus monkeys, and the HP preparation yielded graft survival of 35 days or longer.

A significant difference in graft survival between the two groups was established at 1-year follow-up, when patient entry into the study was stopped. The mean follow-ups are currently 26 months for group A and 25.2 months for group B. Mean graft survivals at 1 year were 78% for group B and 42% for group A (Fig 11). Figures at 2 years were the same. Group A had a significant increase in graft loss from rejection compared with group B. The incidences of clinically significant infection were 28% in group A and 13% in group B; the difference was not statistically significant.

If these results are confirmed, it may be possible to use a preclinical test system to predict the clinical efficacy of an ALG product and eliminate batches of ALG that could be expected to give suboptimal results. Strict quality control of ALG by preclinical primate skin graft testing appears to go a long way toward producing the most effective material.

► [As you can see from Figure 11, the chief influence of antilymphocyte globulin was to improve graft survival by minimizing acute rejection during the first 3 months after transplantation. With a reduction in the use of large doses of steroids to treat rejection crises, the incidence and severity of infectious complications may also have been reduced. Chronic rejection was not avoided.

(1) Lancet 2:671–674, Oct. 1, 1977.

This article contrasts with the one on antithymocyte globulin appearing in the 1977 YEAR BOOK (p. 538), in which treatment did not improve transplant survival. The point made by the present authors is that it is not enough simply to produce antilymphocyte globulin—the product has to be tested for its immunosuppressive potency before use, since the efficacy of different batches may vary widely. Another randomized clinical trial of antilymphocyte globulin carried out by several cooperating centers in Canada also showed a beneficial effect in graft and host during the first 3 months after transplantation (Can. Med. Assoc. J. 115:1205, 1976).—Ed.] ◄

Pseudorejection: Factors Mimicking Rejection in Renal Allograft Recipients. Renal function is affected by factors other than rejection in renal allograft recipients, and many of these may cause an elevation of serum creatinine concentration, leading to an erroneous diagnosis of rejection. Arthur J. Matas, Richard L. Simmons, Carl M. Kjellstrand and John S. Najarian[2] (Univ. of Minnesota) reviewed the courses of 515 patients undergoing renal transplantation in 1969–74 to determine what conditions frequently coincide with an elevated serum creatinine concentration so that rejection is suspected. Six distinct syndromes were found that were associated with greater than 25% elevations in serum creatinine concentration. Patients in this series had nephrectomy and splenectomy before transplantation and received azathioprine, prednisone, antilymphocyte globulin and methylprednisolone for immunosuppression. Those with rejection were treated with local graft irradiation and an increase in the dosage of prednisone.

Nineteen significant creatinine elevations were associated with hyperglycemia in diabetic recipients. The creatinine value returned to normal as the blood sugar concentration was corrected. Two patients with stenosis of the transplant ureter responded to increased steroid administration. Several other patients with ureteral stenosis have not been treated for rejection. Eight documented creatinine elevations were associated with bacterial infection. The creatinine concentration fell with successful treatment of the infection. Viral infections were frequent in this group. Three patients had creatinine elevations in association with perirenal lymph collections. Arterial complications accounted for four creatinine elevations. Three recurrences of focal glomerulosclerosis and 1 possible case of recurrent membranoproliferative glomerulonephritis were encountered.

It is necessary to be aware of the differential diagnosis of elevated serum creatinine concentrations in renal transplant recipients to avoid the morbidity and mortality associated with high-dose steroid administration.

► [The large number of patients with elevated serum creatinine levels due to uncontrolled hyperglycemia is a reflection of the number of diabetics transplanted by Doctor Najarian's group. I would have included overdiuresis for hypertension in this list of conditions that mimic rejection by temporarily worsening renal function. Bear in mind that a big dose of prednisone makes a normal kidney's glomerular filtration rate go up, so a fall in serum creatinine after prednisone is given does not necessarily make the diagnosis of transplant rejection.—Ed.] ◄

Dialysis Dementia: Recovery after Transplantation A syndrome of progressive encephalopathy has been described in patients on chronic hemodialysis. The clinical features include dysarthria with nominal

(2) Ann. Surg. 186:51–59, July, 1977.

aphasia, dementia, myoclonic jerking, grand mal seizures and psychosis. The EEG shows high-voltage delta waves and spike activity with generalized slowing. Death usually occurs 3 – 18 months after onset; no recoveries have been reported. Patrick A. Sullivan, D. J. Murnaghan and N. Callaghan[3] (Cork, Ireland) describe a patient who recovered after transplantation, indicating that this syndrome is potentially reversible once dialysis has ceased and the uremic state has been reversed.

Man, 36, with chronic glomerulonephritis, began home hemodialysis and underwent incomplete parathyroidectomy after 13 months. The serum calcium concentration remained elevated. Transitory episodes of speech difficulty occurred 3 months later, and examination showed dysarthria with nominal aphasia, proximal muscle weakness and blood pressure of 160/100 mm Hg. Tonic-clonic seizures and episodes of nonfluent dysphasia developed 4 weeks later and recurred with increasing frequency. Grand mal seizures also developed, and the patient's speech became unintelligible. He was confused and agitated. He had received propranolol and aluminum hydroxide since starting hemodialysis. Phenytoin was given for the seizures. Cadaver kidney transplantation was performed 6 months after onset of the neurologic syndrome. The tonic-clonic seizures and episodes of mutism ceased, and the speech disturbance gradually subsided. The patient was working full time within a year and had normal findings except for generalized hyperreflexia 18 months after transplantation. The current serum calcium concentration is 9.6 mg/100 ml. The EEG showed considerable improvement; seizure discharges occurred only during photostimulation.

The cause of dialysis dementia is unknown, but high aluminum concentrations have been found in the brains of patients dying of the syndrome, and phosphate depletion has also been implicated. Renal transplantation may be of definite benefit in the management of dialysis dementia.

► [Until this case report, no patients with dialysis dementia had recovered (1977 YEAR BOOK, p. 540) and up to now there was no information on the effects of transplantation. This dramatic recovery certainly sounds hopeful. Why transplantation should help this dreadful disease isn't clear. A. M. Nadel and W. P. Wilson (Neurology 26:1130, 1976) treated 4 patients with dialysis encephalopathy – stuttering speech, dysarthria, mental and EEG changes – with diazepam and noted marked symptomatic improvement. Improvement was also described after subtotal parathyroidectomy in a patient with hypercalcemia (Ball, et al.: J. H., Nephron 18:151, 1977), suggesting that in someone with the peculiar underlying neurologic disorders that sometimes complicate uremia, a variety of systemic, chemical and neurologic influences can play on the brain in such a way as to exacerbate them reversibly. – Ed.] ◄

Complement and Leukocyte-Mediated Pulmonary Dysfunction in Hemodialysis. The transient leukopenia observed in early hemodialysis with cellophane membrane apparatus has been attributed to pulmonary sequestration of leukocytes, somehow provoked by low molecular weight complement components that are activated by dialyzer cellophane. Patients, especially those with antecedent cardiopulmonary dysfunction, are prone to acute cardiopulmonary decompensation during induction of hemodialysis. This and other complications generally are attributed to inadequate volume replacement or excessively rapid induction of blood flow into the dialyzer. Philip R.

(3) Br. Med. J. 2:740, Sept. 17, 1977.

Craddock, Jorg Fehr, Kenneth L. Brigham, Richard S. Kronenberg and Harry S. Jacob[4] performed studies in patients, rabbits and sheep to determine whether the acute cardiopulmonary complications of hemodialysis result from complement-mediated pulmonary vessel leukostasis, respiratory dysfunction and associated arterial hypoxemia.

Severe, transient neutropenia developed in the first 30 minutes of hemodialysis in 34 consecutive patients aged 18 – 65 years with diverse congenital and acquired renal diseases. Monocyte counts also fell. Decrements of 10 – 15 mm Hg in arterial oxygen tension and decreased diffusion efficiency of oxygen lasted 3 or 4 hours longer, as did impaired pulmonary diffusing capacity. The Pa_{CO_2} also declined. Closing volumes increased. Infusion of autologous, cellophane-incubated plasma into rabbits produced acute neutropenia and monocytopenia and significant hypoxemia. Examination of the lungs showed gross intravascular leukostasis, with segmented granulocytes predominating, and prominent interstitial edema. Lung lysozyme levels doubled in parallel with the leukostasis. Studies in sheep also showed neutropenia and pulmonary dysfunction occurring in parallel.

The findings suggest that dialysis-induced hypoxemia results primarily from ventilation-perfusion mismatching due to intravascular leukostasis and secondarily from small airways obstruction and closure, induced by either interstitial edema or reflex constriction. Hypoxemia of the degree observed, with the increment in right ventricular load resulting from pulmonary hypertension and increased cardiac output, may well be a critical challenge to dialyzed uremic patients with antecedent heart or lung disease. Myocardial vascular leukostasis may also occur during dialysis, further compromising cardiopulmonary function.

► [As Kaplow and Goffinet first pointed out 10 years ago (J.A.M.A. 203:1135, 1968), a profound neutropenia rapidly develops during the first 20 minutes of hemodialysis, with leukocyte counts regularly falling to 20% of normal. The mechanism is the activation of complement by dialysis cellophane, which causes the agglutination and margination of leukocytes in pulmonary capillaries. This would be an attractive explanation for the fall in arterial P_{O_2} that also occurs pretty regularly on dialysis. But it turns out that this arterial hypoxemia has a more banal and less worrisome cause – simple reduction of the respiratory drive and consequent hypoventilation. Dialyzed blood loses CO_2 and so arterial P_{CO_2} falls in patients on dialysis, reducing the stimulus to respiration. When the P_{CO_2} of the dialysis broth is kept artificially high, arterial P_{CO_2} does not fall, respiration is not decreased and arterial hypoxemia does not ensue (Aurigemma, N. M., et al.: N. Engl. J. Med. 297:871, 1977). – Ed.] ◄

(4) N. Engl. J. Med. 296:769 – 774, Apr. 7, 1977.

Hypertension and Renin

Estimating Renin Participation in Hypertension: Superiority of Converting Enzyme Inhibitor over Saralasin. Saralasin appears to underestimate true renin dependency, whereas the nonapeptide converting enzyme inhibitor SQ20881 has no pressor activity, and depressor responses correlate well with pretreatment values of plasma renin activity. David B. Case, John M. Wallace, Hans J. Keim, Michael A. Weber, Jan I. M. Drayer, Robert P. White, Jean E. Sealey and John H. Laragh[5] (New York Hosp.-Cornell Med. Center) compared saralasin and the converting enzyme inhibitor in 25 male and 14 female patients, aged 16–57, with different forms of hypertension. Six patients had low, 23 had normal and 10 had high renin activity. Six patients who had undergone bilateral nephrectomy and were on long-term dialysis were also evaluated. Saralasin was infused at a rate of 10 μg/kg per minute for 30 minutes, and, after at least 1 hour, SQ20881 was given as a slow intravenous bolus in a dose of 1 mg/kg.

Saralasin produced an 8.5% increase in blood pressure in low-renin patients, whereas the response to the converting enzyme inhibitor was neutral. Saralasin produced a minimal diastolic pressure response in normal-renin patients, whereas a 10% decline was observed with the inhibitor. High-renin patients had depressor responses to both drugs, but the inhibitor produced slightly greater depressor responses than did saralasin. Decrements in blood pressure for any level of plasma renin activity were greater after the inhibitor than after saralasin, but blood pressure depressor responses correlated well with the pretreatment renin level. Saralasin was pressor in some studies in anephric patients, whereas the inhibitor produced no apparent trend in diastolic pressures. Greater depressor responses were obtained with the inhibitor in matched studies in patients with renovascular hypertension.

The converting enzyme inhibitor appears to be more sensitive than saralasin in exposing renin involvement in blood pressure maintenance at any level of plasma renin activity. The inhibitor appears not to exert a nonspecific hypotensive action related to bradykinin accumulation. Patients should not be receiving other antihypertensive drugs when given saralasin or the inhibitor.

► [It would be nice to have an office procedure capable of identifying rapidly the 15% or so of hypertensive patients in whom plasma renin levels are excessive for their level of sodium intake and in whom, therefore, the origin of hypertension might properly be investigated further. Saralasin, a specific octapeptide antagonist of angiotensin II, was at first thought to fill the bill. However, it has become apparent that saralasin is a partial agonist, attaching to angiotensin II receptors and weakly stimulating them, so that testing with it may grossly underestimate the role of angiotensin II in sustaining blood pressure. For this reason, various maneuvers (low-salt diet, upright position, salt de-

(5) Am. J. Med. 61:790–796, November, 1976.

pletion with furosemide) have been proposed to increase renin secretion as a preliminary to the test injection of saralasin, in order to "make the test more sensitive." The trouble is that with enough volume depletion almost everybody depends on renin to maintain blood pressure. The new inhibitor of converting enzyme that Doctor Case and his colleagues report on gets away from these difficulties and has the convenient feature that it can be given as a single intravenous bolus rather than a prolonged infusion.

Both agents may produce untoward hypotension in patients already receiving other antihypertensive and diuretic agents and in normal subjects on a tilt table after sodium depletion. – Ed.] ◄

► ↓ The following article reports an example of the failure of saralasin to predict curable hypertension, probably because of its agonist effect. – Ed. ◄

Failure of Saralasin to Predict a Response to Surgery in Renovascular Hypertension. Even if an operable renal lesion is found in a hypertensive patient, the response to surgery is difficult to predict. It was hoped that a hypotensive response to intravenous saralasin in patients with renovascular hypertension might predict a successful response to surgery. R. D. Thomas, S. G. Ball and M. R. Lee[6] (Univ. of Leeds) report 2 cases of renovascular hypertension in which a sustained fall in blood pressure followed surgery, despite the lack of a response to saralasin infusion. Both patients had findings of fibromuscular hyperplasia, predominating on one side, and both had elevated renal venous plasma renin activity on the affected side relative to the unaffected kidney.

Case 1. – Man, 30, with a blood pressure of 200/150 mm Hg, had changes suggestive of fibromuscular hyperplasia, mainly involving the right renal artery, and a renal venous renin activity ratio of 1.5. Saralasin infusion led to no change in diastolic blood pressure, but autotransplantation of the right kidney led to normotension. Blood pressure was 140/90 mm Hg without therapy 18 months after surgery.

Case 2. – Woman, 42, with a blood pressure of 230/130 mm Hg, had changes of fibromuscular hyperplasia, mainly affecting the right renal artery. The renal venous renin ratio was 1.8. Saralasin infusion caused no blood pressure changes, but autotransplantation of the right kidney was followed by a blood pressure of 150/90 mm Hg without treatment 4 months after operation.

False negative responses occur in renovascular hypertension after saralasin administration, if a fall in diastolic pressure is taken as the criterion of a positive response. False positive results may also be obtained, and the test is not entirely without hazard. A negative response to saralasin should not necessarily exclude further study of young patients with severe hypertension. There seems to be a range of plasma renin activity in which saralasin infusion will not accurately determine the presence of renovascular disease. The elucidation of such cases would require an antagonist of angiotensin II that is competitive at all dose ratios.

Curable Hypertension with Unilateral Hydronephrosis: Studies on Role of Circulating Renin. Hypertension with unilateral hydronephrosis is rare. Increased renin levels have been found in the venous effluent of the obstructed kidney. Peter Weidmann, Carlo Beretta-Piccoli, David Hirsch, Francois C. Reubi and Shaul G. Massry[7] performed detailed studies in 1 female and 7 male patients, aged

(6) Lancet 1:724–726, Apr. 2, 1977.
(7) Ann. Intern. Med. 87:437–440, October, 1977.

11–66 years, seen in 1966–1976 with unilateral hydronephrosis and hypertension. Six patients presented with recurrent unilateral lumbar pain, lower abdominal pain or urinary symptoms and 2 were asymptomatic and were found to be hypertensive during routine checkups. All patients had mild to moderate hypertension. Four patients had been hypertensive for 1–5 months and the others for 3–20 years. Antihypertension therapy was withdrawn from 3 patients 2–4 weeks before study. In 7 patients the hydronephrotic kidney was removed, and 1 had a pyeloplasty initially. Plasma renin activity was measured by bioassay and radioimmunoassay.

Plasma renin activity was slightly elevated in 1 patient and normal in 6 patients. In 4 patients in whom the ratio of renal venous renin in the two kidneys was over 1.5 and that between the undiseased kidney and the periphery was less than 1.2, blood pressure returned to normal after nephrectomy, as it did in 2 patients in whom renal venous renin values were unavailable. A significant positive correlation was found between postoperative changes in plasma renin activity and blood pressure changes.

Patients with unilateral hydronephrosis may develop persistent hypertension that may resolve after removal of the diseased kidney, suggesting a causal relation between urinary tract obstruction and hypertension. Evidence for both lateralization of renin production in the hydronephrotic kidney and renin suppression in the contralateral kidney may be required for prediction of a favorable effect of surgery on the hypertension.

► [Most patients with hydronephrosis do not develop hypertension. In those who do, the elevated blood pressure may or may not improve when urinary obstruction is relieved. The suggestion here is that reversible hypertension due to hydronephrosis can be diagnosed, like renovascular hypertension, on the basis of differential measurements of renal venous renin. In such patients, blood flow to the kidney is probably compromised by a greatly distended renal pelvis and high intracapsular pressure. – Ed.]

Age and the Renin-Aldosterone System. Age-related changes in the renin-aldosterone system are well documented in patients with essential hypertension. Whether or not similar changes occur in older normotensive subjects is relevant to plasma renin activity (PRA) classification. Robert H. Noth, M. Nathan Lassman, S. Y. Tan, Arturo Fernandez-Cruz, Jr., and Patrick J. Mulrow[8] (Yale Univ.) sought an age effect on PRA in young and older normotensive subjects. Study was made of 17 subjects aged 20–29 years and 19 aged 50–58 years. The normotensive subjects were studied while on their usual diet and on day 4 of a 10-mEq sodium, 75-mEq potassium diet. Several patients in each group received 40 mg furosemide orally on the 1st day of the low-salt diet. Data on 11 young and 15 older patients with essential hypertension were analyzed retrospectively.

Among normal subjects on a normal diet, PRA was significantly lower in the older subjects in the supine position and after 3 or 4 hours of ambulation. On day 4 of the low-sodium diet, PRA was also lower in the older subjects when supine, and the difference was accentuated by ambulation. Among patients with essential hypertension, ambulatory

(8) Arch. Intern. Med. 137:1414–1417, October, 1977.

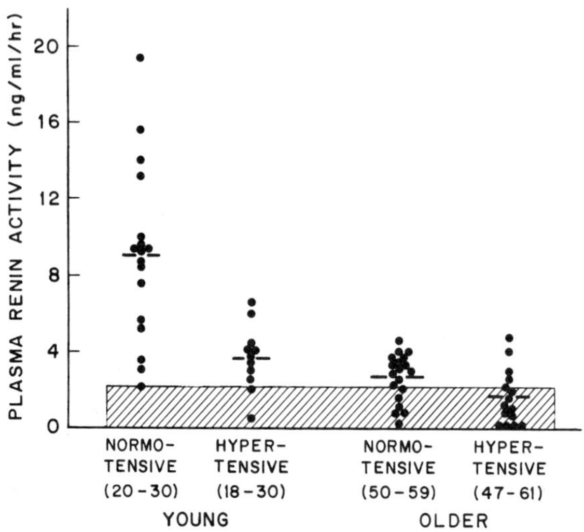

Fig 12.—Age and plasma renin activity (PRA) classification, method 1. Circles represent PRA in normotensive volunteers and patients with essential hypertension determined under set conditions (day 4 of 10-mEq-sodium diet after 4 hours' ambulation). Age range for each group is indicated in parentheses. Shaded area indicates abnormally low range based on data from young normotensives. (Courtesy of Noth, R. H., et al.: Arch. Intern. Med. 137:1414–1417, October, 1977; copyright 1977, American Medical Association.)

PRA values after sodium restriction were lower in the older group despite comparable sodium balances. The incidence of low-renin hypertension increased from 18% to 60% with increasing age (Fig 12). Urinary aldosterone values were comparable in younger and older subjects in both the normotensive and the hypertensive series, and other laboratory values were comparable in younger and older normotensive subjects.

The use of predominantly young control subjects for defining normal limits of PRA may result in an overestimate of the incidence of low-renin hypertension and may contribute to the heterogeneity of low-renin hypertension. Longitudinal data on PRA classification are needed to determine whether the pathogenesis of hypertension differs in the young and in the elderly.

► [The striking decrease in plasma renin with age raises some questions. (1) Is "low-renin hypertension" really a separate entity—or simply an expression of aging? (2) How is this phenomenon related to "hyporeninemic hypoaldosteronism"? (3) What does renin have to do with hypertension anyway? See below.—Ed.] ◄

Chronic One-Kidney Hypertension in Rabbits. III. Renopressin, a New Hypertensive Substance was investigated by Leonard T. Skeggs, Joseph R. Kahn, Melvin Levine, Frederic E. Dorer and Kenneth E. Lentz[9] (Case Western Reserve Univ.). The blood pressure of rabbits with chronic one-kidney hypertension can be reduced to normal by immunization with hog renal cortex preparations that do not contain renin, suggesting a new factor essential for the maintenance of elevated blood pressure. A substance that increases the blood pressure

(9) Circ. Res. 40:143–149, February, 1977.

of normal rabbits over several days, for an indefinite time, has been discovered and termed renopressin. Studies were done in young male rabbits, in some of which hypertension was produced by clipping one renal artery and removing the other kidney. The starting material for all preparations was a crude extract of renal cortex.

Administration of certain cortical extracts to normal rabbits caused a delayed, slow rise in blood pressure and the establishment of a state of moderate, persistent hypertension. The pressure elevation was sustained for at least 94 days after subcutaneous administration of the substance. The hypertension was not blocked by an angiotensin II antagonist. Renopressin did not increase the blood pressure of hypertensive rabbits. The pressure of hypertensive rabbits and of normal rabbits made hypertensive by injection of renopressin was reduced to normal by passive immunization with the same antibody preparation.

The findings are consistent with the possibility that renopressin and the agent causing elevation of blood pressure in hypertensive rabbits are similar or identical. The antibodies produced in hypertensive rabbits by immunization with hog preparations containing renopressin must be directed both toward the substance responsible for elevated pressure in hypertensive rabbits and against the renopressin that elevates the blood pressure of rabbits receiving injections.

► [Keep an eye on this. While our attention has been focused on renin for a long time, the fact is that (1) most patients with essential hypertension have normal or low plasma renin levels and (2) the same is true of most patients with parenchymal kidney disease complicated by hypertension. (Whether the levels of renin they do have are "inappropriate" for their blood pressure and volume status is arguable.) Thus, the time is ripe for a nonrenin renal mechanism to explain high blood pressure. Maybe Doctor Skeggs has a handle on it! – Ed.] ◄

Prostaglandins

► I've included several articles that deal with the effect of prostaglandins on the kidney because this is a new and most exciting field. Prostaglandins and thromboxanes comprise a group of polyunsaturated, hydroxylated, long-chain fatty acids with remarkable biologic actions at extremely low concentrations. These compounds are ubiquitous and appear to be manufactured by all tissues so far examined. A great many of the physiologic effects of essential fatty acids are explained by the fact that they are substrates for prostaglandin biosynthesis. Prostaglandins are rapidly metabolized to inactive forms and generally appear to produce their action in the tissue in which they are synthesized. The first step in their synthesis is usually the release of unsaturated fatty acids (arachidonic acid) from intracellular phospholipid stores by phospholipase A, a reaction that is blocked, interestingly enough, by glucocorticoids. The further processing of arachidonic acid to prostaglandins is inhibited by nonsteroid anti-inflammatory agents.

Prostaglandins of the class "E" are produced in the kidney by the interstitial cells of the renal medulla. Their synthesis appears to be stimulated by renal ischemia or conditions (angiotensin administration, renal nerve stimulation) that predispose to a decrease in renal blood flow. (However, bradykinin, a vasodilating peptide, also stimulates renal prostaglandin.) So far, the following actions on renal function have been documented: (1) An increase in the synthesis of renin. This may be important in the genesis of Bartter's syndrome. (2) Renal vasodilatation and increase in total and renomedullary blood flow. Chronic inhibition of prostaglandin synthesis might therefore contribute to analgesic nephropathy. (3) Antagonism of the antidiuretic effect of vasopressin. This may prove to be the basis of several forms of nephrogenic diabetes insipidus. (4) Salt and water diuresis. This possibly is secondary, in part, to a direct action on the collecting tubule, as suggested by the following article. – Ed. ◄

Inhibition of Sodium Transport by Prostaglandin E_2 across the Isolated, Perfused Rabbit Collecting Tubule. John B. Stokes and Juha P. Kokko[1] (Southwestern Med. School) examined directly the effect of prostaglandin E_2 (PGE_2) on sodium transport, across the in vitro perfused rabbit collecting tubule, to evaluate the possibility that a naturally occurring intrarenal substance could modulate sodium transport by the collecting tubule. Changes in transepithelial potential and isotopic sodium fluxes in response to peritubular PGE_2 were measured in segments of collecting tubules from rabbits. Changes in transepithelial potential of the outer medullary collecting tubule in response to PGE_2 were also measured. Most rabbits received 5 mg deoxycorticosterone acetate (DOCA) daily for 4 – 11 days before study.

Prostaglandin E_2 inhibited the negative transepithelial potential in both the cortical collecting tubule and the outer medullary collecting tubule. It inhibited net sodium transport out of the lumen by inhibiting efflux, whereas backflux was unaffected. Prostaglandin E_2 produced inhibition within 15 minutes; the effects were dose dependent and reversible.

The findings constitute the first evidence that PGE_2 can affect renal tubular sodium transport directly. The evidence that the effect of PGE_2

(1) J. Clin. Invest. 59:1099 – 1104, June, 1977.

is physiologically significant is circumstantial but supported by several studies. Prostaglandin E_2 can inhibit sodium efflux from the lumens of cortical collecting tubules of rabbits stimulated by DOCA. The inhibition is rapid, reversible and dose dependent. Prostaglandin E_2 exerts a similar effect on the outer medullary collecting tubules, greatly enhancing the probability that PGE_2 acts in vivo to inhibit directly sodium reabsorption by the collecting tubule.

► [The effect of prostaglandins to modulate the tubular absorption of sodium in the direction of diuresis may turn out to be most pronounced in sodium-retaining states. Similar experiments by Fine and Trizna (Am. J. Physiol. 232:383, 1977), in which pretreatment with mineralocorticoids was omitted, showed no natriuretic effect of prostaglandin on isolated tubules. Furthermore, prostaglandin inhibition had no effect on sodium excretion during diuresis induced by expansion of the extracellular fluid volume (Kirschenbaum, M. A., and Stein, J. H.: J. Lab. Clin. Med. 90:46, 1977). – Ed.] ◄

Exaggerated Prostaglandin Biosynthesis and Its Influence on Renal Resistance in the Isolated Hydronephrotic Rabbit Kidney. Increasing experimental evidence points to a role for prostaglandins in regulating the renal circulation. Kohei Nishikawa, Aubrey Morrison and Philip Needleman[2] (Washington Univ.) studied the changes in renal prostaglandin (PG) biosynthesis that occur in a ureteral obstruction model of hydronephrosis in rabbits. Renal perfusion was carried out 3 days after ureteral ligation. Isolated assay tissues, including rat stomach strip and chick rectum, were continuously superfused by the renal venous effluent. Renal phospholipids were prelabeled by renal infusion of ^{14}C-arachidonate. Studies were also performed in genetic hydronephrotic rats.

Responsiveness to bradykinin was enhanced in the ureter-obstructed hydronephrotic rabbit kidney at 72 hours. Responses to angiotensin II and norepinephrine were also enhanced. The effect was not explained by reduced PG destruction or decreased renal peptide (bradykinin or angiotensin) inactivation. There was no enhanced PG biosynthesis with exogenous arachidonate. Renal tubular transport of PG from the medulla to the cortex did not appear to be essential for the enhanced PG synthetic response to hormone stimulation. Indomethacin increased basal perfusion pressure in the obstructed kidney and enhanced the renal vasoconstriction produced by angiotensin II in the hydronephrotic kidney. A dose-dependent increase in release of PG-like substance was seen when bradykinin was injected into the isolated perfused rat kidney with genetic hydronephrosis.

Ureteral obstruction initiates an enhanced basal release of prostaglandin E_2, which is further exaggerated by peptide hormone stimulation. The release represents de novo biosynthesis. There is a clear dissociation between renal biosynthesis and the triglyceride content and number of interstitial lipid cell droplets. Local synthesis of PG in cortical resistance vessels may take place. Prostaglandin E_2 may be a protective mechanism initiated to overcome the severe renal vasoconstriction and decrease in glomerular filtration normally associated with chronic hydronephrosis. Enhanced PG synthesis in hydronephrosis may explain the reduction in sodium reabsorption and natri-

(2) J. Clin. Invest. 59:1143–1150, June, 1977.

uresis that are associated with ureteral obstruction and could conceivably be involved in the enhanced sodium excretion that is observed in postobstructive diuresis as well as the reduction in concentrating ability that occurs in obstructive uropathy.

► [Prostaglandins are manufactured by interstitial cells of the renal medulla and might therefore be expected to reach high concentration in the medulla and have special functional effects localized to renal papillary structures. Three such effects have been defined. The first is vascular; prostaglandin E_2 acts as a vasodilator and increases blood flow to the medulla. Second, prostaglandin appears to increase sodium excretion, at least under some circumstances (see the preceding article), by inhibiting sodium transport in the collecting ducts. Third, it antagonizes the action of antidiuretic hormone in medullary collecting ducts (Grantham, J. J., and Orloff, J.: J. Clin. Invest. 47:1154, 1968), and so decreases maximal urinary concentration.

This article shows that hydronephrotic kidneys produce prostaglandins excessively in response to a variety of stimuli. May not, therefore, the well-known salt-wasting tendency, the impaired concentrating ability and the familiar postobstructive diuresis be due, at least in part, to prostaglandin production?

Inhibition of prostaglandin synthesis was recently shown by S. P. Levison and M. E. Levison to reverse the renal concentrating defect in experimental enterococcal pyelonephritis in rats (J. Lab. Clin. Med. 88:958, 1976). It seems as if the role of prostaglandins should be investigated in every disorder of concentrating ability. – Ed.] ◄

Hemodynamic Effects of Potassium Deficiency in the Dog. Potassium deficiency is associated with several hemodynamic changes in both man and experimental animals. The arterial blood pressure is reduced and salt retention occurs, but the cause of the latter change is not clear. Oscar G. Galvez, William H. Bay, Bertram W. Roberts and Thomas F. Ferris[3] (Ohio State Univ.) performed balance studies in potassium-depleted dogs and measured several cardiovascular functions. Angiotensin I was infused before and after hemodialysis with a potassium-free dialysate in 10 female dogs and a potassium-free diet was then given, followed by indomethacin administration for 3 days. Plasma renin activity was measured by radioimmunoassay.

Cumulative sodium retention of 374 mEq occurred with a weight increase of 2.3 kg during 3 weeks of potassium deficiency. The serum potassium fell from 4.5 to 1.8 mEq and remained at 2 – 2.5 mEq/L during this time. Urinary potassium fell to about 5 mEq daily on the potassium-free diet. Serum sodium rose from 146 to 156 mEq/L. No significant change in mean arterial pressure was noted but the cardiac output increased and the peripheral resistance declined. A significant expansion of blood volume and insulin space was observed. There were no significant changes in glomerular filtration rate or para-aminohippuric acid clearance. Plasma renin activity rose from 0.4 to 17.2 ng/ml per hour. There was no significant increase in plasma aldosterone. Changes in urinary prostaglandin E excretion are shown in Figure 13. Saralasin reduced the arterial pressure during the hypokalemic period. Angiotensin sensitivity was partially restored by indomethacin administration. No change in potassium or sodium balance was observed during indomethacin treatment.

Hypokalemia increased urinary prostaglandin E in these studies, with extracellular fluid volume expansion, decreased sensitivity to angiotensin and increased plasma renin activity occurring. The de-

(3) Circ. Res. 40 (Suppl. 1):11 – 16, May, 1977.

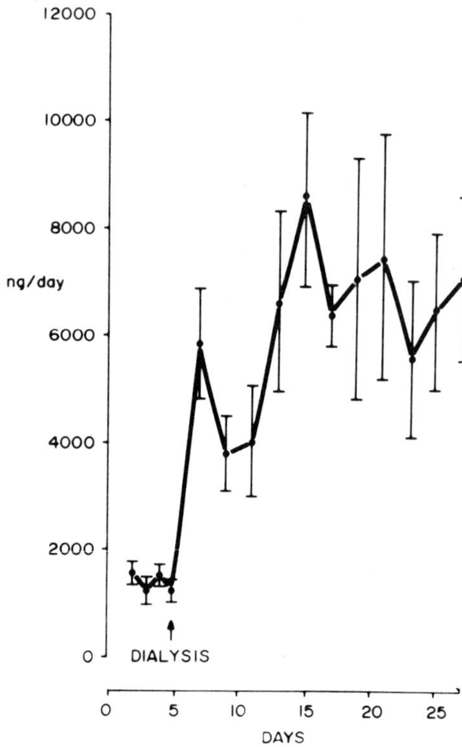

Fig 13.—Urinary prostaglandin E (PGE)-like material in all dogs throughout the study. (Courtesy of Galvez, O. G., et al.: Circ. Res. 40 (Suppl. 1):11–16, May, 1977; by permission of the American Heart Association, Inc.)

creased sensitivity to angiotensin noted with hypokalemia appears to be due to increased prostaglandin E synthesis.

► [The striking increase in production and excretion of prostaglandin E induced by potassium deficiency is major news. It explains a number of heretofore puzzling features of the physiology of potassium depletion. Polyuria that is resistant to vasopressin is a hallmark of advanced potassium deficiency—a result of the antagonism of vasopressin by prostaglandins. In further studies, the renal concentrating defect in these dogs that was produced by potassium depletion was completely reversed by indomethacin treatment.

The tendency to low blood pressure that is also a feature of severe potassium depletion might also be explainable by excessive secretion of the vasodilating prostaglandins. Finally, prostaglandin E has been found to inhibit acute insulin responses and impair glucose tolerance in normal human subjects (Robertson, R. P., and Chen, M.: J. Clin. Invest. 60:747, 1977). Is it possible that this is responsible for the effect of potassium depletion to produce mild diabetes?

It is intriguing to speculate on the relationship of this experiment to Bartter's syndrome of hypokalemic potassium-wasting with elevated plasma renin, angiotensin resistance, high urinary prostaglandin levels and normal blood pressure. Since potassium deficiency alone will increase the production of prostaglandin and renin, the authors suggest that some cases of Bartter's syndrome may represent a primary potassium-wasting disorder of the kidneys. One trouble with this hypothesis is that most patients with Bartter's syndrome have elevated plasma aldosterone levels, whereas potassium deficiency in man or experimental animals does not usually increase the secretion of aldosterone. The low serum potassium present in patients with primary potassium deficiency opposes the stimulatory action of renin on aldosterone production by zona glomerulosa cells of the adrenal cortex (see the article by P. Fredlund et al. in the chapter on Potassium). – Ed.] ◄

Aspirin-Induced Depression of Renal Function. Robert F. Kimberly and Paul H. Plotz[4] (Natl. Inst. of Health) have observed elevations of serum creatinine and blood urea nitrogen and a reduction in creatinine clearance in several patients taking anti-inflammatory doses of aspirin. Increases in serum creatinine of 27–163% and in urea nitrogen of 42–270% were found in 13 of 23 patients with systemic lupus erythematosus (SLE). Sequential creatinine clearance measurements, available in 11 of the 13 patients, showed reductions of up to 58%. Patients with altered renal function were more likely than the others to have active renal disease or hypocomplementemia. Four of 22 patients with rheumatoid arthritis and 2 of 3 normal subjects also showed biochemical changes, but the rate of aspirin-induced change was significantly greater in SLE than in rheumatoid arthritis. Similar changes in renal function were observed in 2 patients with SLE who were receiving indomethacin and in 1 receiving naproxen.

Aspirin and other nonsteroid anti-inflammatory agents can have a major reversible effect on renal function, which may influence interpretations of clinical data. In patients with SLE, the presence of active nephritis or hypocomplementemia appears to predispose to aspirin-induced changes. Changes in renal function have been observed with salicylate concentrations of 20–25 mg/dl, although some patients had higher values. Precise dose-response relations have not been established. Awareness of the potential for aspirin and other medications to alter renal function in clinical situations in which it may influence management decisions is critical for proper diagnostic evaluation and therapeutic intervention.

► [The depression of renal function induced by aspirin in these patients involved changes of serum creatinine within the low measurable range – 0.8–2.4 mg/100 ml – real enough, but not exactly frightening. The interesting thing is that they occurred predominantly in patients with active nephritis. Now, it seems clear that renal secretion of prostaglandins is stimulated when blood flow to the kidneys (renal medulla?) is threatened, and that the local vasodilating action of prostaglandins may serve to maintain renal circulation. It should not be surprising, then, that aspirin and other inhibitors of prostaglandin synthesis seem to decrease renal function selectively in those patients with inflammatory or circulatory threats to the integrity of the circulation to the kidneys.

It is an old observation that edema is occasionally associated with salicylate treatment, an observation that has been echoed more recently in reports of edema with other "anti-inflammatory" agents like phenylbutazone, indomethacin and ibuprofen (J.A.M.A. 237:1716, 1977) and by the finding that prostaglandin inhibitors (aspirin, indomethacin) blunt the diuresis produced by furosemide (Scand. J. Clin. Lab. Invest. 37: 125, 1977). – Ed.] ◄

---

(4) N. Engl. J. Med. 296:418–424, Feb. 24, 1977.

Potassium

Impaired Renal Tubular Potassium Secretion in Systemic Lupus Erythematosus. Impaired renal potassium secretion in the absence of advanced renal insufficiency and with a normal renin-aldosterone axis has only rarely been reported. Ralph A. DeFronzo, C. Robert Cooke, Martin Goldberg, Malcolm Cox, Allen R. Myers and Zalman S. Agus[5] recently encountered 2 patients with systemic lupus erythematosus and only mildly reduced glomerular filtration rates and normal aldosterone secretion, who had persistent hyperkalemia and impaired renal tubular potassium secretion. Ability to increase aldosterone and renin secretion was examined after 2–3 days of a low-sodium diet and furosemide administration. Patients then received fludrocortisone acetate orally for 4–6 days and 1 then received a combination of acetazolamide and sodium bicarbonate.

The observations made in 1 patient are illustrated in Figure 14. Both patients achieved sodium and potassium balance in a 3- to 5-day equilibration period, but constant potassium balance was achieved at the expense of elevated serum potassium levels. Urinary aldosterone excretion increased normally with a normal rise in plasma aldosterone on sodium depletion with furosemide and a low-sodium diet; sodium excretion increased markedly but the plasma renin response was markedly impaired in both subjects. Potassium excretion remained unchanged on fludrocortisone administration. Potassium excretion increased only minimally in the patient given acetazolamide and bicarbonate, despite a marked rise in sodium excretion.

Defective potassium excretion could result from decreased delivery of sodium to distal reabsorptive sites, a defect in aldosterone secretion or a primary defect in tubular potassium secretion. Three of 4 previously described patients with defective tubular potassium secretion in the absence of significant renal impairment of hypoaldosteronism were children and 1 was a patient with systemic lupus. The 2 present patients were among about 50 new patients seen in the past year with systemic lupus erythematosus, a prevalence of about 4%. In both patients the baseline plasma aldosterone was elevated and plasma renin activity failed to increase normally after depletion and volume contraction. These findings probably reflect stimulation of aldosterone secretion and suppression of renin release by persistent hyperkalemia.

► [The defect in renal tubular secretion of potassium seen in these patients is probably related to an interstitial lupus nephritis mediated by immune complexes. The key finding is the failure of potassium excretion to increase under the stimulus of mineralcorticoid administration. This feature and the normal plasma levels of aldosterone distinguish this form of "renal tubular hyperkalemia" from hyporeninemic hypoaldosteronism. One would expect that some deficiency in potassium excretion would be found

(5) Ann. Intern. Med. 86:268–271, March, 1977.

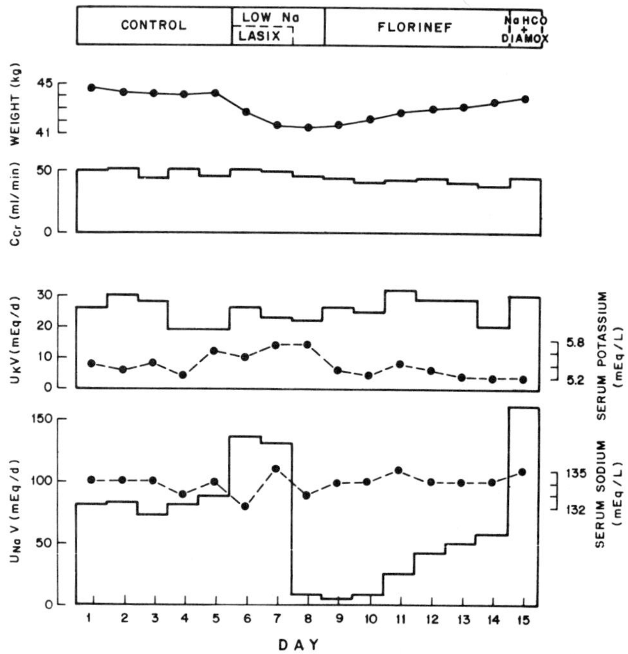

Fig 14. – Changes in urinary sodium and potassium excretion and serum potassium concentration after sodium depletion, furosemide (Lasix), fludrocortisone acetate (Florinef) and acetazolamide (Diamox) plus sodium bicarbonate administration in patient. C_{Cr}, creatine clearance; U_{Na} V, 24-hour urinary sodium excretion; U_KV, 24-hour urinary potassium excretion. (Courtesy of DeFronzo, R. A., et al.: Ann. Intern. Med. 86:268–271, March, 1977.)

frequently in varieties of interstitial nephritis involving the distal tubule and the collecting ducts of the renal papilla, because these are where potassium is secreted. For example, frank hyperkalemia may be seen in medullary cystic disease, especially if salt intake is restricted. Doctor DeFronzo and his colleagues reported at the 10th annual meeting of the American Society of Nephrology that excretion of an intravenous load of potassium is impaired in patients with sickle cell anemia, in whom medullary fibrosis is common. Impaired secretion of potassium may also be apparent after renal transplantation, as in the following article. – Ed.] ◄

Investigations into Mechanisms of Hyperkalemia Following Renal Transplantation. Disorders of renal tubular function have been recognized with increasing frequency after renal transplantation, but hyperkalemia has rarely been described in this setting. Ralph A. DeFronzo, Martin Goldberg, C. Robert Cooke, Clyde Barker, Robert A. Grossman and Zalman S. Agus[6] observed a high rate of hyperkalemia in renal transplantation patients and attempted to define its frequency and to relate it to the presence or absence of rejection and to the development of hyperchloremic acidosis. Data were reviewed on 75 consecutive patients undergoing renal transplantation in 1973–75, and 4 patients who developed hyperkalemia after successful renal transplantation were studied prospectively. The latter patients received a diet containing 22 mEq sodium daily for 3 days and then a high-sodium diet and 9α-fluorohydrocortisone.

---

(6) Kidney Int. 11:357–365, May, 1977.

Hyperkalemia was found in 23 of the 75 patients within 3 months after renal transplantation. It was unrelated to rejection, renal failure, oliguria or acidosis. Patients with hyperkalemia achieved sodium and potassium balance during low sodium intake and furosemide administration but at the expense of significant hyperkalemia (5.3–5.7 mEq/L). Plasma aldosterone concentration and urinary aldosterone excretion rose with sodium restriction in these patients. Treatment with 9α-fluorohydrocortisone when sodium intake was high failed to increase urinary potassium excretion. Neither furosemide nor acetazolamide plus sodium bicarbonate produced a consistent rise in potassium excretion, but hydrochlorothiazide increased urinary potassium excretion in 3 patients, and each had a fall in serum potassium concentration to normal. Three patients had kaliuretic responses to 9α-fluorohydrocortisone and furosemide when restudied with a normal serum potassium concentration.

The findings indicate a reversible defect in urinary potassium excretion after renal transplantation, which is apparently related to an abnormality of renal tubular function. The mechanism of correction with thiazides is unclear. The data do not exclude the possibility that the hyperkalemia is a manifestation of renal tubular rejection.

► [The mild hyperkalemia seen in patients like this should be distinguished from the slightly elevated serum potassium frequently encountered in patients with acidosis or with heart failure, especially when they are on low-salt diets. In those instances, potassium excretion by the kidney is limited for functional reasons. In the patients discussed in this article, excretion of potassium could not be increased by administration of sodium bicarbonate or mineralocorticoids. Thiazide diuretics, however, produced kaliuresis. Presumably there was a distal tubular defect in potassium secretion.

Another reason for persistent hyperkalemia after renal transplantation was illustrated by the case report entitled, "Hyporeninemic Hypoaldosteronism after Renal Transplantation," by G. O. Perez and J. R. Oster (J.A.M.A. 70:363, 1977). In their patient, a defect in adrenal function rather than in the kidney was postulated. – Ed.] ◄

Aldosterone Production by Isolated Glomerulosa Cells: Modulation of Sensitivity to Angiotensin II and ACTH by Extracellular Potassium Concentration. The control of aldosterone secretion at the adrenal level is known to be influenced by changes in plasma concentrations of angiotensin II, ACTH, sodium and potassium, but the mechanisms of control during changes in sodium and potassium balance are uncertain. The use of adrenal cells in vitro under incubation conditions reproducing physiologic changes in electrolyte and peptide hormone concentrations should provide a more complete picture of the interactions between potassium and peptide hormones at the adrenal level. Paul Fredlund, Steven Saltman, Takuma Kondo, Janice Douglas and Kevin J. Catt[7] (Natl. Inst. of Health) used isolated canine glomerulosa cells to investigate the effects of extracellular potassium concentration on the aldosterone responses to angiotensin II and ACTH. Binding properties of ^{125}I-angiotensin II were examined in cultures of collagenase-dispersed canine glomerulosa cells.

Aldosterone production by the cells in response to angiotensin II was highly dependent on the concentration of potassium in the incubation medium. At 2.5×10^{-11}M, the normal circulating level of angiotensin II,

(7) Endocrinology 100:481–486, February, 1977.

aldosterone formation increased fourfold as the medium potassium was increased from 2.5 to 5 mM and sixfold as it was increased from 2.5 to 7.5 mM. Both high-affinity and low-affinity binding sites were present at all potassium concentrations, and association constants did not change significantly with variations in extracellular potassium concentration. Aldosterone production by isolated glomerulosa cells in response to ACTH was also influenced by the medium potassium concentration. The action of ACTH was markedly enhanced when the medium potassium was increased to 5 mM.

The production of aldosterone by isolated canine glomerulosa cells in response to angiotensin II and ACTH is highly dependent on the concentration of potassium in the incubation medium. The findings suggest that potassium-stimulated aldosterone production in vivo could be potentiated by increased sensitivity of the zona glomerulosa to circulating levels of angiotensin II. The precise mechanism of the enhanced sensitivity of the glomerulosa cell to angiotensin II with increasing potassium concentration remains to be determined. The results suggest that the effect of potassium on aldosterone production in vivo is expressed through changes in the sensitivity of glomerulosa cells to peptide hormones, as well as by the direct influence of potassium on steroidogenesis in the zona glomerulosa.

► [These elegant studies of isolated adrenal cells supply the answer to a perplexing question about hyporeninemic hypoaldosteronism. In that condition (1973 YEAR BOOK, p. 635; and 1974 YEAR BOOK, p. 663), low plasma renin is associated with hyperkalemia which elicits an inadequate plasma aldosterone response. Because potassium stimulates the zona glomerulosa of the adrenal directly, rather than through the intermediate offices of renin, why shouldn't a normal adrenal respond to the high serum potassium with enough secretion of aldosterone to bring the level of potassium in serum to normal? The answer is that the adrenal's aldosterone response to angiotensin (or ACTH) is conditioned by the level of potassium, *and the response to potassium is influenced by the level of angiotensin or ACTH.* With abnormally low levels of angiotensin, aldosterone output by normal adrenal cells is reduced at every level of serum potassium.—Ed.] ◄

Amelioration of Metabolic Acidosis with Fludrocortisone Therapy in Hyporeninemic Hypoaldosteronism. Patients with hyperchloremic acidosis associated with hyporeninemic hypoaldosteronism have reduced renal potassium clearance. They have a combined defect in renal tubular secretion of hydrogen ion and potassium. The occurrence of hypoaldosteronism in these patients suggests that the renal dysfunction might be caused by aldosterone deficiency. Anthony Sebastian, Morris Schambelan, Stanley Lindenfeld and R. Curtis Morris, Jr.[8] (San Francisco) studied 4 men with hyporeninemic hypoaldosteronism. Each had stable chronic renal insufficiency (creatinine clearance, 13–44 ml/minute) with persistent hyperkalemia and hyperchloremic metabolic acidosis. Serum potassium was 5.8–6.7 mEq/L, serum bicarbonate 16–21 mEq/L and serum chloride 111–116 mEQ/L. Plasma renin activity was frankly subnormal or low normal and subnormally stimulated by posture and volume depletion. Urinary aldosterone excretion was either frankly subnormal or inappropriately low for the degree of hyperkalemia. The effects of oral fludro-

(8) N. Engl. J. Med. 297:576–583, Sept. 15, 1977.

cortisone were assessed in five balance studies during spontaneous acidosis and the effects of discontinuance of fludrocortisone in two other studies.

Net acid excretion increased during hormone administration, and systemic acidosis was corrected or nearly corrected. Three of the 4 patients required 0.2–0.4 mg fluorohydrocortisone daily. A higher rate of urinary ammonium excretion contributed to the increase in net acid excretion in each study. Urine pH declined when treatment was begun in each study. Urinary potassium excretion increased and the serum potassium concentration declined to normokalemic levels. When fludrocortisone was discontinued, urine pH promptly increased, net acid excretion declined and acidosis recurred.

Mineralocorticoid administration can augment renal hydrogen ion secretion and renal ammonia production and ameliorate metabolic acidosis in patients with hyporeninemic hypoaldosteronism, but this treatment may not be indicated in hypertensive patients or those with limited cardiac reserve. Restriction of dietary potassium and treatment with potassium-binding resins, sodium bicarbonate and loop diuretics may be considered in such patients.

► [As chronic renal insufficiency gradually progresses, the remaining nephrons maintain serum potassium constant in the face of an unchanged dietary load by increasing the tubular secretion of potassium into the urine. One way in which they are enabled to do this is through an increased rate of secretion of aldosterone. If aldactone is given to such patients, hyperkalemia is more pronounced than in normal subjects and acidosis appears. The mechanism of extracellular acidosis is probably twofold: (1) aldosterone directly stimulates H^+ secretion by the kidney, and suppression of its action reduces acid excretion; and (2) hyperkalemia depresses renal production of ammonia and also exchanges with intracellular H^+ to exacerbate acidosis.

What this article suggests is that in certain patients with moderate renal failure, usually with low plasma renin, the adrenal fails to respond to the challenge and secretes suboptimal amounts of aldosterone. The result is hyperkalemic, hyperchloremic metabolic acidosis that can be controlled by supplying the needed additional mineralocorticoid. The amount required is usually larger than that required to maintain an addisonian patient, i.e., more than 0.1 mg fludrocortisone per day. The label "hyporeninemic hypoaldosteronism" may be a misnomer, because some patients have normal plasma renin levels. There is usually, however, an abnormal aldosterone response to a variety of stimuli (like hyperkalemia) that directly stimulate the adrenal gland. In some instances, therefore, a defect may be present at the level of adrenal gland cells.

Diabetic patients with renal disease (sometimes mild, sometimes severe) seem particularly susceptible to hyperkalemia. G. O. Perez et al. (Arch. Intern. Med. 137:852, 1977) point out that the response of plasma aldosterone and plasma renin to the upright posture is severely blunted in diabetes, whether or not hyperkalemia is present. The reason for this isn't clear; it may be related to insulin deficiency or to inapparent diabetic neuropathy involving the sympathetic nervous system. – Ed.] ◄

Diuretics and Potassium Metabolism: Reassessment of the Need, Effectiveness and Safety of Potassium Therapy is presented by Jerome P. Kassirer and John T. Harrington[9] (New England Med. Center Hosp., Boston). An estimated 20 to 30 billion mEq potassium is now prescribed annually. Many studies have shown that the correlation between serum potassium concentration and total body potassium stores is not close, even in the absence of acid-base disturbances. Documentation of depletion of body potassium stores in patients

(9) Kidney Int. 11:505–515, June, 1977.

on long-term diuretic therapy is considerably less definite than observations of serum potassium concentration. At most, a small deficit occurs in hypertensive patients or in normal subjects given oral diuretics. Studies in patients on diuretics have shown little or no alteration in renal function. The major risks of potassium supplementation are hyperkalemic cardiac arrest and small bowel ulceration. Cardiac arrest is the most serious risk.

The lack of clear evidence of clinically significant potassium depletion in nonedematous patients given diuretics and the small risk of life-threatening hyperkalemia lead to the conclusion that neither potassium-sparing diuretics nor potassium supplementation should be routinely given such patients. Rather, the serum potassium concentration should be monitored before treatment and every 1 or 2 months thereafter until a pattern emerges. If the serum potassium concentration remains above 3 mEq/L, there is little reason to attempt to alter it unless symptoms clearly attributable to potassium deficiency develop. In edematous patients the value of restoring potassium balance appears to outweigh the risk of potassium salt or potassium-sparing diuretic treatment. Treatment is probably warranted in patients receiving digitalis and in those susceptible to development of hepatic coma. Potassium chloride and distal blocking agents should be used together only in patients with severe, refractory potassium deficiency, and such treatment requires frequent monitoring of the serum potassium concentration.

► [Very sensible message! The routine use of potassium with diuretics to prevent hypokalemia is unnecessary and also expensive. The cost in Boston of 50 mEq potassium per day, or equivalent therapy in the form of spironolactone, is roughly $8 to $16 per month. In one hospital-based drug surveillance program, these authors note, the frequency of fatal or life-threatening hyperkalemia in hospitalized patients receiving "routine" potassium was 1 in 200. The frequency of hyperkalemia is highest in the elderly and in patients with impaired renal function or diabetes. Large supplements of oral potassium salts are also poorly tolerated in patients with congestive heart failure. – Ed.]

On Mechanism of Polyuria in Potassium Depletion: Role of Polydipsia. The association of hypokalemia with polyuria and a renal concentrating defect has been well established in man and experimental animals, and animal studies have suggested that the derangements may be partly due to a decrease in medullary tonicity. Tomas Berl, Stuart L. Linas, Gary A. Aisenbrey and Robert J. Anderson[1] (Univ. of Colorado) sought to determine whether hypokalemia has a primary effect on thirst and, if so, whether the ensuing polydipsia contributes to the polyuria or to development of the renal concentrating defect or to both. Water intake was compared in rats on potassium-supplemented and potassium-deficient diets. The contributions of polyuria and polydipsia to the concentrating defect in hypokalemia were determined by comparing the urine osmolality of hypokalemic rats allowed free access to water with that of equally hypokalemic rats that were water restricted.

Water intake of rats on a potassium-deficient diet (5 mEq/kg food) became abnormal after 5 days. These rats also consumed less food.

(1) J. Clin. Invest. 60:620–625, September, 1977.

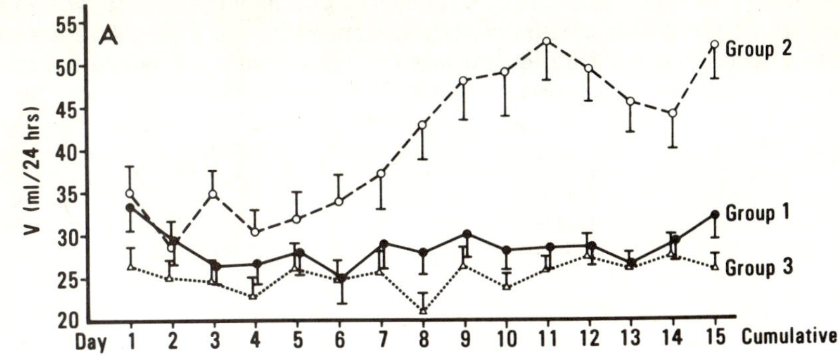

p values

	1	2	3	4	5	6	7	8	9	10	11	12	13	14	15	Cumulative
GROUP 1 VS 2	NS	NS	.05	NS	NS	.05	.05	.005	.001	.001	.001	.001	.001	.001	.001	.001
GROUP 2 VS 3	NS	NS	.01	NS	NS	.05	.01	.001	.001	.001	.001	.001	.001	.001	.001	.001
GROUP 1 VS 3	NS	NS	NS	NS	NS	NS	NS	NS	NS	NS	NS	NS	NS	NS	NS	NS

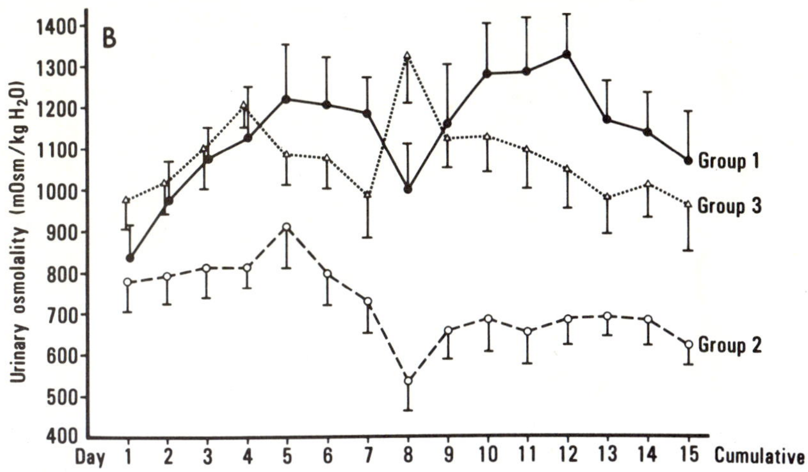

p values

	1	2	3	4	5	6	7	8	9	10	11	12	13	14	15	Cumulative
GROUP 1 VS 2	NS	NS	NS	.01	.05	.05	.0025	.0025	.001	.001	.001	.001	.001	.001	.001	.001
GROUP 2 VS 3	NS	NS	.05	.001	NS	.025	.05	.001	.0025	.0025	.0025	.01	.01	.0025	.0025	.001
GROUP 1 VS 3	NS	NS	NS	NS	NS	NS	NS	.05	NS	NS	NS	.05	NS	NS	NS	NS

Fig 15.—Mean urine flow (**A**) and mean daily urine osmolality (**B**) of rats on normal potassium intake (group 1, n = 12, *solid circles*), potassium-deficient diet and unrestricted access to water (group 2, n = 12, *open circles*) and potassium-deficient diet with water intake matched to that of rats on normal-potassium diet (group 3, n = 14, *open triangles*). (Courtesy of Berl, T., et al.: J. Clin. Invest. 60:620–625, September, 1977.)

Renal concentrating ability was not increased by large doses of vasopressin. The effects of water restriction on urine flow and urine osmolality are shown in Figure 15. The ability of low-potassium rats with restricted water intake to reduce their urine flow and increase urine osmolality was not attributable to intrarenal factors mediated by negative water on extracellular fluid balance. Hypokalemic rats allowed free access to water and water-restricted rats became comparably hypokalemic and developed equally severe defects in urine concentration.

The findings indicate that potassium depletion affects water homeostasis by both central and renal mechanisms. The former is characterized by stimulation of thirst and leads to a primary polydipsia, which is largely responsible for the polyuria observed in this disorder. Further potassium depletion then culminates in deranged renal concentrating ability, which is most likely due to a direct renal effect of hypokalemia.

► [As Dr. Charles Kleeman noted many years ago, certain potassium-deficient patients habitually excrete a urine even more dilute than required by the constraints of their concentrating defect. (The same is true, incidentally, of some patients with lithium-induced nephrogenic diabetes insipidus and others with hypercalcemia.) Injections of vasopressin increase urinary osmolality, though not to normal. The simplest explanation is that thirst is stimulated in some way by the abnormal chemical environment. – Ed.] ◄

Sodium, Water and Acid-Base

Clinical Use of the Anion Gap is discussed by Michael Emmett and Robert G. Narins[2] (Univ. of Pennsylvania). The "anion gap" (AG) is derived from the serum electrolytes and is an important index of acid-base status, as well as a clue to the presence of many potentially fatal diseases. The AG is equal to (Na + K) − (Cl + HCO_3); the K may be neglected because of its minor influence on the AG. Fifty consecutive patients without disease known to alter the AG had values of 12.4 ± 2.0 mEq/L. The normal range has been taken as 8–16 mEq/L.

The finding of an elevated AG is virtually synonymous with the presence of a metabolic acidosis, characterized by the accumulation of organic or inorganic acid in the extracellular space. Uremic acidosis is perhaps the most common form of high-AG metabolic acidosis. The finding of a positive nitroprusside reaction in the serum and urine without abnormality of the serum HCO_3 or AG strongly suggests a high plasma acetone level. Aspirin contributes to elevation of the AG. Intoxication with paraldehyde, methanol or ethylene glycol results in a characteristic clinical syndrome and a severe high-AG metabolic acidosis. A normal-AG metabolic acidosis may be due to gastrointestinal bicarbonate loss, ureteroenterostomy, rapid intravenous hydration or hyperalimentation, the posthypocapnia state or various renal causes including renal tubular acidoses. Acetazolamide, cholestyramine and acidifying agents may also cause a normal-AG metabolic acidosis. Dehydration may lead to a trivial rise in the AG, and the AG may increase on treatment with sodium salts containing "unmeasured" anions. Large doses of carbenicillin or, more rarely, penicillin may increase the AG. A small rise in the AG accompanies respiratory and metabolic alkalosis.

It is not true that random laboratory error is the only cause of a low AG. A reduced concentration of unmeasured anions may cause a decrease in the AG, as in dilution of the extracellular fluid or hypoalbuminemia. Other causes are systematic underestimation of the serum sodium concentration, as in hyperviscosity, and systematic overestimation of the serum chloride concentration, as in bromism. Retained nonsodium cations in multiple myeloma, hypercalcemia, hypermagnesemia or lithium intoxication may be associated with a decreased AG.

► [This readable and useful review is worth perusing in its entirety. Among its pearls are: (1) Most flame photometers underestimate serum sodium in hypernatremia because they are nonlinear above 150 mEq/L. The spuriously low serum sodium results in apparent lowering of the anion gap. (2) In the autoanalyzer colorimetric technique for chloride, bromide reacts more effectively than chloride, causing a deeper color to develop. The result is a spuriously elevated value for the apparent "chloride" concen-

(2) Medicine (Baltimore) 56:38–54, January, 1977.

tration, resulting in an anion gap that is smaller than normal, or even negative, in bromism. (3) In ketoacidosis that is due to starvation, diabetes or alcohol, it is acetoacetate rather than its reduced congener, β-hydroxybutyrate, that reacts with nitroprusside. Accordingly, in anoxia, shock or alcoholism, when ketone bodies are largely in the reduced (β-hydroxybutyrate) form, severe acidosis with a large anion gap may be present with only a weakly positive test for ketones in the serum. – Ed.] ◄

Hyperphosphatemia in Lactic Acidosis. Tranquada reported in 1966 that the serum inorganic phosphorus concentration was elevated in all 10 of 46 patients with lactic acidosis in whom it was measured. Lawrence R. O'Connor, Keith L. Klein and John E. Bethune[3] (Univ. of Southern California) studied the occurrence of hyperphosphatemia in 11 consecutive patients with lactic acidosis. Shock and hypoxia were present in 6, hypoxia alone in 4 and phenformin use in 1. The mean serum lactate concentration was 188.6 mg/dl, compared with 18.8 mg/dl for patients with diabetic ketoacidosis. The serum inorganic phosphorus concentrations were 9.4 mg/dl in the patients with lactic acidosis and 5.5 mg/dl in those with diabetic ketoacidosis, a significant difference. Severity of acidosis was comparable in the two groups. The serum creatinine value was significantly higher in ketoacidosis, probably because it is overestimated by the AutoAnalyzer in the presence of acetoacetate. The serum phosphorus to "serum creatinine" ratio separated the two groups completely (Fig 16). The mean index was 4.45 in lactic acidosis and 1.98 in ketoacidosis.

This study confirmed Tranquada's finding that the serum phosphorus concentration is increased in patients with lactic acidosis. It is unlikely that renal insufficiency explains this finding. When metabolic acidosis is present with an increased anion gap, an elevated serum phosphorus value, in the absence of severe azotemia, may be a clue to the presence of lactic acidosis. A phosphorus-creatinine ratio above 3.0 strongly suggests lactic acidosis if the creatinine is measured by current AutoAnalyzer techniques.

► [The AutoAnalyzer method tends to give falsely high values for serum creatinine in the presence of acetoacetate, as in diabetic acidosis. This source of error (which con-

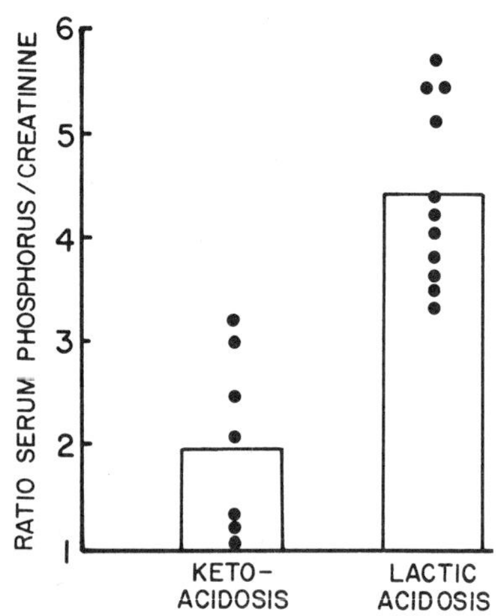

Fig 16. – Calculated serum inorganic phosphate (phosphorus) to serum creatinine ratios for all patients studied. (Courtesy of O'Connor, L. R., et al.: N. Engl. J. Med. 297:707–709, Sept. 29, 1977.)

(3) N. Engl. J. Med. 297:707–709, Sept. 29, 1977.

tributes to the neat separation shown in Figure 16) is minimized in alcoholic ketoacidosis or concomitant lactic acidosis, because acetoacetate is reduced to β-hydroxybutyrate. Under these circumstances the test for acetone in serum and urine may be negative. The high serum phosphate level seen in severe lactic acidosis is thought to be a consequence of the breakdown of high-energy phosphate compounds inside of cells as a result of ischemia. – Ed.] ◄

Bicarbonate Transport by Rabbit Cortical Collecting Tubules: Effect of Acid and Alkali Loads In Vivo on Transport In Vitro. The large pH and bicarbonate gradients between urine and blood have been attributed to transport by the collecting ducts. T. D. McKinney and M. B. Burg[4] (Natl. Inst. of Health) measured bicarbonate transport directly in rabbit cortical collecting tubules in vitro and determined whether prior treatment with alkalinizing or acidifying salts in vivo affected bicarbonate transport measured subsequently in vitro. Bicarbonate was measured in isolated collecting tubules by microcalorimetry as total CO_2. The perfusate and bath were identical solutions containing 25 mM bicarbonate at pH 7.4.

The mean pH of urine in the bladders of untreated rabbits when they were killed was 7.4. Tubules from 10 untreated rabbits absorbed total CO_2 and those from 4 secreted it. The mean rate of total CO_2 transport was not significantly different from zero. The mean urine pH of rabbits treated with ammonium chloride was 5.0. All tubules from such rabbits absorbed total CO_2 and the mean rate of absorption was significantly different from the mean of untreated rabbits. The mean urine pH of rabbits treated with sodium bicarbonate was 8.1. Fifteen tubules from such rabbits secreted total CO_2 and 3 tubules absorbed it. The mean rate of transport was significantly different from those in untreated and ammonium chloride-treated rabbits.

The direction of bicarbonate transport by cortical collecting tubules in this study correlated with the urine pH and was determined by previous treatment of the rabbits with acidifying or alkalinizing salts. The similar cells of the turtle bladder acidify the bladder contents by hydrogen ion secretion. Turtle bladders also secrete bicarbonate, linked to chloride absorption via an electroneutral exchange that is interrupted by inhibitors of metabolism and of carbonic anhydrase. Whether the mechanisms of bicarbonate transport are the same in the turtle bladder and cortical collecting tubule is uncertain.

► [The importance of this article is that it demonstrates a previously unrecognized tubular mechanism that contributes to the regulation of acid-base – secretion of bicarbonate into the urine. Influenced by the powerful contributions of Robert F. Pitts (who died last year), renal physiologists have thought of acid-base excretion primarily in terms of the secretion of hydrogen ions by tubules. Bicarbonate excretion equaled filtered bicarbonate minus bicarbonate reabsorbed through the process of hydrogen ion secretion. Now we will have to take bicarbonate secretion into account. The rabbit probably needs it because of its alkaline-ash diet. – Ed.] ◄

Mechanism of Hypophosphatemia in Acute Heat Stroke. Severe heat stroke may be associated with hypophosphatemia and hypocalcemia. Hypophosphatemia is generally observed within hours after the onset, whereas hypocalcemia usually occurs on the 2d or 3d day, after the hypophosphatemia has spontaneously resolved. James P.

(4) J. Clin. Invest. 60:766 – 768, September, 1977.

Knochel and Jennifer H. Caskey[5] (Univ. of Texas Southwestern Med. School) describe a person who exhibited respiratory alkalosis in the course of severe heat stroke and in whom hypophosphatemia abated spontaneously as metabolic acidosis and acute renal failure supervened and as hypocalcemia became prominent.

Man, 32, a laborer, collapsed while working in the hot sun and was seen in a coma 2½ hours later, with a rectal temperature exceeding 107.9 F. Blood pressure was 70/40 mm Hg on admission and rose after cooling and saline administration. Convulsions occurred during cooling, hyperventilation continued and examination showed dysconjugate gaze and vertical nystagmus. Many severe complications of heat stroke including aspiration of vomitus, pulmonary edema and massive rhabdomyolysis occurred. Myocardial failure, acute oliguric renal failure and hepatocellular damage also complicated the course, as did disseminated intravascular coagulation and gastrointestinal hemorrhage. The patient died on the 3d hospital day.

The hemoglobin concentration was 17.1 gm/dl on admission. An unexplained anion gap of 18 suggested an elevated lactate concentration. A urine test for heme pigment was positive, but the serum was clear. The serum calcium concentration 4 or 5 hours after onset was 11.9 mg/dl and that of phosphorus, 0.9 mg/dl. On the 2d day the calcium concentration was 5.6 mg/dl and that of phosphorus was 4.3 mg/dl. Autopsy showed normal parathyroids. Analysis of a skeletal muscle sample showed a normal 30.7 mM total phosphorus per 100 gm fat-free dry solids and normal values for potassium and sodium.

Accelerated cellular uptake of phosphorus incident to alkalinization of the intracellular contents probably results from increased phosphofructokinase activity. This appears to be adequate to explain acute hypophosphatemia in patients with heat stroke. Evidence suggests that hypophosphatemia in the concentration range observed in this case (below 1 mg/dl), if prolonged, may be responsible for widespread tissue destruction.

► [I have included this article in the YEAR BOOK in order to emphasize the association between respiratory alkalosis and hypophosphatemia first described by Mostellar and Tuttle in 1964 (J. Clin. Invest. 43:138, 1964). It is seen not only in hyperpyrexia but also in hysterical hyperventilation, during hepatic coma and after recovery from diabetic acidosis—all characterized by respiratory alkalosis. Intracellular alkalosis stimulates the activity of the enzyme phosphofructokinase, a gateway to the glycolytic pathway. The inorganic phosphate of extracellular fluid is therefore quickly used up by the necessity to manufacture tricarbon phosphorylated intermediates of glucose metabolism. It is not clear yet whether the profound hypophosphatemia induced by this shift of phosphate from inorganic-extracellular to organic-intracellular has the same deleterious consequences on the physiology of cells as does a low serum phosphate level produced by prolonged phosphate depletion.—Ed.] ◄

(5) J.A.M.A. 238:425–426, Aug. 1, 1977.

Parathyroids and Calcitonin

Urinary Cyclic AMP Analyzed as a Function of Serum Calcium and Parathyroid Hormone in Differential Diagnosis of Hypercalcemia. Up to half of urinary cyclic adenosine monophosphate (UcAMP) is generated in the kidney under the control of parathyroid hormone (PTH). James W. Shaw, Susan B. Oldham, Leonard Rosoff, John E. Bethune and Marshal P. Fichman[6] (Univ. of Southern California) measured UcAMP in normal subjects and in a large number of hypercalcemic patients and correlated it with serum concentrations of calcium and immunoreactive PTH (iPTH) in an effort to improve the diagnostic accuracy of UcAMP determinations in hypercalcemia. Studies were done in 41 normocalcemic controls, 76 patients with hypercalcemia and 5 with hypocalcemia. Fifty-six patients with primary hyperparathyroidism and 16 with nonparathyroid neoplasms and hypercalcemia were studied. All subjects were on a random diet and unrestricted activity. The serum calcium concentration was altered by infusion of 100 or 200 mg calcium gluconate or by infusion of 2 L of 0.9% saline over 2 hours.

No significant circadian variation in UcAMP was seen in the normal subjects. The mean value was 4.42 ± 0.16, as measured by a competitive protein-binding assay. The mean for patients with primary hyperparathyroidism was 8.48 and the mean for those with nonparathyroid neoplasms was 8.36. The 5 hypocalcemic patients had a mean UcAMP of 3.56. In hypercalcemia, a UcAMP above 4.0 was inappropriately high and indicated PTH-mediated hypercalcemia. The UcAMP and serum calcium values were significantly correlated in patients with primary hyperparathyroidism in the PTH-mediated area. A significant negative correlation was found between iPTH and serum calcium concentrations in normal subjects and a significant positive correlation in patients with primary hyperparathyroidism. Serum iPTH and UcAMP values were significantly correlated in the normal subjects but not in hypercalcemic patients. Calcium infusion in 4 patients with primary hyperparathyroidism caused a decrease in UcAMP and iPTH values parallel to that seen in normal subjects.

As long as renal function is adequate, a random UcAMP, expressed as micromoles per gram of creatinine, is a sensitive and accurate reflection of circulating, biologically active PTH. It can be a useful adjunct to radioimmunoassay of PTH in confirming an elevated iPTH value and in determining whether patients with neoplasms have hypercalcemia due to biologically active PTH or to other osteolytic factors.

► [About half of the cyclic AMP excreted by normal human subjects derives from the

(6) J. Clin. Invest. 59:14–21, January, 1977.

influence of circulating titers of parathyroid hormone on the nephrogenous pool of the nucleotide; the rest represents the excretion into the urine of cyclic AMP (cAMP) contained in plasma and filtered at the glomerulus. Urinary cAMP excretion therefore varies with glomerular filtration rate. Patients with disorders of calcium metabolism—hyperparathyroid suspects—tend to have renal impairment and also frequently have muscle wasting, which reduces creatinine excretion. So, in order to refine the usefulness of urinary cAMP measurement as an index of parathyroid activity, it is not only helpful to express it as a function of urinary creatinine, as the present authors do. Even better, say A. E. Broadus et al. (J. Clin. Invest. 60:771, 1977), is to express urinary cAMP as a function of glomerular filtration rate (GFR), the normal range being 1.8–4.6 nanomoles per 100 ml GFR. This should be an interesting and useful way to assess parathyroid activity repeatedly, especially during "suppression tests." The only other clinical condition besides hyperparathyroidism that is known to cause increased urinary cAMP excretion is pheochromocytoma, since, like parathyroid hormone, catechols also activate adenyl cyclase in proximal tubular cells, which leak the nucleotide into the urine. Vasopressin, which activates adenyl cyclase in distal tubular cells, does not regularly increase urinary cAMP since the distal tubular cell membrane is less permeable to nucleotides.

Finally, urinary cAMP should be related to the level of serum calcium, corrected for that portion of calcium bound to serum albumin, to be most useful in the diagnosis of primary hyperparathyroidism (Madsen, S. N., et al.: Acta Med. Scand. 200:195, 1976). —Ed.] ◄

1,25-Dihydroxycholecalciferol: Its Use in Long-Term Management of Idiopathic Hypoparathyroidism in Children is reported by John F. Rosen, Alan R. Fleischman, Laurence Finberg (Albert Einstein College of Medicine, John Eisman and Hector F. DeLuca[7] (Univ. of Wisconsin). The production of 1,25-dihydroxycholecalciferol (1,25$(OH)_2D_3$) is reduced in the absence of parathyroid hormone (PTH), because conversion of 25-hydroxycholecalciferol to 1,25$(OH)_2D_3$ is primarily under PTH control. Three children with previously untreated, undiagnosed, isolated, idiopathic hypoparathyroidism were given 0.4–0.5 μg 1,25$(OH)_2D_3$ per day, orally, for a total of 2,650 treatment days, in an attempt to increase intestinal calcium absorption to normal and maintain normal serum calcium concentrations.

Two children, aged 4 years, achieved and maintained normal serum calcium values after 1–4 days on 0.03 μg 1,25$(OH)_2D_3$ per kg per day (Fig 17). On a low-calcium diet the total serum calcium concentrations fell by 0.8 and 1 mg/dl, respectively, within 2 days. The children have been normocalcemic on a regular diet during 2,300 treatment days. A child who required phenobarbital also responded rapidly, but required 0.16 μg/kg daily, and several brief episodes of hypercalcemia occurred during 350 days of therapy. On each occasion, 1,25$(OH)_2D_3$ was discontinued for 2 days and normocalcemia promptly returned. Pretreatment serum concentrations of 1,25-$(OH)_2D_3$ were 19–51 pg/ml. After treatment for several months, all 3 children showed similar increases in serum levels 4–6 hours after oral dosing and rapid decreases to far below normal values by 16 hours.

This physiologic approach to idiopathic hypoparathyroidism avoids the use of large doses of long-acting vitamin D_3 and its analogues and provides easy dose adjustment. Significant target tissue concentrations of 1,25-$(OH)_2D_3$ may last for a considerable period, and the agent may

(7) J. Clin. Endocrinol. Metab. 45:457–468, September, 1977.

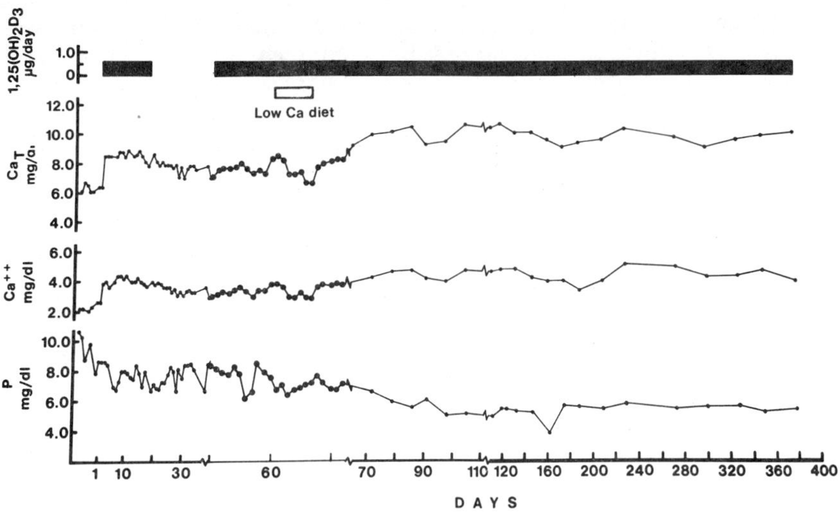

Fig 17.—Effects of small daily oral doses of $1,25(OH)_2D_3$ on serum concentrations of total calcium, ionized calcium and inorganic phosphate in 1 patient. (Courtesy of Rosen, J. F., et al.: J. Clin. Endocrinol. Metab. 45:457–468, September, 1977.)

induce changes at tissue sites that continue long after the hormone is gone.

► [The standard treatment of idiopathic hypoparathyroidism for years has been extremely large doses of vitamin D in the range that would produce intoxication in normal persons. In the absence of parathyroid hormone, the kidney hydroxylates 25-OH-D to the active 1,25 $(OH)_2D_3$ only very slowly. Vitamin D is hydroxylated by the liver at carbon 25 in a normal fashion in such patients, and the enormously high concentrations of 25-OH-D that result presumably stimulate some renal hydroxylation and mobilize calcium via skeleton and intestine by "mass action." The main difficulty in treating patients with the use of ordinary vitamin D is that the difference between a therapeutic and an intoxicating dose of the vitamin can be extremely small. It may take weeks to adjust the dose correctly or to correct overdosage. These disadvantages are overcome by $1,25(OH)_2D_3$—still (but hopefully not for long) an experimental drug. The cheaper analogue, 1α-hydroxycholecalciferol (1977 YEAR BOOK, pp. 561–563), should do equally well.

Elucidation of the role of $1,25(OH)_2D_3$ will become easier with the availability of a simplified and sensitive competitive binding assay for the sterol in plasma (Science 193:1021, 1976). As you would expect, it is absent in nephrectomized subjects and patients with end-stage renal disease.

There is a water-soluble substance in certain South American plants that causes hypercalcemia in cattle that eat too much of it (1975 YEAR BOOK, p. 707). It turns out that it is the glycoside of $1,25(OH)_2D_3$ (ibid. 194:853, 1976), and it might someday conceivably offer some therapeutic advantages over the unconjugated sterol in hypoparathyroid or uremic patients.—Ed.] ◄

Calcium and Phosphorus Homeostasis in Man: Effect of Corticosteroids. An excess of glucocorticoids and their synthetic counterparts can reduce intestinal calcium absorption and produce osteoporosis, and current evidence suggests that the effect is the result of corticosteroid-mediated biochemical or structural changes in intestinal mucosa cells, leading to depressed calcium transport across the mucosal membrane. Barbara P. Lukert and John S. Adams[8] (Univ. of Kan-

(8) Arch. Intern. Med. 136:1249–1253, November, 1976.

sas) found that patients on long-term corticosteroid therapy are capable of normal calcium homeostasis after the effects of secondary hyperparathyroidism are countered by giving calcium intravenously. Studies were done in 9 patients aged 34–67 years with moderate to severe chronic obstructive lung disease, all but 1 of whom were on long-term corticosteroid therapy. Eleven normal subjects were also evaluated. The patients received 10 gm calcium gluconate per day intravenously for 7 days, 6–8 weeks after control studies.

The patients had a higher mean serum calcium concentration than did controls, but the difference was not significant. Serum phosphorus values were also comparable in the two groups. Patients had a significantly higher mean plasma parathyroid hormone level than did controls. Urinary calcium excretion was nearly the same in the two groups, but the patients had a 37% greater mean phosphate excretion rate, and tubular phosphate reabsorption was significantly lower in the patients. Excretion of cyclic adenosine monophosphate (AMP) was also greater in the patients. Calcium infusion increased both serum calcium level and urinary calcium excretion rate in the corticosteroid-treated patients. Serum phosphorus values increased, and the urinary phosphate excretion rate fell substantially. The cyclic AMP-mediated renal tubular response to decreased levels of circulating parathyroid hormone was intact in the corticosteroid-treated patients.

The findings suggest that the effects of secondary hyperparathyroidism in patients maintained on long-term prednisone therapy may be overcome when calcium is given intravenously. Once the intestinal calcium malabsorption-induced effects of secondary hyperparathyroidism are circumvented by intravenous calcium supplementation, corticosteroid-treated patients are capable of normal calcium and phosphorus homeostasis.

► [The level of immunoreactive parathyroid hormone in plasma is elevated in patients who are chronically treated with glucocorticoids (1976 YEAR BOOK, p. 661) and the question is why. One hypothesis is that it is secondary to a calcium-lowering action of glucocorticoids, perhaps an anti-vitamin D effect that diminishes the intestinal absorption of calcium. In that case, intravenous calcium, or for that matter, large quantities of oral calcium, should reverse the process and perhaps help prevent the thin bones of steroid-induced osteoporosis.

A second possibility is that glucocorticoids act directly to stimulate parathyroid secretion. That is suggested by the following article, showing that cortisol stimulated secretion by rat parathyroids in tissue culture. (It might still be possible for calcium to shut off cortisol-induced secretion, but the author of the following article has not yet shown that.) The clear suggestion here is that increased parathyroid hormone activity may play a major role in the osteoporosis of Cushing's syndrome. – Ed.] ◄

Cortisol Stimulation of Parathyroid Hormone Secretion by Rat Parathyroid Glands in Organ Culture. Cortisol and other active glucocorticoid congeners can produce hypocalcemia in parathyroidectomized but not in intact animals, suggesting an interaction between adrenocorticosteroid and parathyroid hormone (PTH) in calcium homeostasis. The rise in serum PTH concentration seen with cortisol administration in intact animals and man has been attributed to an indirect, compensatory response to a postulated transient cortisol-induced hypocalcemia. William Y. W. Au[9] (Univ. of Rochester) re-

(9) Science 193:1015–1017, Sept. 10, 1976.

ports evidence for a direct effect of cortisol in stimulating PTH secretion by rat parathyroids maintained in organ culture. Secretion of rat PTH into the medium was estimated by radioimmunoassay. Glands were obtained from male albino rats and cultured in 5% serum from thyroparathyroidectomized rats.

Low concentrations of calcium (0.75 mM) stimulated and sustained high rates of PTH secretion, whereas high concentrations (1.75 mM) suppressed PTH secretion. Cortisol (10^{-7}M) stimulated a sustained rise in the rate of PTH secretion both in glands exposed to high calcium concentrations and in those already stimulated by exposure to low calcium concentrations. A dose-related response of PTH secretion was obtained for cortisol at $10^{-8}-10^{-6}$M concentrations. Corticosterone also stimulated increases in secretion rates, but deoxycorticosterone and cortexolone did not. Cortexolone did inhibit the stimulatory effect of cortisol. Cortisol increased the uptake of ^{3}H-labeled amino acids by glandular proteins.

Cortisol appears to stimulate the synthesis of proteins and PTH. The findings are consistent with the presence of cortisol receptors in the parathyroid cell. Some of the effects of therapeutic doses of cortisol in reducing bone mass may be mediated through this action. In cortisol-induced osteopenia, the direct stimulation of PTH secretion by cortisol might overcome the inhibitory effect of cortisol on bone resorption. An added effect from secondary stimulation of PTH secretion could result from hypocalcemia produced by cortisol inhibition of gut calcium absorption. The net result would be an increase in plasma PTH concentration, normocalcemia and increased bone resorption in the parathyroid-intact animal treated with cortisol.

► [With a similar technique, G. D. Aurbach and co-workers have been able to show that β-adrenergic agonists also directly stimulate the release of parathyroid hormone from isolated parathyroid cells (Endocrinology 100:1696, 1977). It would be interesting to see what propranolol would do in hyperparathyroidism. —Ed.] ◄

Distribution of Calcitonin-Sensitive Adenylate Cyclase Activity along the Rabbit Kidney Tubule. Calcitonin can stimulate adenylate cyclase activity in preparations of renal cortex and outer medulla, but the preparations used have contained a heterogeneous mixture of membranes from all cell types present in the original tissue. Danièlle Chabardès, Martine Imbert-Teboul, Madeleine Montégut, André Clique and François Morel[1] (Paris) used a micromethod, in which different nephron segments are isolated by microdissection from collagenase-treated rabbit kidneys, and respective enzyme activities are measured in samples containing a single piece of tubule, to determine the distribution of the salmon calcitonin (SCT)-sensitive activity of adenylate cyclase.

Adenylate cyclase sensitivity to SCT was investigated in 11 different segments of the rabbit nephron. In the presence of 0.1 μg synthetic SCT per ml, 8 segments exhibited no hormone sensitivity, whereas maximal responses were induced in 3 segments, including the "bright" portion of the distal convoluted tubule and the cortical and medullary portions of the thick ascending limb of Henle's loop. Sensitivity to cal-

(1) Proc. Natl. Acad. Sci. U.S.A. 73:3608–3612, October, 1976.

citonin of the adenylate cyclase in these segments was extremely high. Half-maximal stimulation corresponded to about 0.3 ng SCT per ml.

The findings suggest that the distal convoluted tubule, as well as the cortical and medullary portions of the thick ascending limb of Henle's loop, represent physiologic target structures of calcitonin action within the kidney. The possibility that the hormone may also act on other segments of the nephron is not excluded. The overall effect of calcitonin on the rabbit kidney has not been fully investigated.

► [These remarkably elegant studies on single portions of renal tubules pinpoint the anatomical locus in the distal tubule for an action of calcitonin on renal function that is not yet precisely known and remains to be demonstrated. The concentrations of calcitonin shown to activate renal tubular adenylate cyclase in these experiments are comparable to those present in human plasma (1976 YEAR BOOK, p. 664). Calcitonin is secreted by thyroid "C" cells in response to hypercalcemia. When injected into animals it increases the excretion of calcium, phosphate and sodium. But is that all it does? This article gives you the feeling that there is something very important there in the distal tubule, waiting to be discovered. – Ed.] ◄

Renal Stones

Treated and Untreated Recurrent Calcium Nephrolithiasis in Patients with Idiopathic Hypercalciuria, Hyperuricosuria or No Metabolic Disorder. Fredric L. Coe[2] (Michael Reese Hosp.) treated 202 recurrent calcium oxalate stone formers with idiopathic hypercalciuria or hyperuricosuria or both for an average of 2.9 years with thiazide, allopurinol or both. Thirty-four untreated and 30 treated patients with no apparent metabolic disorder were also studied. Hypercalciuria over 300 mg/day in men and 250 mg/day in women was controlled with trichlormethiazide; most patients responded to 2 mg twice daily. Allopurinol was given in an initial dosage of 100 mg twice daily and was increased in 50-mg increments until urinary urate excretion fell below 700 mg/24 hours in men or 650 in women. Patients without metabolic

Fig 18 (top left).—Calcium stone formation before and during treatment of definite hypercalciuria with thiazide.

Fig 19 (top right).—Stone formation before and during treatment of marginal hypercalciuria with thiazide.

Fig 20 (bottom left).—Calcium stone formation before and during treatment of hyperuricosuria with allopurinol.

Fig 21 (bottom right).—Calcium stone formation before and during treatment of combined hypercalciuria and hyperuricosuria with thiazide and allopurinol.

(Courtesy of Coe, F. L.: Ann. Intern. Med. 87:404–410, October, 1977.)

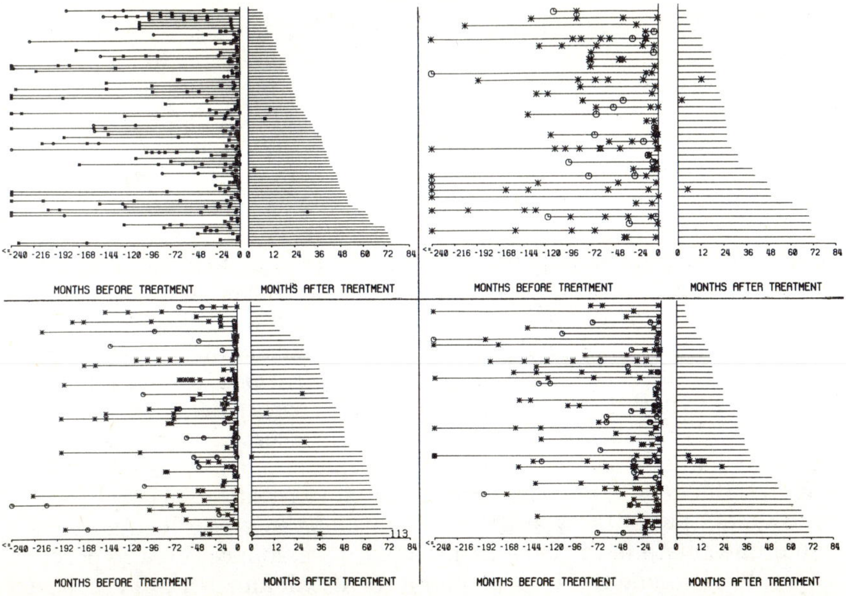

(2) Ann. Intern. Med. 87:404–410, October, 1977.

disorder received 100 mg allopurinol and 2 mg trichlormethiazide twice daily.

Stone formation by hypercalciuric and hyperuricosuric patients was reduced by thiazide and allopurinol therapy as shown in Figures 18–21, in which each patient is represented by a horizontal line, new stones by solid symbols and multiple stones occurring in clusters by open symbols. The reduction in stone occurrence was significant in each metabolic subgroup. Patients with marginal hypercalciuria had nearly the same response to thiazide therapy as those with definite hypercalciuria. Almost as many stones as predicted developed in the untreated patients during follow-up. The patients without metabolic disorder had a reduction in new stone formation during treatment, but the response was less dramatic than in the other groups.

Chronic reversal of idiopathic hypercalciuria and hyperuricosuria with thiazide and allopurinol is an effective way to prevent recurrent calcium oxalate stones. Conservative measures are only marginally effective in treating metabolically normal, stone-forming patients, but thiazide and allopurinol appear to reduce new stone formation.

► [Perhaps one third of patients with calcium stones have hypercalciuria, defined as the excretion of more than 300 mg calcium per day by men and 250 mg by women (Coe, F. L., et al.: The natural history of calcium urolithiasis, J.A.M.A. 238:1519, 1977). Approximately 25% have hyperuricosuria and 12% excrete excessive quantities of both calcium and uric acid. Hyperuricosuria may be important because urates accelerate the crystallization of calcium oxalate from a supersaturated solution. It looks very much as if thiazides and allopurinol can reduce stone formation in these two categories of patients, but the situation is not so clear in the "silent majority" of patients with recurrent stones and no (presently) detectable metabolic abnormality.

Prospective studies in comparison with a placebo or simple hydration should be given the highest priority because of the natural tendency of stone episodes to come in bunches so that any treatment appears effective at least 50% of the time. – Ed.] ◄

On the Pathogenesis of So-called Idiopathic Hypercalciuria. There is no universal view as to the pathogenesis of hypercalciuria in patients with recurrent renal calculi and members of their families. Approximately 60% of hypercalciuric patients have normal urinary calcium when intake is reduced to less than 400 mg/day(type 1). Philippe Bordier, Antoine Ryckewart, Jean Gueris and Howard Rasmussen[3] studied 47 patients identified as having persistent hypercalciuria during a period of low calcium intake (less than 400 mg/24 hours). Type 2 patients had increased and type 3 patients had normal or low serum immunoreactive parathyroid hormone (PTH) values. Type 2a patients responded to either methylchlorothiazide or 25-hydroxyvitamin D_3 with little change in serum calcium, a rise in serum phosphate and a fall in serum PTH concentrations. Type 2b patients responded to both treatments with a rise in serum calcium and no decrease in PTH concentrations. They had successful parathyroid surgery but had persistent postoperative hypercalciuria, and several had suppressible hyperparathyroidism several years after surgery.

In type 3 patients hypercalciuria develops as a result of a primary renal phosphate leak. Type 2a patients have suppressible hyperparathyroidism secondary to a primary renal calcium leak. Type 2b pa-

(3) Am. J. Med. 63:398–409, September, 1977.

tients are also thought to have a long-standing primary renal calcium leak, which leads initially to secondary hyperparathyroidism but eventually to tertiary or nonsuppressible hyperparathyroidism. In some instances a renal phosphate leak may be associated with an increase in 1,25-$(OH)_2$-vitamin D_3 synthesis (type 3 hypercalciuria), whereas in others it leads to no change or to a decrease in 1,25-$(OH)_2$-vitamin D_3 synthesis, i.e., inappropriately low 1,25-$(OH)_2$-vitamin D_3 – vitamin D resistance in adults and children.

► [It looks as if "idiopathic hypercalciuria" is a mixed bag. In all patients, absorption of calcium from the gut is increased, as might be predicted from the fact that their bones are not osteoporotic. If this were the primary event it would tend to suppress parathyroid secretion, but in a minority of patients there is evidence for increased parathyroid hormone activity in the form of an elevated level of immunoreactive hormone in the plasma or an increased excretion of nephrogenous cAMP. In some of those patients, parathyroid adenomas are found (normocalcemic hyperparathyroidism). I suspect that the serum calcium is not entirely normal in such cases, but instead is only intermittently elevated. In others, the chemical signs of parathyroid overactivity disappear when calcium is given or calcium excretion is suppressed by thiazides, and it is in these that a primary renal leak of calcium has been postulated. In still another group of hypercalciuric patients (called "type 3" by the present authors), it has been postulated that renal phosphate wasting is the primary event, the consequent hypophosphatemia stimulating the kidneys to overproduce 1,25$(OH)_2$D which increases intestinal calcium absorption. That interesting hypothesis is discussed further in the following article. From the standpoint of the therapist, it is convenient that thiazides reduce calcium excretion in all forms of hypercalciuria. – Ed.] ◄

Importance of Phosphate in Regulating Plasma 1,25-$(OH)_2$-Vitamin D Levels in Humans: Studies in Healthy Subjects, in Calcium Stone Formers and in Patients with Primary Hyperparathyroidism. Richard W. Gray, Donald R. Wilz, Angela E. Caldas and Jacob Lemann, Jr.[4] (Med. College of Wisconsin) observed an inverse correlation between plasma 1,25-$(OH)_2$-vitamin D and serum phosphate concentrations in normal subjects and in patients with primary hyperparathyroidism or recurrent calcium nephrolithiasis. Studies were done in 48 normal subjects, 26 patients with calcium oxalate or apatite renal stones or both and 9 patients with surgically proved hyperparathyroidism due to adenoma. The effects of dietary phosphate deprivation were evaluated in 8 healthy men and 10 healthy women who took a diet containing 1.8 mM phosphate daily for 11 – 16 days. Plasma 1,25-$(OH)_2$-vitamin D was measured by a chromatin binding assay.

The stone formers exhibited hypophosphatemia and hypercalciuria but normal serum immunoreactive parathyroid hormone (iPTH) levels. Their average serum 25-OH-vitamin D levels were significantly below the normal mean. The average plasma 1,25-$(OH)_2$-vitamin D concentration was significantly elevated in stone formers (Fig 22). The hyperparathyroid patients had high iPTH levels, hypercalcemia, hypophosphatemia and hypercalciuria. Their serum 25-OH-vitamin D levels were significantly below normal, and their plasma 1,25-$(OH)_2$-vitamin D concentration levels were elevated. Plasma 1,25-$(OH)_2$-vitamin D levels rose significantly as the serum phosphate concentrations declined in both the normal and the patient

(4) J. Clin. Endocrinol. Metab. 45:299 – 306, August, 1977.

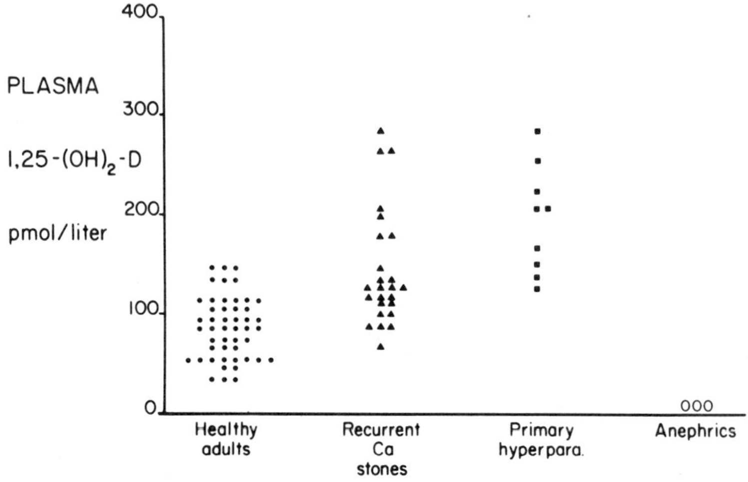

Fig 22.—Plasma 1,25-$(OH)_2$-vitamin D concentrations in healthy subjects, patients with recurrent calcium-containing kidney stones, patients with primary hyperparathyroidism and anephric patients maintained by chronic hemodialysis. (Courtesy of Gray, R. W., et al.: J. Clin. Endocrinol. Metab. 45:299–306, August, 1977.)

groups. Ingestion of a low-phosphate diet was accompanied by a fall in serum phosphate in females only and by a rise in plasma 1,25-$(OH)_2$-vitamin D concentrations in females. Serum iPTH levels fell in both males and females deprived of phosphate.

Reductions in serum phosphate concentrations either directly or indirectly stimulate renal synthesis of 1,25-$(OH)_2$-vitamin D in human subjects. The significant correlation observed between urinary calcium excretion and plasma 1,25-$(OH)_2$-vitamin D concentration is consistent with the augmented intestinal calcium absorption observed in most stone formers and patients with primary hyperparathyroidism and with the observation that urinary calcium reflects the effects of 1,25-$(OH)_2$-vitamin D administered to normal subjects.

► [The serum phosphate tends to be on the low side in many patients with idiopathic hypercalciuria. Renal production of 1,25-$(OH)_2$-vitamin D is enhanced by hypophosphatemia, and therefore it is attractive to think of hypervitaminosis D, stimulated by a renal phosphate leak, as responsible for at least some kinds of hypercalciuria. However, only 8 of the authors' 26 patients with recurrent calcium stones and hypercalciuria had plasma levels of 1,25-$(OH)_2$-vitamin D above the range of normal. You would predict that oral phosphate supplements would restore those high vitamin D levels to normal as well as curing the hypercalciuria, but that remains to be demonstrated. Phosphate treatment did not do very well in a prospective double-blind study of the treatment of recurrent stone formers (1977 YEAR BOOK, p. 566).—Ed.] ◄

Renal Stones and Urinary Infection: Study of Antibiotic Treatment. Some believe that infection is usually the cause rather than the result of stone formation in patients with no metabolic cause for stone formation. It is important to control infection both after operation and when surgery is not advisable. R. H. Chinn, Rosalind Maskell, J. A. Mead and A. Polak[5] evaluated antibiotic therapy in 22 patients in

(5) Br. Med. J. 2:1411–1413, Dec. 11, 1976.

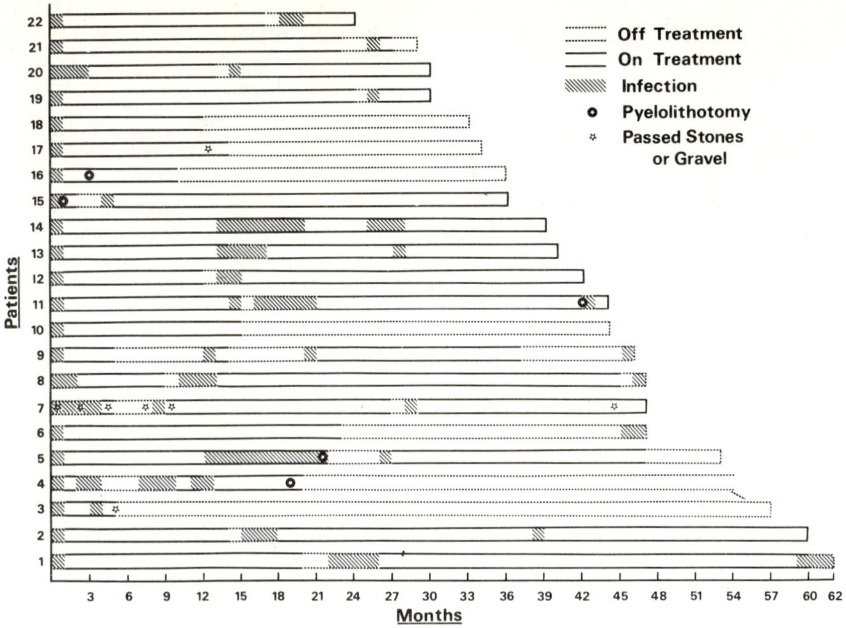

Fig 23.—Treatment and recurrence of infection in 22 patients. (Courtesy of Chinn, R. H., et al.: Br. Med. J. 2:1411–1413, Dec. 11, 1976.)

whom renal calculi and urinary infection were closely associated over 2–5 years. There were 20 women with a mean age of 43 and 2 men in the series. All had well-documented histories of persistent or recurrent urinary tract infection despite intermittent antibacterial therapy. Twenty-one had renal calculi and 1 had passed a stone just before admission; 3 patients had previously passed stones and 4 had had a pyelolithotomy. After completion of a 1-week course of an appropriate agent, usually co-trimoxazole, 20 patients received 1 tablet of co-trimoxazole nightly and 2 received 50 mg nitrofurantoin nightly until the midstream urine was culture negative for 1 year. Recurrences were treated with an appropriate agent for 1 week and prophylaxis then was reinstituted.

Patients were followed for 23–62 months. The most common infecting organisms on admission were *Proteus mirabilis* and *Escherichia coli*. Six patients had an elevated serum creatinine level. Four had bilateral stones. Ureteric catheterization showed renal infection in all 8 patients examined. Recurrences of infection are shown in Figure 23. Eighteen patients had 31 recurrences, 10 while on prophylaxis and 21 off prophylaxis; 15 occurred within 3 months of stopping prophylaxis. No side effects of long-term co-trimoxazole were observed and there were no hematologic changes. Seventeen patients remained symptom free while on successful prophylaxis. Fourteen of 22 patients had no pyuria or hematuria while on successful prophylaxis. Infection recurred after operation in 3 of 5 patients and was successfully controlled with prophylaxis. Two patients had apparently new stones and 2 showed an increase in stone size during successful prophylaxis. The serum creatinine levels declined in 4 of 6 patients in whom it was above 1.4 m/100 ml initially.

Although the urine remained sterile for a long period during antibacterial treatment and prophylaxis, it cannot be assumed that infection in or around calculi was eliminated. Chemotherapy, combined with surgery when appropriate can relieve symptoms and maintain renal function. Antibacterial treatment must be prolonged, possibly indefinitely in some patients. Co-trimoxazole is the agent of choice. Nitrofurantoin is usually ineffective against *Proteus* organisms in vivo. If infection indicates operative treatment, confirmation by a localization procedure is called for.

► [It used to be generally accepted that you could not sterilize the urine in the presence of an infected stone, but co-trimoxazole, a combination of trimethoprim and sulfamethoxazole (marketed in the United States as Bactrim or Septra), seems to have changed that. On long-term prophylaxis, most of these patients felt better, hematuria cleared and they had fewer infections or none, and 4 of 6 patients with an elevated serum creatinine level even improved their renal function. The population of urinary pathogens is reduced in vaginal and fecal flora as well as in the urine, thereby diminishing the risk of reinfection from those sources. In this respect, trimethoprim-sulfamethoxazole seems to do a better job in suppressing *Escherichia coli* than does prophylaxis with nitrofurantoin (Stamey, T. A., et al.: N. Engl. J. Med. 296:780, 1977). It is interesting, however, that in 4 patients stone growth apparently continued even in the presence of sterile urine. – Ed.] ◄

Answers to Current Literature Quiz

The page references direct the reader to the articles containing the answers to the Quiz.

1. Page 37.
2. Page 69.
3. Page 19.
4. Page 57.
5. Page 70.
6. Page 82.
7. Page 39.
8. Page 27.
9. Page 19.
10. Page 55.
11. Page 85.
12. Page 49.
13. Page 92.
14. Page 78.
15. Page 96.
16. Pages 107 and 109.
17. Page 112.
18. Page 128.
19. Page 140.
20. Page 144.
21. Page 148.
22. Page 152.
23. Pages 155–160.
24. Page 167.
25. Page 171.
26. Page 175.
27. Page 181.
28. Page 184.
29. Page 197.
30. Pages 220 and 221.
31. Page 227.
32. Pages 229 and 230.
33. Pages 233–235.
34. Page 237.
35. Pages 238 and 240.
36. Page 241.
37. Page 245.
38. Pages 247 and 249.
39. Page 252.
40. Page 265.
41. Page 268.
42. Pages 270 and 271.
43. Page 279.
44. Page 286.
45. Page 288.
46. Page 289.
47. Page 291.
48. Page 294.
49. Page 296.
50. Page 300.
51. Page 301.
52. Page 303.
53. Page 304.
54. Page 308.
55. Page 313.
56. Page 317.
57. Page 319.
58. Pages 323 and 324.
59. Page 328.
60. Pages 331 and 332.
61. Pages 333 and 334.
62. Page 337.
63. Page 341.
64. Page 343.
65. Page 345.
66. Page 346.
67. Page 349.
68. Page 352.
69. Page 354.
70. Page 357.
71. Page 358.
72. Page 369.
73. Page 376.
74. Page 377.
75. Page 381.
76. Page 385.
77. Page 395.
78. Page 402.
79. Page 405.
80. Page 414.
81. Page 417.
82. Page 427.
83. Page 428.
84. Page 435.
85. Page 456.
86. Page 454.
87. Pages 527 and 528.
88. Page 512.
89. Page 504.
90. Page 531.
91. Page 540.
92. Page 509.
93. Page 529.
94. Page 525.
95. Page 480.
96. Pages 469 and 471.
97. Page 494.
98. Page 506.
99. Page 534.
100. Page 474.
101. Page 479.
102. Page 547.
103. Page 553.
104. Page 554.
105. Page 557.
106. Page 565.
107. Page 567.
108. Pages 573 and 574.
109. Page 581.
110. Page 588.
111. Page 593.
112. Page 594.
113. Page 597.
114. Page 603.
115. Page 606.

Subject Index

B

C

D

H

M

Index to Authors